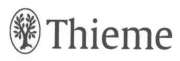

Neurointerventional Surgery

An Evidence-Based Approach

First Edition

Min S. Park, MD, FAANS
Associate Professor
Department of Neurosurgery, University of Virginia Health System
Charlottesville, Virginia, USA

M. Yashar S. Kalani, MD, PhD, MBA, FAANS, FAHA
Associate Professor
Department of Surgery
St. John's Neuroscience Institute/University of Oklahoma School of Medicine
Tulsa, Oklahoma, USA

Michael F. Stiefel, MD, PhD, FAANS
Director
Cerebrovascular and Endovascular Neurosurgery
Department of Neurosurgery, Piedmont Atlanta Hospital
Atlanta, Georgia, USA

219 illustrations

Thieme
New York • Stuttgart • Delhi • Rio de Janeiro

Library of Congress Cataloging-in-Publication Data is available from the publisher.

© 2021 Thieme. All rights reserved.

Thieme Publishers New York
333 Seventh Avenue, New York, NY 10001 USA
+1 800 782 3488, customerservice@thieme.com

Cover design: Thieme Publishing Group
Typesetting by DiTech Process Solutions, India

Printed in USA by King Printing Company, Inc.   5 4 3 2 1

ISBN 978-1-68420-007-8

Also available as an e-book:
eISBN 978-1-68420-008-5

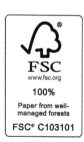

Dedicated to the individuals and families who allow us into their lives during their time of need.

Min S. Park, MD, FAANS

To my mentors and friends, William A. Goddard III, and Roel Nusse.

M. Yashar S. Kalani, MD, PhD, MBA, FAANS, FAHA

A debt of gratitude and appreciation to my mentors, colleagues, friends, and most importantly my family.

Michael F. Stiefel, MD, PhD, FAANS

Contents

Contents

Contents

Contents

Preface

History is rife with novel ideas to solve the vexing problems of the time that ultimately failed in their intended purpose. Medicine is not immune to this process and, in fact, relies upon it to ultimately move the field forward. It is incumbent as practitioners of our particular science and art to critically analyze the basis of our knowledge in order to further our understanding of the disease processes and the modalities designed to treat them.

Neurointerventional Surgery: An Evidence-Based Approach was created to acknowledge the limitations to our understanding of our field and provide a framework for the decisions that we make on a daily basis. The chapters in this textbook are designed to provide the neurointerventional surgeon, whether from a neurosurgical, neurological, or neuroradiological background, the historical literature that underpins our management decisions. This project is particularly well suited to increase the knowledge base of trainees and others with a strong interest in the neurovascular space. The chapter authors selected and critically analyzed the "landmark papers" that we hold as the "gospel truth" and, in that analysis, they established the foundation to our present-day practice.

The necessity of this textbook is clearly illustrated by our rapidly changing understanding of large vessel occlusions in ischemic stroke. Although earlier level 1 evidence studies suggested the futility in mechanical thrombectomy, more recent evidence strongly supported this procedure as a viable and important part of the treatment armamentarium. More and more experience with this procedure led to expanded indications and techniques with countless patients saved from a potentially debilitating event.

Neurointerventional Surgery: An-Evidence Based Approach has benefited from the combined expertise of internationally recognized experts in our field. Without their hard work and dedication, this project would have never come to pass. We hope that you will find some benefit within the pages of this textbook that will help you provide the best possible care to those individuals who have entrusted us with their lives.

Min S. Park, MD, FAANS
M. Yashar S. Kalani, MD, PhD, MBA, FAANS, FAHA
Michael F. Stiefel, MD, PhD, FAANS

Contributors

I. Joshua Abecassis, MD
Department of Neurosurgery
Harborview Medical Center, University of Washington
Seattle, Washington, USA

Peter Abraham, BA
Department of Radiology
University of California San Diego Medical Center
San Diego, California, USA

Nitin Agarwal, MD
Department of Neurological Surgery
University of Pittsburgh Medical Center
Pittsburgh, Pennsylvania, USA

Amin Nima Aghaebrahim, MD
Baptist Primary Stroke Director
Baptist Neurological Institution
Jacksonville, Florida, USA

Erinc Akture, MD
Lyerly Neurosurgery, Baptist Health
Jacksonville, Florida, USA

Felipe Albuquerque, MD
Department of Neurosurgery
Barrow Neurological Institute, St. Joseph's Hospital and
    Medical Center
Phoenix, Arizona, USA

Rami O. Almefty, MD
Department of Neurosurgery
Barrow Neurological Institute, St. Joseph's Hospital and
    Medical Center
Phoenix, Arizona, USA

Arun P. Amar, MD
Director of Endovascular Neurosurgery
University of Southern California Keck School of Medicine;
Stroke Director and Chief of Neurosurgery
LAC+USC Medical Center
Los Angeles, California, United States

Adam S. Arthur, MD, MPH
Professor
Department of Neurosurgery
University of Tennessee Health Sciences Center and
    Semmes-Murphey Clinic
Memphis, Tennessee, USA

Elias Atallah, MD
Department of Neurosurgery
Thomas Jefferson University Hospitals
Philadelphia, Pennsylvania, USA

Lucas Augusto, MD
Lyerly Neurosurgery, Baptist Health
Jacksonville, Florida, USA

Michael B. Avery, MD, MSc
Pacific Neuroscience Institute
Santa Monica, California, USA

Ali Aziz-Sultan, MD
Assistant Professor
Department of Neurosurgery, Cerebrovascular Division
Brigham and Women's Hospital, Harvard Medical School
Boston, Massachusetts, USA

Guilherme Barros, MD
Department of Neurosurgery
Harborview Medical Center, University of Washington
Seattle, Washington, USA

Phillip Bonney, MD
Department of Neurosurgery
University of Southern California Medical Center
Los Angeles, California, USA

Michael G. Brandel, MD
Department of Neurosurgery
University of California San Diego Medical Center
San Diego, California, USA

Marie-Christine Brunet, MD
Department of Neurosurgery & Radiology
University of Miami Miller School of Medicine
Miami, Florida, USA

Stepan Capek, MD
Department of Neurosurgery
University of Virginia Health System
Charlottesville, Virginia, USA

Joseph Carnevale, MD
Department of Neurological Surgery
New York-Presbyterian Hospital, Weill Cornell Medical
    Center
New York, USA

Leonardo Rangel Castilla, MD
Hospital Lomas Internacional
Star Medica Hospital
San Luis Potosi, Mexico

Joshua S. Catapano, MD
Department of Neurosurgery
Barrow Neurological Institute, St. Joseph's Hospital and
    Medical Center
Phoenix, Arizona, USA

Ahmed Cheema, MD
Assistant Professor
Department of Neurosurgery
University of Oklahoma Health Sciences Center
Oklahoma City, Oklahoma, USA

Ching-Jen Chen, MD
Department of Neurological Surgery
University of Virginia Health System
Charlottesville, Virginia, USA

Karen S. Chen, MD
Instructor
Department of Radiology, Interventional Neuroradiology
    Division
Brigham and Women's Hospital, Harvard Medical School
Boston, Massachusetts, USA

Brian M. Corliss, MD
Department of Neurosurgery
University of Florida
Gainesville, Florida, USA

Gustavo Cortez, MD
Lyerly Neurosurgery, Baptist Health
Jacksonville, Florida, USA

Justin E. Costello, DO
Assistant Professor of Radiology
Department of Neuroradiology, Walter Reed National
    Military Medical Center
Bethesda, Maryland, USA

R. Webster Crowley, MD
Associate Professor of Neurosurgery and Radiology
Department of Neurosurgery, Rush University Medical
    Center
Chicago, Illinois, USA

Victor Hugo Da Costa
Department of Cerebrovascular and Endovascular Surgery
Baptist Neurological Institute/Lyerly Neurosurgery
Jacksonville, Florida, USA

Lekhaj C. Daggubati, MD
Department of Neurosurgery
Milton S. Hershey Medical Center, Penn State Health
Hershey, Pennsylvania, USA

Andrew F. Ducruet, MD
Department of Neurosurgery
Barrow Neurological Institute, St. Joseph's Hospital and
    Medical Center
Phoenix, Arizona, USA

Abdullah H. Feroze, MD
Department of Neurosurgery
Harborview Medical Center, University of Washington
Seattle, Washington, USA

Paul M. Foreman, MD
Orlando Health Neuroscience and Rehabilitation Institute
Orlando, Florida, USA

W. Christopher Fox, MD
Department of Neurosurgery
Mayo Clinic in Florida
Jacksonville, Florida, USA

Basavaraj V. Ghodke, MD
Department of Neurosurgery
Harborview Medical Center, University of Washington
Seattle, Washington, USA

Jacob Goldberg, MD
Department of Neurological Surgery
New York-Presbyterian Hospital, Weill Cornell Medical
    Center
New York, USA

L. Fernando Gonzalez, MD
Professor of Neurosurgery
Co-Director Cerebrovascular and Endovascular
    Neurosurgery
Duke University
Durham, North Carolina, USA

Andrew S. Griffin, MD
Department of Neurosurgery
Duke University
Durham, North Carolina, USA

Bradley A. Gross, MD
Department of Neurological Surgery
University of Pittsburgh Medical Center
Pittsburgh, Pennsylvania, USA

Muhamed Hadzipasic, MD, PhD
Department of Neurosurgery
Massachusetts General Hospital
Boston, Massachusetts, USA

Danial K. Hallam, MD
Department of Neurosurgery
Harborview Medical Center, University of Washington
Seattle, Washington, USA

Ricardo Hanel, MD
Department of Cerebrovascular and Endovascular Surgery
Baptist Neurological Institute/Lyerly Neurosurgery
Jacksonville, Florida, USA

Rulon Hardman, MD, PhD
Azura Vascular Care
Malvern, Pennsylvania, USA

Mark R. Harrigan, MD
Department of Neurosurgery
University of Alabama at Birmingham
Birmingham, Alabama, USA

Hans Henkes, Prof, MD, PhD
Medical Director
Neuroradiological Clinic, Katharinenhospital, Klinikum
    Stuttgart
Stuttgart, Germany

Ibrahim Hussain, MD
Resident
Neurological Surgery, Department of Neurological Surgery
New York-Presbyterian Hospital, Weill Cornell Medical
    Center
New York, USA

Troy A. Hutchins, MD
Associate Professor of Radiology
Divisions of Diagnostic and Interventional Neuroradiology
University of Utah Health Sciences Center
Salt Lake City, Utah, USA

Pascal Jabbour, MD
The Angela and Richard T. Clark Distinguished Professor of
    Neurological Surgery
Division Chief
Neurovascular Surgery and Endovascular Neurosurgery,
    Thomas Jefferson University Hospital
Philadelphia, Pennsylvania, USA

Rachel Jacobs, MD
Department of Neurological Surgery
University of Pittsburgh Medical Center
Pittsburgh, Pennsylvania, USA

Brian T. Jankowitz, MD
Department of Neurological Surgery
Cooper Neuroscience Institute
Camden, Pennsylvania, USA

Matthew Johnson, PA-C
Department of Neurosurgery
Maine Medical Center
Portland, Maine, USA

Krishna Chaitanya Joshi, MBBS, MS, MCh
Department of Neurosurgery
Rush University Medical Center
Chicago, Illinois, USA

M. Yashar S. Kalani, MD, PhD, MBA, FAANS, FAHA
Associate Professor
Department of Surgery
St. John's Neuroscience Institute/University of Oklahoma
    School of Medicine
Tulsa, Oklahoma, USA

Claire Kaufman, MD
Department of Radiology, Section of Interventional
    Radiology
University of Utah
Salt Lake City, Utah, USA

Alexander A. Khalessi, MD
Department of Neurosurgery
University of California San Diego Medical Center
San Diego, California, USA

Louis J. Kim, MD
Department of Neurosurgery
Harborview Medical Center, University of Washington
Seattle, Washington, USA

Jared Knopman, MD
Assistant Professor of Neurological Surgery
Director of Cerebrovascular Surgery and Interventional
    Neuroradiology
Department of Neurological Surgery
New York-Presbyterian Hospital, Weill Cornell Medical
    Center
New York, USA

Matthew J. Koch
Department of Neurosurgery
Massachusetts General Hospital
Boston, Massachusetts, USA

Contributors

Jeyan S. Kumar, MD
Department of Neurosurgery
University of Virginia Health System
Charlottesville, Virginia, USA

Wiebke Kurre, MD
Institute of Neuroradiology
University of Frankfurt
Frankfurt, Germany

David Kutler, MD
Associate Professor of Otolaryngology
Department of Otolaryngology
New York-Presbyterian Hospital, Weill Cornell Medical
    Center
New York, USA

Michael R. Levitt, MD
Department of Neurosurgery
Harborview Medical Center, University of Washington
Seattle, Washington, USA

Thomas Link, MD
Department of Neurological Surgery
New York-Presbyterian Hospital, Weill Cornell Medical
    Center
New York, USA

Kenneth C. Liu, MD, FAANS, FACS
Department of Neurosurgery
University of Southern California School of Medicine
Los Angeles, California, USA

Evan Luther, MD
Department of Neurosurgery & Radiology
University of Miami Miller School of Medicine
Miami, Florida, USA

David J. McCarthy, MD
Department of Neurological Surgery
University of Pittsburgh Medical Center
Pittsburgh, Pennsylvania, USA

Alim P. Mitha, MD, SM, FRCSC
Associate Professor of Clinical Neurosciences and Radiology
Faculty of Neuroscience and Biomedical Engineering
Foothills Medical Centre
University of Calgary
Alberta, Canada

Andre Monteiro, MD
Department of Cerebrovascular and Endovascular Surgery
Baptist Neurological Institute/Lyerly Neurosurgery
Jacksonville, Florida, USA

Matias Negrotto, MD
Department of Radiology
Hospital de Clinicas
Montevideo, Uruguay

John D. Nerva, MD
Department of Neurosurgery
University of Florida Health System
Gainesville, Florida, USA

Pedro Norat, MD
Department of Neurological Surgery
University of Virginia Health System
Charlottesville, Virginia, USA

Chesney S. Oravec, MD
Resident Physician
Department of Neurosurgery
Wake Forest Baptist Medical Center
Winston-Salem, North Carolina, USA

J. Scott Pannell, MD
Department of Neurosurgery
University of California San Diego Medical Center
San Diego, California, USA

Min S. Park, MD, FAANS
Department of Neurosurgery
University of Virginia Health System
Charlottesville, Virginia, USA

Aman B. Patel
Director of Cerebrovascular and Endovascular
    Neurosurgery
Department of Neurosurgery
Massachusetts General Hospital
Boston, Massachusetts, USA

Kevin Porras, BS
Department of Neurosurgery
University of California San Diego Medical Center
San Diego, California, USA

Alexander Ramos, MD, PhD
Department of Neurological Surgery
New York-Presbyterian Hospital, Weill Cornell Medical
    Center
New York, USA

Christian Lopez Ramos, MPH
Department of Neurosurgery
University of California San Diego Medical Center
San Diego, California, USA

John F. Reavey-Cantwell, MS, MD
Reynolds Professor
Harold F. Young Neurosurgical Center
Virginia Commonwealth University
Richmond, Virginia, USA

Robert C. Rennert, MD
Department of Neurosurgery
University of California San Diego Medical Center
San Diego, California, USA

Lorenzo Rinaldo, MD, PhD
Department of Neurosurgery
Mayo Clinic
Rochester, Minnesota, USA

Dennis J. Rivet II, MD
Harold J. Nemuth Professor
Harold F. Young Neurosurgical Center
Virginia Commonwealth University
Richmond, Virginia, USA

Nader Sanai, MD
Department of Neurosurgery
Barrow Neurological Institute, St. Joseph's Hospital and
    Medical Center
Phoenix, Arizona, USA

Matthew R. Sanborn, MD
Department of Neurosurgery
Maine Medical Center
Portland, Maine, USA

David R. Santiago-Dieppa, MD
Department of Neurosurgery
University of California San Diego Medical Center
San Diego, California, USA

Alejandro Santillan, MD
Fellow
Interventional Neuroradiology, Department of Neurologi-
    cal Surgery
New York-Presbyterian Hospital, Weill Cornell Medical
    Center
New York, USA

Roberta Santos
Department of Cerebrovascular and Endovascular Surgery
Baptist Neurological Institute/Lyerly Neurosurgery
Jacksonville, Florida, USA

Mithun Sattur
Department of Neurosurgery
Medical University of South Carolina
Charleston, South Carolina, USA

Eric Sauvageau, MD
Department of Cerebrovascular and Endovascular Surgery
Baptist Neurological Institute/Lyerly Neurosurgery
Jacksonville, Florida, USA

Philip G. R. Schmalz, MD
Department of Neurosurgery
University of Alabama at Birmingham
Birmingham, Alabama, USA

Justin Schwarz, MD
Fellow
Interventional Neuroradiology, Department of Neurologi-
    cal Surgery
New York-Presbyterian Hospital, Weill Cornell Medical
    Center
New York, USA

Rajeev Sen, MD
Department of Neurosurgery
Harborview Medical Center, University of Washington
Seattle, Washington, USA

Parampreet Singh, MD
Department of Neurosurgery
University of Southern California Medical Center
Los Angeles, California, USA

Sauson Soldozy, BA
Department of Neurological Surgery
University of Virginia Health System
Charlottesville, Virginia, USA

Alejandro M. Spiotta, MD, FAANS
Professor of Neurosurgery and Neuroendovascular Surgery
Director
Neuroendovascular Surgery Division
Medical University of South Carolina
Charleston, South Carolina, USA

Christopher J. Stapleton
Department of Neurosurgery
Massachusetts General Hospital
Boston, Massachusetts, USA

Robert M. Starke, MD, MSc
Departments of Neurological Surgery and Radiology
University of Miami Health
Miami, Florida, USA

Joel M. Stary, MD, PhD
Department of Neurosurgery
Banner Desert Medical Center
Mesa, Arizona, USA

Jeffrey A. Steinberg, MD
Department of Neurosurgery
University of California San Diego Medical Center
San Diego, California, USA

Michael F. Stiefel, MD, PhD, FAANS
Director of Cerebrovascular and Endovascular
  Neurosurgery
Department of Neurosurgery
Piedmont Atlanta Hospital
Atlanta, Georgia, USA

Arvin R. Wali, MAS
Department of Neurosurgery
University of California San Diego Medical Center
San Diego, California, USA

Melanie Walker, MD
Department of Neurosurgery
Harborview Medical Center, University of Washington
Seattle, Washington, USA

Jeffrey Watkins, BS
Penn State College of Medicine, Milton S. Hershey Medical
  Center, Penn State Health
Hershey, Pennsylvania, USA

Kaan Yağmurlu, MD
Department of Neurosurgery
University of Virginia Health System
Charlottesville, Virginia, USA

1 Introduction to Evidence-Based Medicine

Ching-Jen Chen, M. Yashar S. Kalani, Michael F. Stiefel, and Min S. Park

In response to the growing demands of more evidence-based medicine in the management of cerebrovascular disorders, the American Heart Association (AHA) in conjunction with the American Stroke Association (ASA) has published guidelines on various clinical topics. The purpose of these guidelines is to provide an up-to-date comprehensive set of recommendations for clinicians providing care for patients with cerebrovascular diseases. These guidelines are derived from review of the literature by independent evidence review committees or writing groups comprising topic experts. The AHA/ASA also provides updates of new evidence through focused updates and scientific statements. The clinical topics reviewed range from indications for performing intracranial endovascular neurointerventional procedures to management of acute ischemic stroke and management of aneurysmal subarachnoid hemorrhage.[1,2,3,4,5,6,7]

The recommendation classification system of the AHA/ASA guidelines is adapted from that of the American College of Cardiology (ACC)/AHA clinical practice guidelines developed by the Task Force.[8] The classification system (▶ Fig. 1.1 and ▶ Fig. 1.2) comprise class of recommendation (COR) and level of evidence (LOE). COR is a statement concerning the strength of the recommendation and often serves as the primary guide for clinicians. The choice of COR is dependent upon the effect size or strength, and magnitude of benefit in relation to risk for clinical strategies, interventions, treatments, or diagnostic testing in patient care. The certainty or precision of information in support of the

Fig. 1.1 Classification of recommendations and level of evidence. Reprinted with permission from *Stroke*. 2015;46:2368–2400 ©2015 American Heart Association, Inc.[5]

recommendation is described by the LOE, classified by the type and quality of the evidence.

Class I and III recommendations are considered strong recommendations, based on effect size or strength, and benefit-to-risk es/timates. An intervention is considered a Class I recommendation when its benefits greatly outweigh its risks (benefit > > > risk). The suggested phrases for writing recommendations for Class I recommendation include: should; is recommended; is indicated; and is useful/effective/beneficial. Comparative effectiveness phrases for Class I recommendation include: treatment/strategy A is recommended/indicated in preference to treatment B; and treatment A should be chosen over treatment B. The list of suggested phrases to use when writing recommendations was developed in 2003 by the ACC/AHA Task Force on practice guidelines. It is written such that a recommendation, if separated or presented apart from the rest of the document, would still convey the full intent of the recommendation.

Class III recommendation is further classified into Class III: No Benefit and Class III: Harm. Class III: Harm is a strong recommendation in which the intervention is harmful to patients or incur excessive cost without benefit (benefit < risk). This is usually derived from one or more trials in which the outcomes for intervention were worse compared to that of the control. An intervention is considered a Class III: No Benefit recommendation when evidence suggests that it is no better than the control (benefit = risk). However, it must be noted that such a recommendation is not to be associated with weak evidence of expert opinion (LOE C-LD, C-EO, or C) as randomized trials or carefully conducted observational studies are often required to ascertain lack of benefit.[8] The suggested phrases for writing recommendations for Class III: Harm recommendation include: potentially harmful; causes harm; associated with excessive morbidity/mortality; and should not be performed/administered. The suggested phrases for writing recommendations for Class III: No Benefit recommendation include: is not recommended; is not indicated; should not be performed/administered; and is not useful/beneficial/effective.

Class IIa recommendations are considered intermediate strength recommendations and carry less benefit in comparison to Class I recommendations (benefit > > risk). Suitable phrases for writing recommendations for Class IIa recommendation include: is reasonable; can be useful/effective/beneficial; and is probably recommended or indicated. Comparative effectiveness phrases for Class IIa recommendation include: treatment/strategy A is probably recommended/indicated in preference to treatment B and it is reasonable to choose treatment A over treatment B. Class IIb recommendations are considered to be the weakest among the recommendations and pertain to interventions associated with marginal benefit-to-risk ratios or uncertain outcome advantages (benefit ≥ risk). Hence, additional evidence or studies are necessary to clarify the benefits or risks of the intervention. Suitable phrases for writing recommendations for Class IIb recommendation include: may/might be considered; may/might be reasonable; and usefulness/effectiveness is unknown/unclear/uncertain or not well established.

The precision and quality of the scientific evidence in support of the effect or strength of an intervention is rated by the LOE based upon the type, quantity, consistency, and quality of clinical trials and other relevant sources. The evidence in support of each recommendation is graded based on study type, which may comprise randomized, observational, prospective, or retrospective studies. In addition, the quality of evidence is assessed for potential bias, relevance, and fidelity. In the 2015 update to the COR and LOE classification system (▶ Fig. 1.2), the Task Force has provided additional categories offering greater granularity via distinct categories for randomized and nonrandomized evidence to better define the level and quality of evidence using a graded approach to evidence assessment.

Level A comprises evaluation of multiple populations, with high-quality evidence from more than one randomized controlled trial (RCT), meta-analyses of high-quality RCTs, or one or more RCTs corroborated by high-quality registry studies. Level B comprises limited population evaluation, where data is derived from a single RCT or nonrandomized studies. In the updated 2015 COR and LOE classification system (▶ Fig. 1.2), Level B is further categorized into Level B-R (Randomized) and Level B-NR (Nonrandomized). Level B-R comprises moderate-quality evidence from one or more RCTs or meta-analyses of moderate-quality RCTs. Level B-NR comprises moderate-quality evidence from one or more well-designed, well-executed nonrandomized studies, observational studies, registry studies, or meta-analyses of such studies.

Very limited population evaluation is designated Level C, comprising consensus opinion of experts, case studies, or standard of care. In the updated 2015 COR and LOE classification system (▶ Fig. 1.2), Level C is further categorized into Level C-LD (Limited Data) and Level C-EO (Expert Opinion). Level C-LD comprises randomized or nonrandomized observational or registry studies with limitations of design or execution, meta-analyses of randomized or nonrandomized observational or registry studies with limitations of design or execution, or physiological or mechanistic studies in human subjects. Level C-EO comprises consensus of expert opinion based on clinical experience. It is important to note that a recommendation with LOE C does not imply that the recommendation is weak as many important clinical questions in guidelines do not lend themselves to clinical trials (e.g., due to ethical concerns). Therefore, there may be a very clear clinical consensus that a particular intervention is useful or effective, despite the lack of RCTs.

To lead rather than lag behind clinical practice remains the ongoing challenge for these guidelines, focused updates, and scientific statements. These guidelines strive to maintain rigorous processes and methodology, while at the same time respond to the continually expanding literature in a timely manner. Similarly, the contents and recommendations provided within this book reflect the most up-to-date evidence that was rigorously evaluated at the time of writing. The scope of this book includes recommendations regarding endovascular treatment of cerebrovascular diseases beyond the previous guidelines set forth by the AHA/ASA.

CLASS (STRENGTH) OF RECOMMENDATION

CLASS I (STRONG)   Benefit >>> Risk

Suggested phrases for writing recommendations:
- Is recommended
- Is indicated/useful/effective/beneficial
- Should be performed/administered/other
- Comparative-Effectiveness Phrases†:
  - Treatment/strategy A is recommended/indicated in preference to treatment B
  - Treatment A should be chosen over treatment B

CLASS IIa (MODERATE)   Benefit >> Risk

Suggested phrases for writing recommendations:
- Is reasonable
- Can be useful/effective/beneficial
- Comparative-Effectiveness Phrases†:
  - Treatment/strategy A is probably recommended/indicated in preference to treatment B
  - It is reasonable to choose treatment A over treatment B

CLASS IIb (WEAK)   Benefit ≥ Risk

Suggested phrases for writing recommendations:
- May/might be reasonable
- May/might be considered
- Usefulness/effectiveness is unknown/unclear/uncertain or not well established

CLASS III: No Benefit (MODERATE)   Benefit = Risk
(Generally, LOE A or B use only)

Suggested phrases for writing recommendations:
- Is not recommended
- Is not indicated/useful/effective/beneficial
- Should not be performed/administered/other

CLASS III: Harm (STRONG)   Risk > Benefit

Suggested phrases for writing recommendations:
- Potentially harmful
- Causes harm
- Associated with excess morbidity/mortality
- Should not be performed/administered/other

LEVEL (QUALITY) OF EVIDENCE‡

LEVEL A

- High-quality evidence‡ from more than 1 RCT
- Meta-analyses of high-quality RCTs
- One or more RCTs corroborated by high-quality registry studies

LEVEL B-R   (Randomized)

- Moderate-quality evidence‡ from 1 or more RCTs
- Meta-analyses of moderate-quality RCTs

LEVEL B-NR   (Nonrandomized)

- Moderate-quality evidence‡ from 1 or more well-designed, well-executed nonrandomized studies, observational studies, or registry studies
- Meta-analyses of such studies

LEVEL C-LD   (Limited Data)

- Randomized or nonrandomized observational or registry studies with limitations of design or execution
- Meta-analyses of such studies
- Physiological or mechanistic studies in human subjects

LEVEL C-EO   (Expert Opinion)

Consensus of expert opinion based on clinical experience

COR and LOE are determined independently (any COR may be paired with any LOE).

A recommendation with LOE C does not imply that the recommendation is weak. Many important clinical questions addressed in guidelines do not lend themselves to clinical trials. Although RCTs are unavailable, there may be a very clear clinical consensus that a particular test or therapy is useful or effective.

* The outcome or result of the intervention should be specified (an improved clinical outcome or increased diagnostic accuracy or incremental prognostic information).

† For comparative-effectiveness recommendations (COR I and IIa; LOE A and B only), studies that support the use of comparator verbs should involve direct comparisons of the treatments or strategies being evaluated.

‡ The method of assessing quality is evolving, including the application of standardized, widely used, and preferably validated evidence grading tools; and for systematic reviews, the incorporation of an Evidence Review Committee.

COR indicates Class of Recommendation; EO, expert opinion; LD, limited data; LOE, Level of Evidence; NR, nonrandomized; R, randomized; and RCT, randomized controlled trial.

Fig. 1.2 Classification of recommendations and level of evidence, updated version from August, 2015. Reprinted with permission from *Circulation*. 2014;130:1208–1217 ©2014 American Heart Association, Inc.[8]

References

[1] Meyers PM, Schumacher HC, Higashida RT, et al. American Heart Association. Indications for the performance of intracranial endovascular neurointerventional procedures: a scientific statement from the American Heart Association Council on Cardiovascular Radiology and Intervention, Stroke Council, Council on Cardiovascular Surgery and Anesthesia, Interdisciplinary Council on Peripheral Vascular Disease, and Interdisciplinary Council on Quality of Care and Outcomes Research. Circulation. 2009; 119(16):2235–2249

[2] Saposnik G, Barinagarrementeria F, Brown RD, Jr, et al. American Heart Association Stroke Council and the Council on Epidemiology and Prevention. Diagnosis and management of cerebral venous thrombosis: a statement for healthcare professionals from the American Heart Association/American Stroke Association. Stroke. 2011; 42(4):1158–1192

[3] Connolly ES, Jr, Rabinstein AA, Carhuapoma JR, et al. American Heart Association Stroke Council, Council on Cardiovascular Radiology and Intervention, Council on Cardiovascular Nursing, Council on Cardiovascular Surgery and Anesthesia, Council on Clinical Cardiology. Guidelines for the management of aneurysmal subarachnoid hemorrhage: a guideline for healthcare professionals from the American Heart Association/American Stroke Association. Stroke. 2012; 43(6):1711–1737

[4] Hemphill JC, III, Greenberg SM, Anderson CS, et al. American Heart Association Stroke Council, Council on Cardiovascular and Stroke Nursing, Council on Clinical Cardiology. Guidelines for the management of spontaneous intracerebral hemorrhage: a guideline for healthcare professionals from the American Heart Association/American Stroke Association. Stroke. 2015; 46 (7):2032–2060

[5] Thompson BG, Brown RD, Jr, Amin-Hanjani S, et al. American Heart Association Stroke Council, Council on Cardiovascular and Stroke Nursing, and Council on Epidemiology and Prevention, American Heart Association, American Stroke Association. Guidelines for the management of patients with unruptured intracranial aneurysms: a guideline for healthcare professionals from the American Heart Association/American Stroke Association. Stroke. 2015; 46(8):2368–2400

[6] Derdeyn CP, Zipfel GJ, Albuquerque FC, et al. American Heart Association Stroke Council. Management of brain arteriovenous malformations: a scientific statement for healthcare professionals from the American Heart Association/American Stroke Association. Stroke. 2017; 48(8):e200–e224

[7] Powers WJ, Rabinstein AA, Ackerson T, et al. American Heart Association Stroke Council. 2018 guidelines for the early management of patients with acute ischemic stroke: a guideline for healthcare professionals from the American Heart Association/American Stroke Association. Stroke. 2018; 49 (3):e46–e110

[8] Jacobs AK, Anderson JL, Halperin JL, et al. ACC/AHA TASK FORCE MEMBERS. The evolution and future of ACC/AHA clinical practice guidelines: a 30-year journey: a report of the American College of Cardiology/American Heart Association Task Force on practice guidelines. Circulation. 2014; 130(14): 1208–1217

Section I

Hemorrhagic Stroke

2 Unruptured Cerebral Aneurysms

Min S. Park, M. Yashar S. Kalani, and Michael F. Stiefel

Abstract

The management of unruptured cerebral aneurysms is a fundamental component of most neurointerventional practices. The decision to observe these lesions or offer treatment is predicated on the risk of future rupture of the cerebral aneurysm over the expected remaining lifetime of the patient. The natural history data on unruptured cerebral aneurysms rely on several landmark papers that are well quoted throughout the medical literature; however, it is important to delve closely into the original papers to better understand these results and their limitations. In addition, it is important to have a solid understanding of the evidence that might support neurointerventional management of cerebral aneurysms.

Keywords: cerebral aneurysm, natural history, rupture rate, clipping, coiling, flow diversion

2.1 Goals

1. Review the literature that forms the basis of our understanding of the natural history of cerebral aneurysms.
2. Critically analyze the literature on the natural history of cerebral aneurysms.
3. Review the literature that supports treatment of unruptured cerebral aneurysms versus observation.
4. Critically analyze more recent attempts to quantify the natural history of unruptured cerebral aneurysms and their treatment.

2.2 Case Example

2.2.1 History of Present Illness

A 48-year-old non-Japanese, non-Finnish man presents for initial evaluation after discovery of two incidental cerebral aneurysms on magnetic resonance imaging and angiography (MRI/A) for work-up of a several-year history of cluster-type headaches. He has an extensive history of smoking and alcohol use. He denies any significant neurological complaints including seizures, loss of consciousness, numbness, weakness, or speech/vision difficulty.

Past medical history: Denies history of polycystic kidney disease, collagen vascular disease, prior subarachnoid/intracranial hemorrhage, or hypertension.

Past surgical history: Previous laparoscopic cholecystectomy.

Family history: Denies history of cerebral aneurysms.

Social history: 30 pack/year smoking history.

Review of systems: As per the above.

Neurological examination: Unremarkable.

Imaging studies: See figures.

▶ Fig. 2.1a, b: MRA brain of a 4.5 × 4.5 mm right middle cerebral artery aneurysm and a cerebral angiogram of an irregular 8 × 4 mm left posterior communicating artery aneurysms. Both aneurysms had associated daughter sacs/dome irregularities.

2.2.2 Treatment Plan

The patient agreed to treatment of the incidental aneurysms after he discontinued the use of cigarettes. The recommendation was made for coil embolization of the left posterior communicating artery aneurysm followed by surgical clipping of the right middle cerebral artery aneurysm because of the angiomorphology and accessibility of the respective aneurysms.

2.2.3 Follow-up

The patient did very well after the initial embolization of the posterior communicating artery aneurysm, which had a small residual neck (Raymond 2 occlusion) after the treatment. He underwent uncomplicated clipping of the right middle cerebral artery aneurysm several months later. At his 2-year follow-up visit, he was doing well with a stable, small residual neck of the coiled left posterior communicating artery aneurysm on an MRA brain. Additionally, there was no evidence of recurrence of the right middle cerebral artery aneurysm on computed tomography angiograms of the head.

2.3 Case Summary

1. *What would you report as the rupture risk of the unruptured cerebral aneurysms to this patient?*

   The decision to treat an unruptured cerebral aneurysm is largely predicated on the perceived rupture risk of the aneurysm. We are attempting to improve the long-term outcomes for the patient by reducing the rupture risk of the aneurysm over the patient's lifetime versus the immediate/short-term risk of the treatment.

   Our knowledge of the rupture rate of unruptured cerebral aneurysms has been developed over time by multiple landmark papers that are reviewed in this chapter.[1,2,3,4,5] Additionally, there are multiple factors (patient and aneurysm

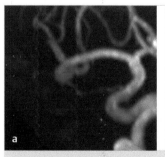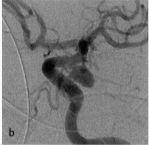

Fig. 2.1(a) Magnetic resonance angiography of the brain demonstrating a 4.5 × 4.5 mm right middle cerebral artery aneurysm. **(b)** Diagnostic cerebral angiogram demonstrating an irregular, 8 × 4 mm left posterior communicating artery aneurysm. Both aneurysms exhibited dome irregularities/daughter sacs.

related) which can be taken into account in the decision-making process. Reported rupture rates can vary widely in the literature based upon the specific study and its methodology. For aneurysms of these sizes in this patient, the rupture rates can be quoted to be as low as < 0.05% per year[5] to as high as approximately 14.5% over 5 years.[4] There are multiple studies that would also place the rupture risk of unruptured cerebral aneurysms at around 1 to 1.5% per year.[3,6]

2. *What patient factors would you consider when deciding on your recommendations for observation or treatment of these unruptured cerebral aneurysms?*

a) Age

Since the risk of cerebral aneurysm rupture is life long, age is an important consideration when counseling patients for either observation or treatment.[7] A recent analysis of three large prospective cohort trials in Japan identified increasing patient age as an independent risk factor for aneurysm rupture[8] corroborating the results of an earlier published meta-analysis.[9] These results, however, are in contradiction to other studies that identified younger patient age as a risk factor for future aneurysm rupture.[3,10] In addition, certain methods of treatment may pose higher risks as patient's age increases.[11]

b) Smoking

Smoking appears to be one modifiable risk factor associated with an increased prevalence of unruptured cerebral aneurysms and, even possibly, with subsequent aneurysm rupture.[4,5,10] Whether or not smoking cessation improves the natural history, however, is unknown.

c) Multiplicity

The presence of multiple aneurysms is found in upwards of 30% of patients with a diagnosis of cerebral aneurysms and may be associated with subsequent aneurysm growth, a strong marker for subsequent rupture.[3,5,6,12] However, other studies suggest that multiplicity of aneurysms is unrelated to future rupture risk.[13]

3. *What aneurysm factors would you consider when deciding on your recommendations for observation or treatment of these unruptured cerebral aneurysms?*

a) Size

Size of an unruptured cerebral aneurysm has been extensively studied in relation to the risk of aneurysm rupture.[1,4,5,6,13] The size cutoff has been set at different levels by different studies. One centimeter was used in earlier studies with subsequent refinement to 7 mm in later studies.[1,4,5] In addition, investigators in Japan identified an increasing risk of rupture with increasing aneurysm size.[6]

b) Vessel location

Likewise, the location of the aneurysm has also been extensively studied in the literature.[4,5,6] Posterior circulation aneurysms have been posited to have a higher rupture rate than anterior circulation aneurysms.[4,5] Interestingly, these studies categorized posterior communicating arteries as posterior circulation aneurysms. The UCAS investigators also found differences in rupture risk based upon location, but only for anterior circulation aneurysms.[6] Aneurysms on the anterior or posterior communicating arteries had a higher rupture risk than aneurysms on the middle cerebral artery. There was no increased rupture risk with posterior circulation aneurysms.

c) Irregularity/daughter sacs

Studies have identified aneurysm irregularities and/or presence of daughter sacs as an independent risk factor for subsequent aneurysm rupture.[6]

4. *What would you recommend for the left posterior communicating artery aneurysm?*

Given the patient's age, smoking history, size, location, and irregularity of the aneurysm, a strong argument can be made for treatment. Studies on the natural history of cerebral aneurysms have suffered from significant selection bias with inclusion of patients who were prescreened for observation over treatment.[1,4,5,6]

Likewise, the method of treatment, either endovascular or surgical, is a decision to be made based upon the expert medical opinion of the practitioner(s) and the patient. Certainly, aneurysm-specific characteristics may preclude treatment by one method over another. In this instance, the aneurysm could be readily treated by either modality. After a lengthy discussion with the patient, he elected for endovascular treatment with balloon-assisted coil embolization. Also, the presence of a second aneurysm factored into the discussion with a strong desire to avoid bilateral open surgeries.

5. *What would you recommend for the right middle cerebral artery aneurysm?*

In this instance, the patient ultimately elected for treatment of this aneurysm for reasons very similar to the ones previously stated. Observation was also a valid option given the smaller size and the location in the anterior circulation/middle cerebral artery. However, the patient's young age and presence of a small daughter sac/dome irregularity weighed more heavily in the decision-making process.

Unlike with the contralateral aneurysm, the middle cerebral artery aneurysm was wide necked, making coil embolization with or without adjunctive techniques a less attractive option. The use of flow diversion has been reported in this location, but the studies have largely been limited to smaller, retrospective, single-center series. In addition, younger patients may do better following surgical clipping than older patients with outcomes comparable to endovascular treatment.[4] Recurrence and retreatment rates following surgical clipping are also lower than with coil embolization.

6. *How would you follow-up these aneurysms with or without treatment?*

There are several methods of following up treated aneurysms with imaging studies: digital subtraction angiography, CT angiography, or MRA. In this instance, we elected to follow up long term with both an MRA and CTA given the different treatment techniques.

2.4 Level of Evidence

Patient's age: Given the patient's relatively young age, treatment of aneurysms, including surgical clipping of the middle cerebral artery aneurysm, is reasonable (Class I, Level of Evidence B).

Smoking history: The patient's extensive smoking history may present a risk for aneurysm development (Class I, Level of Evidence B).

Multiplicity of aneurysms: The patient has middle cerebral and posterior communicating artery aneurysms (Class I, Level of Evidence C).

Angiomorphology and location of the aneurysm: The posterior communicating artery aneurysm was highly irregular with associated daughter sacs (Class I, Level of Evidence C).

Treatment: Surgical clipping may be more durable than endovascular coiling but may be associated with higher procedural morbidity and mortality (Class IIB, Level of Evidence B).

Follow-up of aneurysm: With the small residual neck of the coiled aneurysm, periodic follow-up imaging studies should be performed. In this case, we elected to follow up with MRA studies, which demonstrated stability of the Raymond 2 aneurysm occlusion (Class I, Level of Evidence B).

2.5 Landmark Papers

Wiebers DO, Whisnant JP, O'Fallon WM. The natural history of unruptured intracranial aneurysms. N Engl J Med 1981;304 (12):696–698.

Any discussion of landmark papers on the natural history of unruptured cerebral aneurysms must include the work of Dr. David O. Wiebers and his collaborators at the Mayo Clinic and Mayo Foundation in Rochester, Minnesota.[1] In 1981, they reported on the natural history of 65 patients (22 men and 43 women) with 81 unruptured saccular aneurysms documented by cerebral angiography from 1955 to 1975, who did not undergo surgical treatment and were followed up for a minimum of 5 years after diagnosis or until death. Thirty-six of the patients had angiograms performed due to neurological symptoms (mass effect–like symptoms, ischemic symptoms, and/or headaches), whereas 29 patients had symptoms that were unrelated to the aneurysm.

Over the course of the follow-up period, eight patients experienced aneurysmal rupture, with seven of the eight dying as a result of the intracranial hemorrhage. Wiebers et al performed a multivariate analysis to determine whether patient-related (age, sex, presence of hypertension) and/or aneurysm-related (size, location, number, multilobulated aneurysms, symptoms other than hemorrhage) factors were predictive of future rupture. Their analysis indicated that aneurysm size greater than 10 mm was the most predictive of future rupture. Indeed, four aneurysms between 10 and 20 mm ruptured and four aneurysms greater than 20 mm ruptured, whereas no aneurysms below 10 mm in size ruptured. In addition, four patients with aneurysms ruptured within 2½ months from the initial diagnosis had a mean aneurysm size of 30 mm. The other four patients whose aneurysms ruptured at a later time had a mean size of only 15.7 mm. The authors also noted that aneurysms were unlikely to cause symptoms of mass effect unless they were at least 8 mm in size.

On the basis of their results, the authors concluded that aneurysms less than 10 mm in size had a very low probability of subsequent rupture; however, patients with aneurysms ≥ 10 mm in size should be treated as soon as possible. If aneurysms cause symptoms of mass effect after the initial diagnosis, then it likely indicates enlargement of the aneurysm to greater than 8 mm and, thus, portended a higher likelihood of rupture.

As one of the seminal works on the natural history of cerebral aneurysms, the article by Wiebers et al established the baseline to which all other papers would be compared. Unlike the later series by Juvela et al, there was no reported policy at Wieber et al's institution to not treat incidental, unruptured aneurysms.[3]

This preselection of untreated, unruptured aneurysms potentially introduced an element of selection bias. No information was provided concerning those patients diagnosed with unruptured aneurysms who underwent elective treatment and, thus, were not available for this study. In addition, all of the follow-up was by communication (telephone interviews, records reviews, etc.) rather than by imaging. Thus, the authors were unable to discuss aneurysm growth as a risk factor; other than that the development of symptoms of mass effect over time would suggest aneurysm growth to at least 8 mm in size. The lack of significance of the other studied variables may be related more to the smaller sample size versus a lack of true significance.

Juvela S, Porras M, Heiskanen O. Natural history of unruptured intracranial aneurysms: a long term follow-up study. J Neurosurg 1993;79(2):174–182.

Dr. Seppo Juvela and coauthors published another landmark paper in 1993 in which they followed 142 patients with 181 unruptured cerebral aneurysms in Finland.[3] The basis of this study was an institutional/national policy prior to 1979 of not treating unruptured aneurysms. From 1956 to 1978, 142 patients (66 men and 76 women) with 181 aneurysms were followed up for a total of 1944 patient-years and, on average, 13.7 years per patient.

During the follow-up period, 27 of the 142 (19%) patients ultimately experienced a subarachnoid hemorrhage from an unruptured aneurysm with an approximate annual incidence of aneurysm rupture of 1.4%. The risk of rupture remained fairly constant over the decades of follow-up in their study with the observed cumulative risk of rupture of 32% at 30 years after diagnosis. Although Juvela et al did not find a definitive size cutoff to predict aneurysm rupture as in previous studies, they did note a linear relationship between the risk of rupture and aneurysm size.[2] In addition, they found that all aneurysms which subsequently ruptured increased in size compared with the aneurysms that had not ruptured. De novo aneurysm formation was 2.2% per angiographic follow-up year.

On the basis of their findings, the authors recommended treatment of all cerebral aneurysms, irrespective of size, if technically feasible and if there were no contraindications to surgery from concurrent disease or advanced age.

Although this is easily considered one of the landmark papers on the natural history of unruptured cerebral aneurysms, there is one issue that limits the generalizability of the results. The majority of the patients included in this study had either a symptomatic aneurysm (6 of 142 patients) or a previous subarachnoid hemorrhage from an aneurysm rupture (131 of 142 patients). Only 5 of 142 patients had truly incidental aneurysms. Given the time period of the study (pre-1979) and the lack of advanced, noninvasive imaging studies at that time, this is hardly surprising; however, it does lead to questions concerning the selection bias of this particular cohort and whether their recommendations can be applied to truly incidental aneurysms (i.e., without a prior history subarachnoid hemorrhage). Unlike subsequent and previous studies concerning the natural history, there was no selection bias for treatment since all unruptured aneurysms were managed conservatively.

International Study of Unruptured Intracranial Aneurysms Investigators. Unruptured intracranial aneurysms—risk of rupture and risks of surgical intervention. N Engl J Med 1998;339 (24):1725–1733.

Perhaps one of the most controversial landmark papers on the topic of the natural history of unruptured aneurysms was published in 1998 in the *New England Journal of Medicine*.[5] The International Study of Unruptured Intracranial Aneurysms (ISUIA) involved 2,621 patients in the United States, Canada, and Europe. The investigators retrospectively determined rupture risks in 1,449 patients with 1,937 unruptured aneurysms. About half of these patients (group 1, 727 patients) had no prior history of subarachnoid hemorrhage, while the other half (group 2, 722 patients) did. In addition, they followed up 1,172 patients prospectively who underwent surgical treatment to determine treatment-related morbidity and mortality.

The reported rupture rates for all patients were significantly lower than previously reported. Group 1 patients (no history of subarachnoid hemorrhage) had a rupture risk of < 0.05% per year for aneurysms smaller than 10 mm, whereas group 2 patients had a rupture risk of 0.5% per year for small aneurysms. For aneurysms ≥ 10 mm in diameter, the rupture rates were still less than 1%, although the rupture rate for giant aneurysms (≥ 25 mm) in group 1 was reportedly 6% in the first year. Overall, the rupture rate for all patients, 0.5% per year, was considerably lower than earlier reports. In addition, posterior circulation aneurysms were also noted to have a greater risk of rupture than those in other locations.

The prospective arm of the study also subdivided patients into two groups based on prior history of subarachnoid hemorrhage. The majority of the patients (996 of 1,172 patients) underwent surgical clipping of the aneurysm, with the remainder being treated by "various endovascular procedures." The complications following surgery were considerably higher than previously reported, with combined morbidity and mortality in group 1 patients of 17.5% and 15.7% at 30 days and 1 year, respectively, and 13.6% and 13.1%, respectively, for group 2 patients.

Considering the identified risk of rupture and the combined morbidity and mortality for treatment, the ISUIA investigators stated that it would appear unlikely that the risks of treatment for aneurysms less than 10 mm would improve on the overall natural history of these aneurysms.

Following the publication of what has become known as ISUIA 1, a litany of complaints was voiced by the neurosurgical and neurointerventional community. Most notably, issues were raised concerning the selection bias inherent in these types of studies. Aneurysms that were considered unsuitable for observation were treated, either surgically or endovascularly, and were unavailable for the retrospective component of the study.

Thus, the patients in the retrospective arm would include a preponderance of aneurysms that were deemed "safe" to follow. This resulted in several notable differences in various groups. For example, there was an underrepresentation of larger aneurysms in patients with prior subarachnoid hemorrhage and an overrepresentation of certain types of aneurysms for which most practitioners would not recommend treatment, for example, cavernous internal carotid artery aneurysms. In addition, questions were raised concerning the higher reported complication rates of treated aneurysms as well.

Wiebers DO, Whisnant JP, Huston J III, et al. Unruptured intracranial aneurysms: natural history, clinical outcome, and risks of surgical and endovascular treatment. Lancet 2003;362(9378): 103–111.

The follow-up study to the first ISUIA publication involved a prospective assessment of unruptured aneurysms of 4,060 total patients enrolled over a 7-year period (December 1991 to December 1998).[4] Three groups of patients were involved: 1,692 patients were followed up in the observation arm, 1,917 had open surgery for treatment of their aneurysm, and 451 had endovascular repair. Similar to the original ISUIA publication, the observational arm was divided into two groups based on a prior history of subarachnoid hemorrhage from a separate aneurysm.[4,5]

In the natural history cohort, a total of 51 of 1,692 patients (3%) experienced a confirmed aneurysm rupture within the 5-year follow-up period. Another 36 patients who had both an aneurysm and another potential source for the hemorrhage were excluded from the analysis. This resulted in a more detailed report of 5-year cumulative rupture risks according to the size and location of the aneurysms (▶ Table 2.1). Although groups 1 and 2 were reported separately for aneurysms smaller than 7 mm, they were reported together in all other size categories because of the smaller numbers of patients.

The 5-year natural history of unruptured aneurysms in the observational cohort of what has become known as ISUIA 2 indicated a higher risk of rupture than was reported in ISUIA 1. However, the investigators still contended that aneurysms < 7 mm in size without a prior history of subarachnoid hemorrhage had an exceedingly low rate of rupture (0.1% per year). In addition, the ISUIA investigators included posterior communicating artery aneurysms in the posterior circulation cohort, a rather curious classification given most commonly held anatomical teachings.

The complication rate for open surgical treatment was also reportedly better than in the original study. Combined morbidity

Table 2.1 Five-year rupture rates for aneurysms based on size and location[4]

	<7 mm		7–12 mm	13–24 mm	≥25 mm
	Group 1[a]	Group 2[a]			
Cavernous ICA (n = 210)	0	0	0	3.0	6.4
AC/MC/IC arteries (n = 1,037)	0	1.5	2.6	14.5	40
Posterior/Pcomm (n = 445)	2.5	3.4	14.5	18.4	50

Abbreviations: AC, anterior communicating or anterior cerebral; IC, internal carotid (not cavernous carotid); ICA, internal carotid artery; MC, middle cerebral; Pcomm, posterior communicating artery; SAH, subarachnoid hemorrhage.
[a]Group 1 had no history of previous SAH; Group 2 had a history of previous SAH.
Reprinted from The Lancet, 362(9378), Wiebers DO, Whisnant JP, Huston J, III, et al. International Study of Unruptured Intracranial Aneurysms Investigators. Unruptured intracranial aneurysms: natural history, clinical outcome, and risks of surgical and endovascular treatment, 103–110, 2003, with permission from Elsevier.

and mortality at 1 year in the surgical arm was 12.6% for group 1 patients and 10.1% for group 2 patients, whereas the same rates reported in the initial study were 15.7% and 13.1% for groups 1 and 2, respectively.[4,5] Comparatively, the endovascular complication rates at 1 year were 9.8% and 7.1% for groups 1 and 2, respectively, despite having generally older patients, larger aneurysms, and more posterior circulation aneurysms compared with the surgical arm.

Overall, the risk of aneurysm rupture was similar to the complication rates for treatment, either surgical or endovascular, for an aneurysm of a given size. Thus, recommendations for treatment would concentrate on whether the patient was comfortable with an upfront treatment risk that would be similar to the long-term rupture risk.

Again, the effects of selection bias cannot be eliminated from their findings. The overall cohort was divided into observational and treatment arms based upon the expert opinion of the attending physician at the time of enrollment. Although patients were followed up prospectively in both arms, the initial evaluation led to significant differences in the two cohorts from the start of the study.

A common thread throughout most of the observational studies concerning the natural history of unruptured cerebral aneurysms detailed above and found throughout the medical literature is the influence of selection bias. Generally speaking, the patients who were included for the analysis were those who had been recommended observation over treatment by a medical specialist for their unruptured cerebral aneurysm prior to inclusion in the study. For instance, of the 6,697 aneurysms included in the UCAS prospective registry study in Japan, 3,050 aneurysms were treated prior to rupture and were not included in final rupture risk calculations.[6] In addition, patients who underwent subsequent aneurysm treatment were excluded from the final analysis. The one study where this is not a concern is by Juvela et al.[3] However, this series more accurately represents the natural history of an ethnically homogenous population with the significant majority having a prior history of subarachnoid hemorrhage.

2.6 Recommendations

There is still considerable controversy as to which factors are pertinent when assessing a patient with an unruptured cerebral aneurysm. The American Heart Association/American Stroke Association published guidelines for the evaluation and management of unruptured intracranial aneurysms after an extensive review of the literature from 1977 to 2014.[14] Using the available medical evidence, the working group identified several factors for consideration when designing the management plan for a patient: aneurysm size, location, and morphology; documented growth on serial imaging studies; patient's age; prior history of aneurysmal subarachnoid hemorrhage; multiplicity of aneurysms; family history of aneurysms; and the presence of other cerebrovascular pathology. In the end, however, the guidelines suggested that treatment decisions are largely left to the best judgment of the physician.

Because of these continued questions, multiple attempts have been made to more accurately quantify the natural history of cerebral aneurysms and any recommendations for treatment.

Recently, Greving et al developed the PHASES score to predict the risk of rupture of an aneurysm; their scoring system was based on a pooled analysis of six previously published prospective cohort studies (▶ Fig. 2.2a).[13] The authors identified six predictors of aneurysm rupture: age, hypertension, prior subarachnoid hemorrhage, aneurysm size, aneurysm location, and geographical location of the patient. They created a point system for each of these factors that would provide a predicted 5-year risk of aneurysm rupture to assist with patient counseling and decision making (▶ Fig. 2.2b). However, PHASES, by virtue of its design, also incorporated all of the biases and shortcomings of the six studies used to create the scoring system and has received critical reviews.[15]

Etminan et al developed an Unruptured Intracranial Aneurysm Treatment score (UIATS) using a multidisciplinary consensus model to determine treatment recommendations for unruptured aneurysms.[7] By using a Delphi consensus model, a group of 69 specialists in the fields of neurosurgery, neuroradiology, and neurology identified multiple patient- and aneurysm-related factors that would lead the specialist to recommend conservative management versus treatment. Each factor was weighed based upon the perceived strength of the recommendation for treatment or observation. A scoring system was then created (▶ Fig. 2.3), with the final tabulated score favoring conservative management or treatment. However, there was a third indeterminate category of patients for which a definitive recommendation could not be made. The authors internally and externally validated their study with high reported inter-rater agreements on recommendations.

By nature of its design, the UIATS has a much different goal than the publications previously reviewed in this chapter. The authors reduced the complexities and uncertainties of describing the natural history of aneurysms by relying on expert opinion to guide decision-making. Patient and aneurysm characteristics that the 69 specialists eventually agreed upon using the Delphi consensus were incorporated into the scoring system. This system eliminated the need to statistically compare the risk of aneurysm rupture with the risks inherent with treatment. As the authors stated, the purpose of the UIATS is to assist the practitioner by "indicating how a large group of specialists might manage an individual patient," rather than to provide a statistical risk of the natural history of aneurysms versus the risks of treatment.

Whether we will truly be able to calculate the natural history and rupture risk of all cerebral aneurysms is uncertain. The Trial on Endovascular Aneurysm Management (TEAM) attempted to address this shortcoming in our knowledge.[16,17] It was designed to randomize all patients considered for endovascular treatment of aneurysms to treatment versus observation. With the broad inclusion criteria, the authors attempted to rectify the primary criticism of most previous studies pertaining to selection bias in the observation arm (i.e., observation of patients not preselected for surgery). The study was terminated prematurely secondary to a futility analysis after only 80 patients of the proposed 2,002 patients had been enrolled over a 5-year time frame despite the involvement of 50 international centers. Unfortunately, in addition to the bureaucratic challenges, there was also significant reluctance by participating physicians to enroll patients

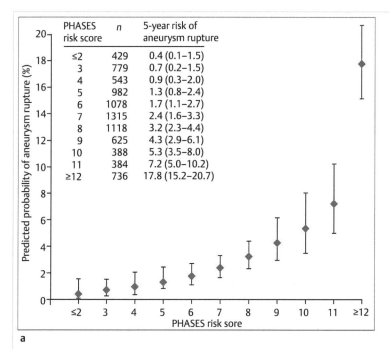

PHASES risk score	n	5-year risk of aneurysm rupture
≤2	429	0.4 (0.1–1.5)
3	779	0.7 (0.2–1.5)
4	543	0.9 (0.3–2.0)
5	982	1.3 (0.8–2.4)
6	1078	1.7 (1.1–2.7)
7	1315	2.4 (1.6–3.3)
8	1118	3.2 (2.3–4.4)
9	625	4.3 (2.9–6.1)
10	388	5.3 (3.5–8.0)
11	384	7.2 (5.0–10.2)
≥12	736	17.8 (15.2–20.7)

a

PHASES aneurysm risk score	Points
(P) Population	
North American, European (other than Finnish)	0
Japanese	3
Finnish	5
(H) Hypertension	
No	0
Yes	1
(A) Age	
<70 years	0
≥70 years	1
(S) Size of aneurysm	
<7.0 mm	0
7.0–9.9 mm	3
10.0–19.9 mm	6
≥20 mm	10
(E) Earlier SAH from another aneurysm	
No	0
Yes	1
(S) Site of aneurysm	
ICA	0
MCA	2
ACA/Pcom/posterior	4

To calculate the PHASES risk score for an individual, the number of points associated with each indicator can be added up to obtain the total risk score. For example, a 55-year-old North American man with no hypertension, no previous SAH, and a medium-sized (8 mm) posterior circulation aneurysm will have a risk score of 0+0+0+3+0+4=7 points. According to figure 3, this score corresponds to a 5-year risk of rupture of 2.4%. SAH=subarachnoid haemorrhage. ICA=internal carotid artery. MCA=middle cerebral artery. ACA=anterior cerebral arteries (including the anterior cerebral artery, anterior communicating artery, and pericallosal artery), Pcom=posterior communicating artery. posterior=posterior circulation (including the vertebral artery, basilar artery, cerebellar arteries, and posterior cerebral artery).

b

Fig. 2.2 (a) PHASES risk prediction charts for aneurysm rupture; **(b)** 5-year risk of aneurysm rupture based upon the total PHASES risks score.[13] Reprinted from The Lancet Neurol, 13(1), Greving JP, Wermer MJ, Brown RD, Jr, et al, Development of the PHASES score for prediction of risk of rupture of intracranial aneurysms: a pooled analysis of six prospective cohort studies, 59–66, 2014, with permission from Elsevier.

in the study and among patients to be enrolled in the study.[18] Whether or not a study to determine the natural history of cerebral aneurysms (vs. the natural history of aneurysms not preselected for treatment) is feasible going forward is questionable.

Likewise, there are no current prospective studies directly comparing endovascular management versus open surgical management of unruptured cerebral aneurysms, unlike with ruptured cerebral aneurysms.[19,20] Existing data support the notion that endovascular treatment has a lower morbidity and mortality rate compared with open surgery but with a higher retreatment/recurrence rate of the aneurysms[4]; however, these studies are largely hampered by the differences in the study population between the two cohorts and/or the retrospective nature of the studies.

Raymond et al proposed the Canadian Unruptured Endovascular versus Surgery (CURES) trial as a pilot study of 260 patients to address this shortcoming.[21] To be eligible for this study, the patient must be a candidate for either surgery or endovascular coiling with or without adjunctive techniques with randomization into either treatment arm. The outcome

measures for this study involve failure of initial treatment, aneurysm recurrence at 1 year, posttreatment hemorrhagic events, and treatment-related morbidity and mortality. The authors expect to compare the clinical outcomes of the two treatment modalities. With the results of the CURES trial, the investigators hope to conduct a larger international, multicenter trial.

While we have a large body of medical literature from which to draw, our knowledge of the natural history of unruptured cerebral aneurysms is incomplete. Furthermore, the advantages of one treatment modality over another (i.e., endovascular coiling vs. surgical clipping) are uncertain, although reviews of multiple administrative data sets point to better outcomes with endovascular treatment.[14] This advantage is tempered by the higher retreatment rates following coil embolization. As an additional confounding variable, the endovascular treatment of aneurysms is advancing at a rapid pace with the introduction of the next generation of coil technology, flow-diverting devices, intrasaccular devices, etc., potentially making the results of ongoing studies obsolete before publication.

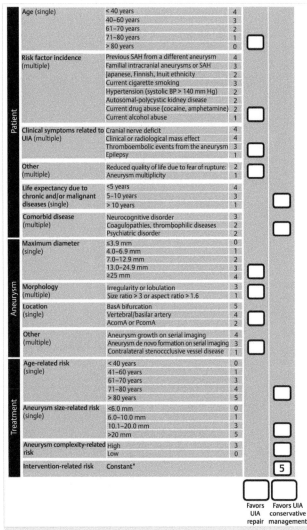

Fig. 2.3 The UIATS scoring sheet.[7]
Reprinted with permission from Etminan N, Brown RD, Jr, Beseoglu K, et al. The unruptured intracranial aneurysm treatment score: a multidisciplinary consensus. Neurology. 2015; 85(10):881–889.

2.7 Summary

1. The understanding of the natural history of unruptured cerebral aneurysms relies on multiple landmark papers,
   which have some inherent limitations largely related to their inclusion criteria.
2. Multiple factors related to the patient and/or the aneurysm can be taken into consideration when evaluating a patient with an unruptured cerebral aneurysm.
3. There is no high-level evidence to support one method of treatment of unruptured cerebral aneurysms over another, although retrospective studies suggest an advantage to endovascular treatment with coil embolization over open surgical clipping in terms of patient outcomes. This must be tempered with the higher retreatment and/or rupture rates following coil embolization.

References

[1] Wiebers DO, Whisnant JP, O'Fallon WM. The natural history of unruptured intracranial aneurysms. N Engl J Med. 1981; 304(12):696–698

[2] Wiebers DO, Whisnant JP, Sundt TM, Jr, O'Fallon WM. The significance of unruptured intracranial saccular aneurysms. J Neurosurg. 1987; 66(1):23–29

[3] Juvela S, Porras M, Heiskanen O. Natural history of unruptured intracranial aneurysms: a long-term follow-up study. J Neurosurg. 1993; 79 (2):174–182

[4] Wiebers DO, Whisnant JP, Huston J, III, et al. International Study of Unruptured Intracranial Aneurysms Investigators. Unruptured intracranial aneurysms: natural history, clinical outcome, and risks of surgical and endovascular treatment. Lancet. 2003; 362(9378):103–110

[5] International Study of Unruptured Intracranial Aneurysms Investigators. Unruptured intracranial aneurysms—risk of rupture and risks of surgical intervention. N Engl J Med. 1998; 339:1725–1733

[6] Morita A, Kirino T, Hashi K, et al. UCAS Japan Investigators. The natural course of unruptured cerebral aneurysms in a Japanese cohort. N Engl J Med. 2012; 366(26):2474–2482

[7] Etminan N, Brown RD, Jr, Beseoglu K, et al. The unruptured intracranial aneurysm treatment score: a multidisciplinary consensus. Neurology. 2015; 85 (10):881–889

[8] Hishikawa T, Date I, Tokunaga K, et al. For UCAS Japan and UCAS II Investigators. Risk of rupture of unruptured cerebral aneurysms in elderly patients. Neurology. 2015; 85(21):1879–1885

[9] Wermer MJ, van der Schaaf IC, Algra A, Rinkel GJ. Risk of rupture of unruptured intracranial aneurysms in relation to patient and aneurysm characteristics: an updated meta-analysis. Stroke. 2007; 38(4):1404–1410

[10] Juvela S, Poussa K, Lehto H, Porras M. Natural history of unruptured intracranial aneurysms: a long-term follow-up study. Stroke. 2013; 44(9):2414–2421

[11] Mahaney KB, Brown RD, Jr, Meissner I, et al. ISUIA Investigators. Age-related differences in unruptured intracranial aneurysms: 1-year outcomes. J Neurosurg. 2014; 121(5):1024–1038

[12] Backes D, Rinkel GJ, Laban KG, Algra A, Vergouwen MD. Patient- and aneurysm-specific risk factors for intracranial aneurysm growth: a systematic review and meta-analysis. Stroke. 2016; 47(4):951–957

[13] Greving JP, Wermer MJ, Brown RD, Jr, et al. Development of the PHASES score for prediction of risk of rupture of intracranial aneurysms: a pooled analysis of six prospective cohort studies. Lancet Neurol. 2014; 13(1):59–66

[14] Thompson BG, Brown RD, Jr, Amin-Hanjani S, et al. American Heart Association Stroke Council, Council on Cardiovascular and Stroke Nursing, and Council on Epidemiology and Prevention, American Heart Association, American Stroke Association. Guidelines for the management of patients with unruptured intracranial aneurysms: a guideline for healthcare professionals from the American Heart Association/American Stroke Association. Stroke. 2015; 46(8):2368–2400

[15] Darsaut TFR, Raymond J. PHASES and the natural history of unruptured aneurysms: science or pseudoscience? J Neurointerv Surg. 2016

[16] Raymond J, Chagnon M, Collet JP, Guilbert F, Weill A, Roy D. A randomized trial on the safety and efficacy of endovascular treatment of unruptured intracranial aneurysms is feasible. Interv Neuroradiol. 2004; 10(2): 103–112

[17] Raymond J, Molyneux AJ, Fox AJ, Johnston SC, Collet JP, Rouleau I, TEAM Collaborative Group. The TEAM trial: safety and efficacy of endovascular treatment of unruptured intracranial aneurysms in the prevention of aneurysmal hemorrhages: a randomized comparison with indefinite deferral of treatment in 2002 patients followed for 10 years. Trials. 2008; 9:43

[18] Raymond J, Darsaut TE, Molyneux AJ, TEAM collaborative Group. A trial on unruptured intracranial aneurysms (the TEAM trial): results, lessons from a failure and the necessity for clinical care trials. Trials. 2011; 12:64

[19] Molyneux A, Kerr R, Stratton I, et al. International Subarachnoid Aneurysm Trial (ISAT) Collaborative Group. International Subarachnoid Aneurysm Trial (ISAT) of neurosurgical clipping versus endovascular coiling in 2143 patients with ruptured intracranial aneurysms: a randomised trial. Lancet. 2002; 360 (9342):1267–1274

[20] McDougall CG, Sr, Spetzler RF, Zabramski JM, et al. The Barrow Ruptured Aneurysm Trial. J Neurosurg. 2012; 116(1):135–144

[21] Darsaut TE, Findlay JM, Raymond J, CURES Collaborative Group. The design of the Canadian UnRuptured Endovascular versus Surgery (CURES) trial. Can J Neurol Sci. 2011; 38(2):236–241

3 Treatment of Ruptured Cerebral Aneurysms

Muhamed Hadzipasic, Matthew J. Koch, Christopher J. Stapleton, and Aman B. Patel

Abstract

The treatment of ruptured cerebral aneurysms has evolved tremendously over the past three decades. Management has shifted from being predominantly open surgery to endovascular intervention. Herein, using a case example of a ruptured anterior communicating artery (ACA) aneurysm, we discuss the current paradigm of surgical versus endovascular management of a ruptured aneurysm. There are reviews of the landmark clinical trials discussing relevant patient factors in selecting a treatment modality, as well as the long-term treatment outcomes. This chapter focuses on the modern thought process of acute neurosurgical intervention for ruptured cerebral aneurysms and the evidence base behind that process.

Keywords: subarachnoid hemorrhage, cerebral aneurysm, coil embolization, microsurgical clipping, vasospasm, flow diversion

3.1 Goals

1. Review the literature of the management of ruptured cerebral aneurysms and understand the strengths and weaknesses of the respective landmark studies.
2. Review the options for treatment of ruptured cerebral aneurysms including the merits of the different treatment strategies.
3. Understand the factors which might favor one treatment modality over another.

3.2 Case Example

3.2.1 History of Present Illness

A 46-year-old right-handed female collapsed at home shortly after complaining of the worst headache of her life. Emergency medical transport was called, but by the time of arrival to the emergency room, the patient's headache had resolved, and she refused further evaluation. That evening, she again became transiently unarousable and was transferred to an outside institution for further evaluation. There, given her waxing and waning mental status, she was intubated for airway protection, head computed tomography (CT) scan was performed, and ultimately was transferred to our hospital.

Past medical history: Opioid abuse currently on methadone; hypertension; migraines.

Past surgical history: None.

Family history: No family history of cerebral aneurysms, connective tissue disorder, or polycystic kidney disease.

Social history: Married, 1 pack per day smoker.

Medications: Methadone.

Physical examination: Pulse 72, temperature 36.4 °C, respiratory rate 18, SpO$_2$ 100%, blood pressure 184/86.

Neurological examination after holding anesthetics for 15 minutes revealed the patient to have a Glasgow Coma Scale of 9 T (E3 VT M6), World Federation of Neurosurgeons score of IV, and a Hunt Hess scale of 3. Extraocular movements were full with bilateral pupils equally reactive to light (contracting from 4 mm to 2 mm) and symmetrical. The patient was able to follow commands in all extremities with symmetric antigravity strength.

Imaging studies: See figures.

▶ Fig. 3.1: Demonstrates subarachnoid hemorrhage (SAH) in the basilar cisterns, bilateral Sylvian fissures, and most prominently in the interhemispheric fissure. Intraventricular hemorrhage is also noted without evidence of intraparenchymal hemorrhage.

▶ Fig. 3.2: CT angiography, coronal reconstructions depict a 2-mm left anterior communicating artery (ACA) projecting medially and anteriorly. This was determined to be the likely source of the patient's SAH.

3.2.2 Treatment Plan

Given the patients intubated status and need for continued intubation/sedation for further evaluation, a right frontal ventriculostomy catheter was placed and the patient was transferred to the neurointerventional suite for angiography and consideration of open versus endovascular intervention.

In ▶ Fig. 3.3a, digital subtraction angiography showed an anteromedially projecting 3-mm ACA aneurysm. Given the configuration of the lesion, coil embolization was chosen as a means of primary treatment. A single 2.5 mm × 4 cm coil was placed

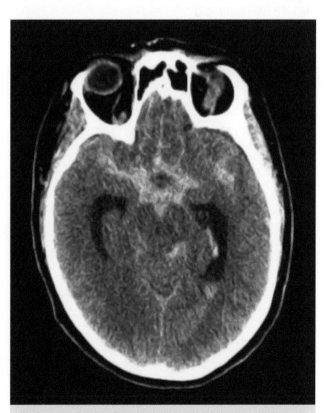

Fig. 3.1 CT head demonstrating diffuse subarachnoid hemorrhage with early signs of hydrocephalus.

3

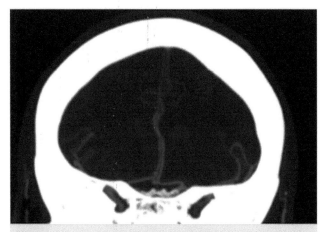

Fig. 3.2 CTA head in the coronal projection demonstrating a small medially directed anterior communicating artery aneurysm.

within the dome of the lesion with a small extraluminal loop of coil noted at the termination of the coil embolization. Follow-up angiography demonstrated slight persistent filling within the coil interstices and the base of the lesion consistent with a modified Ray-Royce classification 3a closure (▶ Fig. 3.3b, c).

Hospital course: Following embolization, the patient was transferred to the neurological intensive care unit for close monitoring. There, she was extubated and maintained on oral Nimodipine. Her external ventricular drain (EVD) was clamped on post–bleed day 2 and removed on post–bleed day 3. On post–bleed day 8, she was noted to have elevated transcranial Doppler values and clinical changes with agitation and confusion. An angiogram demonstrated moderate-to-severe anterior cerebral artery vasospasm bilaterally, which was treated with intra-arterial verapamil. Aneurysm closure improved to mRRC2 on follow-up angiography. She had postprocedural improvement in her mental status and was transferred to rehabilitation on post–bleed day 20.

3.2.3 Follow-up

At 6 months posthemorrhage, the patient presented from home neurologically intact. Follow-up angiography demonstrated improvement to mRRC1 occlusion (▶ Fig. 3.3d).

3.3 Case Summary

1. *What is the time course for the treatment of this lesion?*
   Historically ruptured aneurysms were managed conservatively, and the lesion secured only after some recovery from the initial hemorrhage.[1,2] This evidence predated modern microsurgical and endovascular strategies, and thus, the intervention had to be weighed considering intervention in face of a swollen cortex and the risk of secondary injury from surgery. More recent evidence suggests that the risk of poor outcomes and delayed cerebral ischemia is higher for lesions treated further removed from rupture.[3,4] This, in addition to the ongoing rupture risk following primary rupture, supports treatment within 24 to 48 hours of patient presentation.[5]

2. *What patient factors are considered when selecting an approach?*
   Our patient is a young female who presented with a moderate-grade clinical presentation, HH3, and WFNS IV. When considering open versus endovascular intervention options, consideration is given to the possible complications associated with either treatment modality. The International Subarachnoid Aneurysm Trial (ISAT) demonstrated improved cognitive outcomes with fewer complications in those patients treated with endovascular occlusion compared to open surgical clipping.[6] Further, the brain retraction of acutely injured brain needed for open surgical clipping must be weighed against the ischemic risk of catheterization and coil embolization.[2] On the other hand, the durability of treatment must be considered, given the patient's young age. Surgical clipping, when performed successfully, has a near permanent durability, while endovascular occlusion has a more

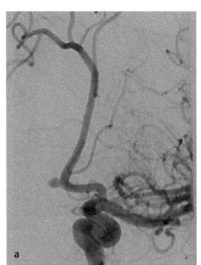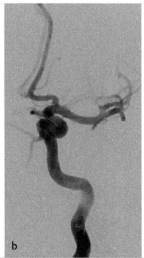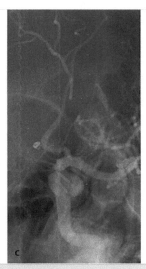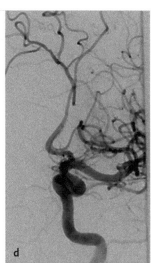

Fig. 3.3 (a) Left internal carotid artery (ICA) angiogram demonstrating the anteromedially-directed, 3 mm ACA aneurysm. (b) Immediate post-embolization angiogram after placement of a single coil demonstrating persistent filling of the aneurysm with a modified Ray-Royce 3a closure. (c) Unsubtracted angiogram demonstrating the single coil placed within the aneurysm. (d) Six-month follow-up angiogram demonstrating complete occlusion of the aneurysm.

variable longevity and requires extended clinical and radiographical follow-up.[4,7]

Our patient is relatively young with minimal cortical atrophy and evidence of cortical injury. In these instances, when technically feasible, we employ a coil-first approach as demonstrated in ▶ Fig. 3.3 with the primary goal of "aneurysm rebleed protection" and the secondary goal of aneurysm occlusion.[8] This is performed with the knowledge that after recovering from their initial injury, permanent occlusion can be achieved with either the use of adjunctive endovascular devices or surgical clipping.

3. *What aneurysm factors are considered in devising a treatment strategy?*

At presentation, a CT angiogram of the head and neck is obtained, which informs the decision regarding the optimal means of treatment. Variables relevant to endovascular intervention, such as aortic arch, cervical, and intracranial anatomy, can be preliminarily assessed. Further, aneurysmal orientation and factors, such as rupture site with respect to aneurysm orientation, accessibility and exposure of aneurysm and aneurysm neck, can be assessed. After this preliminary information, our institution performs an angiogram with 3D angiography to assess, in detail, the aneurysm anatomy to fully evaluate the merits of an endovascular versus an open approach, unless the clinical conditions require more immediate open surgical intervention.

Our patient has a small 2-mm aneurysm with a dome-to-neck aspect ratio of < 2 arising from the left ACA junction which projects medially and anteriorly.[9,10] Although the anterior projection of the lesion indicates this lesion could be addressed with low risk to ACA perforators and the contralateral A2, a left-sided, dominant hemisphere approach would be necessary in order to achieve proximal control.[11] The 3D angiography indicated that the neck may be smaller than demonstrated on 2D projections; thus, primary coiling was selected as the optimal means for approaching the lesion.

4. *Do adjunctive devices play any role in endovascular occlusion of this patient?*

Our patient's lesion does have a mid-range dome-to-neck aspect ratio; thus, adjunct devices could be entertained to assist with treatment. Balloons are often used as both a means to assist coil placement in wide-necked aneurysms and as a safety measure to achieve control should intraprocedural rupture occur. Our practice does not typically use these devices on lesions we perceive to be primarily treatable with coils without the use of a balloon because of the extra thrombogenic risk of an additional requisite catheter.[12,13] Similarly, we typically do not employ stents for the treatment of ruptured lesions, choosing to either use balloon assistance, achieve only dome protection, or alternatively pursue open surgical clipping. This is primarily secondary to the risk of loading a patient with acute hemorrhage on dual antiplatelet therapy, which can lead to both ischemic and hemorrhagic complications.[14,15] Thus, despite mounting literature supporting the acute use of these devices, we presently do not use them routinely unless primary coiling is unachievable and surgical clipping too difficult.[16,17]

5. *How should the patient be followed posttreatment?*

Following the placement of a single coil, filling was no longer visualized at the dome of the lesion consistent with an mRRC3a grading and dome protection.[18] Rather than risking coil dislodgement or rupturing the lesion with recatheterization to achieve a higher packing density, no further coils were added.[19]

Reassurance of the aneurysm's progressive closure was visualized on the patient's vasospasm treatment study. As a protocol, patients are followed up with angiography at 6 months and then interval follow-up is determined based on the stability of the lesion. With a good RRC1 occlusion, we would then repeat angiography at 1.5, 3, and 5 years after which MRA would be used to follow the lesion over time.[18] This follow-up also ensures screening for the 5 to 10% risk of development of a de novo aneurysm.[20]

3.4 Level of Evidence

Timing of treatment: The patient's ruptured aneurysm, young age, and accessibility of lesion warrant intervention for treatment (Class I, Level of Evidence B).

Endovascular intervention: Endovascular intervention may not have the durability of open surgical clipping, but the present evidence supports endovascular embolization when feasible to minimize secondary brain injury (Class IIB, Level of Evidence B).

Nimodipine: Class I Level of Evidence A.

Follow-up: Given filling within the coil loops at treatment conclusion and at the aneurysm neck at vasospasm follow-up, a 6-month follow-up angiogram is warranted in order to evaluate whether further treatment is needed (Class I, Level of Evidence B).

3.5 Landmark Papers

Molyneux AJ, Kerr RS, Birks J, et al; ISAT Collaborators. Risk of recurrent subarachnoid haemorrhage, death, or dependence and standardised mortality ratios after clipping or coiling of an intracranial aneurysm in the International Subarachnoid Aneurysm Trial (ISAT): long-term follow-up. Lancet Neurol 2009;8(5): 427–433.[6]

Molyneux A, Kerr R, Stratton I, et al; International Subarachnoid Aneurysm Trial (ISAT) Collaborative Group. International Subarachnoid Aneurysm Trial (ISAT) of neurosurgical clipping versus endovascular coiling in 2143 patients with ruptured intracranial aneurysms: a randomized trial. J Stroke Cerebrovasc Dis 2002;11(6):304–314.[21]

Motivated by the development and widespread adoption of endovascular techniques for the occlusion of intracranial aneurysms, the International Subarachnoid Aneurysm Trial (ISAT) was a landmark, multicenter, randomized control study that sought to compare morbidity and mortality of coiling with conventional craniotomy/aneurysm clipping for ruptured cerebral aneurysms. Specifically, starting in 1994 the trial began enrolling patients with CT- or lumbar puncture (LP)-proven SAH with a CT- or angiographically proven aneurysmal culprit, who, on the basis of angiographic anatomy (as adjudicated by a neurosurgeon and endovascular specialist), would be suitable for clipping or coiling (with equipoise as to the optimal modality). The study was powered to detect a 25% reduction in the proportion of patients dead or dependent (as defined by modified Rankin scale 3–6) at 1 year in the coiling group, with additional intent to compare rates of rebleeding from the treated aneurysm, quality of life at 1 year, frequency of epilepsy, cost-effectiveness, and neuropsychological outcomes in coiling versus clipping groups. The study also intended to examine the long-term outcome of treatment in terms of frequency of further hemorrhage and to assess the significance of angiographic results in the context of long-term follow-up.

Out of 9,559 patients assessed, 2,143 were randomized to either endovascular coiling using detachable platinum coils or conventional craniotomy/clipping with 801 and 793 analyzed at 1 year, respectively. The authors found a significant decrease in dependency or death at 1 year in the coiling group (23.7% vs. 30.6% in the clipping group) corresponding to an absolute risk reduction of 22.6% (dependency) and 6.9% (death). Furthermore, after 1 year, at the time of the initial ISAT report, there were only two recorded delayed rebleeding events (both in the endovascular group). From this initial report, the authors concluded that with ruptured intracranial aneurysms suitable for both endovascular and open treatment, endovascular treatment was more likely to result in disability-free survival at 1-year follow-up.

Detailed analysis and longer term follow-up were reported in subsequent papers. Specifically, in 2005, ISAT2 presented a randomized comparison of effects on survival, dependency, seizures, rebleeding, subgroups, and aneurysmal occlusion in the coiling versus microsurgical clipping groups. The results confirmed the initially reported survival benefit as maintained up to at least 7 years, also adding that the risk of epilepsy was lower in patients initially allocated to endovascular treatment with the caveat of a higher (albeit slightly higher) risk of late rebleeding.

The ISAT studies were landmark analyses addressing an increasingly relevant topic; hence, the conclusions were intensely debated. The main criticism of ISAT involves the large number of patients treated at trial centers throughout the study, who were ultimately not included in the trial. These exclusions were primarily due to the motivation to include only cases in which the optimal treatment (clipping vs. coiling) was unclear, resulting in almost 80% of initially evaluated patients being screened out. Hence, the general applicability of the results to patients presenting with aneurysmal rupture was questioned.

Other criticisms concerned a potential lack of experience of ISAT practitioners performing microsurgical clipping. Also, given the difference in rebleeding before treatment observed in the ISAT group assigned to clipping (23 vs. 14 in the endovascular group), it is questioned whether outcomes in the clipping group could have been better if more expedient surgery had been performed.

Regardless of these criticisms, ISAT provided a foundation upon which to address the question of whether to coil or clip a ruptured aneurysm equally amenable to either modality. In this scenario, the results clearly favored coiling with respect to functional independence with the caveat of higher risk of rebleeding.

Spetzler RF, McDougall CG, Zabramski JM, et al. The Barrow Ruptured Aneurysm Trial: 6-year results. J Neurosurg 2015;123 (3):609–617.[7]

Molyneux A, Kerr R, Birks J. Barrow ruptured aneurysm trial. J Neurosurg 2013;119(1):139–141.[22]

Spetzler RF, McDougall CG, Albuquerque FC, et al. The Barrow Ruptured Aneurysm Trial: 3-year results. J Neurosurg 2013;119 (1):146–157.[23]

Building on the evidence put forth by the ISAT study, the Barrow Ruptured Aneurysm Trial (BRAT) set out to compare coiling and clipping in a more easily generalizable manner. Specifically, the trial set out to evaluate the null hypothesis that no difference in outcomes exists between endovascular coiling and microsurgical clipping in the context of ruptured cerebral aneurysms. Patients with SAH were randomly assigned a modality of treatment with ultimate outcome assessed by modified Rankin score (mRS). Specifically, 725 patients with SAH were screened resulting in 500 eligible patients; 238 and 233 of whom were assigned to clipping and coiling, respectively.

Because the goal of BRAT was to reflect "real-world practicalities of ruptured aneurysm treatment in North America," a patient was assigned to a given surgeon with an intended modality of treatment, but the assigned surgeon had the "right of refusal," meaning they would consider the case and could either perform the intended treatment or cross the patient over. In either case, intention to treat analysis was performed so that neither modality would benefit from crossing over certain types of patients. In this manner, by understanding which patients were treated with each technique when the a priori policy was biased toward a given modality, the authors of BRAT aimed to improve the understanding of the applicability of ISAT findings.

At 1-year follow-up, a poor outcome (mRS > 2) was observed in 33.7% of patients initially assigned to clipping, and 23.2% of patients initially assigned to coiling, leading to an odds ratio (OR) of 1.68 favoring endovascular coiling. This result remained significant after adjustment for age greater than 50 years, as well as Hunt Hess score > II (both of these parameters were significantly associated with a poor outcome at 1 year irrespective of initial assigned treatment modality).

Importantly, a secondary analysis was conducted which confirmed better outcomes in patients actually receiving coiling, regardless of the initially assigned modality, compared with those undergoing clipping, regardless of initially assigned modality (20.4% vs. 33.9%, OR 2.01 in favor of coiling). Of note, there were 75 patients who crossed over from coiling to clipping. While there were no differences in the clinical grade of patients crossing over from coil embolization to clipping, their aneurysms tended to be small and arise from the anterior circulation (other common reasons for crossing over to clipping were for simultaneous evacuation of coexisting clot, uncertainty as to which of several aneurysms bled, wide-based aneurysm neck, or presence of a branch vessel).

The follow-up results of BRAT at 3 and 6 years have been reported. At 3 years, there was no longer a statistically significant benefit to coiling in terms of mRS scores. Also, patients undergoing clipping had a significantly higher degree of aneurysm obliteration and lower rate of recurrence and retreatment. Therefore, these results suggested no difference in risk between clipping and coiling and also supported clipping as resulting in better occlusion and less need for follow-up with lower rates of rebleeding. These results were reinforced at the 6-year follow-up; no difference in patients with mRS > 2 existed between the coiling and clipping groups. Importantly, it was observed that a high number of patients with anterior circulation aneurysms assigned to coiling crossed over to clipping. When anterior circulation aneurysms were analyzed separately, no difference was observed in outcomes between clipping and coiling (except at a 6-month time point which favored coiling). This was not the case for posterior circulation aneurysms for which coiling displayed significantly higher mRS scores at both the 3- and 6-year follow-up time points (although the authors point out that this is likely confounded by an unexpectedly high number of posterior inferior cerebellar artery [PICA] aneurysms randomized to clipping, as well as the overall small numbers of posterior circulation aneurysms studied).

Overall, while the study design of BRAT set out with the goal of making its results more generalizable, long-term follow-up revealed the complex role aneurysmal location, anatomy, and treatment modality undoubtedly play in patient outcomes.

Koivisto T, Vanninen R, Hurskainen H, Saari T, Hernesniemi J, Vapalahti M. Outcomes of early endovascular versus surgical treatment of ruptured cerebral aneurysms. A prospective randomized study. Stroke 2000;31(10):2369–237.[24]

"Outcomes of early endovascular versus surgical treatment of ruptured cerebral aneurysms" was a single-center prospective, randomized trial comparing clipping and coiling outcomes for treatment of aneurysmal SAH (aSAH) with respect to Glasgow Outcome Scale (GOS) score, neuropsychological outcomes, and radiographic occlusion rate in Finland. Of 242 consecutive patients with proven aSAH, 109 aSAH patients were randomized to either early (< 72 h) surgical or endovascular treatment arms (57 surgical, 52 endovascular). The primary end points were rebleeding and death, with secondary end points defined as refilling of the aneurysm prompting additional treatment. The primary outcomes were 12-month clinical, neuropsychological, and radiological results. Neuropsychological outcomes (comprehensive evaluation including tests of general intelligence, memory, language, attention, and flexibility in mental processing) were measured at 3 and 12 months, MRI was performed at 12 months, and follow-up angiography was performed at 3 months (and 12 months if a remnant was found) in the clipping group, and at 3 and 12 months in the endovascular group.

Of the initial 242 patients considered, the most common exclusion criteria were large hematoma (26% of excluded patients), followed by aneurysm morphology not conducive to clipping (25%). Only two patients (1.5%) were excluded due to their aneurysm not being suitable for treatment. The locations of excluded aneurysms with respect to ACA, middle cerebral artery (MCA), internal carotid artery (ICA), and vertebrobasilar artery (VBA) territories were somewhat evenly distributed at 26, 59, 27, and 11%, respectively. Of note, crossover from the endovascular to surgical group was significantly higher than the converse (12 vs. 4).

Importantly, there was no significant difference in cumulative survival times between endovascular and surgical groups with mean survival days totaling 1,575 and 1,572, respectively. No late rebleeding events occurred. Angiography identified refilling aneurysms in both the groups, with an 86% rate of complete occlusion in clipped aneurysms versus a 77% rate for coiled lesions at 1 year.

The 12-month clinical outcomes as assessed by GOS score did not differ significantly between surgical and endovascular groups (with 79% of endovascular vs. 75% of surgical patients having good or moderate recovery as assessed by GOS), while Hunt-Hess grade, postoperative symptomatic vasospasm, need for permanent shunt creation, Fisher grade, size of aneurysm, age, size of aneurysmal neck, and preintervention hydrocephalus were all significantly associated with poorer overall clinical outcome. Neuropsychological testing also did not reveal significant differences between endovascular and surgical clipping, with both groups improving performance between 3- and 12-month time points.

Radiological results revealed by MRI indicated that both superficial retraction deficits and ischemic lesions in the territory of the ruptured aneurysm were significantly more frequent in the surgically treated group. Radiographic size of the ischemic lesion in the parental artery territory, deficit due to preoperative intracerebral hematoma, and higher ventricular-intracranial width ratio were associated with poor clinical outcomes irrespective of the group. While superficial brain retraction injury was noted in many surgical patients, it showed no correlation with outcome.

Hence, the Finnish study concluded that outcomes from endovascular treatment of ruptured cerebral aneurysms were equal to those from surgical clipping. Furthermore, while endovascular treatment had lower risk of ischemic retraction injury, it also achieved lower rates of aneurysm occlusion. Due to only a 1-year follow-up, the study obviously left open questions of endovascular durability, as well as long-term risks of re-rupture with either technique. A relatively small number of patients in the study also raises the concern that it was underpowered to detect differences between the two techniques. However, the study did establish the notion of endovascular treatment as being an alternative to clipping in patients presenting with SAH, laying the groundwork for the larger studies that followed.

Li ZQ, Wang QH, Chen G, Quan Z. Outcomes of endovascular coiling versus surgical clipping in the treatment of ruptured intracranial aneurysms. J Int Med Res 2012;40(6):2145–2151.[25]

Published in 2012, the "Outcomes of endovascular coiling versus surgical clipping in the treatment of ruptured intracranial aneurysms" was a prospective randomized clinical trial of surgical clipping versus endovascular coil embolization for treatment of SAH from ruptured aneurysms.

Between 2005 and 2009, 192 patients were entered into the study with 96 randomized to both endovascular and surgical clipping groups. Of note, Hunt-Hess grades, location of target aneurysm, and time interval between aSAH and treatment procedure were not significantly different between groups. Patients underwent CT scans on admission, 24 to 48 hours after treatment, and on the day of discharge. Cerebral angiography was performed between day 4 and 14 following SAH.

Symptomatic vasospasm occurred among 22/94 (23%) versus 34/92 (37%) of the patients in the endovascular and surgical groups, respectively, a significant difference corresponding to an OR of 1.24. There was a significantly lower number of new cerebral infarctions observed in the endovascular group as well (12/94 [12%] vs. 20/92 [21%] in the clipping group). Of these new infarctions, the number related to vasospasm was also significantly lower in the endovascular group (8/12 or 66% vs. 17/20 or 85%). Imaging follow-up revealed a higher rate of residual aneurysm after treatment for patients treated with coiling (12/94 or 12.8% vs. 4/92 or 4% in the clipping group). Similarly, incidence of complete aneurysm occlusion was lower following endovascular treatment versus surgery. Clinical outcomes at 1-year follow-up: overall morbidity between the groups was not significantly different (10.6% for endovascular vs. 15.2% for clipping), and there was no significant difference in the number of patients achieving a good outcome (i.e., mRS < 3; 75% in the endovascular vs. 67% in the surgical groups).

From this data, the authors concluded that advantages of endovascular treatment (less symptomatic vasospasm and cerebral infarction) generally outweighed the disadvantages (lower rates of complete occlusion which had an unknown effect on re-rupture rate and did not seem to affect overall outcome). Therefore, the authors seem to suggest that endovascular treatment represents a sensible alternative to open surgery and should be strongly considered (if not preferred) for first-line treatment of aSAH.

3.6 Recommendations

The advent of the Guglielmi detachable coil (GDC coil) fundamentally changed the landscape of treatment of ruptured intracranial aneurysms. Since 1991, there has been fervent debate and research into the optimal management of ruptured cerebral aneurysms. To date, there have been four randomized trials exploring this debate.[6,7,24,25] The largest and only multicentered trial, ISAT demonstrated superior primary patient outcomes in patients treated with coil embolization in those lesions where there was clinical equipoise between clipping and coiling.[6] These findings have been called into question with the BRAT[7] and other studies, demonstrating overall similar outcomes between the two groups with persistent questions regarding the durability of treatment.

Inherent in ISAT[6] as well as Finnish et al[24] and Chinese study[25] is the lesion selection bias. All of these studies were based on groups of patients with lesions that could be addressed surgically or endovascularly. This introduces a definite bias as to which patients are included in these studies and the overall generalizability. This bias is even further complicated by what in fact qualifies in current clinical practice as a "coilable" lesion. This definition ranges from aneurysms amenable to complete primary occlusion (therefore, not requiring further treatment) to those simply amenable to "dome protection" (indicating further treatment would likely be required after recovery). The BRAT study attempted to address this bias by randomizing all patients with aneurysmal SAH and performing intention to treat analysis when crossovers occurred following treatment.[7]

The commonality among these studies is the overwhelming bias toward the evaluation of anterior circulation lesions. Thus, the available grade 1 evidence is best applied to lesions of the anterior circulation, which, with limitations in mind, indicates that for a given anterior circulation aneurysm causing SAH that can be equally well treated with open surgery or endovascular intervention, coiling is the preferred treatment with notable caveats.

Durability is a known limitation of endovascular treatment; thus, the need for close follow-up and potential retreatment must be weighed against the risk of secondary injury from brain retraction, higher risk of intraoperative complication, and the longer procedure associated with a craniotomy. Thus, in younger patients with better grade lesions (indicating potentially less injured/swollen brain parenchyma) that are readily anatomically accessible, surgery still remains a primary consideration. This is especially true in wide-necked lesions and larger lesions which the above trials demonstrated had a higher risk, and risk of recurrence associated with coiling. Of note, this must be reconciled with the ever-expanding armamentarium of endovascular devices to treat wide-necked lesions. Presently, the majority of these devices require dual antiplatelet therapy, making them unattractive for ruptured patients.

Of late, the notion of "dome-protection" (which requires a need for future treatment and using either adjunctive devices or even open surgery at a later date) has been proposed. Unlike repeat open surgery, repeat endovascular intervention is not associated with significantly elevated risks compared to primary treatment. Although this methodology has been borne out in clinical practice, a trial to compare and quantitate the additional risks or benefits has not yet been performed.

Intraparenchymal hemorrhage has traditionally been considered a potential indication for open surgical versus endovascular intervention, with improved outcomes demonstrated with hematoma evacuation. Presently, with improvements in endovascular technology decreasing procedure time, intraparenchymal hemorrhage does not need to be a primary factor in treatment planning. Series have demonstrated the safety of endovascular embolization followed by surgical hemorrhage evacuation. Thus, treatment decisions for these lesions can continue to be made based on applicability, safety, and ease of treatment.

Posterior circulation aneurysms are underrepresented in currently available clinical trials. This may be due to the equipoise of treatment biasing these lesions toward trial exclusion and endovascular intervention. Yet, the available data does strongly suggest an even more significant benefit to primary endovascular treatment of these lesions. This is augmented by currently available series demonstrating improved outcomes and a lower complication profile for the endovascular treatment of posterior circulation lesions.

Given the inherently complex decision-making process required to effectively treat these lesions, regardless of lesion location or outstanding patient characteristics, SAH patients are best handled in high-volume centers equipped with open and endovascular surgeons. Thus, patients get the best available treatment from experienced providers as opposed to the only available treatment from less-experienced practitioners.

3.7 Future Directions

Endovascular therapy continues to improve and innovate, further pushing the limits of what constitutes a "treatable" lesion. Unlike open surgery, endovascular devices continue to improve at a faster pace. As practitioners gain experience with newer generation intravascular devices and coil adjuvants improve (perhaps negating the necessity for dual antiplatelet therapy), lesions requiring open surgery will continue to diminish.

3.8 Summary

1. Ruptured cerebral aneurysms are neurosurgical emergencies that require expeditious management to ensure the best possible outcomes.

2. The clinical presentation of the patient and aneurysm morphology are important factors to consider when discussing treatment options.

3. Both surgical and endovascular treatment options should be considered in the decision making process.

4. If there is equipoise with either treatment option, endovascular treatment may result in improved clinical outcomes when compared with surgical treatment.

5. Surgical clipping of a ruptured aneurysm is more durable with less residual/recurrent aneurysms following initial treatment when compared with coil embolization.

References

[1] The International Cooperative Study on the Timing of Aneurysm Surgery. J Neurosurg. 1990; 73(1):37–47

[2] Öhman J, Heiskanen O. Timing of operation for ruptured supratentorial aneurysms: a prospective randomized study. J Neurosurg. 1989; 70(1):55–60

[3] Baltsavias GS, Byrne JV, Halsey J, Coley SC, Sohn MJ, Molyneux AJ. Effects of timing of coil embolization after aneurysmal subarachnoid hemorrhage on procedural morbidity and outcomes. Neurosurgery. 2000; 47(6):1320–1329, discussion 1329–1331

[4] Dorhout Mees SM, Molyneux AJ, Kerr RS, Algra A, Rinkel GJE. Timing of aneurysm treatment after subarachnoid hemorrhage: relationship with delayed cerebral ischemia and poor outcome. Stroke. 2012; 43(8):2126–2129

[5] Naidech AM, Janjua N, Kreiter KT, et al. Predictors and impact of aneurysm rebleeding after subarachnoid hemorrhage. Arch Neurol. 2005; 62(3):410–416

[6] Molyneux AJ, Kerr RS, Birks J, et al. ISAT Collaborators. Risk of recurrent subarachnoid haemorrhage, death, or dependence and standardised mortality ratios after clipping or coiling of an intracranial aneurysm in the International Subarachnoid Aneurysm Trial (ISAT): long-term follow-up. Lancet Neurol. 2009; 8(5):427–433

[7] Spetzler RF, McDougall CG, Zabramski JM, et al. The Barrow Ruptured Aneurysm Trial: 6-year results. J Neurosurg. 2015; 123(3):609–617

[8] Waldau B, Reavey-Cantwell JF, Lawson MF, et al. Intentional partial coiling dome protection of complex ruptured cerebral aneurysms prevents acute rebleeding and produces favorable clinical outcomes. Acta Neurochir (Wien). 2012; 154(1):27–31

[9] Gonzalez N, Sedrak M, Martin N, Vinuela F. Impact of anatomic features in the endovascular embolization of 181 anterior communicating artery aneurysms. Stroke. 2008; 39(10):2776–2782

[10] Brinjikji W, Cloft HJ, Kallmes DF. Difficult aneurysms for endovascular treatment: overwide or undertall? AJNR Am J Neuroradiol. 2009; 30(8):1513–1517

[11] Rhoton AL, Jr. Aneurysms. Neurosurgery. 2002; 51(4) Suppl:S121–S158

[12] Layton KF, Cloft HJ, Gray LA, Lewis DA, Kallmes DF. Balloon-assisted coiling of intracranial aneurysms: evaluation of local thrombus formation and symptomatic thromboembolic complications. AJNR Am J Neuroradiol. 2007; 28(6): 1172–1175

[13] Shapiro M, Babb J, Becske T, Nelson PK. Safety and efficacy of adjunctive balloon remodeling during endovascular treatment of intracranial aneurysms: a literature review. AJNR Am J Neuroradiol. 2008; 29(9):1777–1781

[14] Walcott BP, Koch MJ, Stapleton CJ, Patel AB. Blood flow diversion as a primary treatment method for ruptured brain aneurysms—concerns, controversy, and future directions. Neurocrit Care. 2017; 26(3):465–473

[15] Hudson JS, Prout BS, Nagahama Y, et al. External ventricular drain and hemorrhage in aneurysmal subarachnoid hemorrhage patients on dual antiplatelet therapy: a retrospective cohort study. Neurosurgery. 2018; yy127–nyy127

[16] Linfante I, Mayich M, Sonig A, Fujimoto J, Siddiqui A, Dabus G. Flow diversion with Pipeline Embolic Device as treatment of subarachnoid hemorrhage secondary to blister aneurysms: dual-center experience and review of the literature. J Neurointerv Surg. 2017; 9(1):29–33

[17] Nagahama Y, Allan L, Nakagawa D, et al. Dual antiplatelet therapy in aneurysmal subarachnoid hemorrhage: association with reduced risk of clinical vasospasm and delayed cerebral ischemia. J Neurosurg. 0(0):1–9

[18] Mascitelli JR, Moyle H, Oermann EK, et al. An update to the Raymond–Roy Occlusion Classification of intracranial aneurysms treated with coil embolization. J Neurointerv Surg. 2014; 011258

[19] Gupta V, Chugh M, Jha AN, Walia BS, Vaishya S. Coil embolization of very small (2 mm or smaller) berry aneurysms: feasibility and technical issues. AJNR Am J Neuroradiol. 2009; 30(2):308–314

[20] Kemp WJ, III, Fulkerson DH, Payner TD, et al. Risk of hemorrhage from de novo cerebral aneurysms. J Neurosurg. 2013; 118(1):58–62

[21] Molyneux A, Kerr R, Stratton I, et al. International Subarachnoid Aneurysm Trial (ISAT) Collaborative Group. International Subarachnoid Aneurysm Trial (ISAT) of neurosurgical clipping versus endovascular coiling in 2143 patients with ruptured intracranial aneurysms: a randomized trial. J Stroke Cerebrovasc Dis. 2002; 11(6):304–314

[22] Molyneux A, Kerr R, Birks J. Barrow ruptured aneurysm trial. J Neurosurg. 2013; 119(1):139–141

[23] Spetzler RF, McDougall CG, Albuquerque FC, et al. The Barrow Ruptured Aneurysm Trial: 3-year results. J Neurosurg. 2013; 119(1):146–157

[24] Koivisto T, Vanninen R, Hurskainen H, Saari T, Hernesniemi J, Vapalahti M. Outcomes of early endovascular versus surgical treatment of ruptured cerebral aneurysms. A prospective randomized study. Stroke. 2000; 31(10): 2369–2377

[25] Li ZQ, Wang QH, Chen G, Quan Z. Outcomes of endovascular coiling versus surgical clipping in the treatment of ruptured intracranial aneurysms. J Int Med Res. 2012; 40(6):2145–2151

3

4 Mycotic Aneurysms: Incidence, Natural History, and Treatment Strategies

Lorenzo Rinaldo and Leonardo Rangel Castilla

Abstract

Mycotic aneurysms (MA) are rare entities that present daunting clinical challenges due to the medical complexity of the harboring patient population. The morbidity and mortality associated with the presence and rupture of these lesions are significant, though favorable neurologic outcomes are achievable in patients who are not moribund from a disseminated infection. Understanding the indications for screening and treatment of MAs is essential to obtaining a successful outcome. Herein, available evidence on the incidence, natural history, and treatment outcomes of MAs is reviewed to detail the basis for management algorithms of these complex vascular lesions.

Keywords: angiography, infective endocarditis, intracranial hemorrhage, mycotic aneurysm, screening

4.1 Goals

1. Review the literature detailing the incidence of and risk factors for MA formation.
2. Review the literature describing the natural history of MAs.
3. Review the literature detailing the risks of cardiac surgery in the setting of a known MA.
4. Review the literature forming the basis of treatment algorithms for MAs.

4.2 Case Example

4.2.1 History of Present Illness

A 30-year-old male with a history of a bicuspid aortic valve and associated aortic regurgitation presented to the emergency department with transient episodes of left-sided face and arm sensory disturbances. The patient's symptoms were characterized by tingling of the mouth and tongue as well as his left arm. These episodes lasted for approximately 10 seconds, during which he also experienced difficulty speaking. He denied any alteration in consciousness or upper or lower extremity weakness. Computed tomography (CT) of the head demonstrated a small focus of traumatic subarachnoid hemorrhage in the posterior right temporal lobe (▶ Fig. 4.1a), with CT angiography (CTA) demonstrating a 4- to 5-mm likely aneurysm along the right frontal convexity (▶ Fig. 4.2a). Follow-up magnetic resonance imaging (MRI) revealed multifocal punctate infarcts in the right posterior temporal and frontal lobes (▶ Fig. 4.1b, c). The patient was also noted to have multiple renal and splenic infarcts on abdominal imaging. Subsequent cardiac ultrasound demonstrated 1.0- and 1.6-cm vegetation on his aortic and mitral valves, respectively, and severe aortic regurgitation with associated heart failure. Blood cultures were obtained and found to be positive for *Cardiobacterium hominis*.

Past medical history: Anemia, bicuspid aortic valve, aortic regurgitation.

Past surgical history: None.

Family history: Uncle with bicuspid aortic valve.

Social history: Endorses use of chewing tobacco and denies intravenous drug use, recent foreign travel, or sick contacts.

Review of systems: Endorses fatigue, night sweats, and 15-lb weight loss over the 3 months preceding presentation.

Neurologic examination: Mild dysarthria, otherwise unremarkable.

Imaging studies: See figures.

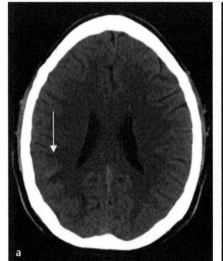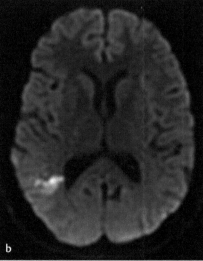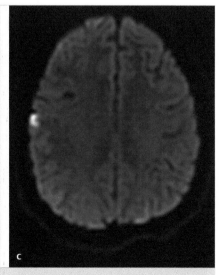

Fig. 4.1 Initial computed tomography (CT) and magnetic resonance (MR) imaging. Initial head CT demonstrates a subtle focus of subarachnoid blood in the right posterior temporal lobe (a). Follow-up MRI demonstrates areas of restricted diffusion in the right posterior temporal (b) and frontal (c) lobes, consistent with embolic infarction.

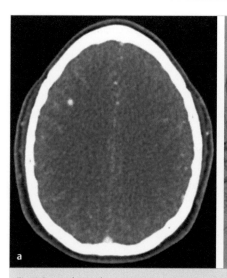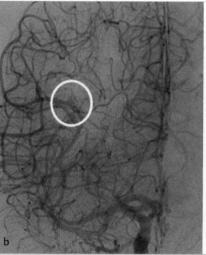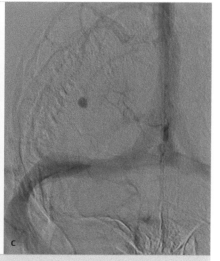

Fig. 4.2 Initial vascular imaging. Computed tomography (CT) angiography demonstrates a focus of enhancement in the right frontal lobe **(a)**. Formal angiography revealed an aneurysm located on the branch of the middle cerebral artery **(b)** that filled well into the venous phase **(c)**.

4.2.2 Treatment Plan

The patient's clinical presentation was consistent with infective endocarditis (IE) complicated by septic cerebrovascular thromboemboli causing multifocal infarctions and formation of a distal right middle cerebral artery (MCA) mycotic aneurysm (MA). The patient was started on a third-generation cephalosporin, ceftriaxone, administered intravenously. The patient's sensory episodes were indicative of partial seizures; he was initiated on an antiepileptic medication and experienced no further recurrence of his spells. He was evaluated by cardiovascular surgery and deemed to require urgent aortic valve replacement. Prior to surgery, a cerebral angiogram was obtained, which demonstrated the previously seen distal right MCA aneurysm (▶ Fig. 4.2a). Aneurysm filling was seen well into the venous phase, suggestive of intra-aneurysmal stasis (▶ Fig. 4.2b, c). Given the aneurysm's unruptured status, it was determined to continue medical management with antibiotics and proceed with aortic valve replacement on day 5 after initial presentation.

4.2.3 Follow-up

The patient's aortic valve replacement proceeded uneventfully. He was given intravenous heparin intraoperatively and subsequently reversed with protamine sulfate at the conclusion of the procedure. Postoperatively, he was noted to be at his neurologic baseline but soon developed a dense left-sided hemiplegia and right-sided gaze deviation. A head CT demonstrated a right frontal intraparenchymal hemorrhage (IPH) with intraventricular extension (▶ Fig. 4.3a). Due to early hydrocephalus, a left-sided ventriculostomy was placed. Shortly after placement of the ventriculostomy, the patient became acutely comatose and was found to have a fixed and dilated left pupil. He was taken emergently for a repeat CT scan, which demonstrated expansion of the patient's IPH and IVH, now with complete casting of the right lateral ventricle (▶ Fig. 4.3b, c). Significant right-to-left midline shift was noted; thus, the patient was taken for a decompressive right-sided hemicraniectomy, hematoma evacuation, and resec-

tion of the known MA. Intraoperatively, the aneurysm was localized via ultrasound and found to be thrombosed; it was resected using microsurgical technique. Postoperative CT/CTA demonstrated partial intraparenchymal and intraventricular hematoma evacuation and a de novo aneurysm off the distal anterior cerebral artery (▶ Fig. 4.3d); given the relative locations of the aneurysm and hematoma, this new aneurysm was deemed responsible for the patient's postoperative hemorrhage. The patient was subsequently taken for endovascular Onyx embolization of the ACA aneurysm with good angiographic result (▶ Fig. 4.4a–d).

After an initial recovery period, the patient returned to his preoperative cognitive baseline, though he remained with a dense left-sided hemiplegia. He was initiated on anticoagulation for his aortic valve without adverse effects. A cranioplasty was performed approximately 2 months after his decompressive surgery that proceeded without complication. Serial blood cultures after initiation of antibiotics remained negative for growth. Prior to dismissal, an echocardiogram was performed that demonstrated good functioning of his prosthetic valve. The patient was ultimately dismissed to an inpatient rehabilitation facility.

4.3 Case Summary

1. *Which predisposing risk factor for MA formation was present in this patient?*

   MAs are rare entities that occur most frequently in the setting of IE, with less common etiologies including meningitis, sinusitis, skull osteomyelitis, sepsis, and general immunocompromised state.[1,2,3,4,5] Causative microbial organisms are generally bacterial, usually Streptococcus or Staphylococcus species, though viral and fungal etiologies are not uncommon.[1,2,4,5,6,7] MAs have a predilection for distal branches of the anterior or posterior circulation,[1,6,8,9] though aneurysms resulting from meningitis or other local infections may occur more frequently at proximal locations.[4,5] In a large series of patients with IE undergoing cerebral angiography, the reported incidence of MAs ranges from 2.0 to 8.9% (Mean: 4.5%, Standard Deviation: 3.2%).[7,10,11,12] Criteria for screening patients with

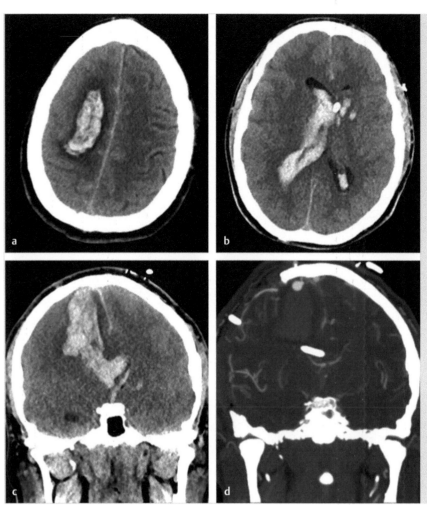

Fig. 4.3 Imaging after cardiac surgery. On the evening after cardiac surgery, a head computed tomography (CT) was obtained in response to neurologic deterioration that demonstrated a right frontal intraparenchymal hemorrhage **(a)**. After placement of a left-sided ventriculostomy, repeat imaging demonstrated enlargement of the hemorrhage with intraventricular extension and casting of the right lateral ventricle **(b,c)**. Postoperative vascular imaging after decompressive hemicraniectomy, clot evacuation, and middle cerebral artery (MCA) aneurysm resection demonstrated a new aneurysm off the anterior cerebral artery adjacent to the hematoma **(d)**.

IE are not well-defined. Though MAs may be present in a minority of patients with intracranial hemorrhage,[13] intraparenchymal or subarachnoid hemorrhage is predictive of MAs and should prompt vascular imaging.[4,10,12] The utility of screening in patients with IE and focal neurologic deficits is less clear, given the similar frequency of neurologic deficits noted in patients with and without MAs, yet may nevertheless be warranted given the morbidity associated with MA rupture.[12] Screening neurologically asymptomatic patients is likely to be of low yield and to have an unfavorable risk-to-benefit ratio.[7] Both CT and MR angiography have limited sensitivity for MAs; thus, all patients in whom the diagnosis of MA is suspected should undergo formal angiography.[10,14]

2. *What is the natural history of patients with MAs treated with appropriate antibiotics?*

In the presented case, the patient's distal MCA aneurysm was unruptured, with his neurologic symptoms on presentation instead attributable to multifocal cerebral infarctions resulting from septic thromboemboli. Given the unruptured status and prolonged filling of the aneurysm visualized on initial angiography (▸ Fig. 4.2b, c), this aneurysm was deemed likely to spontaneously thrombose and was not treated. The patient unfortunately experienced an intracranial hemorrhage from rupture of a de novo aneurysm forming sometime between initial angiography and cardiac surgery. In general, available evidence suggests that conservative management of unruptured MAs is reasonable, with multiple series describing no instances of rupture and high frequency of spontaneous resolution in patients with unruptured MAs treated with antibiotics alone,[1,3,5,8,15] though rupture of initially unruptured MAs despite medical therapy has been reported.[2,6] Unruptured MAs should nevertheless be monitored with serial imaging to ensure stability or resolution as aneurysm growth during medical therapy can occur[3,6,8] and has preceded fatal hemorrhage.[6] In contrast to noninfectious aneurysms, ruptured MAs typically present with IPH.[4,5,9] Ruptured MAs have a high rate of rebleeding with significant associated morbidity and mortality and thus should be treated if technically feasible.[4,6,9] Data on the rate of de novo aneurysm formation while on antibiotic therapy is limited, though available literature suggests it is uncommon.[8,16]

3. *How would you counsel the patient regarding the risks of cardiac surgery in the setting of a known MA?*

Cardiac surgery for valve replacement is often necessary in patients with IE complicated by heart failure.[17] Reported mortality rates after valve replacement in the setting of known cerebrovascular complications are high but also variable, ranging from 0.0 to 25.0% in available case series (Mean: 9.7%, SD: 8.4%).[18,19,20,21,22,23] Shorter interval between onset of neurologic symptoms and cardiac surgery is strongly associated with higher rates of neurologic morbidity and mortality, with respective rates of 43.8 and 31.3%

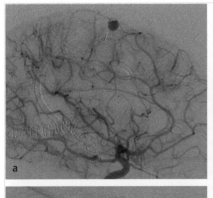
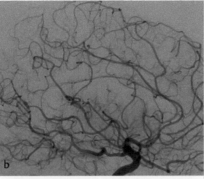
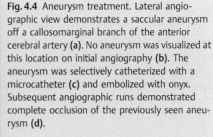

Fig. 4.4 Aneurysm treatment. Lateral angiographic view demonstrates a saccular aneurysm off a callosomarginal branch of the anterior cerebral artery (**a**). No aneurysm was visualized at this location on initial angiography (**b**). The aneurysm was selectively catheterized with a microcatheter (**c**) and embolized with onyx. Subsequent angiographic runs demonstrated complete occlusion of the previously seen aneurysm (**d**).

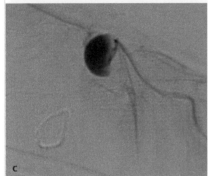
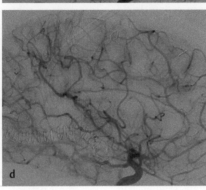

4

observed in a large case series when valve replacement was performed within 7 days of initial neurologic injury.[18] Valve replacement should thus be delayed in patients with intracranial hemorrhage, with a suggested time interval of 4 weeks between presentation and surgery.[18,22] As was the case in our patient, however, such delays are not always feasible in the presence of decompensated heart failure. In patients requiring urgent surgery, the risk of morbidity and mortality with valve replacement is exceedingly high and patients should be counseled as such. Data specific to the management of MAs in the setting of IE requiring valve replacement are limited, but available evidence suggests that treatment of MAs, if warranted, can be safely performed in the interval between presentation and cardiac surgery.[20,23,24,25,26] If cardiac surgery must precede aneurysm treatment, the risk of rehemorrhage from an unsecured ruptured MA is likely substantial.[22]

4. *What are the treatment options for MAs and how do they compare in terms of efficacy and outcome?*
As evidenced in the presented case, MAs can be amenable to either surgical or endovascular therapy. Previously reported surgical treatment options include clipping, wrapping, or trapping with either subsequent resection or bypass.[3,27] Endovascular options include parent vessel occlusion, saccular occlusion with coils or liquid embolic agents, or stenting with or without coil embolization.[28,29,30,31] Distal aneurysms located in noneloquent cortex can be safely treated with trapping and resection, while direct clipping or bypass after trapping may be necessary for aneurysms in eloquent cortex.[3] Similarly, simple parent vessel occlusion with either coils or liquid embolic agents is an effective and durable endovascular option for distal aneurysms in noneloquent cortex.[28,30,31] In eloquent cortex, direct aneurysmal embolization is preferable if feasible, but not always possible in instances of fusiform or dissecting morphology.[3] Treatment-related

morbidity, as well as recurrence and rebleeding rates, appears to be low after surgical therapy, though data are limited to small case series.[3,6,8,9] A systematic review analyzing the outcomes of endovascular treatment of 86 MAs quoted procedure-related morbidity and mortality rates of 12.6 and 6.1%, respectively, with recurrence and rebleeding rates after treatment of 7.9 and 5.8%, respectively.[32] Comparative studies of surgical versus endovascular therapies would be of interest; however, these are likely to be technically difficult, given the rarity of MAs and medical complexity of the patient population. Several authors advocate a multimodal approach to treatment of MAs, with selection of medical, surgical, or endovascular therapy dependent on both clinical circumstances and aneurysm characteristics. For example, for unruptured aneurysms, Chun and colleagues advocate medical treatment with appropriate antibiotics followed by serial angiography. For ruptured aneurysms in noneloquent cortex, endovascular treatment is recommended and if unsuccessful followed by microsurgery. Finally, ruptured aneurysms in eloquent cortex are treated initially with microsurgery. If a hematoma is present causing elevated intracranial pressure, microsurgery is favored regardless of aneurysm location.[3]

4.4 Level of Evidence

Screening: Patients with IE presenting with intracranial hemorrhage should undergo screening with formal angiography for the detection of MA (Class IV, Level of Evidence A). Patients presenting with neurologic symptoms should undergo screening for MAs with formal angiography (Class IV, Level of Evidence C).

Treatment of unruptured MAs: Patients with unruptured MAs should be treated with appropriate antibiotics and monitored with serial angiography to assess for aneurysm enlargement despite therapy (Class IV, Level of Evidence B).

Treatment of ruptured MAs: Patients with ruptured MAs should undergo treatment with open surgery or endovascular therapy (Class IV, Level of Evidence B).

Timing of cardiac surgery: Patients with IE requiring valve replacement and a ruptured MA should undergo a procedure to secure the MA prior to cardiac surgery, if feasible (Class IV, Level of Evidence B).

4.5 Landmark Papers

Salgado AV, Furlan AJ, Keys TF. Mycotic aneurysm, subarachnoid hemorrhage, and indications for cerebral angiography in infective endocarditis. Stroke 1987;18:1057–1060.

At the time of publication of Salgado and colleagues' article, neither the incidence of MAs in the setting of IE nor the typical clinical presentation that preceded or accompanied MA rupture was well defined. As such, evidence-based criteria for the screening of patients with IE were largely absent. In addition, upon identification of an MA, consensus on appropriate management, particularly for unruptured MAs, was minimal. The efficacy of appropriate antibiotic therapy in the treatment of MAs was unproven, and given the morbidity and mortality associated with MA rupture, certain studies had advocated the treatment of unruptured MAs immediately after diagnosis.[2] In this context, Salgado and colleagues endeavored to address three basic questions. First, what clinical and radiographic characteristics predict the presence of MAs in patients with IE? Second, what is the risk of intracranial hemorrhage from an unruptured MA in patients treated solely with antibiotics? By better characterizing the clinical presentation of patients with MAs and defining the risk of rupture from an undiagnosed, unruptured MA treated with appropriate antibiotics, the authors could address their third question: what are indications for diagnostic angiography in patients with IE?

The authors retrospectively reviewed the clinical course of 150 patients treated for IE at their institution. Within this cohort, there were three patients with MAs confirmed by angiography. The total number of patients who underwent angiography within the cohort was not defined. The authors also reviewed the literature and collected information on the clinical presentation of 68 patients with angiographically confirmed MAs. Characteristics of patients with MAs were compared to those of patients without MAs treated at the authors' institution. While patients with MAs were younger, older, and showed a female-predominance relative to patients without MAs, there were no significant differences in the clinical presentation between patients with and without MAs. Most surprisingly, there were roughly equal percentages of patients presenting with a focal neurologic deficit in both groups. The most common neurologic prodrome preceding MA detection, however, was nevertheless a focal deficit consistent with embolic infarction. As expected, the incidence of subarachnoid hemorrhage or IPH was much greater in the cohort with MAs (57.4 vs. 0.0%). Apart from the association of intracranial hemorrhage with an underlying MA, these results suggested that there were no defining clinical features, even with regard to neurologic symptomatology, which predicted MA formation.

The follow-up data of patients treated for IE at the authors' institution were then reviewed. The authors reasoned that as a very small minority of patients treated for IE underwent formal angiography, it was possible that some of these patients harbored undiagnosed, asymptomatic MAs. Defining the risk of MA rupture in this population would aid in determining how aggressively MAs should be sought in patients with IE. There were 25 patients who died during admission and 3 who were lost to follow-up, leaving 122 patients with long-term follow-up data. Among these patients, one experienced a fatal intracranial hemorrhage in the setting of oral anticoagulation use and supratherapeutic coagulation parameters. There were no instances of subarachnoid or intracranial hemorrhage in the remainder of patients during a mean follow-up period of 40.1 months. Taken together, these results suggested that the risk of intracranial hemorrhage from an undiagnosed, unruptured MA was low.

Synthesizing their results, the authors then proposed criteria for the angiographic screening of patients with IE. Unsurprisingly, all patients with intracranial hemorrhage were recommended to undergo screening. Determining the proper course of action for patients with neurologic symptoms but no intracranial hemorrhage was more difficult, given the limited specificity of neurologic symptoms for MAs in their series. Nevertheless, most patients with MAs presented with neurologic symptoms, and given the morbidity associated with MA rupture, the authors recommended that patients with neurologic symptoms receive angiographic screening. Finally, for neurologically asymptomatic patients without evidence of intracranial hemorrhage, after treatment with appropriate antibiotics the likelihood of neurologic morbidity from rupture of an undiagnosed aneurysm was thought to be low. As such, screening in this population was deemed to be unnecessary. Regarding actual screening protocols, recommendation included angiography 48 hours after initial presentation and again at the termination of antibiotic therapy (given rupture of 2/68 aneurysms despite antibiotics).

Chun JY, Smith W, Halbach VV, Higashida RT, Wilson CB, Lawton MT. Current multimodality management of infectious intracranial aneurysms. Neurosurgery 2001;48:1203–1214.

The advent and evolution of endovascular technology allowed for a new treatment modality in the management of MAs. The rarity of MAs, however, again precluded consensus on the appropriate role of endovascular therapy relative to surgical and medical management. To address this issue, Chun and colleagues published a retrospective case series of MAs treated at their institution over a period of 10 years. The authors proposed a management algorithm informing treatment selection on the basis of patient and aneurysm characteristics. Specifically, all unruptured aneurysms were initially managed medically, with serial angiography performed to monitor for growth. Ruptured aneurysms in noneloquent cortex were treated with endovascular therapy, while aneurysms in eloquent cortex were treated with microsurgery. In instances of elevated intracranial pressure from a space-occupying IPH, microsurgery for aneurysm resection and hematoma evacuation was favored regardless of aneurysm location.

There were 20 patients with a total of 27 MAs included for analysis. A majority of aneurysms were located distally on branches of the MCA and had fusiform or dissecting morphology. Fifteen aneurysms were ruptured, five of which had resulted in an intraparenchymal hematoma. Medical management was favored for all unruptured aneurysms, as well as for two initially ruptured aneurysms. In these latter cases, one patient suffered from severe combined immunodeficiency syndrome resulting in a disseminated fungal infection and was deemed medically unfit for intervention. The second patient had a fusiform aneurysm located on the distal superior cerebellar artery. Invasive treatment of this aneurysm was considered to carry too great a risk for brainstem infarction. No medically managed aneurysms, including the initially ruptured aneurysms, hemorrhaged while on antibiotic therapy. After diagnostic angiography, patients underwent repeat angiography 1 week after the initial study. Further angiography was performed at the discretion of the managing team and was influenced mostly by aneurysm morphology. Two aneurysms subsequently enlarged and required treatment.

Endovascular therapy was attempted in six patients and completed in five. In one case, the procedure was aborted due to inability to access the aneurysm with a microcatheter. This patient was instead treated with microsurgery. As stated previously, endovascular therapy was favored for MAs located in noneloquent cortex. Eloquence was assessed during diagnostic angiography via Amytal injection and subsequent serial neurologic examinations in an awake patient. The authors favored direct aneurysm coiling whenever feasible as opposed to parent vessel sacrifice; however, two aneurysms were treated with parent vessel occlusion due to fusiform or dissecting morphology. Procedure-related morbidity occurred in two patients: the first suffered a brainstem infarction after vertebral artery occlusion despite intraprocedural tolerance of balloon-test occlusion, and the second suffered a cortical infarction after coiling of a distal MCA aneurysm. No aneurysm recurrences or rehemorrhages were observed after initial treatment.

Microsurgery treatment was selected in 11 patients for the treatment of 16 aneurysms. Aneurysm trapping and resection was the most common treatment modality ($n = 6$) but was reserved for aneurysms in noneloquent cortex. Two aneurysms in eloquent cortex were treated with trapping and subsequent bypass. Direct clipping was performed for four aneurysms. The use of direct clipping for the treatment of MAs is controversial, given the increased friability of aneurysm tissue relative to noninfectious aneurysms and perceived increased risk of vessel wall tears and resultant catastrophic hemorrhage. In this series, clipping was reserved for unruptured aneurysms and ruptured aneurysms that had been treated with antibiotics for a minimum of 2 weeks prior to surgery. No intraoperative complications occurred during clipping. In one patient, three unruptured fusiform aneurysms located on the M1 segment were treated with wrapping; none of these aneurysms hemorrhaged during follow-up lasting 7 years. Finally, a single patient underwent surgical exploration, but no aneurysm could be found. No procedural-related morbidity was incurred. One patient experienced parent vessel occlusion after direct clipping; however, the patient remained asymptomatic. The four patients with intraparenchymal hematomas underwent hematoma evacuation at the time of aneurysm treatment.

Overall, 15 of 20 patients experienced a good neurologic outcome as assessed by the Glasgow Outcome Scale. Treatment-related morbidity was incurred in 2 of 15 patients, both of whom underwent endovascular therapy. Though based on a small number of patients, this study provided a workable framework for approaching the management of MA in the setting of multiple treatment options.

Petr O, Brinjikji W, Burrows AM, Cloft H, Kallmes DF, Lanzino G. Safety and efficacy of endovascular treatment for intracranial infectious aneurysms: a systematic review and meta-analysis. J Neuroradiol 2016;43:309–316.

Data on the safety and efficacy of the endovascular treatment of MAs is limited mostly to small case series, and thus a realistic estimate of the procedural risk associated with this treatment modality has been difficult to discern from available literature. Petr and colleagues attempted to address this issue by performing a systematic review and meta-analysis of studies examining the complications and outcomes of endovascular treatment of MA. This study provides a valuable reference point as well as a benchmark for proceduralists managing this complex clinical problem.

Eleven studies detailing the outcomes after treatment of 86 MAs were included for analysis. A majority of aneurysms were located in the anterior circulation (93.2%) and were ruptured (85.5%), with 64.4% of ruptured aneurysms resulting in an intraparenchymal hematoma. A majority of aneurysms were treated with parent vessel occlusion (60/86; 69.8%). Liquid embolization with Onyx was the most common treatment modality ($n = 47$, 54.7%), followed by coil embolization ($n = 17$, 19.8%); treatment modality was not defined for 22 patients (25.6%). Complete aneurysm occlusion was observed in 95.3% of all patients. Procedure-related morbidity occurred in 12.6% of patients, with 5.3% and 5.4% experiencing intraprocedural aneurysm rupture and perioperative stroke, respectively. Mortality related to endovascular intervention occurred in 6.1% of patients. Aneurysm recurrence was seen in 7.9% of patients, with 5.8% experiencing recurrent hemorrhage. Overall, 68.0% of patients experienced a good neurologic outcome.

The results of the review by Petr and colleagues suggest that endovascular treatment is effective in the treatment of MAs; however, the risks do not appear to be minimal. These results stress the importance of multimodal treatment strategies in the management of the complex vascular lesions.

4.6 Recommendations

As is evident on review of the literature, current strategies for the management of MAs are based primarily on the results of small case series, with no randomized evidence available to guide treatment decisions. Nevertheless, there appears to be sufficient evidence to reach a consensus on basic management questions, mainly on when screening for MAs is appropriate and indications for invasive treatment.

In patients with IE, the presence of either subarachnoid hemorrhage or IPH is predictive of MAs and should prompt angiography.[7,10,12] Neurologic deficits are not uncommon in patients with IE and have been shown to occur with relatively equal frequency in patients with and without MAs,[12] and thus recommending angiography for all patients presenting with neurologic symptoms is somewhat controversial. Moreover, the likelihood of subsequent hemorrhage from an undiagnosed, unruptured MA treated with appropriate antibiotics appears to be low.[12] Nevertheless, enlargement and subsequent rupture of unruptured MAs despite antibiotic therapy has been observed and is associated with high mortality.[3,6,8] As such, angiography in patients presenting with neurologic symptoms may be beneficial, though an estimate on the number needed to screen to prevent a single hemorrhage is unavailable due to lack of evidence. Screening should be performed with formal angiography as noninvasive vascular imaging modalities have been shown to have low sensitivity for MAs.[10,14] Indications for screening patients with etiologies other than IE are even less defined; however, angiography is likely prudent in patients with invasive cranial or disseminated infections presenting with intracranial hemorrhage.

The decision to treat MAs hinges primarily on whether the aneurysm is ruptured or unruptured. There is ample evidence to suggest that administration of appropriate antibiotics results in the stabilization or regression of a majority of unruptured, and even some ruptured, MAs.[1,3,5,8,12,15,16] Patients managed medically should nevertheless undergo serial angiography during therapy to monitor for MA growth, and invasive treatment should be pursued for enlarging aneurysms.[3,8,16] Given the high rate of rehemorrhage and resultant morbidity and mortality, ruptured MAs should be treated.[4,6,9] MAs are amenable to either surgical or endovascular therapies, and currently no comparative data exist comparing the safety and efficacy of these two modalities. The most common endovascular treatment method is parent vessel occlusion with either coils or liquid embolic agents. Saccular occlusion is preferable; however, it is not always possible in the setting of fusiform morphology. Available literature suggests that the technical success rate of endovascular therapy is high, but that the complication, recurrence, and rehemorrhage rates after treatment are not insignificant,[32] which should be considered when determining treatment strategy. Multimodal approaches, in which the choice of surgical versus endovascular therapy depends on clinical circumstances, have been shown to result in favorable outcomes.[3]

Finally, in the setting of IE, patients harboring MAs will not uncommonly require cardiac valve replacement for the treatment of heart failure. In patients with preexisting neurologic complications of IE, including MAs, the rate of exacerbation of neurologic morbidity appears to be inversely correlated to the amount of time elapsed between onset of neurologic symptoms and cardiac surgery,[18,23] with neurologic morbidity and mortality rates approaching 50% when valve replacement is performed within 7 days. If the patient's heart failure is compensated, studies have suggested a time interval between presentation and cardiac surgery of 4 weeks.[18] If feasible, ruptured MAs should be treated in this interval.

4.7 Summary

1. Patients with IE, or other systemic infections, presenting with neurologic symptoms or intracranial hemorrhage are at a risk of harboring an MA and should undergo a formal angiography.
2. Unruptured MAs should be treated medically with appropriate antibiotics. Serial imaging should be performed to assess for response to medical therapy, and enlarging aneurysms should be treated.
3. Ruptured MAs should be treated, with treatment selection dependent upon both clinical and aneurysm characteristics.

4. In the setting of IE, patients with a ruptured MA who also require valve replacement should first undergo aneurysm treatment if feasible due to the substantial risk of postcardiac surgery neurologic complications.

References

[1] Allen LM, Fowler AM, Walker C, et al. Retrospective review of cerebral mycotic aneurysms in 26 patients: focus on treatment in strongly immunocompromised patients with a brief literature review. AJNR Am J Neuroradiol. 2013; 34(4):823–827

[2] Bohmfalk GL, Story JL, Wissinger JP, Brown WE, Jr. Bacterial intracranial aneurysm. J Neurosurg. 1978; 48(3):369–382

[3] Chun JY, Smith W, Halbach VV, Higashida RT, Wilson CB, Lawton MT. Current multimodality management of infectious intracranial aneurysms. Neurosurgery. 2001; 48(6):1203–1213, discussion 1213–1214

[4] Kannoth S, Iyer R, Thomas SV, et al. Intracranial infectious aneurysm: presentation, management and outcome. J Neurol Sci. 2007; 256(1–2):3–9

[5] Matsubara N, Miyachi S, Izumi T, et al. Results and current trends of multimodality treatment for infectious intracranial aneurysms. Neurol Med Chir (Tokyo). 2015; 55(2):155–162

[6] Brust JC, Dickinson PC, Hughes JE, Holtzman RN. The diagnosis and treatment of cerebral mycotic aneurysms. Ann Neurol. 1990; 27(3):238–246

[7] Monteleone PP, Shrestha NK, Jacob J, et al. Clinical utility of cerebral angiography in the preoperative assessment of endocarditis. Vasc Med. 2014; 19 (6):500–506

[8] Corr P, Wright M, Handler LC. Endocarditis-related cerebral aneurysms: radiologic changes with treatment. AJNR Am J Neuroradiol. 1995; 16(4):745–748

[9] Venkatesh SK, Phadke RV, Kalode RR, Kumar S, Jain VK. Intracranial infective aneurysms presenting with haemorrhage: an analysis of angiographic findings, management and outcome. Clin Radiol. 2000; 55(12):946–953

[10] Hui FK, Bain M, Obuchowski NA, et al. Mycotic aneurysm detection rates with cerebral angiography in patients with infective endocarditis. J Neurointerv Surg. 2015; 7(6):449–452

[11] Salaun E, Touil A, Hubert S, et al. Intracranial haemorrhage in infective endocarditis. Arch Cardiovasc Dis. 2018; 111(12):712–721

[12] Salgado AV, Furlan AJ, Keys TF. Mycotic aneurysm, subarachnoid hemorrhage, and indications for cerebral angiography in infective endocarditis. Stroke. 1987; 18(6):1057–1060

[13] Hart RG, Kagan-Hallet K, Joerns SE. Mechanisms of intracranial hemorrhage in infective endocarditis. Stroke. 1987; 18(6):1048–1056

[14] Walkoff L, Brinjikji W, Rouchaud A, Caroff J, Kallmes DF. Comparing magnetic resonance angiography (MRA) and computed tomography angiography (CTA) with conventional angiography in the detection of distal territory cerebral mycotic and oncotic aneurysms. Interv Neuroradiol. 2016; 22(5):524–528

[15] Phuong LK, Link M, Wijdicks E. Management of intracranial infectious aneurysms: a series of 16 cases. Neurosurgery. 2002; 51(5):1145–1151, discussion 1151–1152

[16] Bingham WF. Treatment of mycotic intracranial aneurysms. J Neurosurg. 1977; 46(4):428–437

[17] Pant S, Patel NJ, Deshmukh A, et al. Trends in infective endocarditis incidence, microbiology, and valve replacement in the United States from 2000 to 2011. J Am Coll Cardiol. 2015; 65(19):2070–2076

[18] Eishi K, Kawazoe K, Kuriyama Y, Kitoh Y, Kawashima Y, Omae T. Surgical management of infective endocarditis associated with cerebral complications: multi-center retrospective study in Japan. J Thorac Cardiovasc Surg. 1995; 110(6):1745–1755

[19] Gillinov AM, Shah RV, Curtis WE, et al. Valve replacement in patients with endocarditis and acute neurologic deficit. Ann Thorac Surg. 1996; 61 (4):1125–1129, discussion 1130

[20] Jara FM, Lewis JF, Jr, Magilligan DJ, Jr. Operative experience with infective endocarditis and intracerebral mycotic aneurysm. J Thorac Cardiovasc Surg. 1980; 80(1):28–30

[21] Takagi Y, Higuchi Y, Kondo H, et al. The importance of preoperative magnetic resonance imaging in valve surgery for active infective endocarditis. Gen Thorac Cardiovasc Surg. 2011; 59(7):467–471

[22] Fukuda W, Daitoku K, Minakawa M, Fukui K, Suzuki Y, Fukuda I. Infective endocarditis with cerebrovascular complications: timing of surgical intervention. Interact Cardiovasc Thorac Surg. 2012; 14(1):26–30

[23] Fukuda W, Daitoku K, Minakawa M, Fukui K, Suzuki Y, Fukuda I. Management of infective endocarditis with cerebral complications. Ann Thorac Cardiovasc Surg. 2014; 20(3):229–236

[24] Fujita W, Daitoku K, Taniguchi S, Fukuda I. Infective endocarditis with cerebral mycotic aneurysm: treatment dilemma. Gen Thorac Cardiovasc Surg. 2010; 58(12):622–625

[25] Asai T, Usui A, Miyachi S, Ueda Y. Endovascular treatment for intracranial mycotic aneurysms prior to cardiac surgery. Eur J Cardiothorac Surg. 2002; 21(5):948–950

[26] Erdogan HB, Erentug V, Bozbuga N, Goksedef D, Akinci E, Yakut C. Endovascular treatment of intracerebral mycotic aneurysm before surgical treatment of infective endocarditis. Tex Heart Inst J. 2004; 31(2):165–167

[27] Day AL. Extracranial-intracranial bypass grafting in the surgical treatment of bacterial aneurysms: report of two cases. Neurosurgery. 1981; 9(5):583–588

[28] Dhomne S, Rao C, Shrivastava M, Sidhartha W, Limaye U. Endovascular management of ruptured cerebral mycotic aneurysms. Br J Neurosurg. 2008; 22 (1):46–52

[29] Ding D, Raper DM, Carswell AJ, Liu KC. Endovascular stenting for treatment of mycotic intracranial aneurysms. J Clin Neurosci. 2014; 21(7):1163–1168

[30] Esenkaya A, Duzgun F, Cinar C, et al. Endovascular treatment of intracranial infectious aneurysms. Neuroradiology. 2016; 58(3):277–284

[31] Grandhi R, Zwagerman NT, Linares G, et al. Onyx embolization of infectious intracranial aneurysms. J Neurointerv Surg. 2014; 6(5):353–356

[32] Petr O, Brinjikji W, Burrows AM, Cloft H, Kallmes DF, Lanzino G. Safety and efficacy of endovascular treatment for intracranial infectious aneurysms: a systematic review and meta-analysis. J Neuroradiol. 2016; 43(5):309–316

4

5 Traumatic Brain Aneurysms

Krishna Chaitanya Joshi and R. Webster Crowley

Abstract

Traumatic intracranial aneurysms are rare and account for less than 1% of intracranial aneurysms. They can have a myriad of presentations and are often not initially apparent. Most of these traumatic aneurysms are actually pseudoaneurysms that are formed due to direct or indirect stress on the vessel walls. Various treatment options exist and can be tailored based on the presentation and angioarchitecture of the aneurysm. While there are generally numerous endovascular options, these may be somewhat limited by an inability or reluctance to use antiplatelets as the traumatic nature of the injury often means that most of these patients have concomitant musculoskeletal or internal visceral injuries. There is no consensus on the natural history and behavior of these subsets of aneurysms, and the evidence in the literature is scarce. Therefore, a broad understanding of the various treatment options is essential before treating these aneurysms.

Keywords: cerebral aneurysm, traumatic aneurysm, pseudoaneurysm, vessel sacrifice, coiling

5.1 Goals

1. Understand the epidemiology and pathophysiology of traumatic intracranial aneurysms (TICAs).
2. Review the literature to understand the various types of TICAs and their clinical presentations.
3. Critically analyze the timing and role of computed tomography angiography (CTA) versus catheter angiogram in diagnosis and management of TICA.
4. Review the literature for various treatment options currently available for the treatment of TICAs.

5.2 Case Example

5.2.1 History of Present Illness

A man in his thirties presents to the emergency department (ED) with a severe traumatic head injury after his car collided with a snowplow. He appeared to have sustained severe maxillofacial injuries and lost consciousness en route to the hospital. History was obtained from family.

Past medical history: No significant history, including no past history of aneurysms or polycystic kidney disease.

Family history: Denies history of cerebral aneurysms.

Social history: Has smoked one to two packs of cigarettes/day for at least 15 years.

Neurological examination: Drowsy and confused. Oriented to person only. Severe periorbital edema on the right side and right pupillary size could not be assessed. No other cranial nerve palsy was observed at that time. He was moving all four limbs equally in response to pain. There was no evidence of cerebrospinal fluid (CSF) leakage from his nose or the scalp wound.

Imaging studies: CT scan and subsequent cerebral angiogram revealed extensive subarachnoid hemorrhage and a traumatic wide-necked aneurysm of the clinoidal segment of the internal carotid artery. See ▶ Fig. 5.1 and ▶ Fig. 5.2.

5.2.2 Treatment Plan

The patient was treated with endovascular coiling to occlude the aneurysm as well as the segment of the right internal carotid artery (ICA) that incorporated the aneurysm. The aneurysm neck was deemed too wide and the aneurysm likely too fragile to treat using intrasaccular coils alone (▶ Fig. 5.2a). Stent or flow diverter placement was felt to be suboptimal due to the

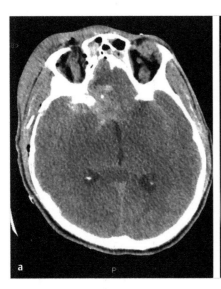
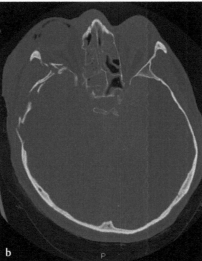

Fig. 5.1 (a,b) Computed tomography (CT) brain showing a comminuted fracture of the right temporal bone, the lateral wall of orbit, and medial wall of orbit extending into the ethmoid sinus. There is severe subarachnoid hemorrhage, predominantly in the basal cisterns and extending into the right Sylvian fissure.

5

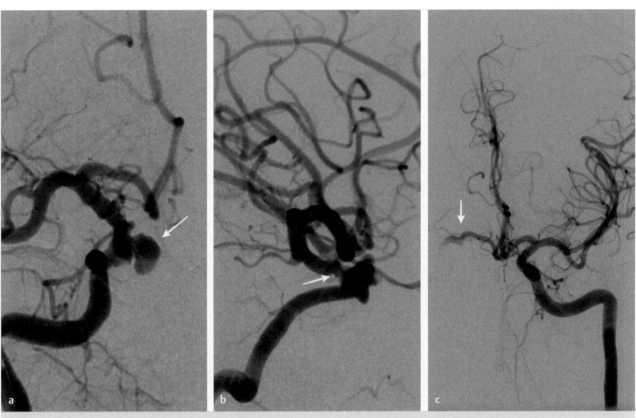

Fig. 5.2 Angiographic images. (**a**) Anteroposterior (AP) view—wide-necked, irregular-walled aneurysm in the clinoidal segment of the right internal carotid artery (ICA). (**b**) Lateral view—there is postaneurysmal narrowing of the vessel. The aneurysm is directed medially and inferiorly. (**c**) AP view, contralateral ICA injection showing reasonable collateral flow into the right anterior cerebral and middle cerebral arteries despite concurrent flow through the right ICA.

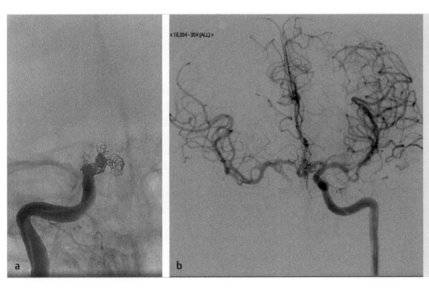

Fig. 5.3 (**a**) Anteroposterior (AP) view—postcoiling images of the right internal carotid artery (ICA) and pseudoaneurysm, showing complete occlusion of the parent artery. (**b**) AP view—injection from the left ICA showing collateral flow across the anterior communicating artery.

need for antiplatelet therapy in the setting of the patient's extensive intracranial blood and concomitant injuries. The patient tolerated the occlusion due to the presence of collateral flow from the contralateral ICA (▶ Fig. 5.3b).

5.2.3 Follow-up

Following the embolization, the patient eventually required decompressive hemicraniectomy for elevated intracranial pressure

(ICP) as a result of his traumatic brain injury. However, he did not experience any negative sequelae of the carotid sacrifice. At 2-year follow-up, he was doing well, with intact cognition and only slight weakness and sensory disturbance on the side contralateral to the aneurysm, a neurological deficit felt to be secondary to his initial injury.

5.3 Case Summary

1. *What is the pathophysiology of traumatic intracranial aneurysms (TICAs)?*

   TICAs are rare and account for < 1% of all cerebral aneurysms.[1] They are reported to occur in 3.2% of civilian penetrating craniofacial injuries[2] and in 42% of patients with gunshot wounds and missile head injuries.[3] They are more commonly seen in patients younger than 18 years.[1,4,5] This is possibly secondary to higher rates of traffic accidents and other trauma in this age group. The etiology can be variable and can range from seemingly trivial head injury to severe penetrating head injury. They are associated with severe mortality and morbidity when left untreated.[6]

   Histologically, they can be classified into true, false (pseudoaneurysms), and mixed aneurysms.[7] True aneurysms occur either due to direct impact or indirect transmission of force to the vessel wall, leading to an area of focal vessel weakness. Further flow dynamics across this weak wall leads to the formation of an aneurysm with the adventitia intact over it. False aneurysms, otherwise known as pseudoaneurysms, are far more common[4,7] and are due to rupture of all three layers of the vessel wall and formation of a contained hematoma. This leads to the formation of a false lumen and persistent flow into the false lumen which creates an aneurysmal dilatation.[4,8,9] Pseudoaneurysms are usually associated with penetrating or stab injuries. Mixed aneurysms are true aneurysms that have a contained rupture and subsequently form a pseudoaneurysm. The term "mixed aneurysms" are also occasionally used interchangeably with dissecting aneurysms.[10,11]

2. *What are the common sites of TICAs?*

   Although TICAs are seen in both the anterior and posterior circulations, they are predominantly found in the anterior circulation and are more frequent in the distal cerebral branches. The most frequent sites are the peripheral branches of the middle cerebral artery (MCA), followed by the branches of the pericallosal artery.[12,13] These are usually associated with penetrating injuries, in which the missile impact has scattered numerous fragments of bone or metal in diverging trajectories.[8] Pseudoaneurysms can also be associated with closed head injuries and are caused secondary to shearing forces. One common site in children is the pericallosal aneurysm formed by the impact of the pericallosal artery against the falx margin.[8,14] TICAs on more proximal intracerebral arteries are commonly located in the supraclinoid ICA.[15]

   The clinical presentation of TICAs can vary based on the location of the aneurysm. Supraclinoid TICAs can present with massive subarachnoid hemorrhage, delayed intracerebral hemorrhage, or progressive cranial neuropathies.[4,16,17] The average time from trauma to aneurysmal hemorrhage is approximately 21 days, and these lesions carry a mortality of almost 50%.[7,17] Infraclinoidal aneurysms often present as massive or recurrent epistaxis, cranial neuropathies, diabetes insipidus, or headaches.[18,19,20,21]

   Patients with distal branch TICAs usually present with delayed ICH. They can also present with seizures, can be diagnosed incidentally on routine radiographic follow-up, or in the evaluation of patients with growing skull fractures.[22,23]

3. *Do TICAs vary based on the mechanism of injury?*

   Blunt trauma is a frequent cause of TICAs in children. The cranium is softer and the relatively mobile cerebral content is more prone to shearing forces which may cause greater harm to the delicate vessels.[4,24] Another proposed mechanism is arterial injury due to cranial base fracture, which can result in the development of an intracavernous aneurysm, similar to traumatic carotid-cavernous fistula (CCF) development.[7,23] These aneurysms usually present in a delayed fashion. TICAs can also develop as a result of missile or gunshot injuries. These present commonly on the distal branches of the MCA and are a result of full-thickness tear in the vessel wall due to the fragments. They present with recurrent bleeding and ICH. These patients generally tend to be sicker due to associated brain injury, and therefore, one should have a low threshold for screening these patients with an emergent angiogram.[3,26]

4. *What is the best timing of doing a cerebral angiogram to diagnose TICAs?*

   CT is a widely used primary screening tool in patients with a traumatic brain injury, but it has a very low sensitivity for cerebrovascular injuries. Neurological deterioration due to unexplained ICH, massive epistaxis, and new cranial neuropathies should raise a suspicion for TICAs and warrant further investigation.[4,7] CTA is a noninvasive tool that is helpful in detecting vascular lesions. It has the added benefit of providing vessel wall information as compared to conventional angiography. It is, however, important to recognize that CTA is particularly inaccurate in aneurysms 5 mm or smaller and for those in the region of the anterior communicating artery.[7,27]

   Digital subtraction angiography (DSA) remains the gold standard diagnostic modality for intracranial aneurysms.[27,28] DSA generates high-resolution images of up to 0.1 to 0.2 mm and provides two-dimensional projection images, which is often enhanced by rotational angiography with three-dimensional image reconstruction, which appears to enhance its sensitivity and specificity.[29]

   There are currently no existing guidelines for the timing of angiography in TICAs. Isolated case reports and some case series have previously reported that most aneurysms after blunt traumatic injury present in a delayed fashion and suggest that the first angiography should be performed approximately 10 days to 2 weeks after the injury to avoid missed diagnoses.[7,8,9,30] However, the immediate risk of rupture is much higher in penetrating brain injuries, and there is a higher chance of harboring a pseudoaneurysm in these patients.[31,32] Therefore, a more emergent angiography as well as follow-up angiography 2 weeks later may be reasonable. Of course, patients with subarachnoid hemorrhage are at an increased risk for cerebral vasospasm, and repeat angiography at an earlier time interval may be necessary if signs and symptoms of vasospasm arise, with additional attention paid to investigating for the interval development of a pseudoaneurysm.

5. *What are the various treatment modalities available for TICAs?*

Conservative management of TICAs has a reported mortality of 41%. Thus, most cases should be treated, either with open surgery or endovascular methods. The treatment of far distal aneurysms can typically be successfully managed with endovascular occlusion of the parent artery, either with coils or liquid embolic agents. In select cases, coiling of the aneurysm with preservation of the parent vessel may be possible; however, if a pseudoaneurysm is suspected, this is generally avoided.[33]

The advent and subsequent improvement of flow diverters have also made treatment of more distal aneurysms with parent vessel preservation feasible using flow diversion.[34] This may be particularly attractive for patients in whom it is felt that vessel sacrifice would not be tolerated, or when the aneurysm is discovered in a delayed fashion without an acute rupture. Delayed presentation often negates many of the concerns of using antiplatelet therapy that exist in the acute setting. Flow diversion can be considered in acutely ruptured aneurysms; however, the risks of antiplatelet therapy must be considered again. One must remember that flow diversion does not typically occlude an aneurysm immediately, and therefore, it may not be ideal for particularly fragile or actively bleeding aneurysms.

Open surgery may increase the possibility of clipping the aneurysm with preservation of parent vessel but involves longer anesthesia duration, bleeding risks, and possible difficult dissection secondary to dense adhesions or brain swelling in the setting of trauma. However, curative surgical treatment, particularly of a pseudoaneurysm, may require trapping and sacrifice of the injured segment. In this case, endovascular occlusion is likely equally effective as open surgical ligation. If it is felt that the patient is unlikely to tolerate parent vessel sacrifice, bypass in combination with aneurysm trapping is an option (i.e., superficial temporal artery bypass for an MCA aneurysm or A3-A3 bypass for anterior cerebral artery aneurysms). Given that many of these lesions are a result of trauma, including penetrating injuries, the planned bypass vessel may also be injured and should be identified prior to surgery.

Proximally located aneurysms are perhaps more technically challenging to treat, largely due to the greater territory at risk for hypoperfusion and subsequent stroke, should occlusion be required. Surgical options usually require sacrificing the parent vessel as reconstructing the parent vessel when a pseudoaneurysm is present is fairly risky and with low likelihood of success. When time permits, a thorough evaluation using balloon test occlusion can be done to test the collateral circulation. If the patient passes the balloon test occlusion, endovascular sacrifice of the artery may be reasonable. If occlusion is not felt to be a tolerated option, surgical options are generally limited to parent vessel sacrifice with high flow bypass or com-

plex reconstruction of the vessel with a series of clips or wrapping which may be associated with high morbidity. Endovascular treatment options that preserve the parent artery may include coiling or placement of a stent graft/ covered stent.[33] More recently, flow-diverting stents have been reported as useful and relatively safe in the treatment of carotid pseudoaneurysms.[35] Again, it is important to note that placement of stents requires antiplatelet therapy, and the risks and benefits must be weighed carefully in the acute trauma setting. The initiation of antiplatelet therapy is much less of a concern for traumatic aneurysms that are seen in a delayed fashion and have not bled. However, as experience accumulates, flow diversion has become the treatment of choice for TICAs in many centers, even in the setting of acute bleed.

5.4 Landmark Papers

Cohen JE, Gomori JM, Segal R, et al. Results of endovascular treatment of traumatic intracranial aneurysms. Neurosurgery 2008; 63(3):476–486.

The literature on treatment of TICAs has been limited to isolated case reports and a few case series. The rarity of these lesions in the civilian population and high mortality have made it difficult to have more elaborate studies on this entity.

Cohen et al, for the first time, presented a series on endovascular-treated TICAs. Of the 34 patients with traumatic brain injury who underwent angiography (25 penetrating brain injuries, 9 blunt injuries), 13 TICAs were diagnosed (10 penetrating brain injuries, 3 blunt injuries). The Glasgow Coma Scale score at diagnosis ranged from 5 to 15. Angiography was performed for screening in eight patients and for clinical indications in five patients; 11 TICAs were diagnosed before rupture. Seven aneurysms were located on branches of the MCA, two on pericallosal branches of the anterior cerebral artery, and four on the ICA. No recanalization was detected in 12 patients. One patient treated with a bare stent and coiling had a growing intracavernous pseudoaneurysm; therefore, ICA occlusion with extracranial-intracranial microvascular bypass was performed. Six patients refused angiographic follow-up, but CTA failed to show recanalization. No patient presented with delayed bleeding (mean follow-up, 2.6 y). There were no procedure-related complications or mortality.

Two main subgroups of lesions requiring different treatments emerged: proximal lesions, which may be obliterated with preservation of the parent vessel, and lesions distal to the first cerebral artery segments, which usually required vessel sacrifice by liquid embolic agents. Using this endovascular approach, they reported zero mortality and low levels of morbidity. Their results are impressive, given the natural history of these lesions without intervention.

Surgical management of these types of aneurysms is technically demanding and carries a higher surgical risk and should be only considered when the endovascular approach is not indicated. Cohen et al very articulately describe the complete range of techniques that can be used in the endovascular armamentarium from the sacrifice of parent vessel to reconstruction using stent grafts.

5

They recommend early angiographic diagnosis and endovascular treatment of TICAs and conclude that the endovascular approach offers a valuable alternative to surgery for the treatment of TICAs. Different techniques can be selected for specific cases, allowing the early treatment of TICAs with excellent results.

Mao Z, Wang N, Hussain M, et al. Traumatic intracranial aneurysms due to blunt brain injury—a single center experience. Acta Neurochirurgica 2012;154(12): 2187–2193.3.[36]

In this retrospective series from the Department of Neurosurgery, Xuanwu Hospital, Beijing, their aneurysm database from 2005 to 2011 was reviewed, and patients with TICAs secondary to blunt brain injury were analyzed. Variables assessed included age, sex, causes of blunt brain injury, skull fracture, location, classification, clinical presentation, time elapsed to arrive at diagnosis, treatment, and eventual outcome.

Fifteen patients (0.64%) with TICAs secondary to blunt brain injury were identified. Motor vehicle accidents (MVAs) were observed to be the most common cause of injury (10 patients, 66.7%), followed by TICAs sustained after falls (5 patients, 33.3%). The most common symptom at presentation was epistaxis (6 patients, 40%), followed by ophthalmic problems (6 patients, 40%), with both presentations seen in 1 patient. The most common diagnostic modality used was DSA in 12 patients (80%) followed by CTA in 2 patients (13.3%). Infraclinoid TICAs were seen in 9 patients (60%), whereas supraclinoid TICAs were seen in 5 patients (33.3%), with perifalcine TICAs seen in 1 patient. Endovascular intervention therapies were performed in 11 patients (73.3%), bypass surgery and trapping in 2 patients (13.3%), and transnasal endoscopic approach in combination with balloon-assistance in 2 patients. At discharge, 2 patients had poor clinical outcomes (13.3%), 5 had fair (33.3%), and 8 resulted with good outcomes (53.3%).

This series highlights TICAs secondary to blunt head injury, which are very different in presentation and behavior compared to penetrating head injuries. Infraclinoid ICA seems to be the most common location followed by supraclinoid ICA and the arteries in the perifalcine region. Based on the analysis of clinical presentations of TICAs, they conclude that traumatic patients presenting with recurrent epistaxis, oculomotor nerve palsy, and delayed intracranial hemorrhage should receive cerebral angiography as soon as possible. An early diagnosis and proper treatment could prove to be helpful in terms of improving the final clinical outcome.

5.5 Recommendations

Due to the relative rarity of this entity and the varied presentations, there are no set guidelines for the treatment of TICAs. A high degree of suspicion is required, especially in atypical cases. They are found more commonly after penetrating or shrapnel injuries, and early cerebral angiography is recommended in these cases. There is currently no recommendations for CTA in cases with blunt head injury. Cerebral vascular imaging is recommended after delayed hemorrhage, epistaxis, or development of new cranial neuropathies in patients with blunt head injury, especially so in children. In cases with vasospasm on initial angiogram, a repeat angiogram is recommended.

Treatment of TICAs may vary on a case-to-case basis. Endovascular techniques are considered as the first-line treatment,

with surgical treatment reserved for cases where endovascular therapy has failed. Peripherally placed aneurysms can be treated with vessel sacrifice using coils or liquid embolic agents. Larger aneurysms with favorable neck dome ratios and with large proximal arteries may be treated with coil embolization with preservation of the parent vessel. Proximal ICA aneurysms can be treated with proximal ligation and trapping after confirming adequate collateral status using balloon test occlusion. Stent grafts or covered grafts have also been used with mounting evidence supporting the use of flow-diverting stents. It is very important to carefully weigh the risks of using antiplatelet agents in acute trauma setting before using stents.

5.6 Summary

1. TICAs are rare and constitute < 1% of intracranial aneurysms. They are more commonly found in war injuries and secondary to MVAs. They are also found more commonly in young adults.
2. TICAs are a heterogeneous entity and can have a myriad of presentations based on the mechanism of injury and location of the aneurysm.
3. A high index of suspicion is required, especially in patients with gunshot or missile injury and in patients presenting with delayed hemorrhage, epistaxis, and cranial neuropathies.
4. Endovascular treatment appears to be safe and preferred over surgical options in most cases. However, a case-by-case approach is prudent and the final decision is based on the angioarchitecture of the aneurysm, as well as the perceived tolerance for parent artery occlusion or antiplatelet therapy.

References

[1] Harbaugh RE. Unruptured intracranial aneurysms: decision making & management. Contemp Neurosurg. 1991; 13(12):1
[2] Levy ML, Rezai A, Masri LS, et al. The significance of subarachnoid hemorrhage after penetrating craniocerebral injury: correlations with angiography and outcome in a civilian population. Neurosurgery. 1993; 32(4): 532–540
[3] Jinkins JR, Dadsetan MR, Sener RN, Desai S, Williams RG. Value of acute-phase angiography in the detection of vascular injuries caused by gunshot wounds to the head: analysis of 12 cases. AJR Am J Roentgenol. 1992; 159(2):365–368
[4] Buckingham MJ, Crone KR, Ball WS, Tomsick TA, Berger TS, Tew JM, Jr. Traumatic intracranial aneurysms in childhood: two cases and a review of the literature. Neurosurgery. 1988; 22(2):398–408
[5] Ventureyra EC, Higgins MJ. Traumatic intracranial aneurysms in childhood and adolescence: case reports and review of the literature. Childs Nerv Syst. 1994; 10(6):361–379
[6] Fleischer AS, Patton JM, Tindall GT. Cerebral aneurysms of traumatic origin. Surg Neurol. 1975; 4(2):233–239
[7] Larson PS, Reisner A, Morassutti DJ, Abdulhadi B, Harpring JE. Traumatic intracranial aneurysms. Neurosurg Focus. 2000; 8(1):e4
[8] Amirjamshidi A, Rahmat H, Abbassioun K. Traumatic aneurysms and arteriovenous fistulas of intracranial vessels associated with penetrating head injuries occurring during war: principles and pitfalls in diagnosis and management. A survey of 31 cases and review of the literature. J Neurosurg. 1996; 84 (5):769–780
[9] Kieck CF, de Villiers JC. Vascular lesions due to transcranial stab wounds. J Neurosurg. 1984; 60(1):42–46
[10] Nass R, Hays A, Chutorian A. Intracranial dissecting aneurysms in childhood. Stroke. 1982; 13(2):204–207

[11] Patel H, Smith RR, Garg BP. Spontaneous extracranial carotid artery dissection in children. Pediatr Neurol. 1995; 13(1):55–60

[12] Benoit BG, Wortzman G. Traumatic cerebral aneurysms: clinical features and natural history. J Neurol Neurosurg Psychiatry. 1973; 36(1):127–138

[13] Nakstad P, Nornes H, Hauge HN. Traumatic aneurysms of the pericallosal arteries. Neuroradiology. 1986; 28(4):335–338

[14] Holmes B, Harbaugh RE. Traumatic intracranial aneurysms: a contemporary review. J Trauma. 1993; 35(6):855–860

[15] Jung S-H, Kim S-H, Kim T-S, Joo S-P. Surgical treatment of traumatic intracranial aneurysms: experiences at a single center over 30 years. World Neurosurg. 2017; 98:243–250

[16] Yang T-C, Lo Y-L, Huang Y-C, Yang S-T. Traumatic anterior cerebral artery aneurysm following blunt craniofacial trauma. Eur Neurol. 2007; 58(4):239–245

[17] Cogbill TH, Moore EE, Meissner M, et al. The spectrum of blunt injury to the carotid artery: a multicenter perspective. J Trauma. 1994; 37(3):473–479

[18] Uzan M, Cantasdemir M, Seckin MS. Traumatic intracranial carotid tree aneurysms. J Vasc Interv Radiol. 1999; 10(6):840

[19] Dubey A, Sung W-S, Chen Y-Y, et al. Traumatic intracranial aneurysm: a brief review. J Clin Neurosci. 2008; 15(6):609–612

[20] Türeyen K. Traumatic intracranial aneurysm after blunt trauma. Br J Neurosurg. 2001; 15(5):429–431

[21] Yazbak PA, McComb JG, Raffel C. Pediatric traumatic intracranial aneurysms. Pediatr Neurosurg. 1995; 22(1):15–19

[22] Almeida GM, Pindaro J, Plese P, Bianco E, Shibata MK. Intracranial arterial aneurysms in infancy and childhood. Childs Brain. 1977; 3(4):193–199

[23] Endo S, Takaku A, Aihara H, Suzuki J. Traumatic cerebral aneurysm associated with widening skull fracture: report of two infancy cases. Childs Brain. 1980; 6(3):131–139

[24] Casey ATH, Moore AJ. A traumatic giant posterior cerebral artery aneurysm mimicking a tentorial edge meningioma. Br J Neurosurg. 1994; 8(1):97–99

[25] Gemmete JJ, Elias AE, Chaudhary N, Pandey AS. Endovascular methods for the treatment of intracranial cerebral aneurysms. Neuroimaging Clin N Am. 2013; 23(4):563–591

[26] Benzel EC, Day WT, Kesterson L, et al. Civilian craniocerebral gunshot wounds. Neurosurgery. 1991; 29(1):67–71, discussion 71–72

[27] Bederson JB, Connolly ES, Jr, Batjer HH, et al. American Heart Association. Guidelines for the management of aneurysmal subarachnoid hemorrhage: a statement for healthcare professionals from a special writing group of the Stroke Council, American Heart Association. Stroke. 2009; 40(3):994–1025

[28] Brisman JL, Song JK, Newell DW. Cerebral aneurysms. N Engl J Med. 2006; 355(9):928–939

[29] Pradilla G, Wicks RT, Hadelsberg U, et al. Accuracy of computed tomography angiography in the diagnosis of intracranial aneurysms. World Neurosurg. 2013; 80(6):845–852

[30] Aarabi B. Traumatic aneurysms of brain due to high velocity missile head wounds. Neurosurgery. 1988; 22(6 Pt 1):1056–1063

[31] Armonda RA, Bell RS, Vo AH, et al. Wartime traumatic cerebral vasospasm: recent review of combat casualties. Neurosurgery. 2006; 59(6):1215–1225, discussion 1225

[32] du Trevou MD, van Dellen JR. Penetrating stab wounds to the brain: the timing of angiography in patients presenting with the weapon already removed. Neurosurgery. 1992; 31(5):905–911, discussion 911–912

[33] Cohen JE, Gomori JM, Segal R, et al. Results of endovascular treatment of traumatic intracranial aneurysms. Neurosurgery. 2008; 63(3):476–485, discussion 485–486

[34] Durst CR, Hixson HR, Schmitt P, Gingras JM, Crowley RW. Endovascular treatment of a fusiform aneurysm at the M3-M4 junction of the middle cerebral artery using the pipeline embolization device. World Neurosurg. 2016; 86:511.e1–511.e4

[35] Sami MT, Gattozzi DA, Soliman HM, et al. Use of Pipeline™ embolization device for the treatment of traumatic intracranial pseudoaneurysms: case series and review of cases from literature. Clin Neurol Neurosurg. 2018; 169:154–160

[36] Mao Z, Wang N, Hussain M, et al. Traumatic intracranial aneurysms due to blunt brain injury—a single center experience. Acta Neurochirurgica. 2012; 154(12):2187–2193

5

6 Cerebral Vasospasm

Michael B. Avery and Alim P. Mitha

Abstract

Cerebral vasospasm is a phenomenon that can occur after subarachnoid hemorrhage, most notably after aneurysm rupture. It represents a significant cause of morbidity and mortality in an already devastating disease. Much research has been conducted to understand the pathophysiology and to use this information to develop targeted therapies to both prevent and treat this disease. Despite this, there are very few effective options available. The rapid onset and significant sequelae mean that the treating physician must have a thorough understanding of the current state of therapeutic options to be able to act quickly and mitigate the effects of vasospasm-induced ischemia.

Keywords: vasospasm, delayed cerebral ischemia, subarachnoid hemorrhage, aneurysm, angioplasty, triple-H therapy

6.1 Goals

1. Define cerebral vasospasm and differentiate it from other potential causes of neurological decline in the setting of aneurysmal subarachnoid hemorrhage (SAH).
2. Review the literature that has been paramount to developing our current clinical management strategy of cerebral vasospasm.
3. Discuss recent therapeutic interventions.

6.2 Case Example

6.2.1 History of Present Illness

A 45-year-old male experienced a sudden onset of severe headache with no loss of consciousness but elected to present to the hospital 3 days later with persistent headache but neurologically intact. Computed tomography (CT) of the head demonstrated diffuse SAH throughout the anterior basal cisterns, and CT angiography revealed a broad-based blister aneurysm of the right supraclinoid internal carotid artery (ICA) (▶ Fig. 6.1a). The patient was started on nimodipine, as well as aspirin and

clopidogrel prior to undergoing uncomplicated placement of a flow-diverting stent from the right ICA into the middle cerebral artery (MCA) (▶ Fig. 6.1b). Postoperatively, he developed hypoxia requiring an intensive care unit admission. Imaging studies revealed significant bilateral pulmonary edema. On SAH day 7, the patient's level of consciousness suddenly deteriorated.

Past medical history: Noncontributory.

Family history: Noncontributory.

Social history: Occasional social alcohol. No smoking history.

Review of systems: Tachypnea and increased work of breathing. S3 noted on auscultation.

Neurological examination: Glasgow Coma Scale (GCS)—$E_3V_4M_6$; drowsy and disoriented; weak left arm.

Imaging studies: CT and digital subtraction angiography (DSA) (see ▶ Fig. 6.1 and ▶ Fig. 6.2).

6.2.2 Treatment Plan

The patient initially did well after the flow-diverting stent was placed across the aneurysm. Intravenous crystalloid was infused to maintain euvolemia and normotension. Shortly after the treatment, he developed neurogenic pulmonary edema and required supplemental oxygen as well as diuretic therapy. The hypoxia was short lived and he was successfully weaned off of oxygen. Daily transcranial Doppler (TCD) studies were performed beginning on the date of admission, which showed progressively increasing velocities in the proximal right MCA. On post-SAH day 8, the patient developed a decreased level of consciousness and left arm weakness consistent with symptoms of cerebral vasospasm. Plain CT and CT angiography were performed that confirmed significant vasospasm of the right MCA, but no obvious infarction. He was immediately started on a norepinephrine infusion. Despite reaching a systolic blood pressure of 200 mmHg, his symptoms persisted. He was then brought to the angiography suite where an angiogram redemonstrated the severe right proximal MCA stenosis, distal to the flow-diverting stent (▶ Fig. 6.2a). Balloon angioplasty was performed by partial inflation of a 4-mm compliant balloon system, followed by the selective administration of 3 mg of verapamil into the MCA. The procedure resulted in clinical improvement, but not angio-

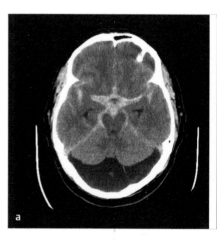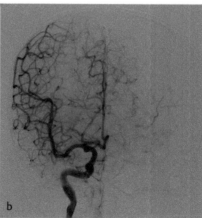

Fig. 6.1 (a) Unenhanced computed tomography (CT) head of a patient with significant aneurysmal subarachnoid hemorrhage. An incidental finding of a large posterior fossa cyst was made. **(b)** Anteroposterior view of a right internal carotid artery (ICA) injection angiogram demonstrating a right supraclinoid ICA ruptured broad-based blister aneurysm. The aneurysm was treated with a flow-diverting stent placed from the right ICA into the ipsilateral middle cerebral artery (MCA).

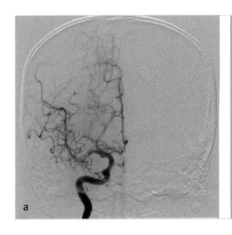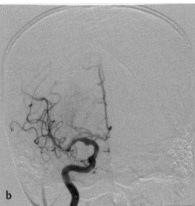

Fig. 6.2 **(a)** Anteroposterior view of a right internal carotid artery (ICA) injection angiogram showing severe right middle cerebral artery (MCA) vasospasm distal to the flow-diverting stent. **(b)** Similar angiogram performed immediately postballoon angioplasty and selective arterial injection of 3 mg of verapamil. Vasospasm has improved but is still present.

graphic resolution, of the vasospasm (▶ Fig. 6.2b). His symptoms subsequently resolved and his level of consciousness returned to baseline while being maintained on a norepinephrine infusion. The patient was gradually weaned off the vasopressor infusion and was discharged home on post-SAH day 18.

6.2.3 Follow-up

The patient was discharged home in a good condition with slight residual left arm weakness. He was seen in the clinic for a follow-up 6 weeks later with a normal neurological examination. DSA at 6 months demonstrated complete parent vessel remodeling with no filling of the blister aneurysm.

6.3 Case Summary

1. *What is the definition of cerebral vasospasm and is it synonymous with delayed cerebral ischemia (DCI)?*

   Cerebral vasospasm is defined as the prolonged radiographic narrowing of cerebral arteries and can be seen in several pathologies, most notably aneurysmal SAH. The peak incidence in this scenario is between 4 and 14 days postrupture, and radiographic vasospasm is estimated to have an overall incidence of approximately 43%.[1] However, radiographic vasospasm does not imply symptomatology, and thus, it should be differentiated from symptomatic vasospasm, which is estimated to occur in about 33%. The pathogenesis of vasospasm appears to be multifactorial and remains elusive. Several mechanistic processes have been described, including endothelial injury, vascular smooth muscle contraction, and inflammatory cascade activation.[2] Endothelial injury is thought to largely occur in an outside-in fashion, beginning with oxyhemoglobin found in the subarachnoid blood-inducing hydroxyl radical and lipid peroxide formation.[3,4] These are thought to diffuse through the arterial wall and disrupt both the vascular smooth muscle cells and the endothelium, by upregulating endothelin-1 (vasoconstrictor) and downregulating nitric oxide production (vasodilator), respectively.[5,6] Acute arterial smooth muscle cell contraction is dependent on adenosine triphosphate, while the chronic vasospasm condition appears not to be. Instead, research has shown that after short-term smooth muscle contraction occurs, various contractile proteins are activated (including rho-kinase, protein kinase C, and protein tyrosine kinase),

leading to sustained muscle shortening independent of intracellular calcium stores.[7] Finally, various inflammatory proteins are upregulated postaneurysmal SAH in both serum and cerebrospinal fluid and are suspected to play a role in inducing vasospasm.[2,8,9]

DCI, on the other hand, is a more encompassing term for neurological decline and includes other etiologies, including microthrombi, cortical spreading depression, distal microvascular constriction, etc. The literature is fraught with inconsistent terminology, and in an effort to standardize research efforts, a group recently proposed a unifying definition of DCI: "The occurrence of focal neurological impairment, or a decrease of at least 2 points on the Glasgow Coma Scale. This should last for at least 1 hour, is not apparent immediately after aneurysm occlusion, and cannot be attributed to other causes by means of clinical assessment, CT or MRI scanning of the brain, and appropriate laboratory studies."[10] DCI is, therefore, a diagnosis of exclusion and should be reserved for situations where other potential causes for neurological decline, such as hyponatremia, hydrocephalus, infection, and others, have been ruled out. In the example case, the patient was suffering from DCI secondary to vasospasm of the proximal right MCA as other potential causes were ruled out and an angiogram revealed severe stenosis of a culprit artery.

2. *Are there any predictive factors for the onset of cerebral vasospasm?*

   The original Fisher grading scale aimed to predict the onset of symptomatic vasospasm after aneurysmal SAH, allowing practitioners to implement protective measures in anticipation.[11] Using CT, the authors found that thick SAH and intraventricular blood were associated with symptomatic vasospasm. Later, Frontera et al published a modification of the Fisher grading scale which better predicted the onset (▶ Table 6.1).[12] Our patient had a modified Fisher grade 3 SAH and thus would be quoted a 33% chance of developing symptomatic vasospasm.

   Other predictors of symptomatic vasospasm have more recently been identified, which include prolonged clearance of cisternal blood, smoking history, hyperglycemia, systemic inflammatory response syndrome, and hydrocephalus.[13,14] Furthermore, there is some evidence that female gender, hypertension, initial loss of consciousness, and perhaps others may portend a higher risk.[13]

6

Table 6.1 Modified Fisher scale for aneurysmal SAH

Grade	Description	Symptomatic vasospasm rate (%)
0	No SAH or IVH	0
1	Focal or diffuse thin SAH, no IVH	24
2	Focal or diffuse thin SAH, IVH present	33
3	Thick SAH, no IVH	33
4	Thick SAH, IVH present	40

Abbreviations: IVH, intraventricular hemorrhage; SAH, subarachnoid hemorrhage.
Note: Thin SAH < 1 mm < thick SAH.

3. *Are there any prophylactic measures that can be taken?*
   To date, nimodipine is the only therapeutic intervention aimed at preventing cerebral vasospasm that has been shown to improve outcomes. It is a dihydropyridine calcium channel blocker which primarily acts upon the cerebral vasculature and has minimal effects on the cardiac conduction system. Administered 60 mg orally every 4 hours (or 30 mg every 2 h if hypotension is encountered) has been shown in a meta-analysis to improve the vasospasm-induced deficit and mortality rates (odds ratio [OR]: 0.46–0.58).[15] However, no reduction in incidence of cerebral vasospasm has been found.
   It is important to also implement general medical measures including maintaining euvolemia; avoiding hyponatremia, hypotension, anemia, and high intracranial pressure; optimizing ventilation and oxygenation; and avoiding surgical clipping during the period of peak vasospasm incidence.[2,16,17] Syndrome of inappropriate antidiuretic hormone (SIADH) secretion and cerebral salt wasting are potential complications that must be managed aggressively without compromising the aforementioned physiological parameters. For instance, a patient with SIADH should not be fluid restricted, as is the standard treatment. Instead, patients should receive hypertonic saline as needed. During vasospasm, oral fludrocortisone 0.3 mg per day may be used as well.[18] In the example case, our patient received nimodipine 60 mg orally every 4 hours and tolerated the dosing without an issue. Furthermore, neurogenic pulmonary edema occurred, requiring prompt treatment.
   Many experimental therapies have been trialed in humans with limited success as some have reduced the incidence of angiographic vasospasm but have had no significant effect on clinical outcome. These include strategies to improve subarachnoid blood clearance (intracisternal thrombolytics), prophylactic balloon angioplasty, endothelin-1A receptor antagonists (CONSCIOUS-1, 2, and 3 trials), intrathecal vasodilators, magnesium infusion (MASH and MASH-2 trials), statins (STASH trial), and many others.[14,19,20,21,22,23,24,25,26]

4. *How would you monitor for the development of vasospasm?*
   It is important to remember the distinction between symptomatic vasospasm and radiographic vasospasm. Of course, symptomatic vasospasm requires clinical deterioration or alteration and is one etiology of DCI. Radiographic cerebral vasospasm may be diagnosed using several different modalities. TCD measures blood flow velocity, which increases during vasospasm, and is a feasible method of noninvasive bedside monitoring. The transtemporal window is most frequently used but limits the assessment to the proximal intracerebral arteries. While blood velocity trends in all arteries may be useful, parameters have been established for predicting MCA and basilar artery (BA) vasospasm. Blood velocities greater than 200 cm/s for the MCA and 85 cm/s for the BA are highly predictive of vasospasm.[27] However, these increased velocities may be indicative of a hyperemic state, so the Lindegaard ratio was developed to minimize false positives by normalizing velocity by dividing by the proximal arterial velocity (ICA for MCA velocity, and extracranial vertebral artery for BA velocity). A Lindegaard ratio greater than 3 is highly suggestive of vasospasm. While TCD may be used to monitor for vasospasm, other imaging modalities are used for diagnosis and include CT angiography, CT perfusion, magnetic resonance angiography (MRA), MR perfusion, positron emission tomography (PET), and single-photon emission computed tomography (SPECT). DSA, although the most invasive, remains the gold standard for diagnosing cerebral vasospasm. Two-dimensional DSA exhibits a nearly 100% sensitivity and specificity. Mills et al recently published a thorough review comparing the advantages and disadvantages of these various modalities.[28] More invasive monitoring techniques are also available, which include microdialysis and brain tissue oxygenation. Microdialysis can only provide a highly specific regional alteration in metabolism, with increased lactate and glutamate occurring approximately 24 hours prior to clinical ischemia.[29] Similarly, brain tissue oxygenation is only measured in one region but can detect tissue hypoxia with an oxygen tension below 15 mmHg.
   Finally, electroencephalography can be used to predict vasospasm. Studies have shown that the alpha wave to delta wave ratio and percent alpha wave variability can predict vasospasm and often precedes the onset by approximately 2 days.[30]
   Our patient developed gradually increasing velocities in the right MCA territory. As the patient remained asymptomatic initially, we elected to observe carefully. At our center, we do not routinely rely on perfusion imaging at the onset of symptoms. Instead, we generally confirm TCD results with CT angiography, then perform DSA with an intention to treat, after other potential causes of neurological decline have been ruled out.

5. *What factors would you consider when deciding whether or not to treat cerebral vasospasm in this patient?*
   As mentioned previously, a distinction must be made between radiographic and symptomatic vasospasm. Neurological symptoms appear to occur in approximately half of the patients demonstrating angiographic large artery narrowing.[31] Treatment of cerebral vasospasm, whether through medical or interventional means, should not be performed if the patient is asymptomatic. However, it may be prudent to consider treatment in patients who are comatose and demonstrate severe angiographic vasospasm if a reliable neurological examination is not available. In this case, our patient was not comatose but demonstrated a decreased level of consciousness and focal neurological deficits attributable to the vasospastic artery. With good neurological function prior to his decline, and minimal lag time after symptom onset, we elected to treat swiftly and aggressively.

6. *What options are available for treatment?*

Once the diagnosis of symptomatic cerebral vasospasm has been made, there are several treatment options available. Prior to endovascular therapy, triple-H therapy was the mainstay treatment, theorized to improve rheology to optimize cerebral blood flow and oxygen transport. This regimen consists of hemodilution, hypervolemia, and hypertension. Expansion of the effective circulating volume using an infusion of isotonic crystalloid effectively addresses the former two; however, there is evidence that cerebral blood flow does not change between a hypervolemic state and a euvolemic state.[17] A hypervolemic state is associated with potential complications in those with cardiorespiratory comorbidities and thus euvolemia should be targeted. Furthermore, excessive hemodilution may be detrimental to blood's oxygen-carrying capacity. Perhaps a more important strategy is to achieve relative hypertension only, as it may be more beneficial than hemodilution and hypervolemia.[32,33] Hypertension should be aggressively achieved using inotropic infusions, but care should be taken in the setting of an unsecured aneurysm.

In the setting of symptomatic vasospasm with correlating angiographic findings, angioplasty may be employed as early as possible if inducing hypertension and maintaining euvolemia fail to resolve symptoms. The prophylactic use of angioplasty is not indicated.[19] Angioplasty is generally performed on affected proximal arteries only with a carefully sized balloon for the artery of interest. Distal arterial balloon angioplasty (beyond M1 or A1 segments) has traditionally been thought to incur a high risk of rupture given the thinner wall. However, this notion has been challenged.[34] For proximal artery vasospasm, success rates have improved since the technique's inception, with a recent study demonstrating approximately a 97% success rate in relieving radiographic vasospasm with a complication rate of 1%.[35] The rate of clinical improvement appears to be slightly lower. Local intra-arterial infusions of vasodilators, including nicardipine (dihydropyridine calcium channel blocker), verapamil (non-dihydropyridine calcium channel blocker), and milrinone (phosphodiesterase-III inhibitor), have been studied for treating more distal arterial vasospasm with mixed results.[36,37,38,39,40,41] Intravenous milrinone infusions have also been investigated due to the drug's inotropic and vasodilational effects.[42] Although many centers employ intra-arterial infusion of vasodilators, including our own, at this time there is insufficient evidence to recommend the routine use of these therapies.

Several other investigational therapies for symptomatic vasospasm are undergoing animal and human trials, including endothelin-1A receptor antagonists, magnesium, nitric oxide, statins, and others.[2,43] Thus far, no other successful therapeutic strategies have been borne out of these trials.

We rapidly initiated vasopressor therapy upon symptom onset and did not have target blood pressure limitations due to cardiorespiratory comorbidities. Despite achieving a systolic blood pressure of 200 mmHg, our patient did not demonstrate symptom resolution; thus, we brought him to the angiography suite for immediate assessment of the vasculature and treatment of vasospasm with balloon angioplasty and selective intra-arterial verapamil administration.

6.4 Level of Evidence

Cerebral vasospasm prophylaxis: Currently, nimodipine is the only intervention that may minimize the risk of developing symptomatic cerebral vasospasm (does not reduce the risk of developing angiographic vasospasm). Nimodipine should be administered 60 mg every 4 hours, or 30 mg every 2 hours if hypotension occurs (Class I, Level of Evidence A). Euvolemia should be maintained as there is evidence to suggest that not doing so can be detrimental (Class I, Level of Evidence B). Other prophylactic measures, including inducing hypervolemia or angioplasty, should not be performed (Class III, Level of Evidence B).

Monitoring for vasospasm: TCD is a convenient and relatively reliable way to monitor regularly for vasospasm (Class IIa, Level of Evidence B). Perfusion imaging (CT or MRI) can be used in suspected or confirmed vasospasm (Class I, Level of Evidence B).

Treating symptomatic vasospasm: Should symptoms arise in the setting of angiographic vasospasm, initial treatment should be prompt and include inducing hypertension with vasopressors (Class I, Level of Evidence B). Care should be taken with regards to the patient's ability to tolerate relative hypertension (i.e., cardiorespiratory comorbidities) and the status of the aneurysm. An unsecured aneurysm may require more conservative blood pressure goals. If a rapid response to medical management is not achieved, it is recommended to proceed with angioplasty with or without selective intra-arterial vasodilator administration (Class IIa, Level of Evidence B). If the offending artery is fairly distal, it may be technically challenging or relatively risky to perform angioplasty, in which case selective intra-arterial vasodilator administration alone may be considered.

6.5 Landmark Papers

Fisher CM, Kistler JP, Davis JM. Relation of cerebral vasospasm to subarachnoid hemorrhage visualized by computerized tomographic scanning. Neurosurgery 1980;6(1):1–9.

Prior to this publication, clinicians had no reliable way of predicting the onset of cerebral vasospasm after aneurysmal SAH. Fisher and colleagues undertook a retrospective analysis of 47 patients who had a CT scan performed within 5 days of SAH and subsequently developed angiographically confirmed cerebral vasospasm.[11] Four grades of CT results were described, including none to focal thin subarachnoid blood (Grade 1); diffuse, thin blood collection not greater than 1 mm (Grade 2); localized subarachnoid clot or thick layer greater than 1 mm (Grade 3); and any amount of SAH but with either an intraparenchymal hematoma or intraventricular blood (Grade 4). Vasospasm was categorized as either none, slight-to-moderate, or severe based on angiographic arterial measurements. No patient with slight-to-moderate vasospasm developed clinical findings.

The authors found that 2 out of 11 (18.1%) Grade 1 patients developed severe vasospasm, while 23 out of 24 (95.8%) Grade 3 patients did. None of the Grade 1 patients, but all of the Grade 3 patients, with severe vasospasm demonstrated clinical signs and symptoms. No Grade 2 or Grade 4 patients developed severe angiographic vasospasm.

The results of this study were incorporated into clinical practice and prompted investigators to determine whether any prophylactic measures could be performed in these high-risk patients to prevent or minimize the onset and effects of delayed ischemia secondary to cerebral vasospasm. To date, oral nimodipine is the only evidence-based strategy clinically indicated for vasospasm prophylaxis.[15]

Modern imaging modalities have substantially higher resolutions than the modalities used at the time of this manuscript. A modified Fisher grading scale was developed by Frontera et al in 2006.[12] They studied 1,355 patients from a prospectively collected database and redefined 5 groups based on initial CT imaging (▶ Table 6.1). All patients with radiographic evidence of SAH or intraventricular hemorrhage appear to be at the risk of symptomatic vasospasm, with a 40% risk for those with thick SAH and intraventricular blood.

Kassel NF, Peerless SJ, Durwood QJ, et al. Treatment of ischaemic deficits from vasospasm with intravascular volume expansion and induced arterial hypertension. Neurosurgery 1982;11:337–343.

In 1976, Kosnik and Hunt first reported the use of hypertension to reverse new neurological deficits secondary to cerebral vasospasm occurring several days after aneurysmal SAH.[44] Kassell et al then performed a retrospective series analysis investigating the use of both induced hypertension and hypervolemia to treat patients with symptomatic vasospasm, which was the first study to do so.[45]

The study consisted of a single arm of 58 patients who had SAH (56 had confirmed aneurysms) with angiography-confirmed symptomatic cerebral vasospasm. The onset of symptoms occurred prior to securing the aneurysm in some. Symptoms were promptly treated first by hypervolemia through the infusion of blood products and/or colloid, to achieve a target central venous pressure of 10 mmHg and pulmonary artery wedge pressure of 18 to 20 mmHg. Crystalloid infusion was administered to maintain normal electrolyte levels. If hypervolemia was insufficient to reverse neurological deficits, vasopressors were administered, with fludrocortisone as needed. Maximal systolic blood pressure in patients with secured aneurysms was 240 mmHg; 160 mmHg in those with unsecured aneurysms. Once deficits were reversed from hypervolemia and hypertension, the blood pressure was allowed to fall to the minimum required to prevent the return of symptoms.

Reversal of vasospasm-induced deficits occurred within 1 hour in 81% of patients, with therapy being required for anywhere between 12 hours and 8 days. Permanent symptom relief was achieved in 74%. Iatrogenic complications most commonly encountered were aneurysmal rebleeding (19%) and pulmonary edema (17%).

This study was important as it resulted in the development of a medical protocol for treating symptomatic vasospasm. Hemodilution was added to hypervolemia and hypertension later, coining the term "triple-H therapy." As is discussed in Question 6 of the Case Summary section, further studies have suggested that the original triple-H protocol be revised to simply maintain euvolemia and induce relative hypertension with vasopressors to medically treat symptomatic cerebral vasospasm.[17,32,33]

Pickard JK, Murray GD, Illingworth R, et al. Effect of oral nimodipine on cerebral infarction and outcome after subarachnoid haemorrhage: British aneurysm nimodipine trial. BMJ 1989;298:636–642.

While not the first prospective randomized controlled trial studying the prophylactic use of nimodipine for cerebral vasospasm in post-aneurysmal SAH patients, it is the largest.[46] The British group randomized 554 SAH patients (confirmed by either CT or lumbar puncture; no angiographic confirmation of an aneurysm was required) within 96 hours of the onset of symptoms to either nimodipine (60 mg orally every 4 h) or placebo. Treatment continued until posthemorrhage day 21. Nimodipine dosing was changed to 30 mg every 2 hours if hypotension developed. Patients were monitored for deterioration, defined as new focal neurological deficit(s), or a decrease in GCS score by at least one for more than 6 hours. This led to obtaining a CT scan when able to determine the etiology of deterioration. The primary outcome was the rate of cerebral infarction, rebleeding, or poor outcome after at least 3 months based on the Glasgow Outcome Scale.

The trial reported that 22% of the patients taking prophylactic nimodipine developed a cerebral infarction, compared to 33% of the patients in the placebo group ($p = 0.014$), with poor outcomes after 3 months occurring in 20% versus 33%, respectively ($p < 0.001$). Mortality was not statistically different between the two groups.

The authors of this trial based their design on the previous studies, including the first study investigating nimodipine in this setting by Allen et al.[47] Interestingly, compared to the placebo group, the nimodipine group had a larger number of patients presenting with poor prognostic signs, including nuchal rigidity, hypertension, and nonreactive pupils. Despite this, the nimodipine group had improved outcomes, suggesting that the effect size could potentially be falsely small in this study. Regardless, this landmark paper had a significant impact on the management of SAH, prompting centers around the world to adopt the nimodipine protocol. Other similar studies, including a meta-analysis by Barker et al, came to similar conclusions.[15]

6.6 Recommendations

Cerebral vasospasm has long been recognized as a major source of morbidity and mortality with SAH. While commonly associated with aneurysms, it may also be encountered with subarachnoid blood from any nonaneurysmal source, including after trauma. Much research has gone into understanding this devastating disease phenomenon, leading to the development of clinical tools with which to identify patients at increased risk, and to monitor and identify the onset of vasospasm. Despite many interventions being studied, very few have made an impact on patient outcomes, with overall vasospasm outcomes being relatively stagnant over several decades.

Promising advances in understanding the specific pathogenesis of vasospasm have been made. Researchers have begun to characterize the signaling pathways involved, including the differing mechanisms responsible for the onset and maintenance of arterial wall contraction. For example, after the initial arterial smooth muscle contraction occurs in the presence of subarachnoid blood breakdown products, maintenance of contraction is achieved in a calcium-independent fashion through the activity of several contractile proteins, including rho-kinase, protein kinase C, and protein tyrosine kinase. Fasudil is a rho-kinase inhibitor that has been found to significantly decrease the incidence of vasospasm (both angiographic and symptomatic), cerebral infarction, and poor outcome in patients with aneurysmal SAH based on a systematic review and meta-analysis.[48] The studies analyzed include largely small series and the authors comment that several clinical details were unavailable, leaving several potential sources of bias. Thus, more research must be done prior to recommending this agent and other similar ones. Regardless, there may be therapeutic potential in inhibiting new molecular targets in the vasospasm cascade, as our understanding of the pathophysiology progresses.

Until then, the current management paradigm for cerebral vasospasm involves medical optimization and administration of prophylactic nimodipine. Specific strategies include achieving euvolemia and eunatremia with crystalloid infusions, avoiding hypoxia and body temperature alterations, and maintaining cerebral perfusion pressure greater than 70 mmHg with the use of external ventricular drainage as needed. Frequent neurological checks and daily TCD studies should be performed to assess for signs of vasospasm. Particular attention should be paid to patients without a reliable neurological examination, such as comatose patients. Increases in arterial velocities should trigger close monitoring for signs of symptomatic ischemia and may be confirmed with angiography or perfusion imaging as needed.

Should neurological deterioration occur, it is prudent to determine the likely etiology, as vasospasm is but one possible cause. Other entities to rule out include rehemorrhage, seizure, increased intracranial pressure, electrolyte alterations (SIADH or cerebral salt wasting), hypoxia, etc. Once symptomatic vasospasm has been identified as the cause of neurological decline, urgent medical interventions, such as crystalloid and vasopressors, must be implemented to increase blood pressure sufficiently to alleviate symptoms. Potential complications, including pulmonary edema, myocardial ischemia/infarction, or congestive heart failure, should be monitored.

An unsecured aneurysm may be at risk of rehemorrhage with induced hypertension and should be managed cautiously. If neurological decline is not mitigated with medical management, urgent endovascular strategies should be utilized. For focal, proximal intracranial arterial vasospasm, balloon angioplasty may be performed with a carefully selected and sized balloon. An undersized balloon may not achieve the desired results, while an oversized balloon increases the risk of arterial rupture. Similarly, a hypercompliant balloon may not exert sufficient outward radial force at the location of greatest vasospasm, while a less compliant balloon must be inflated cautiously so as not to overdistend the artery. Selective intra-arterial vasodilators may be utilized as well, particularly for diffuse or distal vasospasm. Repeat procedures may be warranted if vasospasm worsens or progressively involves more arteries. Some centers advocate for leaving the endovascular access sheath in situ for the sake of repeated vasodilator infusions and quicker access if required.

Endovascular surgery is a rapidly progressing field with new devices being introduced on a continual basis. Devices are becoming smaller and able to reach further into the arterial tree. This may prove highly beneficial as the treatment of vasospasm may improve with more distal access and safer angioplasty technology. However, perhaps the key to successful outcomes in cerebral vasospasm lies in the development of effective primary preventive strategies, as opposed to reactionary ones.

6.7 Summary

1. Cerebral vasospasm is a complex clinical entity induced by blood in the subarachnoid space that may lead to neurological deterioration and must be differentiated from other causes of DCI.
2. The current management paradigm for cerebral vasospasm has changed over the past few decades and involves maintenance of euvolemia and nimodipine, with induced hypertension upon the development of clinical vasospasm. Endovascular therapies are to be employed upon failure of medical management and involve balloon angioplasty and/or selective intra-arterial vasodilator administration.
3. Many novel therapeutic agents, based on our increasing understanding of vasospasm pathophysiology, have been studied in animal models and in humans, thus far with limited efficacy.

References

[1] Dorsch NW, King MT. A review of cerebral vasospasm in aneurysmal subarachnoid haemorrhage. Part I: Incidence and effects. J Clin Neurosci. 1994; 1 (1):19–26

[2] Findlay JM, Nisar J, Darsaut T. Cerebral vasospasm: a review. Can J Neurol Sci. 2016; 43(1):15–32

[3] Ohta T, Satoh G, Kuroiwa T. The permeability change of major cerebral arteries in experimental vasospasm. Neurosurgery. 1992; 30(3):331–335, discussion 335–336

[4] Foley PL, Takenaka K, Kassell NF, Lee KS. Cytotoxic effects of bloody cerebrospinal fluid on cerebral endothelial cells in culture. J Neurosurg. 1994; 81 (1):87–92

[5] Iuliano BA, Pluta RM, Jung C, Oldfield EH. Endothelial dysfunction in a primate model of cerebral vasospasm. J Neurosurg. 2004; 100(2):287–294

[6] Chow M, Dumont AS, Kassell NF. Endothelin receptor antagonists and cerebral vasospasm: an update. Neurosurgery. 2002; 51(6):1333–1341, discussion 1342

[7] Koide M, Nishizawa S, Ohta S, Yokoyama T, Namba H. Chronological changes of the contractile mechanism in prolonged vasospasm after subarachnoid hemorrhage: from protein kinase C to protein tyrosine kinase. Neurosurgery. 2002; 51(6):1468–1474, discussion 1474–1476

[8] Dumont AS, Dumont RJ, Chow MM, et al. Cerebral vasospasm after subarachnoid hemorrhage: putative role of inflammation. Neurosurgery. 2003; 53 (1):123–133, discussion 133–135

[9] Mack WJ, Ducruet AF, Hickman ZL, et al. Early plasma complement C3a levels correlate with functional outcome after aneurysmal subarachnoid hemorrhage. Neurosurgery. 2007; 61(2):255–260, discussion 260–261

[10] Vergouwen MD, Vermeulen M, van Gijn J, et al. Definition of delayed cerebral ischemia after aneurysmal subarachnoid hemorrhage as an outcome event in clinical trials and observational studies: proposal of a multidisciplinary research group. Stroke. 2010; 41(10):2391–2395

[11] Fisher CM, Kistler JP, Davis JM. Relation of cerebral vasospasm to subarachnoid hemorrhage visualized by computerized tomographic scanning. Neurosurgery. 1980; 6(1):1–9

[12] Frontera JA, Claassen J, Schmidt JM, et al. Prediction of symptomatic vasospasm after subarachnoid hemorrhage: the Modified Fisher Scale. Neurosurgery. 2006; 59(1):21–27, discussion 21–27

[13] de Rooij NK, Rinkel GJ, Dankbaar JW, Frijns CJ. Delayed cerebral ischemia after subarachnoid hemorrhage: a systematic review of clinical, laboratory, and radiological predictors. Stroke. 2013; 44(1):43–54

[14] Amin-Hanjani S, Ogilvy CS, Barker FG, II. Does intracisternal thrombolysis prevent vasospasm after aneurysmal subarachnoid hemorrhage? A meta-analysis. Neurosurgery. 2004; 54(2):326–334, discussion 334–335

6

[15] Barker FG, II, Ogilvy CS. Efficacy of prophylactic nimodipine for delayed ischemic deficit after subarachnoid hemorrhage: a metaanalysis. J Neurosurg. 1996; 84(3):405–414

[16] McGirt MJ, Blessing R, Nimjee SM, et al. Correlation of serum brain natriuretic peptide with hyponatremia and delayed ischemic neurological deficits after subarachnoid hemorrhage. Neurosurgery. 2004; 54(6):1369–1373, discussion 1373–1374

[17] Lennihan L, Mayer SA, Fink ME, et al. Effect of hypervolemic therapy on cerebral blood flow after subarachnoid hemorrhage : a randomized controlled trial. Stroke. 2000; 31(2):383–391

[18] Mori T, Katayama Y, Kawamata T, Hirayama T. Improved efficiency of hypervolemic therapy with inhibition of natriuresis by fludrocortisone in patients with aneurysmal subarachnoid hemorrhage. J Neurosurg. 1999; 91(6):947–952

[19] Zwienenberg-Lee M, Hartman J, Rudisill N, et al. Balloon Prophylaxis for Aneurysmal Vasospasm (BPAV) Study Group. Effect of prophylactic transluminal balloon angioplasty on cerebral vasospasm and outcome in patients with Fisher grade III subarachnoid hemorrhage: results of a phase II multicenter, randomized, clinical trial. Stroke. 2008; 39(6):1759–1765

[20] Macdonald RL, Kassell NF, Mayer S, et al. CONSCIOUS-1 Investigators. Clazosentan to overcome neurological ischemia and infarction occurring after subarachnoid hemorrhage (CONSCIOUS-1): randomized, double-blind, placebo-controlled phase 2 dose-finding trial. Stroke. 2008; 39(11):3015–3021

[21] Wang J, Alotaibi NM, Akbar MA, Ayling OG, Ibrahim GM, Macdonald RL, SAHIT collaborators. Loss of consciousness at onset of aneurysmal subarachnoid hemorrhage is associated with functional outcomes in good-grade patients. World Neurosurg. 2017; 98:308–313

[22] Macdonald RL, Higashida RT, Keller E, et al. Randomized trial of clazosentan in patients with aneurysmal subarachnoid hemorrhage undergoing endovascular coiling. Stroke. 2012; 43(6):1463–1469

[23] Kramer AH, Fletcher JJ. Locally-administered intrathecal thrombolytics following aneurysmal subarachnoid hemorrhage: a systematic review and meta-analysis. Neurocrit Care. 2011; 14(3):489–499

[24] Wong GK, Chan MT, Boet R, Poon WS, Gin T. Intravenous magnesium sulfate after aneurysmal subarachnoid hemorrhage: a prospective randomized pilot study. J Neurosurg Anesthesiol. 2006; 18(2):142–148

[25] Dorhout Mees SM, Algra A, Vandertop WP, et al. MASH-2 Study Group. Magnesium for aneurysmal subarachnoid haemorrhage (MASH-2): a randomised placebo-controlled trial. Lancet. 2012; 380(9836):44–49

[26] Kirkpatrick PJ, Turner CL, Smith C, Hutchinson PJ, Murray GD, Collaborators S, STASH Collaborators. Simvastatin in aneurysmal subarachnoid haemorrhage (STASH): a multicentre randomised phase 3 trial. Lancet Neurol. 2014; 13 (7):666–675

[27] Naqvi J, Yap KH, Ahmad G, Ghosh J. Transcranial Doppler ultrasound: a review of the physical principles and major applications in critical care. Int J Vasc Med. 2013; 2013:629378

[28] Mills JN, Mehta V, Russin J, Amar AP, Rajamohan A, Mack WJ. Advanced imaging modalities in the detection of cerebral vasospasm. Neurol Res Int. 2013; 2013:415960

[29] Spiotta AM, Provencio JJ, Rasmussen PA, Manno E. Brain monitoring after subarachnoid hemorrhage: lessons learned. Neurosurgery. 2011; 69(4):755–766, discussion 766

[30] Claassen J, Hirsch LJ, Kreiter KT, et al. Quantitative continuous EEG for detecting delayed cerebral ischemia in patients with poor-grade subarachnoid hemorrhage. Clin Neurophysiol. 2004; 115(12):2699–2710

[31] Connolly ES, Jr, Rabinstein AA, Carhuapoma JR, et al. American Heart Association Stroke Council, Council on Cardiovascular Radiology and Intervention, Council on Cardiovascular Nursing, Council on Cardiovascular Surgery and Anesthesia, Council on Clinical Cardiology. Guidelines for the management of aneurysmal subarachnoid hemorrhage: a guideline for healthcare professionals from the American Heart Association/American Stroke Association. Stroke. 2012; 43(6):1711–1737

[32] Raabe A, Beck J, Keller M, Vatter H, Zimmermann M, Seifert V. Relative importance of hypertension compared with hypervolemia for increasing cerebral oxygenation in patients with cerebral vasospasm after subarachnoid hemorrhage. J Neurosurg. 2005; 103(6):974–981

[33] Dankbaar JW, Slooter AJ, Rinkel GJ, Schaaf IC. Effect of different components of triple-H therapy on cerebral perfusion in patients with aneurysmal subarachnoid haemorrhage: a systematic review. Crit Care. 2010; 14(1):R23

[34] Santillan A, Knopman J, Zink W, Patsalides A, Gobin YP. Transluminal balloon angioplasty for symptomatic distal vasospasm refractory to medical therapy in patients with aneurysmal subarachnoid hemorrhage. Neurosurgery. 2011; 69(1):95–101, discussion 102

[35] Chalouhi N, Tjoumakaris S, Thakkar V, et al. Endovascular management of cerebral vasospasm following aneurysm rupture: outcomes and predictors in 116 patients. Clin Neurol Neurosurg. 2014; 118:26–31

[36] Feng L, Fitzsimmons BF, Young WL, et al. Intraarterially administered verapamil as adjunct therapy for cerebral vasospasm: safety and 2-year experience. AJNR Am J Neuroradiol. 2002; 23(8):1284–1290

[37] Linfante I, Delgado-Mederos R, Andreone V, Gounis M, Hendricks L, Wakhloo AK. Angiographic and hemodynamic effect of high concentration of intra-arterial nicardipine in cerebral vasospasm. Neurosurgery. 2008; 63(6):1080–1086, discussion 1086–1087

[38] Badjatia N, Topcuoglu MA, Pryor JC, et al. Preliminary experience with intra-arterial nicardipine as a treatment for cerebral vasospasm. AJNR Am J Neuroradiol. 2004; 25(5):819–826

[39] Albanese E, Russo A, Quiroga M, Willis RN, Jr, Mericle RA, Ulm AJ. Ultrahigh-dose intraarterial infusion of verapamil through an indwelling microcatheter for medically refractory severe vasospasm: initial experience. Clinical article. J Neurosurg. 2010; 113(4):913–922

[40] Fraticelli AT, Cholley BP, Losser MR, Saint Maurice JP, Payen D. Milrinone for the treatment of cerebral vasospasm after aneurysmal subarachnoid hemorrhage. Stroke. 2008; 39(3):893–898

[41] Shankar JJ, dos Santos MP, Deus-Silva L, Lum C. Angiographic evaluation of the effect of intra-arterial milrinone therapy in patients with vasospasm from aneurysmal subarachnoid hemorrhage. Neuroradiology. 2011; 53(2):123–128

[42] Lannes M, Teitelbaum J, del Pilar Cortés M, Cardoso M, Angle M. Milrinone and homeostasis to treat cerebral vasospasm associated with subarachnoid hemorrhage: the Montreal Neurological Hospital protocol. Neurocrit Care. 2012; 16(3):354–362

[43] Tallarico RT, Pizzi MA, Freeman WD. Investigational drugs for vasospasm after subarachnoid hemorrhage. Expert Opin Investig Drugs. 2018; 27 (4):313–324

[44] Kosnik EJ, Hunt WE. Postoperative hypertension in the management of patients with intracranial arterial aneurysms. J Neurosurg. 1976; 45(2):148–154

[45] Kassell NF, Peerless SJ, Durward QJ, Beck DW, Drake CG, Adams HP. Treatment of ischemic deficits from vasospasm with intravascular volume expansion and induced arterial hypertension. Neurosurgery. 1982; 11(3):337–343

[46] Pickard JD, Murray GD, Illingworth R, et al. Effect of oral nimodipine on cerebral infarction and outcome after subarachnoid haemorrhage: British aneurysm nimodipine trial. BMJ. 1989; 298(6674):636–642

[47] Allen GS, Ahn HS, Preziosi TJ, et al. Cerebral arterial spasm: a controlled trial of nimodipine in patients with subarachnoid hemorrhage. N Engl J Med. 1983; 308(11):619–624

[48] Liu GJ, Wang ZJ, Wang YF, et al. Systematic assessment and meta-analysis of the efficacy and safety of fasudil in the treatment of cerebral vasospasm in patients with subarachnoid hemorrhage. Eur J Clin Pharmacol. 2012; 68 (2):131–139

7 Nonaneurysmal Subarachnoid Hemorrhage

Sauson Soldozy, Kaan Yağmurlu, Pedro Norat, Michael F. Stiefel, Min S. Park, and M. Yashar S. Kalani

Abstract

In 1985, van Gijn et al[1] were the first to report the existence of a variant of subarachnoid hemorrhage (SAH) characterized by negative angiography and focal bleeding in the prepontine cistern, referred to as nonaneurysmal perimesencephalic subarachnoid hemorrhage (PMSAH). Early prospective series revealed that patients with PMSAH had superior clinical outcomes when compared with aneurysmal or classic bleeding patterns on computed tomography (CT) that were also angiographically unremarkable, including reduced rebleeding and neurologic deficits.[2,3] These findings prompted the need for developing a diagnostic paradigm for angiographically occult patients with SAH, especially in those patients with classic SAH patterns on CT with no evidence of aneurysm rupture.

Keywords: subarachnoid hemorrhage, angiographically negative hemorrhage, perimesencephalic hemorrhage, nonaneurysmal hemorrhage, catheter-based angiography

7.1 Goals

1. Evaluate the natural history of patients with nonaneurysmal subarachnoid hemorrhages (SAHs).
2. Explore the basis for the evaluation and management of patients with nonaneurysmal SAHs.
3. Understand the results of repeated testing for nonaneurysmal SAHs.

7.2 Case Example

7.2.1 History of Present Illness

A 65-year-old female with a history of coronary artery disease status postbypass graft, hypertension, hyperlipidemia, and diabetes mellitus presented to the emergency department with sudden onset 10/10 bitemporal and occipital headache with altered mental status, confusion, nausea, vomiting, photophobia, and weakness. Her blood pressure was 229/89 on admission, and she was started on a nicardipine drip and intravenous labetalol. She was well oriented and responsive but appeared distressed. Noncontrast computed tomography (CT) head demonstrated spontaneous SAH of unknown origin, and the patient was transferred to the Neurological Interventional Care Unit.

Past medical history: Angina pectoris; coronary artery disease status post bypass graft; diabetes mellitus; high cholesterol; hypertension; migraine headache.

Past surgical history: Cardiac catheterization (×2); cardiac ablation of ventricular tachycardia and premature ventricular contraction; coronary artery bypass graft; vascular surgery.

Allergies: Phenergan; Levaquin (rash); Penicillins (rash); Percocet (anxiety).

Medications: Acetaminophen; ascorbic acid, calcium carbonate-vitamin D; clobetasol; desoximetasone; fexofenadine; fish oil; furosemide; detemir; lispro; levothyroxine; lisinopril; multivita-min; nitroglycerin; nystatin-hydrocortisone-zinc oxide; rosuvastatin; tramadol.

Family history: Mother—diabetes; father—stroke age 62, lung cancer age 72; brother—myocardial infarction age 60, history of drug abuse; brother—myocardial infarction age unknown, history of drug abuse.

Social history: Married; works as a bookkeeper; former smoker 20 pack-years, quit date January 1, 1970; rare alcohol consumption.

Physical examination: Pulse 89, temperature 36.2 °C, respiratory rate 12, SpO_2 98%, blood pressure 229/89.

Glasgow Coma Scale (GCS) of 15, Hunt and Hess grade 1. Cranial nerves were intact, no pronator drift, 5/5 strength, and sensation intact to light touch in all extremities.

Imaging studies: See ▶ Fig. 7.1.

7.2.2 Treatment Plan

Given the continued need for monitoring and the appearance of early hydrocephalus on the CT scan, a right frontal ventriculostomy catheter was placed, and the patient was transferred to the

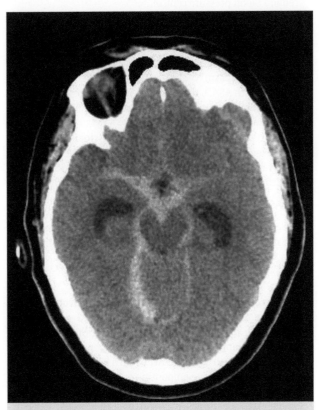

Fig. 7.1 CT head demonstrating subarachnoid hemorrhage with the greatest burden in the prepontine cisterns (Fisher grade 4). There is also a moderate burden of subarachnoid hemorrhage in the suprasellar cistern and also along the right tentorial leaflet extending to the posterior fossa. Small intraventricular hemorrhage layering in the posterior occipital horns is also present. There are enlarged temporal horns demonstrating early hydrocephalus.

Neurosurgical Intensive Care Unit. A six-vessel diagnostic cerebral angiogram the following morning was negative for any source of the diffuse SAH.

7.2.3 Hospital Course

The patient was admitted to the Neurointensive Care Unit. The patient received serial transcranial Doppler studies and repeat angiography was performed 1 week later, which did not show clear pathology explaining the SAH. The external ventricular drain (EVD) was discontinued during the course of her hospitalization, and the patient was discharged to an acute rehabilitation facility. A follow-up computed tomography angiography (CTA) head performed after 6 weeks was negative for any significant vascular pathology.

7.3 Case Summary

1. *What is the time course for the treatment of nonaneurysmal SAH?*

   Care for nonaneurysmal SAH (NASAH) is generally the same as aneurysmal SAH (ASAH), in that both are treated as an acute emergency. Neurologic decompensation occurs in up to 35% of patients within 24 hours of symptom onset.[4] In addition, patients presenting in a hypertensive state often require blood pressure control.

   The amount of subarachnoid blood present, neurologic status on admission, and volume and blood pressure status are predictors of delayed cerebral ischemia (DCI).[5] Nimodipine is administered to minimize the complications secondary to cerebral vasospasm. While it is the standard of care for patients with ASAH, there are no formal studies showing benefit of nimodipine in perimesencephalic subarachnoid hemorrhage (PMSAH) or NASAH.

   Some studies suggest that the reduced incidence of vasospasm in this cohort argues against nimodipine use.[6] Triple H therapy is another method used to address vasospasm. Triple H therapy represents induced hypertension, hypervolemia, and hemodilution therapy. Cardiac complications, such as transient left ventricular dysfunction (TLVD) in SAH, are also contributing factors to DCI.[7] While vasospasm is the most critical side effect of SAH to address, hyponatremia, deep venous thrombosis (DVT), hyperglycemia, anemia, and fever are other medical complications that may arise.

2. *How do different hemorrhage patterns impact treatment and patient outcomes?*

   The specific bleeding pattern is useful in guiding clinical decision making and predicting overall prognosis in patients who present with SAH. PMSAH pattern is characterized by blood restricted to the prepontine or interpeduncular cistern with limited extension into the Sylvian fissure.[8] PMSAH are angiographically negative with an unclear etiology. Other bleeding patterns include convex, intraventricular, or interhemispheric, although less is known with respect to clinical course and outcomes in this cohort of patients without a defined source of the hemorrhage.[9]

   Patients with NASAH should continue to have their symptomatic needs met as they would in the setting of an ASAH.

Once an aneurysmal source is definitively ruled out with repeat angiography, minor treatment modifications can be implemented. For instance, some studies suggest the discontinuation of nimodipine in angiographically negative SAH given both the reduced incidence and clinical significance of vasospasm in this population.[10,11] The timeline for the reinstatement of anticoagulation in patients following a nonaneurysmal SAH continues to remain unclear. It is well known that patients previously on antiplatelet or anticoagulant therapy who present with SAH often fare worse than patients not on these medications.[12] Considering the reduced rebleed rate in NASAH when compared to ASAH, the argument for resuming anticoagulation earlier in these patients has been proposed. However, continuing anticoagulation therapy within the first few days of hemorrhage incurs rebleeding in patients with NASAH similar to those with ASAH.[13] Therefore, both hemorrhage patterns should be treated the same in this respect. Generally, nonaneurysmal SAHs are regarded as "benign" variants of spontaneous SAH with a better prognosis, lower risk of vasospasm, and reduced hospital stay.[6,14]

7.4 Level of Evidence

Nimodipine administration: The patient received nimodipine throughout her hospitalization despite the absence of a ruptured cerebral aneurysm. While there is Class I, Level of Evidence B support for the use of nimodipine for aneurysmal SAH, its utility in nonaneurysmal SAH is not as well established (Class IIB, Level of Evidence C).

Utility of follow-up imaging: The patient received follow-up imaging both during and approximately 6 weeks following her initial hospitalization (Class IIB, Level of Evidence C).

7.5 Landmark Papers

Elhadi AM, Zabramski JM, Almefty KK, et al: Spontaneous subarachnoid hemorrhage of unknown origin: hospital course and long-term clinical and angiographic follow-up. J Neurosurg 2015;122:663–670.

Little AS, Garrett M, Germain R, et al: Evaluation of patients with spontaneous subarachnoid hemorrhage and negative angiography. Neurosurgery 2007;61:1139–1150.

Of the 472 patients enrolled in the Barrow Ruptured Aneurysm Trial (BRAT),[15] 100 patients were initially identified with an unknown etiology of hemorrhage.[16] In those patients with no evidence of aneurysm rupture, angiography was repeated 1 week later in addition to magnetic resonance imaging (MRI) and magnetic resonance angiography (MRA) of the brain and cervical spine. Patients underwent outpatient follow-up vascular imaging, including CTA, MRA, or catheter-based angiography at 4 to 6 weeks posthemorrhage if no identifiable lesion was detected during hospitalization. Other elements of the diagnostic protocol consisted of laboratory investigations and medical history.[16]

Little et al[16] stratified these patients into four groups: (1) CT negative with xanthochromia on lumbar puncture; (2) aneurysmal (classical) hemorrhage pattern; (3) perimesencephalic hemorrhage characterized by prepontine cistern bleeding with no evidence of basal, interhemispheric, or Sylvian cistern hemorrhage as defined by published criteria[2,17]; and (4) convexity hemorrhage. Of the 44 patients found to have a classic hemorrhage pattern on CT, 7 patients (16%) were found to have a cause of SAH requiring either endovascular or surgical intervention.

For other bleeding patterns, the yield of further diagnostic work-up was shown to be low. In patients with CT negative SAH, there were no reports of positive repeat angiography. For patients with perimesencephalic bleeding patterns, repeat angiography showed a recanalized anterior inferior cerebellar artery (AICA) aneurysm in one case.[16] Of the 25 patients with convexity SAH, vasculitis was identified as a cause of bleed in one patient on repeat imaging, with laboratory studies, relevant history, and pharmacological considerations aiding in determining bleeding etiology in another two patients. Overall, further imaging and work-up revealed 17 patients (out of 100) with an identifiable cause of hemorrhage.

In 2014, Elhadi et al[18] evaluated 57 of the 83 remaining patients from the BRAT who had no underlying pathology on angiography despite repeat imaging and diagnostic work-up. The goal of this study was to provide insight on and explore the utility of long-term angiographic and clinical follow-up at 6 months, 1 year, and 3 years. Patients were stratified similarly to those in the previous study,[16] with the exception of convexity hemorrhage, which was not assessed in this series. In addition, patients were graded based on a modified Fisher scale, with the presence of intraventricular hemorrhage (IVH) being reported separately.[18] Thirty-two (57%) patients had classic SAH pattern, 13 (23%) with PMSAH, and 11 (20%) with CT negative SAH. Sixteen (29%) patients were observed to have IVH.

Among the 57 patients, one 67-year-old woman with a Fisher grade 2 hemorrhage was found to have a 2- to 3-mm basilar trunk aneurysm on CTA at 6 weeks posthemorrhage follow-up. The remaining patients had no source of hemorrhage identified during any of the follow-ups. Four (7%) patients with classic SAH experienced DCI. Of these patients, one was found to have a left PCA ischemic stroke due to vasospasm. This was not identified in the other groups. Sixteen (29%) patients required EVD placement for treatment of hydrocephalus, with four of these patients requiring placement of a ventriculoperitoneal (VP) shunt. Patients with classic SAH and those with an IVH were significantly more likely to require an EVD ($p = 0.0028$; $p < 0.0001$, respectively).

Long-term outcomes were available in 45 of 56 patients. At discharge, 29 of the 45 patients had a GOS of 5, and 34 patients had a GOS of 5 at 6-months follow-up. The number of patients remained unchanged at 1- and 3-year follow-up, suggesting that follow-up after 6 months in angiographically occult SAH patients has little clinical utility, regardless of initial hemorrhage pattern. Limitations of this study include the small number of patients, the retrospective nature of the data analysis, and the loss of 10 patients to follow-up.

Geng B, Wu X, Brackett A, Malhotra A. Meta-analysis of recent literature on utility of follow-up imaging in isolated perimesencephalic hemorrhage. Clin Neurol Neurosurg 2019;180:111–116.

Kalra VB, Wu X, Matouk CC, Malhotra A. Use of follow-up imaging in isolated perimesencephalic subarachnoid hemorrhage. Stroke 2015;46:401–406.

A meta-analysis by Karla et al[19] was performed in 2015 that evaluated studies published between 2008 and 2014.

It assessed a total of 1,031 patients with follow-up imaging, including CTA, MRA, and digital subtraction angiography (DSA) over 40 studies. All studies included were retrospective analyses. Inclusion criteria were patients with perimesencephalic SAH on initial noncontrast CT undergoing CTA, DSA within 24 hours of admission, and additional follow-up angiographic imaging. History of trauma, diffuse SAH, thick blood above the perimesencephalic cistern, and IVH were all exclusion criteria. Studies lacking follow-up, less than five patients with PMSAH, and those with CT negative SAH were also excluded.

Of the 1,031 patients included in this meta-analysis, a total of 8 aneurysms in 8 patients were discovered on follow-up imaging in a total of 6 studies. An aneurysm detection rate of 0.90% (95% CI, 0.18–1.62%) was reported for initial DSA, with a detection rate of 1.64% (95% CI, 0–3.89%) for initial DSA and CTA combined. Initial CTA alone did not detect any aneurysms. In addition, follow-up CTA and combined follow-up DSA and CTA also failed to identify aneurysms. A two-way ANOVA test found no significant difference for the three initial diagnostic modalities ($p = 0.353$) or three follow-up strategies ($p = 0.701$).

Another meta-analysis performed by the same group provided a more recent perspective with respect to follow-up imaging and PMSAH by evaluating retrospective studies published between the years 2014 and 2017.[20] A total of 13 studies with 588 patients were included. Inclusion criteria were the same as their previous study.[19] Of the 588 patients, an aneurysm was found in 3 patients, with an aneurysm detection rate of 0.10% (95% CI, 0–0.81%). Similar to the previous meta-analysis, the authors concluded that patients with PMSAH might not require repeat imaging.

7.6 Recommendations

1. ICU admission.
2. Placement of EVD as needed.
3. CT angiography head and neck.
4. MRI brain and cervical spine with and without contrast.
5. Formal cerebral angiography.
6. Repeat angiography at 7 days.
7. Close ICU observation.

7.7 Summary

Based on the current evidence available, the clinical approach to patients presenting with PMSAH, when compared to ASAH, differs mostly concerning diagnostic studies and imaging. Medically, the approach to symptomatic management and stabilization is similar. While a consensus on the utility of follow-up imaging has yet to be reached, it is imperative to consider all factors when deciding upon the appropriate management strategy for this subset of SAH patients.

References

[1] van Gijn J, van Dongen KJ, Vermeulen M, Hijdra A. Perimesencephalic hemorrhage: a nonaneurysmal and benign form of subarachnoid hemorrhage. Neurology. 1985; 35(4):493–497

[2] Rinkel GJ, Wijdicks EF, Hasan D, et al. Outcome in patients with subarachnoid haemorrhage and negative angiography according to pattern of haemorrhage on computed tomography. Lancet. 1991; 338(8773):964–968

7

[3] Rinkel GJ, Wijdicks EF, Vermeulen M, Hageman LM, Tans JT, van Gijn J. Outcome in perimesencephalic (nonaneurysmal) subarachnoid hemorrhage: a follow-up study in 37 patients. Neurology. 1990; 40(7):1130–1132

[4] Long B, Koyfman A, Runyon MS. Subarachnoid hemorrhage: updates in diagnosis and management. Emerg Med Clin North Am. 2017; 35(4):803–824

[5] van Gijn J, Kerr RS, Rinkel GJ. Subarachnoid haemorrhage. Lancet. 2007; 369 (9558):306–318

[6] Mensing LA, Vergouwen MDI, Laban KG, et al. Perimesencephalic hemorrhage: a review of epidemiology, risk factors, presumed cause, clinical course, and outcome. Stroke. 2018; 49(6):1363–1370

[7] Temes RE, Tessitore E, Schmidt JM, et al. Left ventricular dysfunction and cerebral infarction from vasospasm after subarachnoid hemorrhage. Neurocrit Care. 2010; 13(3):359–365

[8] Nesvick CL, Oushy S, Rinaldo L, Wijdicks EF, Lanzino G, Rabinstein AA. Clinical complications and outcomes of angiographically negative subarachnoid hemorrhage. Neurology. 2019; 92(20):e2385–e2394

[9] Akcakaya MO, Aydoseli A, Aras Y, et al. Clinical course of nontraumatic nonaneurysmal subarachnoid hemorrhage: a single institution experience over 10 years and review of the contemporary literature. Turk Neurosurg. 2017; 27(5):732–742

[10] Prat D, Goren O, Bruk B, Bakon M, Hadani M, Harnof S. Description of the vasospasm phenomena following perimesencephalic nonaneurysmal subarachnoid hemorrhage. BioMed Res Int. 2013; 2013:371063

[11] Wijdicks EF, Schievink WI, Miller GM. Pretruncal nonaneurysmal subarachnoid hemorrhage. Mayo Clin Proc. 1998; 73(8):745–752

[12] Rinkel GJE, Prins NEM, Algra A. Outcome of aneurysmal subarachnoid hemorrhage in patients on anticoagulant treatment. Stroke. 1997; 28(1):6–9

[13] van der Worp HB, Fonville S, Ramos LMP, Rinkel GJE. Recurrent perimesencephalic subarachnoid hemorrhage during antithrombotic therapy. Neurocrit Care. 2009; 10(2):209–212

[14] Tsermoulas G, Flett L, Gregson B, Mitchell P. Immediate coma and poor outcome in subarachnoid haemorrhage are independently associated with an aneurysmal origin. Clin Neurol Neurosurg. 2013; 115(8):1362–1365

[15] McDougall CG, Spetzler RF, Zabramski JM, et al. The Barrow Ruptured Aneurysm Trial. J Neurosurg. 2012; 116(1):135–144

[16] Little AS, Garrett M, Germain R, et al. Evaluation of patients with spontaneous subarachnoid hemorrhage and negative angiography. Neurosurgery. 2007; 61(6):1139–1150, discussion 1150–1151

[17] Ruigrok YM, Rinkel GJE, Van Gijn J. CT patterns and long-term outcome in patients with an aneurysmal type of subarachnoid hemorrhage and repeatedly negative angiograms. Cerebrovasc Dis. 2002; 14(3–4):221–227

[18] Elhadi AM, Zabramski JM, Almefty KK, et al. Spontaneous subarachnoid hemorrhage of unknown origin: hospital course and long-term clinical and angiographic follow-up. J Neurosurg. 2015; 122(3):663–670

[19] Kalra VB, Wu X, Matouk CC, Malhotra A. Use of follow-up imaging in isolated perimesencephalic subarachnoid hemorrhage: a meta-analysis. Stroke. 2015; 46(2):401–406

[20] Geng B, Wu X, Brackett A, Malhotra A. Meta-analysis of recent literature on utility of follow-up imaging in isolated perimesencephalic hemorrhage. Clin Neurol Neurosurg. 2019; 180:111–116

7

8 Unruptured Cerebral Arteriovenous Malformations

Marie-Christine Brunet, Evan Luther, David J. McCarthy, and Robert M. Starke

Abstract

The management of unruptured cerebral arteriovenous malformations (AVMs) is a difficult topic that remains controversial. The decision to manage these lesions conservatively or intervene depends largely on patient's age, presentation, lesion size, and location. Even with ideal circumstances for intervention, some argue for conservative management. There remains insufficient knowledge regarding the lifetime hemorrhage risk of AVMs, and studies supporting conservative therapy over intervention often provide only early results. To manage these patients appropriately, it is imperative to understand the implications and limitations of these studies, AVM hemorrhage risk factors, and risks and benefits of various treatment options.

Keywords: arteriovenous malformations, embolization, radiosurgery, risk management

8.1 Goals

1. Analyze the literature regarding the natural history of arteriovenous malformations (AVMs).
2. Assess studies that investigate treatment of unruptured AVMs versus observation.
3. Briefly review AVM treatment options, risks, and success rates.

8.2 Case Example

8.2.1 History of Present Illness

A 41-year-old previously healthy female presents for initial evaluation complaining of progressively worsening right-sided headaches, right orbital pain, and "visual difficulties."

Past medical history: Denies any prior relevant history.

Past surgical history: None.

Family history: Denies history of any vascular disease.

Social history: Nonsmoker, drinks socially.

Review of systems: As per the above.

Neurological examination: With detailed examination, she was found to have a left-homonymous hemianopsia.

Imaging studies: See figures.

▶ Fig. 8.1 (a,b) Brain cerebral angiogram demonstrated a Spetzler–Martin grade IV right temporo-occipital AVM with a maximum diameter of 40.1 mm, primarily fed by the middle cerebral artery with an associated 8.0 × 6.9 mm perinidal aneurysm and both superficial and deep venous drainage.

8.2.2 Treatment Plan

The patient agreed to treatment of the symptomatic AVM. The recommendation was made for neoadjuvant embolization of the deep feeder to ease the surgical removal of the AVM. Postoperative angiogram seen in ▶ Fig. 8.2a, b demonstrates no residual AVM.

8

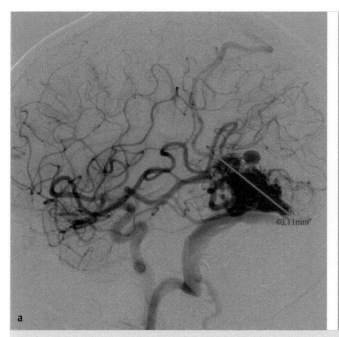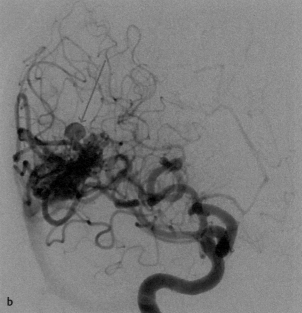

Fig. 8.1 Brain angiogram **(a,b)** showing a Spetzler–Martin grade IV right arteriovenous malformation (AVM) with a maximum diameter of 40.1 mm, primarily fed by the middle cerebral artery, with an associated 8.0 × 6.9 mm perinidal aneurysm (*arrow* in **b**).

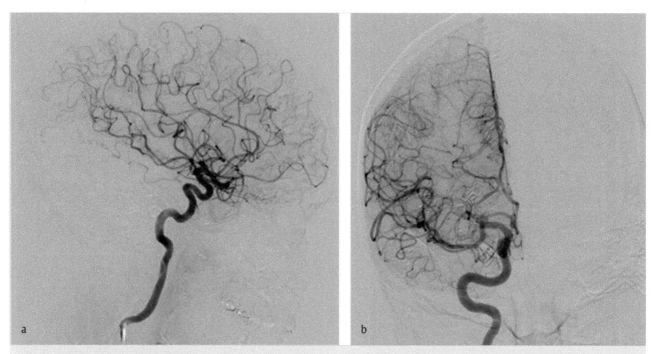

Fig. 8.2 (a,b) Six-month follow-up angiogram of the brain demonstrating complete arteriovenous malformation (AVM) obliteration.

8.2.3 Follow-up

The patient did very well after the embolization and microsurgical resection. As expected she had initial worsening of her homonymous hemianopsia. At her 6-month follow-up visit, angiogram demonstrated complete AVM obliteration (▸ Fig. 8.2b) as well as subjective and objective improvement of her homonymous hemianopsia. Only a trace homonymous hemianopsia residual was noted on physical examination, which was not perceptible to patient. She returned to work fully functional.

8.3 Case Summary

1. *What would you consider the rupture risk of the unruptured AVM in this patient?*

    Our knowledge, with regard to the natural risk of AVM rupture, is limited to prospective and retrospective cohorts. Later in this chapter, we will review the largest of these studies and the strengths and limitations of each one. The most recent meta-analyses report the annual rupture risk for unruptured brain AVMs to be 1.3 to 2.2%, but the overall literature supports an annual risk of 1 to 4%.[1,2]

2. *What patient factors would you consider when deciding on your recommendations for observation or treatment of these unruptured cerebral AVMs?*

    a) Age

       Since it is believed that the annual risk of hemorrhage for AVMs remains constant, younger patients have a higher lifetime risk of hemorrhage; therefore, there is more precedent for treatment. Conversely, younger patients may have to live longer with deficits incurred due to complications of an intervention. It is imperative to weigh the risks of treatment versus conservative management as we will discuss later.

       In elderly patients with low-risk lesions, it may be better to intervene as opposed to observation since increasing age has been identified as a possible risk factor for rupture in some meta-analysis. Other studies failed to reach the same conclusion, and this may be due to lead time, selection, and follow-up bias.[1,3,4,5,6]

    b) Patient symptoms

       Other than hemorrhage, brain AVMs may present with a variety of complaints and neurological alterations. Often unruptured AVMs can cause focal or secondary seizures, with a reported 5-year risk of seizure estimated around 8%.[7,8] Younger age, temporal location, cortical involvement, and nidus diameter > 3 cm increase the risk of seizure.[3,8] It is not certain that intervention reduces seizure risk; however, a meta-analysis reported that microsurgery had the highest seizure reduction rate (78.3%), followed by stereotactic radiosurgery (SRS) (62.8%), and embolization (49.3%).[9]

       Unruptured AVMs may present with headaches and other variable symptoms, such as focal weakness or visual alterations. There is no evidence showing that AVM intervention reduces headaches.[10] However, in our case example, the patient had almost complete resolution of symptoms.

3. *What AVM factors would you consider when deciding on your recommendations for observation or treatment?*

    a) Prior hemorrhage

       While our patient never suffered a hemorrhage, the largest risk factor for future hemorrhage of an AVM is a prior hemorrhage.[3]

    b) AVM location

       It has been shown that deep and infratentorial AVM locations are independent risk factors for hemorrhage.[1,2,3,4,5,6]

c) Various angioarchitecture characteristics
There are several AVM angioarchitectural characteristics that increase its risk of hemorrhage. In short, venous outflow limited to deep venous structures, associated arterial aneurysms (pre- or intranidal), single draining veins, venous varices, and venous stenosis are all considered independent risk factors.[2,3,6,11,12,13,14] Our patient had a large perinidal aneurysm, increasing her risk for future hemorrhage.

4. *How would you follow this AVM with or without treatment?*
There are several methods for following treated AVMs with imaging studies: digital subtraction angiography, computed tomography angiography, or magnetic resonance angiography. Depending on the method of treatment, intensive imaging follow-up may be necessary. It has been reported that magnetic resonance angiography follow-up offers similar accuracy in lesions greater than 1 cm.[15] All patients should have an angiogram at some point to ensure complete obliteration. In this instance, we elected to follow up with digital subtraction angiography.

8.4 Level of Evidence

Patient's age, symptoms, and AVM grade: Given the Spetzler–Martin grade IV AVM, surgical treatment poses significant risks; however, since the patient was young, had neurological deficit, and a perinidal aneurysm, we elected to proceed with intervention (Class IIb, Level of Evidence B).

Risk of future hemorrhage: The patient was young and had a large perinidal aneurysm (Class IIa, Level of Evidence A).

Treatment: Due to the large size of the lesion, we decided against SRS treatment (Class I, Level of Evidence B). We decided to perform preoperative embolization to decrease the morbidity and mortality associated with the surgery resection (Class IIa, Level of Evidence B).

Follow-up of aneurysm: We followed this lesion with digital subtraction angiography (Class I, Level of Evidence B).

8.5 Hemorrhage Risk in Unruptured AVMs

8.5.1 Natural History

The natural history of unruptured brain AVMs remains a controversial topic. Our current understanding is based on studies analyzing the clinical course of untreated patients; however, there has yet to be a prospective clinical study that aims to describe rupture risk in a population that is without selection bias.[3] Based on the available data, it is generally accepted that the annual risk of rupture in untreated unruptured AVMs is between 1 and 4%.[3,4,6,16,17,18]

In 1990, Ondra et al published a retrospective series on the natural history of 166 patients with known brain AVMs who did not undergo surgical treatment. The follow-up rate was very high (96%), and the patients were monitored for a mean of 24 years. This cohort demonstrated a 4% annual rupture risk and 1% annual mortality rate. However, these results were based on composite outcomes that included previously ruptured brain AVMs, leaving the true rate of hemorrhage for unruptured AVMs unknown.[18]

More recently, Halim et al performed a prospective analysis of 790 patients with brain AVMs diagnosed between 1961 and 2001. Beginning with the date of initial AVM diagnosis (including AVMs presenting with hemorrhage), patients were followed until subsequent rupture, initiation of treatment, or last available follow-up appointment.[4] The dropout rate was similar to Ondra's study, but follow-up time was significantly less. In the patient cohort who did not present with rupture, the annual rupture risk was found to range from 0.3 to 4% and decreased over time. In 2006, Stapf et al published a similar prospective study on 622 patients with brain AVMs. Again, the patients were followed from initial diagnosis until onset of treatment.[6] With a mean follow-up time of 2.3 years, the annual rupture risk was 1.3%, similar to that of Halim's cohort. The short follow-up times are limitations to both studies, but they did provide some further insight into the natural history of unruptured AVMs. In 2008, Hernesniemi et al published another prospective study that followed 238 patients with brain AVMs for a mean follow-up period of 13.5 years. During this period, they found that the average rupture risk of unruptured AVMs was 1.6%.[5] These studies all indicated that the annual rupture risk for well-selected unruptured AVMs might in fact be lower than previously described. More recently, several meta-analyses have reported an annual rupture risk of 1.3 to 2.2% for unruptured AVMs.[1,2] All of these studies suffer from selection bias and suggest that rupture risk is dependent on a number of identifiable clinical and morphological features.

8.5.2 Predictors of Hemorrhage

The most important and consistently demonstrated clinical characteristic that has been found to increase the risk of hemorrhage in AVMs is rupture at initial presentation.[3] Increasing age has also been identified as a possible risk factor for rupture in some meta-analyses, but this has not been confirmed in other studies.[1,3,4,5,6] Anatomic features that have been identified in meta-analyses and observational cohorts as independent risk factors for hemorrhage are deep and infratentorial locations.[1,2,3,4,5,6] Several studies have also been performed to analyze the various angioarchitectural characteristics that contribute to hemorrhage in unruptured AVMs. These included venous outflow limited to deep venous structures, associated arterial aneurysms (pre- or intranidal), single draining veins, venous varices, and venous stenosis.[2,3,6,11,12,13,14] AVM size has also been identified as a possible predictor, but results have been inconsistent.

8.6 Management: Conservative versus Intervention

In 2010, Ross and Al-Shahi Salman conducted a systematic review to identify randomized clinical studies comparing outcomes following different unruptured AVM management.[7] No completed study met their inclusion criteria; however, they identified the ARUBA study[17] as the only ongoing study investigating this important question.

8

Mohr JP, Parides MK, Stapf C, et al. Medical management with or without interventional therapy for unruptured brain arteriovenous malformations (ARUBA): a multicentre, non-blinded, randomised trial. The Lancet 2014;383:614–621.

From 2007 to 2013, Mohr et al screened 1,740 patients for trial eligibility, ultimately randomizing 226 patients to either intervention (*n* = 116) or medical management (*n* = 110). Patients were assessed for eligibility if they were older than 18 years, had neurovascular image confirmed AVM, and no prior hemorrhage or treatment attempt. Interventions included radiosurgery, microsurgery, endovascular intervention, or any combination of these procedures. Primary outcome was time until any-cause death or symptomatic stroke, defined as any new neurological focal deficit, headache, or seizure with associated image findings (blood or low-density ischemic lesions). Secondary outcome was functional dependency at 5 years, defined as modified Rankin scale of 2 or higher.[19]

Originally designed to enroll 800 patients, sample size was reduced to 400 patients following slow patient accrual in the first 18 months. The ARUBA trial was prematurely halted when conservative management reached a predetermined efficacy, for the prevention of stroke or death, in an interim analysis. A total of 223 patients were randomized, with a mean follow-up of 33.3 months (IQR 16.3–49.8 months). The final statistical analysis was conducted with 53% of the anticipated data (of the 400-patient sample size). Under both intention-to-treat and as-treated analyses, investigators found that conservative management had a significantly lower risk for primary outcome event than intervention. In addition, the risk of death or neurological disability was significantly lower in the conservatively managed cohort. Further analysis demonstrated that primary event occurrence remained similar regardless of Spetzler–Martin (S-M) grade in the medically managed arm; however, it occurred more frequently in patients with an S-M grade II or III in the intervention arm.

The ARUBA study reached the controversial conclusion that the risk of death or stroke in patients with unruptured AVMs was higher for patients undergoing intervention versus conservatively managed for 33 months of follow-up. In 2017, Magro et al conducted a systematic review of all the published critiques and comments involving ARUBA and identified 31 published critiques.[20] While the ARUBA trial addressed a paramount question, the trial design and possible biases limited the external validity of the study. Regarding study design, the academic community has critiqued the study's end points, selection criteria, and absent treatment arm standardization.

Many stated that the end points were "soft" and favored conservative management.[20] The primary end point of the trial labeled a stroke as any postoperative new or worsening neurological focal deficit, headache, or seizure with associated imaging findings (blood or low-density ischemic lesions). Practitioners argue that a headache or an initial worsening of symptoms with contrast leakage often transiently occurs following an endovascular intervention. This argument was supported by an unusually high primary outcome incidence of 30.7% in the intervention arm, most of which occurred during the first 6 months following intervention. Furthermore, the AVM obliteration rate was not reported—a relevant statistic considering that partial AVM embolization does not necessarily reduce hemorrhage risk.[3]

Authors did not specify if endovascular embolization was performed with cyanoacrylate-based liquid embolic agents or Onyx, each of which have different success rates.[3]

The ARUBA trial was also subjected to selection bias. During its enrollment period, investigators screened 1,740 patients, of which only 226 were ultimately enrolled. The remaining patients were split as followed: 1,014 were not eligible due to prior hemorrhage, 323 refused participation, and 177 patients had the clinician select treatment outside randomization. Most high-volume centers (treating more than 50 patients per year) enrolled one to two patients per year. It is imperative to appreciate these numbers when interpreting the results. For 177 patients to have been selected for treatment outside of randomization, it implies that for each of those patients the clinician felt uncomfortable to randomize the patient to conservative treatment. This calls into question ARUBA's equipoise and leads to the next commonly discussed pitfall of ARUBA, lack of standardization of the intervention arm.

In the intervention arm, 66 patients received single treatment therapy; 30 had embolization, 31 radiosurgeries, and 5 microsurgeries. The remainder of the intervention arm received embolization prior to radiosurgery (*n* = 15), surgery (*n* = 12), and both surgery and radiosurgery (*n* = 1). Critics often point out that surgical therapy is underrepresented.[3,20] The reported rates of surgical risk with Spetzler–Martin grades I-II are around 0.7% and incur high obliteration success.[21] In most circumstances, experts feel that for grade I-II lesions in well-selected patients intervention is warranted and there is no equipoise regarding treatment. While we are uncertain of what treatment options were taken with the aforementioned 177 patients who were excluded from the study, due to the low surgical representation in ARUBA it is possible that these patients fell into this low surgical risk category, implying that the treating physicians felt ethically obliged to exclude them from randomization. Bervini et al's analysis of their prospectively maintained cohort of 377 unruptured AVMs supports this presumption.[22] They found that the 5-year rupture risk was 11.5% for an unruptured AVM, whereas only 1.6% of the Spetzler–Ponce class A AVMs treated by surgery had a risk for a permanent neurological deficit leading to an mRS score > 1. Their results showed that surgical treatment is favorable in these low-graded AVMs.

One might argue that many of the complications following AVM intervention impose a "front-loaded" risk, or occur shortly following the surgery, whereas AVM hemorrhage risk is believed to be a compounding risk, or similar year-after-year risk or hemorrhage. This leads to another main pitfall of the ARUBA study, short follow-up time. Literature regarding unruptured AVM management with a mean follow-up of 33 months leaves room for misinterpretation of the main results. Even with the original planned follow-up for 15 to 20 years, the study may be underpowered as a pretrial analysis with 400 patients demonstrated that 10 to 20 years would be necessary before the intervention curve would cross the nonintervention curve. The ARUBA investigators plan on following the patients for five additional years to address this concern; however, a longer follow-up may be necessary to answer the question.

Some additional critiques of the ARUBA trial include the slow study enrollment and the premature interruption of enrollment.[20] However, these two critiques are somewhat unavoidable. Trial investigators designed a prior safety threshold to halt the trial and patient accrual was slower than anticipated; thus, the study was repowered accordingly.

Regardless of the outcome and critiques, ARUBA investigators conducted an ethically difficult trial that challenged the standard of care, ultimately opening discussion to a crucial question that requires further elucidation. Often practitioners consider RCTs to be the highest level of evidence. However, in circumstances where ethics and equipoise make conducting RCTs technically challenging, observational studies may be conducted. While ARUBA has been the only RCT to date investigating conservative versus interventional management for AVMs, important observational studies have been conducted.

Al-Shahi Salman R, White PM, Counsell CE, et al. Outcome after conservative management or intervention for unruptured brain arteriovenous malformations. JAMA 2014;311:1661–1669.

One of the more influential observational studies, regarding AVM treatment, was published a few months after ARUBA by the Scottish Audit of Intravascular Malformations (SIVMS). Al-Shahi et al conducted a prospective observational study of 204 Scotland residents who were diagnosed with unruptured AVM between the years 1999–2003 and 2006–2010.[23] Patients were included if they were 16 years or older with a radiographically confirmed unruptured AVM and no distant cerebral aneurysms. Interventions were any combination of embolization (glue or coil), radiosurgery, and microsurgery. Decision to pursue intervention or conservative treatment was left up to the patients and their treating physicians. Patients were followed from the time of diagnosis (conservative treatment) or from the time of treatment for the patients who underwent intervention. The primary outcome was first occurrence of handicap, defined as Oxford Handicap Scale 2–5, that was sustained for at least 2 years or any-cause death. Secondary outcome was death, due to intervention or AVM, or nonfatal symptomatic stroke.

During the study period, 101 patients with AVMs were managed conservatively and 103 patients underwent intervention. Due to the observational nature of the study, patients who received intervention were younger, more likely to present with seizure, more likely to have angiogram, and less likely to have maximum AVM diameter greater than 6 cm. Sixty-eight patients underwent single treatment: 28 radiosurgeries, 22 endovascular embolizations, and 18 microsurgeries. Thirty-five patients underwent multimodality treatment: 20 embolization and radiosurgery, 12 embolization and microsurgery, 2 radiosurgery and embolization, and 1 had all the 3 treatments. Overall AVM obliteration rate was 66%.

Median follow-up was 6.8 years (IQR 4–11 y), accounting for a total of 1,479 person-years. For the first 4 years, the risk of primary outcome was greater in the intervention group than the conservatively managed group (HR 0.59, 95% CI 0.35–0.99). However, in the subsequent time periods, 4 to 8 and 8 to 12 years, no significant difference in primary outcome was observed. The overall 12-year death rate was higher in the conservatively managed group (31 vs. 10 deaths); however, this was attributable to deaths from other causes and statistical significance disappeared after adjusting for age. Due to a large incidence of symptomatic stroke following intervention, the risk for progression to secondary outcome was significantly lower in the conservatively managed patients over the entirety of the study (HR 0.37, 95% CI 0.19–0.72).

The SIVMS investigation was an observational study that ultimately had comparable results to those of the ARUBA trial. While the SIVMS study circumvented many of the critiques that ARUBA received, it was not without limitations. Due to the observational nature of the study, patients treated with interventions were naturally younger, more likely to present with seizure, and had smaller AVM nidal diameter. Furthermore, since the intervention cohort was younger, more patients suffered non-AVM death in the conservatively managed arm, rendering the primary outcome difficult to interpret beyond the first 4 years of the study. Like ARUBA, critics argue that further follow-up of the SIVMS cohort is warranted to assess if the reduced risk associated with conservative management persists.

More than ever, the ARUBA and SIVMS studies call upon our code of "first do no harm." While both studies have significant limitations and flaws, they investigate an important topic that still required further elucidation. One must use their clinical judgment and critical understanding of the published literature, in addition to specific patient and AVM characteristics when deciding to intervene or conservatively manage unruptured AVMs. As such, many centers have further refined their patient selection criteria especially for high-risk patients leading to decreased morbidity and mortality.

8.7 Recommendations and Treatment Modalities

When considering treatment of cerebral AVMs, three main treatment modalities are available and are often complementary: microsurgical resection, endovascular embolization, and SRS. Cerebral AVMs treatment goal should be complete obliteration of the nidus and elimination of the arteriovenous shunt. Partial nidus obliteration should be avoided as it does not appear to reduce hemorrhagic risk.[24] In rare complex cases, palliative treatment can be considered to improve neurological symptoms related to hemodynamic changes or to target high-risk features of the malformation.[25,26]

8.7.1 Microsurgical Resection

Microsurgical resection via craniotomy is a widely used approach to cure brain AVMs. Microsurgical resection of AVM nidus can be performed primarily or after adjuvant endovascular embolization or stereotaxic radiosurgery. The following surgical steps are executed in specific order: (1) craniotomy and exposure of the malformation, (2) subarachnoid dissection and elimination of feeding arteries, (3) circumferential dissection of the nidus in the cerebral parenchyma, (4) transection of venous drainage and removal of the lesion, and (5) hemostasis and closure of the wound.

Therapeutic decision-making is a complex process requiring analysis of multiple factors including age of the patient, natural history of hemorrhage from AVM and suggested hemorrhage risk factors, patient expectations, and treatment risk associated with surgical removal of the malformation. The ability to estimate the treatment risk for an individual patient with a brain AVM is extremely challenging due to the heterogeneous complexity of AVMs. As a result, numerous grading systems have been developed. The most widely utilized system used to

Table 8.1 Spetzler-Martin AVM grading classification

Spetzler–Martin grading	Points	Supplementary grading
Size (cm)		Age (y)
<3	1	<20
3–6	2	20–40
>6	3	>40
Venous drainage		Bleeding
No	0	Yes
Yes	1	No
Eloquence		Compactness
No	0	Yes
Yes	1	No
Total	5	

perform a relative surgical risk analysis was reported by Spetzler and Martin in 1986 (▶ Table 8.1). Their grading system is based on three criteria: AVM size (small [< 3 cm], medium [3–6 cm], or large [> 6 cm]), pattern of venous drainage (superficial or deep), and neurological eloquence of adjacent brain regions (sensorimotor, language, and visual cortex; hypothalamus and thalamus; internal capsule; brain stem; cerebellar peduncles, and deep cerebellar nuclei are considered eloquent).[27] The prospective evaluation of the Spetzler–Martin grading system reported by Hamilton and Spetzler[28] identified permanent postsurgical major neurological deficits for grades I-III were 0%, increasing to 21.9 and 16.7% in patients with grade IV and V lesions, respectively. Based on those results, grade I and II lesions are generally considered safe and favorable for surgical resection, whereas grade IV and V lesions are frequently accompanied with significant morbidity and are considered unfavorable surgical candidates. Grade III lesions are in a gray zone, representing a group of very heterogeneous lesions, each possessing varied surgical risk. As suggested by Lawton, grade III–AVMs (S1V1E1) have a surgical risk like that of low-grade AVMs and can be safely treated with microsurgical resection. Grade III + AVMs (S2V0E1) have a surgical risk like that of high-grade AVMs and are best managed conservatively. Grade III AVMs (S2V1E0) have intermediate surgical risks and require judicious selection for surgery.[29]

A supplementary grading system was developed recently by Lawton et al to improve selection of patients with cerebral AVMs for surgery considering three new factors: patient's age, hemorrhagic presentation, and compactness of the lesion.[30] Hemorrhagic presentation not only indicates AVMs with high risk of rehemorrhage but also facilitates surgery.[31] Hematomas help separate AVMs from adjacent brain; evacuation of hematoma creates working space around the AVM that can minimize transgression of normal brain or access a deep nidus that might otherwise have been unreachable. AVM hemorrhage and microsurgery can injure brain tissue; however, youth and plasticity can enhance a patient's ability to recover neurological function. Compact AVMs with tightly woven arteries and veins often have distinct borders that separate cleanly from the adjacent brain, whereas diffuse AVMs with ragged borders and intermixed brain force the neurosurgeon to establish dissection planes that can extend into normal brain.

Reported outcomes of angiographic cure rates following surgical resection of brain AVMs are very high, 95 to 99%.[32,33] Complications include new seizures in 6 to 15% of the patients with supratentorial AVMs, new neurologic deficits, and intraparenchymal hemorrhage in the postoperative period. Intraparenchymal hemorrhage in the immediate postoperative period may be a consequence of incomplete hemostasis, residual AVM nidus, or normal perfusion pressure breakthrough (NPPB). While NPPB theory remains controversial, it refers to hemodynamic changes that are induced once an AVM is removed, which lead to postoperative hemorrhage because of long-term diminished perfusion of adjacent brain created by a steal phenomenon.

8.7.2 Endovascular Management

Therapeutic embolization of a brain AVM was first described in 1960 by Luessenhop and Spence utilizing flow-directed steel spheres covered with methyl methacrylate injected directly into a surgically accessed cervical internal carotid artery.[34] This technique relied on the proportionately greater degree of blood flow to the AVM compared with normal cerebral branches to direct the embolic agents into the AVM nidus. Accidental embolization of normal cerebral vessels resulting in cerebral infarction was a potential problem. In 1976, Kerber described the use of a microcatheter with a calibrated-leak balloon to selectively catheterize the cerebral vasculature.[35] The novel device overcame previous problems of nontarget embolization; in addition, Kerber used a liquid embolic agent, isobutyl-2-cyanoacrylate. Over the past several decades, the development of smaller microcatheters, microguidewires, and novel embolic materials has led to technical achievements in AVM embolization and solidified its role as a valuable tool in the treatment of brain AVMs. Currently, endovascular embolization is used as adjuvant therapy before definitive microsurgery or radiosurgery, as palliative therapy for inoperable AVMs, and as primarily curative therapy.

Definitive cure of brain AVMs by endovascular embolization is found to be desirable in a minority of cases; the angioarchitecture of the AVM must permit solid casting of the AVM nidus with permanent embolic material such that the draining vein is occluded only after the nidus is completely occluded. Failure to completely occlude the nidus before casting the draining vein can lead to disastrous bleeding complications. In published series, success rates of curative embolization range from 5 to 20%, and complete obliteration was achieved in 13% of the cases in a recent meta-analysis.[33] Despite the low cure rate in the majority of these published series, Valavanis and Yaşargil demonstrated greater success, with cure rates of 40% in their large series of 387 patients.[36] AVM characteristics that favor endovascular curative treatment include: a nidus that is accessible with the tip of the catheter, three or fewer arterial feeders, and a nidus of 3 cm or less.[37] These characteristics are also common to S-M grade I and IIb AVMs, which can be treated safely with surgery. Other concerns with curative embolization include the durability of the embolic materials used and the length of follow-up required to ascertain a definitive cure. There are several case reports of AVM recurrence after initially complete angiographic obliteration.[38]

Preoperative embolization is the most widely used application of endovascular therapy for AVM treatment. The goal of preoperative embolization is to facilitate surgical removal of the

AVM by decreasing operative time, blood loss, and morbidity and mortality associated with the surgery.[3,39] Pasqualin et al demonstrated that patients treated with embolization prior to surgery experienced fewer postoperative neurological deficits, fewer deaths, and had a lower incidence of postoperative epilepsy when compared with patients who had surgery alone.[40] Embolization strategies include occlusion of deep-feeding arteries not easily accessible during surgery and stepwise occlusion and penetration of the AVM nidus over multiple sessions. Weber et al[41] and Natarajan et al[42] demonstrated the efficacy of preoperative embolization when they reported that it reduced the mean nidus volume 84 and 74%, respectively. The timing of preoperative embolization in relation to surgery is uncertain, with no high-level evidence supporting either the immediate presurgical or delayed surgical approach.

Embolization therapy before radiosurgery has two major goals: reducing overall AVM size to a volume suitable for SRS and treating high-flow fistulas and associated aneurysms less likely to respond to SRS.[43] In 1996, Gobin et al published their experience with pre-SRS embolization with n-butyl cyanoacrylate (nBCA), reporting that it decreased AVM nidal size sufficiently for SRS in 76% of lesions.[44] Despite the obvious benefits of size reduction, there is some concern that embolization may result in lower rates of obliteration during the latency period.[45,46] This may be the result of inaccurate targeting of the lesion secondary to the radiopaque embolic material artifact. Although embolization has more commonly been performed prior to radiosurgery, embolization following radiosurgery remains an option that may be useful. The primary goal of post-SRS embolization is obliteration of residual AVM when radiosurgery fails to achieve cure.

Targeted embolization of an AVM consists of obliteration of high-risk features of an AVM in which complete cure is not considered possible. These high-risk features may include high-flow fistulas or intranidal and flow-related aneurysms. Palliative embolization relies on the idea that high-flow AVMs may become symptomatic by stealing blood flow from normal brain. When these particular AVMs are considered incurable, partial palliative embolization may lessen the flow demand of the AVM, with subsequent amelioration of their symptoms.[43]

Since the use of methyl methacrylate embolospheres, Gelfoam, and pieces of muscle a few decades ago, substantial advances in the embolic materials utilized for AVMs' embolization have been made. Cyanoacrylate polymers are low-viscosity liquid agents that immediately polymerize on contact with free hydrogen ions in blood (the delivery catheter needs to be rinsed with dextrose to prevent premature initiation of the polymerization). While several cyanoacrylates have been used for the treatment of brain AVMs, nBCA has widely become the cyanoacrylate of choice in most centers. In the late 1980s, ethyl alcohol-dimethyl sulfoxide (Onyx-DMSO) was first used for the embolization of cerebral AVMs. Unlike nBCA, which is adhesive, Onyx is a cohesive liquid agent that polymerizes as the solvent, dimethyl sulfoxide, dissipates. Its cohesive nature decreases its risk of adherence to the microcatheter. This confers the ability to start and stop the injection when reflux occurs or if the Onyx is coursing in an undesirable fashion. Despite the predominance of those liquid embolics, other options are available including detachable coils and polyvinyl alcohol.[43]

The two most common complications of embolization are intracerebral hemorrhage and ischemic stroke. The causes of ischemic stroke include thromboembolic complications of catheterization and nontarget embolization. Brain hemorrhage may occur from vessel perforation caused by devices, catheter adhesion, AVM rupture, draining vein occlusion, or intranidal aneurysm rupture.[47] Typically, neurological deficits occur in 10 to 14% of the patients, disabling deficits in 2 to 5% and death in approximately 1%.[37,48]

8.7.3 Stereotactic Radiosurgery

SRS is typically performed to achieve obliteration of bAVMs that are deemed too risky for resection because of anatomic factors or unfavorable patient baseline health status. SRS leads to endothelial cell proliferation, progressive concentric vessel wall thickening, and eventually luminal closure. Radiosurgery is typically recommended for AVMs that are small (< 2–3 cm diameter), unruptured, and surgically inaccessible.[47] Many series with long-term follow-up demonstrate obliteration of 70 to 80% of AVMs after SRS,[49,50] although a recent meta-analysis showed only 38% of AVM cure with SRS.[33] Unlike microsurgery or embolization, the beneficial and adverse effects of SRS may not be apparent for several years following treatment. Furthermore, there is a risk of hemorrhage during the latency period, before AVM obliteration and after SRS.[51] During this latency period, the risk of hemorrhage is ≈1 to 3% per year and does not appear to be appreciably altered from the natural history of bAVMs.[52] Other factors, including prior embolization, history of hemorrhage, and patient's age, have also been demonstrated to affect the outcome of SRS for AVMs, and thus, these factors frequently affect the decision-making process concerning AVM management with SRS. Kano et al demonstrated that pre-SRS embolization was associated with a lower rate of total obliteration ($p = 0.028$) in comparison to radiosurgery alone.[53]

Radiosurgery can also be performed prior to surgical removal as adjunctive therapy. As demonstrated by Sanchez-Mejia et al, radiosurgery prior to surgery reduced mean AVM volumes by 78% and the use of preoperative embolization by 56%. Radiosurgery also facilitates AVM surgical resection with reduction in the length of the surgery and blood loss.[54]

Potential adverse effects following radiosurgery include radiation-induced necrosis, edema, and cyst formation. Symptomatic changes attributable to adverse radiation effects occur in ≈10% of patients, but this risk varies by bAVM location, target volume, and margin dose (dose to surrounding normal tissue). Corticosteroids and, less frequently, bevacizumab have been used to ameliorate symptomatic adverse radiation effects.[55,56] Permanent neurological changes from adverse radiation effects are seen in 2 to 3% of patients. When additional treatment may be advised, repeated SRS might be an option if it is performed ≥ 3 years after the initial treatment.[57,58]

8.8 Summary

1. The understanding of the natural history of unruptured AVMs relies largely on meta-analyses of retrospective and prospective cohorts, all of which have inherent limitations.

2. Multiple factors related to the patient and AVM must be taken into consideration when evaluating a patient with an unruptured AVM.

3. The high-level evidence supporting conservative management over intervention has serious caveats and should not be generalized to every unruptured AVM.

4. There are many modalities for the treatment of unruptured AVMs, each of which has certain indications and associated complications.

5. When evaluating a patient with an unruptured AVM, you must use your clinical judgment to synthesize evidence regarding natural AVM history, patient and AVM risk factors, available treatments, and their respective risks in order to decide whether to treat, and if so how to treat, a patient's unruptured AVM.

References

[1] Kim H, Al-Shahi Salman R, McCulloch CE, Stapf C, Young WL, MARS Coinvestigators. Untreated brain arteriovenous malformation: patient-level meta-analysis of hemorrhage predictors. Neurology. 2014; 83(7):590–597

[2] Gross BA, Du R. Natural history of cerebral arteriovenous malformations: a meta-analysis. J Neurosurg. 2013; 118(2):437–443

[3] Derdeyn CP, Zipfel GJ, Albuquerque FC, et al. American Heart Association Stroke Council. Management of brain arteriovenous malformations: a scientific statement for healthcare professionals from the American Heart Association/American Stroke Association. Stroke. 2017; 48(8):e200–e224

[4] Halim AX, Johnston SC, Singh V, et al. Longitudinal risk of intracranial hemorrhage in patients with arteriovenous malformation of the brain within a defined population. Stroke. 2004; 35(7):1697–1702

[5] Hernesniemi JA, Dashti R, Juvela S, Väärt K, Niemelä M, Laakso A. Natural history of brain arteriovenous malformations: a long-term follow-up study of risk of hemorrhage in 238 patients. Neurosurgery. 2008; 63(5):823–829, discussion 829–831

[6] Stapf C, Mast H, Sciacca RR, et al. Predictors of hemorrhage in patients with untreated brain arteriovenous malformation. Neurology. 2006; 66(9):1350–1355

[7] Ross J, Al-Shahi Salman R. Interventions for treating brain arteriovenous malformations in adults. Cochrane Database Syst Rev. 2010(7):CD003436

[8] Josephson CB, Leach JP, Duncan R, Roberts RC, Counsell CE, Al-Shahi Salman R. Scottish Audit of Intracranial Vascular Malformations (SAIVMs) steering committee and collaborators. Seizure risk from cavernous or arteriovenous malformations: prospective population-based study. Neurology. 2011; 76 (18):1548–1554

[9] Baranoski JF, Grant RA, Hirsch LJ, et al. Seizure control for intracranial arteriovenous malformations is directly related to treatment modality: a meta-analysis. J Neurointerv Surg. 2013:010945

[10] Steiger H-J, Etminan N, Hänggi D. Epilepsy and headache after resection of cerebral arteriovenous malformations: trends in neurovascular interventions. Springer; 2014:113–115

[11] Pollock BE, Flickinger JC, Lunsford LD, Bissonette DJ, Kondziolka D. Factors that predict the bleeding risk of cerebral arteriovenous malformations. Stroke. 1996; 27(1):1–6

[12] Lv X, Wu Z, Jiang C, et al. Angioarchitectural characteristics of brain arteriovenous malformations with and without hemorrhage. World Neurosurg. 2011; 76(1–2):95–99

[13] Sahlein DH, Mora P, Becske T, et al. Features predictive of brain arteriovenous malformation hemorrhage: extrapolation to a physiologic model. Stroke. 2014; 45(7):1964–1970

[14] Alexander MD, Cooke DL, Nelson J, et al. Association between venous angioarchitectural features of sporadic brain arteriovenous malformations and intracranial hemorrhage. AJNR Am J Neuroradiol. 2015; 36(5):949–952

[15] O'Connor TE, Friedman WA. Magnetic resonance imaging assessment of cerebral arteriovenous malformation obliteration after stereotactic radiosurgery. Neurosurgery. 2013; 73(5):761–766

[16] Wong J, Slomovic A, Ibrahim G, Radovanovic I, Tymianski M. Microsurgery for ARUBA Trial (A Randomized Trial of Unruptured Brain Arteriovenous Malformation)–eligible unruptured brain arteriovenous malformations. Stroke. 2017; 48(1):136–144

[17] Mohr JP, Parides MK, Stapf C, et al. International ARUBA Investigators. Medical management with or without interventional therapy for unruptured brain arteriovenous malformations (ARUBA): a multicentre, non-blinded, randomised trial. Lancet. 2014; 383(9917):614–621

[18] Ondra SL, Troupp H, George ED, Schwab K. The natural history of symptomatic arteriovenous malformations of the brain: a 24-year follow-up assessment. J Neurosurg. 1990; 73(3):387–391

[19] van Swieten JC, Koudstaal PJ, Visser MC, Schouten HJ, van Gijn J. Interobserver agreement for the assessment of handicap in stroke patients. Stroke. 1988; 19(5):604–607

[20] Magro E, Gentric JC, Darsaut TE, et al. Responses to ARUBA: a systematic review and critical analysis for the design of future arteriovenous malformation trials. J Neurosurg. 2017; 126(2):486–494

[21] Davidson AS, Morgan MK. How safe is arteriovenous malformation surgery? A prospective, observational study of surgery as first-line treatment for brain arteriovenous malformations. Neurosurgery. 2010; 66(3):498–504, discussion 504–505

[22] Bervini D, Morgan MK, Ritson EA, Heller G. Surgery for unruptured arteriovenous malformations of the brain is better than conservative management for selected cases: a prospective cohort study. J Neurosurg. 2014; 121(4):878–890

[23] Al-Shahi Salman R, White PM, Counsell CE, et al. Scottish Audit of Intracranial Vascular Malformations Collaborators. Outcome after conservative management or intervention for unruptured brain arteriovenous malformations. JAMA. 2014; 311(16):1661–1669

[24] Lv X, Wu Z, Li Y, Yang X, Jiang C. Hemorrhage risk after partial endovascular NBCA and ONYX embolization for brain arteriovenous malformation. Neurol Res. 2012; 34(6):552–556

[25] Krings T, Hans FJ, Geibprasert S, Terbrugge K. Partial "targeted" embolisation of brain arteriovenous malformations. Eur Radiol. 2010; 20(11):2723–2731

[26] Kusske JA, Kelly WA. Embolization and reduction of the "steal" syndrome in cerebral arteriovenous malformations. J Neurosurg. 1974; 40(3):313–321

[27] Bruno CA, Jr, Meyers PM. Endovascular management of arteriovenous malformations of the brain. Intervent Neurol. 2013; 1(3–4):109–123

[28] Hamilton MG, Spetzler RF. The prospective application of a grading system for arteriovenous malformations. Neurosurgery. 1994; 34(1):2–6, discussion 6–7

[29] Lawton MT, UCSF Brain Arteriovenous Malformation Study Project. Spetzler-Martin Grade III arteriovenous malformations: surgical results and a modification of the grading scale. Neurosurgery. 2003; 52(4):740–748, discussion 748–749

[30] Lawton MT, Kim H, McCulloch CE, Mikhak B, Young WL. A supplementary grading scale for selecting patients with brain arteriovenous malformations for surgery. Neurosurgery. 2010; 66(4):702–713, discussion 713

[31] Lawton MT, Du R, Tran MN, et al. Effect of presenting hemorrhage on outcome after microsurgical resection of brain arteriovenous malformations. Neurosurgery. 2005; 56(3):485–493, discussion 485–493

[32] Spetzler RF, Ponce FA. A 3-tier classification of cerebral arteriovenous malformations. Clinical article. J Neurosurg. 2011; 114(3):842–849

[33] van Beijnum J, van der Worp HB, Buis DR, et al. Treatment of brain arteriovenous malformations: a systematic review and meta-analysis. JAMA. 2011; 306(18):2011–2019

[34] Luessenhop AJ, Spence WT. Artificial embolization of cerebral arteries. Report of use in a case of arteriovenous malformation. JAMA. 1960; 172:1153–1155

[35] Kerber C. Balloon catheter with a calibrated leak. A new system for superselective angiography and occlusive catheter therapy. Radiology. 1976; 120 (3):547–550

[36] Valavanis A, Yaşargil MG. The endovascular treatment of brain arteriovenous malformations. Adv Tech Stand Neurosurg. 1998; 24:131–214

[37] Starke RM, Komotar RJ, Connolly ES. 71 – Surgical decision making, techniques, and periprocedural care of cerebral arteriovenous malformations. In: Mohr JP, Wolf PA, Grotta JC, Moskowitz MA, Mayberg MR, von Kummer R, eds. Stroke (Fifth Edition). Saint Louis: W.B. Saunders; 2011:1358–1365

[38] Bauer AM, Bain MD, Rasmussen PA. Onyx resorbtion with AVM recanalization after complete AVM obliteration. Interv Neuroradiol. 2015; 21(3):351–356

[39] Starke RM, Komotar RJ, Otten ML, et al. Adjuvant embolization with N-butyl cyanoacrylate in the treatment of cerebral arteriovenous malformations: outcomes, complications, and predictors of neurologic deficits. Stroke. 2009; 40 (8):2783–2790

8

[40] Pasqualin A, Scienza R, Cioffi F, et al. Treatment of cerebral arteriovenous malformations with a combination of preoperative embolization and surgery. Neurosurgery. 1991; 29(3):358–368

[41] Weber W, Kis B, Siekmann R, Jans P, Laumer R, Kühne D. Preoperative embolization of intracranial arteriovenous malformations with Onyx. Neurosurgery. 2007; 61(2):244–252, discussion 252–254

[42] Natarajan SK, Ghodke B, Britz GW, Born DE, Sekhar LN. Multimodality treatment of brain arteriovenous malformations with microsurgery after embolization with onyx: single-center experience and technical nuances. Neurosurgery. 2008; 62(6):1213–1225, discussion 1225–1226

[43] Crowley RW, Ducruet AF, McDougall CG, Albuquerque FC. Endovascular advances for brain arteriovenous malformations. Neurosurgery. 2014; 74 Suppl 1:S74–S82

[44] Gobin YP, Laurent A, Merienne L, et al. Treatment of brain arteriovenous malformations by embolization and radiosurgery. J Neurosurg. 1996; 85(1):19–28

[45] Schwyzer L, Yen CP, Evans A, Zavoian S, Steiner L. Long-term results of gamma knife surgery for partially embolized arteriovenous malformations. Neurosurgery. 2012; 71(6):1139–1147, discussion 1147–1148

[46] Lee CC, Chen CJ, Ball B, et al. Stereotactic radiosurgery for arteriovenous malformations after Onyx embolization: a case-control study. J Neurosurg. 2015; 123(1):126–135

[47] Starke RM, Yen CP, Ding D, Sheehan JP. A practical grading scale for predicting outcome after radiosurgery for arteriovenous malformations: analysis of 1012 treated patients. J Neurosurg. 2013; 119(4):981–987

[48] Baharvahdat H, Blanc R, Termechi R, et al. Hemorrhagic complications after endovascular treatment of cerebral arteriovenous malformations. AJNR Am J Neuroradiol. 2014; 35(5):978–983

[49] Pollock BE. Stereotactic radiosurgery for arteriovenous malformations. Neurosurg Clin N Am. 1999; 10(2):281–290

[50] Starke RM, Kano H, Ding D, et al. Stereotactic radiosurgery for cerebral arteriovenous malformations: evaluation of long-term outcomes in a multicenter cohort. J Neurosurg. 2017; 126(1):36–44

[51] Bollet MA, Anxionnat R, Buchheit I, et al. Efficacy and morbidity of arctherapy radiosurgery for cerebral arteriovenous malformations: a comparison with the natural history. Int J Radiat Oncol Biol Phys. 2004; 58(5): 1353–1363

[52] Yen CP, Sheehan JP, Schwyzer L, Schlesinger D. Hemorrhage risk of cerebral arteriovenous malformations before and during the latency period after GAMMA knife radiosurgery. Stroke. 2011; 42(6):1691–1696

[53] Kano H, Kondziolka D, Flickinger JC, et al. Stereotactic radiosurgery for arteriovenous malformations after embolization: a case-control study. J Neurosurg. 2012; 117(2):265–275

[54] Sanchez-Mejia RO, McDermott MW, Tan J, Kim H, Young WL, Lawton MT. Radiosurgery facilitates resection of brain arteriovenous malformations and reduces surgical morbidity. Neurosurgery. 2009; 64(2):231–238, discussion 238–240

[55] Deibert CP, Ahluwalia MS, Sheehan JP, et al. Bevacizumab for refractory adverse radiation effects after stereotactic radiosurgery. J Neurooncol. 2013; 115(2):217–223

[56] Williams BJ, Park DM, Sheehan JP. Bevacizumab used for the treatment of severe, refractory perilesional edema due to an arteriovenous malformation treated with stereotactic radiosurgery. J Neurosurg. 2012; 116(5):972–977

[57] Yen CP, Jain S, Haq IU, et al. Repeat γ knife surgery for incompletely obliterated cerebral arteriovenous malformations. Neurosurgery. 2010; 67(1):55–64, discussion 64

[58] Kano H, Kondziolka D, Flickinger JC, et al. Stereotactic radiosurgery for arteriovenous malformations, Part 3: outcome predictors and risks after repeat radiosurgery. J Neurosurg. 2012; 116(1):21–32

8

9 Carotid-Cavernous Fistulas

Joel M. Stary, John F. Reavey-Cantwell, and Dennis J. Rivet II

Abstract

Carotid-cavernous fistulas (CCFs) are rare, potentially life-threatening, conditions that often threaten vision. Their presentation and classification is central to the diagnosis and treatment of these lesions. As understanding of the pathology and natural history of CCFs progressed, new avenues of intervention developed and evolved. A number of neurointerventional techniques have been developed to safely and effectively treat these complex lesions.

Keywords: carotid-cavernous fistula, direct, indirect, dural, neurointerventional, endovascular, flow diversion, coil embolization, liquid embolics

9.1 Goals

1. Review clinical presentation of carotid-cavernous fistulas (CCFs) and discuss factors impacting diagnosis.
2. Review indications for treatment.
3. Review classification schemes and their role in determining treatment modality.
4. Critically analyze current and future treatment options.

9.2 Case Example

9.2.1 History of Present Illness

A 53-year-old Caucasian female presented to the neuro-ophthalmology clinic for evaluation of retro-orbital pain, diplopia, and periorbital swelling following the sudden onset of left-sided headache 6 months prior. She complained of transient tingling in the left V2 distribution along with tinnitus. The symptoms were all exacerbated by strenuous exercise. She denied a history of trauma, seizures, or recent illnesses/infections. A computed tomography angiography (CTA) of the head revealed asymmetric enhancement of the cavernous sinus and a dilated left superior ophthalmic vein. She was referred to neurosurgery for evaluation.

Past medical history: Depression.

Past surgical history: None.

Family history: No known family history of vascular disorders or lesions.

Social history: 15 pack-year history. Weekly social use of alcohol and caffeine. No recreational drug use.

Review of systems: Positive for ringing in the left ear, transient diplopia, left eye swelling, and facial tingling.

Examination: Physical examination noted swollen and injected conjunctiva OS without proptosis. Her neurologic and physical examinations were otherwise normal and included a funduscopic examination and complete evaluation of extraocular muscles. Prior testing by neuro-ophthalmology also revealed no visual deficits and mildly asymmetric, but not elevated, intraocular pressure.

Imaging: The CTA demonstrated asymmetric avid enhancement of the left cavernous sinus (▶ Fig. 9.1a). In addition, a dilated superior ophthalmic vein was identified (▶ Fig. 9.1b) connecting with the angular vein (▶ Fig. 9.1c).

9.2.2 Treatment Plan

Due to the concerns for a CCF, arrangements were made for a digital subtraction angiogram (DSA). A six-vessel DSA was performed, and it demonstrated fistulous filling of the left cavernous sinus during (▶ Fig. 9.2a) selective left external carotid artery (ECA) injection, (▶ Fig. 9.2b) selective right internal carotid artery (ICA) injection, and (▶ Fig. 9.2c) selective left ICA injection. Venous outflow was via the superior ophthalmic vein to the angular and facial veins without evidence of retrograde cortical venous drainage.

Based upon the imaging findings, the recommendation was made for transvenous embolization of the fistula. The CCF was treated with transvenous coil embolization via the inferior

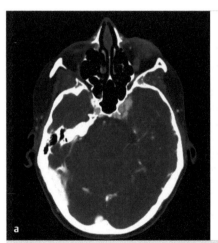 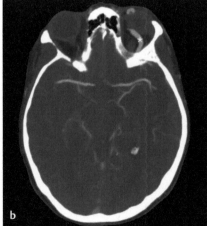 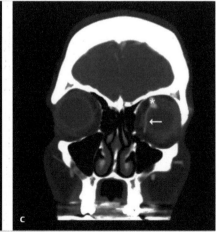

Fig. 9.1 CT angiogram demonstrating **(a)** axial views of asymmetric avid enhancement of the LEFT cavernous sinus, **(b)** dilated superior ophthalmic vein (*asterisk*) and multiplanar reconstruction demonstrating **(c)** the superior ophthalmic (*asterisk*) and the angular veins (*white arrow*).

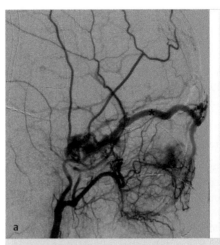
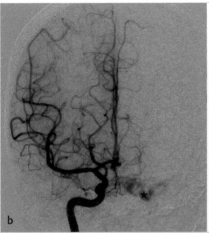
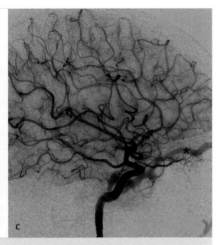

Fig. 9.2 Selected angiographic images demonstrating fistulous filling of the left cavernous sinus and superior ophthalmic vein (*asterisk*) from **(a)** left external carotid artery injection in the lateral projection, **(b)** right internal carotid artery injection in the AP projection, and **(c)** left internal carotid artery injection in the lateral projection.

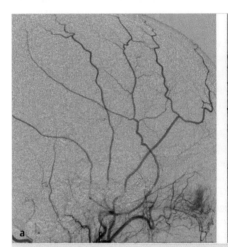
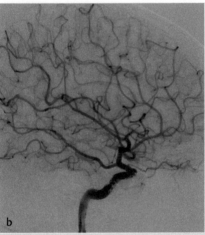
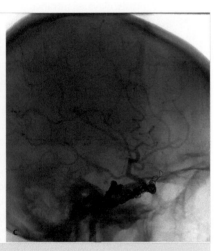

Fig. 9.3 Selected angiographic images after coil embolization demonstrating no definitive filling of the left cavernous sinus from **(a)** left external carotid artery injection in the lateral projection, **(b)** left internal carotid artery injection in the lateral projection, and **(c)** native view of the coil mass in the lateral projection.

petrosal sinus; coiling was directed from the confluence of the left superior ophthalmic vein and cavernous sinus in a retrograde manner to the posterior cavernous sinus. Complete obliteration of the CCF was achieved without complications.

9.2.3 Follow-up

The patient remained neurologically intact and was discharged home on postoperative day 1 with resolution of all presenting symptoms. However, the patient returned on postoperative day 4 with a partial left abducens palsy. A CTA demonstrated near complete resolution of the previously dilated left superior ophthalmic vein. A repeat DSA demonstrated no fistulous connections to the cavernous sinus (► Fig. 9.3a, b) with a stable coil mass (► Fig. 9.3c). A follow-up angiogram 6 months postoperatively demonstrated continued obliteration of the fistulous connections. The partial abducens palsy had resolved.

9.3 Case Summary

1. *How can this carotid-cavernous fistula be classified?*
   After the seminal 1985 publication,[1] the Barrow classification became the most widely used scheme to describe CCFs. This classification system was based on angioarchitecture, and it categorized CCFs into four distinct types.
   Type A direct CCFs have a direct connection between the cavernous ICA and the cavernous sinus usually due to a rupture in the carotid wall. These CCFs are high-flow lesions and have a low chance of resolving without intervention. The high-flow characteristics and their rapidly progressive nature make type A CCFs more likely to lead to vision loss.
   Types B, C, and D are known as indirect or dural fistulas and arise from connections between the cavernous sinus and meningeal branches from the ICA (type B), meningeal branches from the ECA (type C), or both (type D). Type B, C, and D CCFs are less common than type A CCFs. For our

patient, the imaging showed supply from bilateral internal and ipsilateral external carotid arteries (type D).

2. *Which patient factors aid in determining conservative management versus treatment?*

In 60 to 90% of cases, symptoms involve the orbit (conjunctival injection, chemosis, proptosis, glaucoma, diplopia, orbital hemorrhage, retro-orbital pain, and visual changes including vision loss). Less frequently, there can be progressive pain in the trigeminal distribution most commonly involving the V2 distribution. More rare presentations include intracranial hemorrhage, subarachnoid hemorrhage, epistaxis, or otorrhagia. CCFs can also present with headaches or tinnitus. While the decision to treat type A CCFs is straightforward, type B-D CCFs require more consideration given the greater likelihood of spontaneous resolution. While any threat to vision warrants treatment, patients with only headaches and/or tinnitus may require more nuanced discussions.

In this instance, the patient had 6 months of intermittent diplopia, conjunctival injection, headaches, V2 sensory changes, and persistent tinnitus. She did not have hemorrhage, proptosis, elevated intraocular pressure, or vision changes; however, the symptoms were significantly impacting her quality of life. The treatment decision was elective and based on consideration of the risks, benefits, and alternatives.

3. *How did both the type of fistula play a role in determining treatment modality?*

There are multiple management options for CCFs: serial imaging, conservative treatment with manual external carotid compression, embolization, radiosurgery, and open surgery. However, endovascular treatment is the preferred treatment modality and includes the largest range of treatment options. Current endovascular modalities include detachable coils, liquid embolic agents (N-butyl cyanoacrylate [NBCA] and ethylene vinyl alcohol copolymer [EVOH]), covered stents, and flow diverting stents. Depending on the specific characteristics of the CCF, the lesion can be accessed via transvenous, transarterial, or combined approaches. Because this indirect CCF was fed from both ICA and ECA branches, we elected to proceed with transvenous coil embolization of the cavernous sinus.

4. *What manner of follow-up is appropriate for these lesions?*

Cross-sectional imaging of all types is limited in the ability to detect fistulous connections. Therefore, a follow-up DSA should be performed to confirm successful treatment. There is no definitive recommendation for the timing of a follow-up study, but treatment modality and symptomatology can influence the time frame. However, the most common strategy described in the literature is a 6-month follow-up angiogram with the option for an additional 1-year follow-up angiogram.

9.4 Level of Evidence

The current level of evidence for endovascular treatment of CCF is Level C due to the lack of randomized controlled trials or other data to support a higher level. This is not unexpected, given the relative infrequency of presentation and the changing treatment modalities over the past several decades. There are a large number of studies indicating benefit of endovascular intervention. However, these studies are almost entirely composed of cohort studies, retrospective analyses, and case reports. So while the level of evidence is low, treatment recommendations can be considered strong (Class IIa) due to the amount of published data and the anticipated natural history of CCFs.

9.5 Landmark Papers

Surgeries for pulsating exophthalmos have been performed since the early 1800s. If conservative measures failed, surgeons often proceeded to ligation of the common or internal carotid artery. Treatment modalities changed with the introduction of detachable balloon catheters by Serbinenko in 1974.[2] The papers below give an abbreviated history on the classification of CCFs and how treatments have evolved since the 1980s. Beyond these select articles, there are many additional papers that have significantly contributed to the body of knowledge.[3,4,5]

Barrow DL, Spector RH, Braun IF, et al. Classification and treatment of spontaneous carotid-cavernous sinus fistulas. J Neurosurg. 1985;62:248–256.[1]

Previously, CCFs were classified according to three criteria: (1) traumatic or spontaneous, (2) high-flow or low-flow, and (3) direct or dural flow on angiography. These were applied in a variable manner in prior studies. Barrow et al posited that angiography actually demonstrated only four distinct types of CCFs, direct shunting and three variants of dural shunting. The classification proposed by Barrow et al effectively combined prior classifications and offered a four-part scheme. Type A CCFs with direct flow from the ICA generally have higher flow and are frequently traumatic in nature. Type B CCFs were determined to have indirect flow into the cavernous sinus from branches off the ICA, were slower flow states, and were most often spontaneous in origin. Type C CCFs had indirect flow from ECA branches and were spontaneous in origin. Finally, type D CCFs had indirect flow from both ICA and ECA branches and were more frequently spontaneous in origin. Treatment decisions could now be made based upon the CCFs classification.

This classification has become the most widely used schema for evaluating and determining treatment course. The effectiveness of the classification stems primarily from its assessment of the CCF's angioarchitecture which has the greatest influence on the choice of therapeutic modality. The study also highlights the importance of cerebral angiography in the work-up of these patients. Despite the small sample sizes used to create the classification system, the results have held true in multiple subsequent studies.

Cognard C, Gobin YP, Pierot L, et al. Cerebral dural arteriovenous fistulas: clinical and angiographic correlation with a revised classification of venous drainage. Radiology. 1995;194(3):671–680.[6]

In 1978, Rene Djindjian proposed a classification of purely meningeal fistulae into four types based on angioarchitecture and venous drainage.[7] Using this classification system, Cognard et al evaluated a consecutive series of 205 patients with the intention to validate and expand upon the original description. While their results closely mirrored those of Djindjian, they expanded and clearly defined the categories of indirect CCFs.

9

A Cognard type I fistula drained into the sinus with normal antegrade flow. Type II fistulas were subdivided into three categories: type IIa drained into a sinus with retrograde flow within the sinus; type IIb drained into the sinus via retrograde flow through cortical veins with anterograde sinus drainage; and type IIa + b had retrograde drainage in both the cortical veins and the sinus. Type III fistulas drained directly into cortical veins with no demonstrated ectasia, while type IV fistulas demonstrated ectatic veins. Type V fistulas drained directly into spinal perimedullary veins. Thirty-three patients in their series had CCFs, and all were classified as type I, type IIb, or type IIa + b.

Recently, Griauzde et al[8] argued against using the Barrow classification for indirect CCFs. They stated that direct CCFs are distinct entities from indirect CCFs and should be considered separately. The Cognard classification system was better able to identify high-risk fistulas requiring treatment by the identification of cortical venous reflux. In addition, Griauzde et al found that presentation with ocular symptoms had an association with Cognard groups IIa and IIa + b. Despite their arguments, however, the Barrow classification still remains the most widely implemented.

Debrun GM, Vinuela F, Fox AJ, et al. Indications for treatment and classification of 132 carotid-cavernous fistulas. Neurosurgery. 1988;22(2):285–289.[9]

Debrun et al applied the Barrow classification to their series of 132 CCFs and detailed the frequency of each type of fistula and demonstrated the utility of the Barrow classification to guide treatment.

The authors found that type A fistulas were the most common and most often associated with trauma. Of the 100 patients with type A CCFs, 95 were traumatic in origin. Ninety-two patients were treated with detachable balloons, and ICA patency was maintained in approximately 70% of the cases. Three patients required repeat endovascular treatment and four required open surgery after initial endovascular treatment. The complication rate was 30% and included transient and permanent oculomotor nerve palsies.

The authors also found that types C and D were dural arteriovenous fistulas with flow characteristics and angioarchitecture as described by Barrow et al—slow flow, spontaneous in origin, and originating from the branches of the ECA (type C) and a combination of the ECA and ICA (type D). Type D CCFs were more common than type C CCFs. No type B CCFs were seen in their series. With the exception of three type D patients who spontaneously resolved, all had endovascular treatment. All 4 type C and 25 of 28 type D patients were treated initially via particle embolization and/or liquid embolic agents through the ECA feeding vessels. This proved curative for the type C CCFs, but only 12 of 25 type D patients had complete obliteration even after several rounds of embolization. Several patients had transvenous balloon occlusion, and one required surgical exposure of the cavernous sinus for definitive fistula obliteration. These results reflected the more complex nature of type D CCFs.

Their series provided a wealth of corroborating information that was in accordance with the Barrow classification. The absence of type B CCFs in this group suggested that these lesions were uncommon. In addition, they demonstrated the ability of detachable balloons to treat type A fistulas without

sacrifice of the ICA and the role of a multimodal approach in the treatment of persistent type D fistulas.

Meyers PM, Halbach VV, Dowd CF, et al. Dural carotid cavernous fistula: Definitive endovascular management and long-term follow-up. Am J Ophthal. 2002;134(1):85–92.[10]

In this retrospective analysis of 135 patients with indirect CCFs, 133 patients had endovascular treatment including 101 transvenous embolizations. They demonstrated the safety and efficacy of the transvenous approach with a 90% angiographic cure rate, 96% symptom improvement/resolution rate, and a 6% complication rate. With long-term clinical and angiographic follow-up, Meyers et al demonstrated the long-term efficacy of their treatments.

Ducruet AF, Albuquerque FC, Crowley RW, McDougall CG. The evolution of endovascular treatment of carotid cavernous fistulas: a single-center experience. World Neurosurg. 2013;80 (5):538–548.[11]

Ducruet et al reported managing 100 direct and indirect CCFs over an approximately 17-year period. In this timespan, endovascular treatments went through significant changes including the removal of the detachable balloon from the US market in 2004. These changes led to the use of coils as the mainstay for embolization. The data reflected both the changing treatments and the improvement in outcomes as endovascular techniques and tools evolved.

Detachable balloons were used to successfully treat 18 of the 42 type A CCFs. An additional 12 patients were treated with coil embolization. While ICA occlusion was necessary in 50% of the detachable balloon cases, only 25% of patients treated with coil embolization required ICA occlusion. The transvenous approach was used when either the transarterial approach was not possible or the transarterial approach failed to treat the fistula.

Coil embolization from the venous side was performed with a transarterial balloon or stent deployed within the ICA for protection. They reported a 10% complication rate (one death) for treatment of type A CCFs with an estimated 90% of patients demonstrating resolution or improvement in their symptoms.

Indirect CCFs were treated via the transvenous approach for 42 of the 48 patients in their series; 41 coil embolization cases and one liquid embolic case. Six patients underwent transarterial treatment and an additional five had combined approaches. Liquid embolics were utilized (seven with NBCA and four with EVOH) with the transarterial approach. The complication rate for indirect fistulas was ~8% (no deaths) and > 80% experienced improvement or resolution of their symptoms.

This paper demonstrates an institution's evolution in treatment of CCFs highlighting the innovations in endovascular equipment and advances in technique. The authors transitioned from transarterial balloon occlusion and ICA sacrifice to transvenous. By the time of publication, the authors were utilizing endovascular treatments as a first-line therapy with open surgery reserved for salvage therapy.

9.6 Recommendations

The classic signs and symptoms of diplopia, chemosis, proptosis, and conjunctival injection remain the most common presenting symptoms of CCF. However, vision loss, headaches, ocular pain, retinal hemorrhage, transient ischemic attacks (TIAs), stroke, epistaxis, otorrhagia, ptosis, glaucoma, ophthalmoplegia, tinnitus, paresthesias, intracranial hemorrhages, and seizures can also occur.[12] A history of trauma with any of the aforementioned signs and symptoms should raise the index of suspicion for a CCF.

While an MRA or a CTA does not allow for appropriate evaluation of the angioarchitecture of the fistulous connection, it is often obtained during the initial workup and can demonstrate indirect signs of the presence of a CCF. The constellation of classic symptoms and imaging findings will often be sufficient to determine the need for diagnostic cerebral angiography.

Cerebral angiography is still considered the gold standard for diagnosis of CCFs. Regardless of the classification system employed, a six-vessel cerebral angiogram will afford the necessary evaluation of the angioarchitecture of the fistula, as well as the flow patterns associated with it.

While many of the angiographic suites in use today are capable of high frame-rates for detailed evaluation of fistula architecture, angiographic assessment of very high-flow lesions can prove difficult. Several techniques have been developed to better assess the CCF. The Heuber maneuver[13] requires an ipsilateral posterior communicating artery (PCOM). During compression of the ipsilateral carotid artery, an angiogram is performed through a vertebral artery; the fistula then fills via retrograde flow through the PCOM. In addition, the Mehringer–Hieshima maneuver[14] is performed with subtotal compression of the ipsilateral carotid artery during an ipsilateral angiogram. Flow through the CCF is decreased due to the manual compression.

Balloon test occlusion (BTO) was previously an integral component prior to intervention for any type of CCF in anticipation of possible artery sacrifice. Today, the need for carotid occlusions are more limited, but more commonly seen in emergent interventions for unstable, traumatic fistulas. A BTO remains a diagnostic option when carotid sacrifice seems possible.

The decision for intervention should be based on patient presentation, initial imaging findings, and CCF characteristics. External bleeding/intracranial hemorrhage, the acute onset of cranial nerve palsies, proptosis/exophthalmos, rapidly progressive vision loss, and/or TIA/stroke are symptoms more likely to warrant urgent or emergent intervention.[15] Patients presenting with headaches and/or a slow progression of symptoms can be evaluated for intervention on an elective basis. If imaging demonstrates an aneurysm/pseudoaneurysm, large cavernous varix, cortical edema, acute/subacute hemorrhage, high-flow fistula, retrograde cortical venous drainage, or thrombosed cortical veins, then earlier intervention is warranted. Low-flow fistulas without venous reflux or retrograde flow and Barrow type B, C, or D CCFs can be managed electively.

Treatments include conservative management including external manual compression, endovascular embolization or flow diversion, radiosurgery, and open surgery. Endovascular treatment remains the mainstay for those CCFs requiring treatment. External compression of the carotid artery is likely a safe option for low-flow CCFs with mild symptoms and has a reported response rate ranging from 20 to 60%.[5,11,16,17] Radiosurgery may also be safely recommended for low-risk CCFs. However, there is an expected delay of 6 to 18 months for clinical resolution of symptoms following treatment.[17,18,19] Open surgery is increasingly rare and has become the salvage option

when all possible endovascular interventions fail. In addition, surgery can be used as part of a multimodal treatment to facilitate access for embolization; surgical, transorbital cannulation of the superior or inferior ophthalmic vein[20,21,22,23,24,25]; or a small craniotomy for access to the cerebral vasculature and the cavernous sinus.[26,27]

Coil embolization has been used for treatment of CCF for several decades[10,28,29] and can be performed via either the transarterial or transvenous approach. The liquid embolic agents (NBCA and EVOH) have been employed via transvenous and transarterial approaches.[3,10,11,17,30] The transvenous approach is used for all types of CCFs oftentimes with temporary balloon occlusion of the cavernous ICA to prevent egress of the embolic agents into the carotid circulation. Because liquid embolics can penetrate the interstices of the cavernous sinus, it is very useful when employed in conjunction with coil embolization to accelerate fistula occlusion.[31] The transarterial approach is used less frequently in the ICA distribution due to the risk of distal ICA embolization. However, ECA branches can often be safely occluded with these agents.

Since minimally porous, covered endovascular stent grafts were first used for treatment of traumatic CCFs in 2001,[32] there has been progressive development and improvement of intracranial stents.[33,34,35,36,37,38] Recent experience demonstrates the efficacy of flow diverting stents for treatment of type A CCFs. Stents are also used as an adjunct to coil embolization to maintain ICA patency and prevent coil herniation, while flow diverting stents may facilitate thrombosis and fistula closure.[38] Depending on the stent type, these devices may exhibit relatively poor navigability and oftentimes require dual antiplatelet medications to prevent stent thrombosis.

9.7 Summary

1. CCFs are rare but potentially morbid lesions. Diagnosis relies on multimodal evaluation with digital subtraction angiography as the gold standard.
2. While early treatments often relied on open surgery, the current mainstay of treatment is endovascular intervention. There is no high-level evidence involving treatment due to the relative rarity of the lesion, the heterogeneity in classes and treatment, and the constantly evolving treatment options. Despite this, endovascular intervention has resulted in a concomitant decrease in the morbidity and mortality of these lesions.
3. Any treatment should be carefully considered and tailored to the patient, their symptoms, and the characteristics of CCFs.

References

[1] Barrow DL, Spector RH, Braun IF, Landman JA, Tindall SC, Tindall GT. Classification and treatment of spontaneous carotid-cavernous sinus fistulas. J Neurosurg. 1985; 62(2):248–256

[2] Serbinenko FA. Balloon catheterization and occlusion of major cerebral vessels. J Neurosurg. 1974; 41(2):125–145

[3] Higashida RT, Halbach VV, Tsai FY, et al. Interventional neurovascular treatment of traumatic carotid and vertebral artery lesions: results in 234 cases. AJR Am J Roentgenol. 1989; 153(3):577–582

[4] Lewis AI, Tomsick TA, Tew JM, Jr. Management of 100 consecutive direct carotid-cavernous fistulas: results of treatment with detachable balloons. Neurosurgery. 1995; 36(2):239–244, discussion 244–245

9

[5] Wu Z, Zhang Y, Wang C, Yang X, Li Y. Treatment of traumatic carotid-cavernous fistula. Interv Neuroradiol. 2000; 6(4):277–289

[6] Cognard C, Gobin YP, Pierot L, et al. Cerebral dural arteriovenous fistulas: clinical and angiographic correlation with a revised classification of venous drainage. Radiology. 1995; 194(3):671–680

[7] Djindjian R, Merland J-J. Meningeal arteriovenous fistulae. In: Super-selective arteriography of the external carotid artery. Berlin, Heidelberg: Springer; 1978:405–536

[8] Griauzde J, Gemmete JJ, Pandey AS, Chaudhary N. Dural carotid cavernous fistulas: endovascular treatment and assessment of the correlation between clinical symptoms and the Cognard classification system. J Neurointerv Surg. 2017; 9(6):583–586

[9] Debrun GM, Viñuela F, Fox AJ, Davis KR, Ahn HS. Indications for treatment and classification of 132 carotid-cavernous fistulas. Neurosurgery. 1988; 22(2):285–289

[10] Meyers PM, Halbach VV, Dowd CF, et al. Dural carotid cavernous fistula: definitive endovascular management and long-term follow-up. Am J Ophthalmol. 2002; 134(1):85–92

[11] Ducruet AF, Albuquerque FC, Crowley RW, McDougall CG. The evolution of endovascular treatment of carotid cavernous fistulas: a single-center experience. World Neurosurg. 2013; 80(5):538–548

[12] Zanaty M, Chalouhi N, Tjoumakaris SI, Hasan D, Rosenwasser RH, Jabbour P. Endovascular treatment of carotid-cavernous fistulas. Neurosurg Clin N Am. 2014; 25(3):551–563

[13] Huber P. A technical contribution of the exact angiographic localization of carotid cavernous fistulas. Neuroradiology. 1976; 10(5):239–241

[14] Mehringer CM, Hieshima GB, Grinnell VS, Tsai F, Pribram HF. Improved localization of carotid cavernous fistula during angiography. AJNR Am J Neuroradiol. 1982; 3(1):82–84

[15] Halbach VV, Hieshima GB, Higashida RT, Reicher M. Carotid cavernous fistulae: indications for urgent treatment. AJR Am J Roentgenol. 1987; 149(3):587–593

[16] Wang W, Li YD, Li MH, et al. Endovascular treatment of post-traumatic direct carotid-cavernous fistulas: a single-center experience. J Clin Neurosci. 2011; 18(1):24–28

[17] Rodrigues T, Willinsky R, Agid R, TerBrugge K, Krings T. Management of dural carotid cavernous fistulas: a single-centre experience. Eur Radiol. 2014; 24(12):3051–3058

[18] Barcia-Salorio JL, Soler F, Barcia JA, Hernández G. Stereotactic radiosurgery for the treatment of low-flow carotid-cavernous fistulae: results in a series of 25 cases. Stereotact Funct Neurosurg. 1994; 63(1–4):266–270

[19] Gemmete JJ, Chaudhary N, Pandey A, Ansari S. Treatment of carotid cavernous fistulas. Curr Treat Options Neurol. 2010; 12(1):43–53

[20] Benndorf G, Bender A, Campi A, Menneking H, Lanksch WR. Treatment of a cavernous sinus dural arteriovenous fistula by deep orbital puncture of the superior ophthalmic vein. Neuroradiology. 2001; 43(6):499–502

[21] White JB, Layton KF, Evans AJ, et al. Transorbital puncture for the treatment of cavernous sinus dural arteriovenous fistulas. AJNR Am J Neuroradiol. 2007; 28(7):1415–1417

[22] Dashti SR, Fiorella D, Spetzler RF, Albuquerque FC, McDougall CG. Transorbital endovascular embolization of dural carotid-cavernous fistula: access to cavernous sinus through direct puncture: case examples and technical report. Neurosurgery. 2011; 68(1) Suppl Operative:75–83, discussion 83

[23] Luo B, Zhang X, Duan CZ, et al. Surgical cannulation of the superior ophthalmic vein for the treatment of previously embolized cavernous sinus dural arteriovenous fistulas: serial studies and angiographic follow-up. Br J Neurosurg. 2013; 27(2):187–193

[24] Luo CB, Teng MMH, Chang FC, Guo WY, Chang CY. Transorbital direct puncture of the posterior cavernous sinus through the internal carotid artery for embolization of isolated cavernous sinus dural arteriovenous fistula. J Neurointerv Surg. 2013; 5(2):e1

[25] Phan K, Xu J, Leung V, et al. Orbital approaches for treatment of carotid cavernous fistulas: a systematic review. World Neurosurg. 2016; 96:243–251

[26] Chaudhary N, Lownie SP, Bussière M, Pelz DM, Nicolle D. Transcortical venous approach for direct embolization of a cavernous sinus dural arteriovenous fistula: Technical case report. Neurosurgery. 2012; 70(2, Suppl Operative):343–348

[27] Akamatsu Y, Sato K, Endo H, Matsumoto Y, Tominaga T. Single-session hematoma removal and transcranial coil embolization for a cavernous sinus dural arteriovenous fistula: a technical case report. World Neurosurg. 2017; 104:1046.e7–1046.e12

[28] Bavinzski G, Killer M, Gruber A, Richling B. Treatment of post-traumatic carotico-cavernous fistulae using electrolytically detachable coils: technical aspects and preliminary experience. Neuroradiology. 1997; 39(2):81–85

[29] Lu X, Hussain M, Ni L, et al. A comparison of different transarterial embolization techniques for direct carotid cavernous fistulas: a single center experience in 32 patients. J Vasc Interv Neurol. 2014; 7(5):35–47

[30] Goto K, Hieshima GB, Higashida RT, et al. Treatment of direct carotid cavernous sinus fistulae. Various therapeutic approaches and results in 148 cases. Acta Radiol Suppl. 1986; 369:576–579. Accessed July 26, 2018

[31] de Castro-Afonso LH, Trivelato FP, Rezende MT, et al. Transvenous embolization of dural carotid cavernous fistulas: the role of liquid embolic agents in association with coils on patient outcomes. J Neurointerv Surg. 2018; 10(5):461–462

[32] Redekop G, Marotta T, Weill A. Treatment of traumatic aneurysms and arteriovenous fistulas of the skull base by using endovascular stents. J Neurosurg. 2001; 95(3):412–419

[33] Gomez F, Escobar W, Gomez AM, Gomez JF, Anaya CA. Treatment of carotid cavernous fistulas using covered stents: midterm results in seven patients. AJNR Am J Neuroradiol. 2007; 28(9):1762–1768

[34] Wang C, Xie X, You C, et al. Placement of covered stents for the treatment of direct carotid cavernous fistulas. AJNR Am J Neuroradiol. 2009; 30(7):1342–1346

[35] Li J, Lan ZG, Xie XD, You C, He M. Traumatic carotid-cavernous fistulas treated with covered stents: experience of 12 cases. World Neurosurg. 2010; 73(5):514–519

[36] Yin B, Sheng HS, Wei RL, Lin J, Zhou H, Zhang N. Comparison of covered stents with detachable balloons for treatment of posttraumatic carotid-cavernous fistulas. J Clin Neurosci. 2013; 20(3):367–372

[37] Li K, Cho YD, Kim KM, Kang HS, Kim JE, Han MH. Covered stents for the endovascular treatment of a direct carotid cavernous fistula: single center experiences with 10 cases. J Korean Neurosurg Soc. 2015; 57(1):12–18

[38] Ogilvy CS, Motiei-Langroudi R, Ghorbani M, Griessenauer CJ, Alturki AY, Thomas AJ. Flow diverters as useful adjunct to traditional endovascular techniques in treatment of direct carotid-cavernous fistulas. World Neurosurg. 2017; 105:812–817

9

10 Dural Arteriovenous Fistulas

Lucas Augusto, Andre Monteiro, Erinc Akture, Gustavo Cortez, Ricardo Hanel, and Eric Sauvageau

Abstract

The contemporary management of dural arteriovenous fistulas relies heavily on endovascular therapy. Excellent understanding of the clinical manifestations, natural history, and therapeutic approaches is fundamental to obtain the best results. The current endovascular armamentarium allows for a personalized approach to treat the fistulas using the arterial or venous routes, but it remains important to recognize specific circumstances where surgical approaches remain safer and quite effective. While the rarity and the heterogeneity of these lesions remain problematic, a review of the literature allows one to obtain a good grasp to optimize management.

Keywords: dural arteriovenous fistula, endovascular, embolization, management, Borden, Cognard

10.1 Goals

1. Review the literature of dural arteriovenous fistulas (dAVFs) and explain the importance of the angioarchitecture pattern on the natural history.
2. Review the endovascular strategies available to treat dAVFs.
3. Review the roles of the other treatment modalities available for the treatment of dAVFs.

10.2 Case Example

10.2.1 History of Present Illness

A 61-year-old female is seen in consultation in the context of right retroauricular pain with pulsatile tinnitus for approximately 6 months. The patient spontaneously mentioned that manual compression behind her right ear decreased the intensity of the bruit. The patient was initially assessed by an ENT who referred the patient for suspicion of a dAVF. The patient had a recent computed tomography (CT) head and magnetic resonance imaging (MRI) brain without contrast which was negative for any significant pathology.

The patient denied any significant neurological complaints.
Past medical history: Hyperlipidemia, hypertension, gastroesophageal reflux disease (GERD).
No significant history of trauma.
No past medical/surgical ENT or neurological history.
Neurological examination: Unremarkable.
Imaging studies: See ▶ Fig. 10.1 and ▶ Fig. 10.2.

10.2.2 Treatment Plan

Treatment options were discussed and the patient elected to proceed with transvenous obliteration of the fistulas.

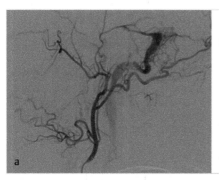
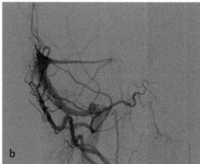

Fig. 10.1 Cerebral angiogram anteroposterior (AP) and lateral images. Lateral **(a)** and AP oblique **(b)** views of external carotid artery injections showing dural arteriovenous fistula (dAVF) feeders from posterior meningeal artery and occipital feeders. Multiple venous tributaries to transverse-sigmoid sinus junction with prominent cortical venous reflux can be visualized.

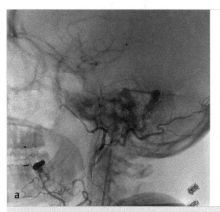
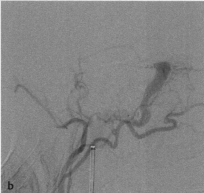
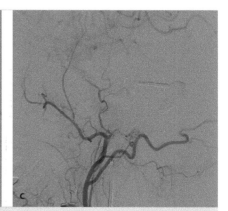

Fig. 10.2 Endovascular procedure steps: microcatheter in place via transvenous approach **(a)**, initial coils placed showing that there is still filling of the sinus **(b)**, and final result after completion of embolization **(c)**.

A lateral angiogram obtained with a transvenous microcatheter positioned within the superior petrosal sinus demonstrated cortical venous reflux. Treatment proceeded with embolization via the superior petrosal sinus to eliminate this reflux. After embolization of the superior petrosal sinus, fistulous connections still existed draining into the transverse sigmoid junction. After coiled embolization of the transverse sigmoid junction, the dAVF was obliterated.

10.2.3 Follow-up

The patient did very well after the treatment. The final angiographic run after treatment confirmed complete obliteration. The tinnitus resolved after treatment.

A follow-up angiogram 18 months later confirmed no recurrence or residual shunting.

10.3 Case Summary

1. *This patient was found to have a symptomatic unruptured dAVF. No clear abnormalities were documented on CT and MRI. Does negative noninvasive imaging rule out the diagnosis of dAVF?*

   Catheter-based digital subtraction angiography (DSA) is the mainstay of diagnosis for dAVFs. A six-vessel angiography is necessary for these lesions as the feeding vessels can be bilateral, intra- or extra-cranial, and/or arise from the anterior or posterior circulation. The study of the venous phase is of paramount importance. Although MRI, magnetic resonance angiography (MRA), or computed tomography angiography (CTA) can give valuable diagnostic information, a negative CT or MRI does not exclude the diagnosis of a dAVF. Noninvasive modalities can be helpful adjuncts to DSA, such as detecting hydrocephalus or white matter edema. Also, noninvasive modalities can be the first imaging modality suspecting the presence of a dAVF with detection of prominent pial vessels or tortuous, enlarged veins.

2. *What is the expected natural history on this patient?*

   Patients can present with pulsatile tinnitus, retroauricular pain, intracranial hypertension, venous dementia, seizures, venous infarctions, and intracerebral hemorrhage. Intracerebral hemorrhage is the most dreaded presentation with a case fatality of 20%. The overall risk of annual hemorrhage from dAVF is 1.8%. However, angioarchitecture is the main determinant of the hemorrhage risk. In conservatively managed malformations, 12.5% spontaneously regressed and 4% progressed to higher grade.[1] However, the reported spontaneous regression rate for lesions with cortical venous reflux is 3%.[2] The two most commonly used classification systems today are Borden and Cognard classification systems. These systems mainly focus on venous drainage patterns and aid in establishing natural history and decision making in treatment. Most Borden type I and Cognard type I and IIa lesions have benign clinical courses, whereas higher grade lesions with cortical venous reflux have higher risks of rupture. In one of the largest series for dAVFs with cortical reflux, the annual rupture rate for untreated lesions was 13%. The same study reported that presence of venous ectasia increased the rupture risk by sevenfold (3.5% no ectasia vs. 27% with ectasia).[3]

3. *Should treatment be considered in this patient?*

   The decision to treat a dAVF is largely based on the presentation and angioarchitecture (mainly presence of cortical venous drainage). The goal of therapy should be aimed at reducing the risk of rupture or re-rupture. Quality of life improvement can also be a factor in the decision to treat low-risk lesions causing tinnitus. This patient had cortical venous reflux and symptomatic pulsatile tinnitus. The treatment decision was made to eliminate or decrease the annual hemorrhage risk and provide symptomatic relief.

4. *If no cortical venous drainage is present, should treatment still be offered?*

   In patients without cortical venous drainage (Borden I and Cognard 1 and IIa), observation is a viable option. However, treatment may be considered in certain cases. Venous hypertension and related complications such as dementia, hydrocephalus, and intracranial hypertension may necessitate treatment. If possible, complete cure should be the goal of treatment when feasible and safe. However, in selected cases, focused treatments such as addressing a venous sinus stenosis or decreasing overall flow in the lesion by selective arterial embolization can revert the symptoms caused by increased venous pressures. Also, treatment can be considered if symptoms such as pulsatile tinnitus or retroauricular pain are disabling.

5. *What treatment alternatives are available to address this entity?*

   Conservative management, endovascular therapies, open surgery, and radiosurgery are the main options for treatment of these lesions. Asymptomatic or minimally symptomatic lesions without cortical venous reflux can be managed conservatively. Intermittent manual arterial compression could be discussed with limited expectation for asymptomatic/minimally symptomatic lesions without cortical venous reflux. Endovascular treatment options are currently the mainstay of treatment of dAVFs. Transvenous and transarterial routes are the two main options in endovascular management of these lesions. Regardless the route chosen, specific occlusion of the fistulous point with the draining vein offers the best chance for complete cure. Occlusion of only the arterial feeders with intact venous outflow can result in recruitment of new feeders and recurrence of the fistula, though venous occlusion should not be at the expense of normal venous drainage.

   Although endovascular therapies should be considered the first-line treatment, open surgery remains a viable option. Currently, the main goal for surgery is to occlude the draining vein when the anatomy allows. Surgery could also be an adjunct to endovascular treatment via accessing the draining vein or sinus for transvenous endovascular treatment. Radiosurgery can also be a viable tool in the armamentarium in the management of dAVFs not amenable to endovascular or surgical treatment. A meta-analysis of the radiosurgical literature reported a rate of obliteration of 63%. Lesions with cortical venous drainage had worse obliteration rate (56%) compared to the ones without (75%).[4] Also, it should be kept in mind that radiosurgery has a latency period for dAVF obliteration.

6. *Would you follow this lesion after treatment? How would you follow a lesion that is not treated?*

There are no set guidelines for follow up for dAVFs. There are few reports citing angiographic change in these lesions to a higher angiographic grade. Partially treated lesions can recruit new feeders and change over time. Even after complete angiographic cure, these lesions can recur. In our practice, we perform diagnostic cerebral angiography on treated dAVFs 12 to 18 months after treatment.

10.4 Level of Evidence

Natural history: The natural history of her dAVF with cortical venous reflux is well described through retrospective series (Class I, Level of Evidence C).

Endovascular treatment: The decision to proceed initially with endovascular embolization for a symptomatic, high-grade dAVF is reasonable (Class I, Level of Evidence C).

Follow-up: Angiographic follow-up of treated dAVFs is reasonable, given the recurrence rate of these lesions (Class IIA, Level of Evidence C).

10.5 Landmark Papers

Borden JA, Wu JK, Shucart WA. A proposed classification for spinal and cranial dural arteriovenous fistulous malformations and implications for treatment. J Neurosurg 1995;82(2):166–179.

Borden et al proposed a classification that unified spinal and cranial dural arteriovenous fistulous malformations (AVFMs) and organized them in three main types that could provide a rationale for treatment. The authors associated each type with higher or lesser risk of hemorrhage and neurological deficits based upon the pattern of venous drainage and direction and intensity of flow.[5] Type I fistulas drained directly into dural sinuses or meningeal veins in an anterograde direction and are often asymptomatic but can present with cranial nerve deficits or pulsatile tinnitus when cranial, or with myelopathy, bruits, and epidural hematomas when spinal. Type II lesions also drained into the dural sinuses, but the arterialized blood flow reversed (retrograde) into the subarachnoid veins, usually presenting with neurological deficits or hemorrhage secondary to venous hypertension. Type III lesions drained directly into the subarachnoid veins or indirectly to it, when the fistula occurs through a segment of dural sinus that is thrombosed on both sides, creating an isolated compartment. Type III fistulas frequently presented with hemorrhage or neurological sequelae secondary to superficial or deep venous hypertension. Subtypes of each dAVFs are also described by Borden in this same study. Treatment is discussed for each type. However, this study was published prior to the significant increase in sophistication of endovascular treatments. Regardless, this study forms the basis for our understanding of dAVFs.

Cognard C, Gobin YP, Pierot L, et al. Cerebral dural arteriovenous fistulas: clinical and angiographic correlation with a revised classification of venous drainage. Radiology 1995;194(3):671–680.[6]

Cognard et al reviewed 258 patients with dAVFs from their institution. Two hundred and five patients had enough clinical and angiographic data and 120 had follow-up information (mean time = 52 months). The purpose of this study was to correlate the progression associated with each kind of venous pattern seen on angiography. The authors chose to base their

Table 10.1 Cognard grading scale for dAVF[6]

Type I	Antegrade drainage into a sinus or meningeal vein
Type IIa	As type I but with retrograde flow
Type IIb	Reflux into cortical veins
Type IIa + b	Reflux into both sinus and cortical veins
Type III	Direct cortical venous drainage without venous ectasia
Type IV	Direct cortical venous drainage with venous ectasia
Type V	Spinal venous drainage

observation in the classification proposed by Djindjian but expanded it to five types as seen in ▶ Table 10.1.

Type I dAVFs almost never progressed to more severe types and did not require aggressive treatment attempts. Type IIa lesions could be treated with arterial embolization with particles and, when necessary, with glue and transvenous occlusion in certain locations. Types IIb and II a + b have a high risk of bleeding. Occlusion was mandatory in these high-grade lesions and could be done by arterial embolization, transvenous occlusion, or surgical resection of the sinus. Types III to V are very aggressive lesions with a high risk of hemorrhage, which does not change with partial obliteration, requiring therapies such as complete endovascular occlusion, radiosurgery, surgery, or combination of these.

Cognard C, Januel AC, Silva NA Jr, Tall P. Endovascular treatment of intracranial dural arteriovenous fistulas with cortical venous drainage: new management using Onyx. AJNR Am J Neuroradiol 2008;29(2):235–241. Epub 2007 Nov 7.

Cognard et al presented a novel use for the new liquid embolic agent Onyx. Thirty patients were prospectively included from 2003 to 2006 to undergo embolization of dAVFs. Ten patients were type II, 8 were type III, and 12 were type IV. Of the 25 patients who had never been embolized previously, cure was achieved in 23. Only one patient of the five who had been previously embolized achieved cure. Obliteration was confirmed with follow-up angiography. Of the six patients who achieved partial occlusion, two were successfully cured with surgery and two more with radiosurgery. One cured patient rebled 2 days after embolization, secondary to thrombosis of a draining vein. One patient had transient cranial nerve palsy. The authors considered Onyx a reasonable alternative for treatment of dAVFs and suggested a reconsideration of the global treatment strategies for these fistulas.

Davies MA, TerBrugge K, Willinsky R, Coyne T, Saleh J, Wallace MC. The validity of classification for the clinical presentation of intracranial dural arteriovenous fistulas. J Neurosurg 1996;85(5):830–837.[7]

This study is a very interesting analysis demonstrating the reliability of both Borden and Cognard classifications in predicting the presenting behavior of dAVFs. Ninety-eight patients were assessed at a single institution. Hemorrhage and nonhemorrhagic neurological deficits were considered to be an aggressive presentation. When analyzed according to the Borden classification, aggressive presentation was present in 2% of type I, 39% of type II, and 79% of type III (p < 0.0001) dAVFs. When the Cognard classification was used, aggressive presentation was seen in 0% of type I, 7% of type IIa, 38% of type IIb, 40%

of type IIa + b, 69% of type III, 83% of type IV, and 100% of type V lesions (*p* < 0.0001).

10.6 Recommendations

Catheter angiography is the gold standard diagnostic test for dAVFs. A negative CTA or MRI/MRA does not exclude the diagnosis. Decision-making in the management of these lesions heavily depend on natural history, which in turn is dictated by angioarchitecture of the lesion. Borden and Cognard classification systems provide a good basis for categorizing angioarchitecture. Cortical venous reflux is associated with increased risks of hemorrhage. Venous ectasia also increases bleeding risk significantly.

Treatment decision for lesions without cortical venous reflux should be made on a case-by-case basis. If manifestations of increased venous pressure such as hydrocephalus, venous infarcts, cerebral edema, and/or dementia are present, low-grade lesions should be treated. If complete cure is not feasible or risky, low-grade lesions can simply be managed by reducing the venous pressures. Venous outflow obstructions can be addressed for symptomatic management. Flow reduction strategies with selective arterial embolization could also be applied. Low-grade lesions with debilitating tinnitus or retro auricular pain can also warrant treatment. There are no set guidelines for follow up for low-grade lesions. Some studies suggest that low-grade lesions can become high grade over time.[5] This raises a question for routine follow-up for Borden Grade I or Cognard grade I and IIa lesions. Development of new symptoms or worsening of symptoms could warrant a repeat study. Intermittent manual occlusion could be presented to the patients as an option for lesions fed by favorable vessels.

Lesions with cortical venous reflux have an unfavorable natural history. These lesions should be treated with the goal of total cure. Complete venous outflow takedown with preservation of normal venous drainage offers the best chance for total cure. This goal can be achieved by endovascular means (transarterial or transvenous) or by open surgery.

dAVFs presenting with hemorrhage carry significant rehemorrhage risks, and these lesions should be treated in a timely fashion. Reported rates of annual hemorrhage are 46% in Borden type I and II fistulas presenting with hemorrhage versus 3% for those lesions presenting without hemorrhage.[2] Early rebleeding within 20 days is reported as high as 35%.[8]

The most effective treatment of dAVFs is occlusion of the draining vein. Treatment is aimed at complete elimination of the arteriovenous shunt. A proximal arterial occlusion is not sufficient to cure the dAVF as the fistulous site will still be patent and recruit a new arterial supply over time. This could lead to a possible redirection of the venous outflow and an increased risk of hemorrhage.[9,10] Embolization of the arterial feeders alone can be used as a palliative measure in benign fistulas without cortical reflux. Advantages of transvenous embolization (TVE) include the relative simplicity of retrograde venous access to the fistulous site and the ability to close the fistula in one session. TVE is particularly valuable for dAVFs with multiple arterial feeders of small size or tortuous course for which complete or practical treatment by transarterial embolization is not achievable.[11]

The endovascular treatment can be accomplished by use of embolic agents such as n-BCA glue (TRUFILL n-Butyl Cyanoacrylate;

DePuy, Warsaw, Indiana, USA) or Onyx (ev3/Covidien, Plymouth, Minnesota, USA).[10]

Onyx embolization is reportedly superior to nBCA and coil embolization in obliteration of dAVFs, with a lesser need for postembolization surgery.[12] Despite its advantages, Onyx embolization has its pitfalls. Unwanted embolization, microcatheter retention, cranial neuropathy, as well as failure to penetrate the fistulous connections and draining veins or failure to deliver the embolic agent due to difficult tortuous arteries have been described.[11,13,14] Onyx injection should be avoided into vessels known to supply the lower cranial nerves (petrosal branch of the middle meningeal artery, jugular branch of the ascending pharyngeal artery, and stylomastoid branch of the posterior auricular and occipital arteries), and catheter retention can be avoided by limiting reflux around the catheter tip and positioning the catheter tip in a relatively straight vessel segment.[9] If an intra-arterial approach is chosen, goal for such embolization should be progressive and controlled occlusion of the fistula including the venous pouch with liquid embolic agents for a total cure. Care must be taken to prevent ischemic injury to cranial nerves and their ganglia in certain anatomical locations.

Venous embolization is also a viable strategy in the endovascular management of dAVFs. Coils or liquid embolic agents can be used to occlude the draining vein. Care should be taken to occlude the vein as close to the fistula as possible. In some cases, endovascular sinus sacrifice can be considered using coils and/or embolic agents. Care must be taken to ensure that alternative drainage pathways for the brain remain preserved. Transarterial venous sinus occlusion using Onyx is safe, effective, and durable in the treatment of extensive dAVFs of codominant or nondominant transverse and sigmoid sinuses.[15] The decision to occlude the transverse or sigmoid sinus in a patient is multifactorial. The sufficiency of venous drainage of the normal brain must be evaluated with late venous phases on angiography. In dAVFs of the transverse and sigmoid sinuses, identification of the vein of Labbé and inferior cerebellar vein, which both drain into the transverse sinus, is necessary to avoid venous infarctions of the temporo-occipital lobe and posterior fossa. If both already have alternative pathways for venous drainage and/or are involved in the cortical venous reflux, then it can be assumed that the transverse sinus may be closed safely. In 39% of dAVFs involving the transverse and sigmoid sinuses, the venous sinuses are isolated or compartmentalized because of previous thrombosis.[16] Also, venous sinus occlusion can be considered when a lesion is determined to have extensive involvements in circumference or length of the sinus wall with cortical venous drainage. dAVFs that involve a focal segment of sinus, a specific leaflet of the sinus, or cortical vein adjacent to a sinus can usually be embolized without sinus closure.[17]

Most published series of transverse-sigmoid dAVF embolizations, with both combined transarterial and transvenous or transvenous-only embolizations report good results. High angiographic cure rates (55–87.5%) and symptom improvement or resolution (90–96%) with low-transient (10–15%) and permanent (0–5%) complication rates are reported.[18,19,20]

For many years, surgery has been considered the treatment of choice in most tentorial and anterior fossa dAVFs that are known to carry a significant risk for complications when managed endovascularly. Particularly, ethmoidal dAVFs were considered almost exclusively surgical lesions because of the danger of unintended embolization of the ophthalmic artery, inability to achieve a distal microcatheter position, and the relative ease of the surgical exposure and ligation of these lesions. Endovascular techniques and technology continue to evolve and, in selected patients, endovascular treatment may be an option. However, surgical ligation continues to have an important role in the management of these lesions.[21] There are various microsurgical management strategies proposed. Venous and arterial feeder anatomy is important in surgical decision making. Lesions in the anterior cranial fossa or around the foramen of magnum could be difficult for endovascular access, and dangerous anastomotic networks could make these lesions high risk for arterial embolization. Microsurgical clipping of the draining vein in such areas is a safe and feasible option. Combining microsurgery with presurgical arterial embolization results in a total occlusion rate of 87 to 100%. However, the treatment-related mortality and morbidity rates are still relatively high.[22,23] A variety of hybrid surgical/endovascular procedures have evolved as well, including surgical exposure for microcatheter embolization of the superior ophthalmic vein or petrosal vein for access to the cavernous and petrosal sinus, respectively.[24,25]

The major limitation of radiosurgery is the latency from treatment until cure. Until completion of vessel thrombosis, the hemorrhage risk remains elevated, and therefore, it is usually recommended only for dAVFs without evidence of cortical venous reflux and in locations that are difficult to reach (e.g., vein of Galen, tentorial incisura). In a systematic review of stereotactic radiosurgery (SRS) for dAVFs, complete obliteration was observed in 56 and 75% of patients with and without cortical venous reflux, respectively.[4] SRS may be an excellent and safe adjunctive therapy for inaccessible or incompletely treated dAVFs. In a recent multicenter study, the results following Gamma Knife radiosurgery (GKRS) of cerebral dAVFs demonstrated an effective obliteration rate of 68.4%. Female sex, absent venous ectasia, and carotid cavernous sinus location were predictors of post-GKRS dAVF obliteration. A middle fossa or tentorial location and mean peripheral radiation dose greater than 23 Gy were predictors of unfavorable outcome.[26]

Recurrence following initial angiographic cure of dAVF is not uncommon. Incomplete penetration of the embolic material into the proximal portion of the venous outlet may lead to late recurrence. Hence, it is essential to follow these patients closely with serial angiography for the first 2 years.[27]

10.7 Summary

1. Understanding of the natural history of dAVFs is of utmost importance to appropriately manage dAVFs.
2. The clinical presentation and the angioarchitecture of these lesions are key in developing a suitable treatment plan.
3. Conventional cerebral angiography remains the gold standard to rule out and evaluate a dAVF.
4. The aggressive natural history of dAVF with cortical venous drainage who present with hemorrhage or other associated neurological deficit warrant treatment.

5. Treatment is also advisable in asymptomatic fistulas with cortical venous drainage.
6. Dural AVF without aggressive features may be treated if they develop intolerable symptoms. Changes in symptoms should prompt angiographic reassessment.

References

[1] Kim DJ, terBrugge K, Krings T, Willinsky R, Wallace C. Spontaneous angiographic conversion of intracranial dural arteriovenous shunt: long-term follow-up in nontreated patients. Stroke. 2010; 41(7):1489–1494

[2] Gross BA, Du R. The natural history of cerebral dural arteriovenous fistulae. Neurosurgery. 2012; 71:594–602; discussion -3

[3] Bulters DO, Mathad N, Culliford D, Millar J, Sparrow OC. The natural history of cranial dural arteriovenous fistulae with cortical venous reflux: the significance of venous ectasia. Neurosurgery. 2012; 70(2):312–318, discussion 318–319

[4] Chen CJ, Lee CC, Ding D, et al. Stereotactic radiosurgery for intracranial dural arteriovenous fistulas: a systematic review. J Neurosurg. 2015; 122(2):353–362

[5] Borden JA, Wu JK, Shucart WA. A proposed classification for spinal and cranial dural arteriovenous fistulous malformations and implications for treatment. J Neurosurg. 1995; 82(2):166–179

[6] Cognard C, Gobin YP, Pierot L, et al. Cerebral dural arteriovenous fistulas: clinical and angiographic correlation with a revised classification of venous drainage. Radiology 1995;194(3):671–680

[7] Davies MA, TerBrugge K, Willinsky R, Coyne T, Saleh J, Wallace MC. The validity of classification for the clinical presentation of intracranial dural arteriovenous fistulas. J Neurosurg 1996;85(5):830–837

[8] Duffau H, Lopes M, Janosevic V, et al. Early rebleeding from intracranial dural arteriovenous fistulas: report of 20 cases and review of the literature. J Neurosurg. 1999; 90(1):78–84

[9] Gandhi D, Chen J, Pearl M, Huang J, Gemmete JJ, Kathuria S. Intracranial dural arteriovenous fistulas: classification, imaging findings, and treatment. AJNR Am J Neuroradiol. 2012; 33(6):1007–1013

[10] Sorkin GC, Hopkins LN. Endovascular role in dural arteriovenous fistula management. World Neurosurg. 2013; 80(6):e219–e220

[11] Elhammady MS, Wolfe SQ, Ashour R, et al. Safety and efficacy of vascular tumor embolization using Onyx: is angiographic devascularization sufficient? J Neurosurg. 2010; 112(5):1039–1045

[12] Hu YC, Newman CB, Dashti SR, Albuquerque FC, McDougall CG. Cranial dural arteriovenous fistula: transarterial Onyx embolization experience and technical nuances. J Neurointerv Surg. 2011; 3(1):5–13

[13] Nyberg EM, Chaudry MI, Turk AS, Turner RD. Transient cranial neuropathies as sequelae of Onyx embolization of arteriovenous shunt lesions near the skull base: possible axonometric traction injuries. J Neurointerv Surg. 2013; 5 (4):e21

[14] Cognard C, Januel AC, Silva NA, Jr, Tall P. Endovascular treatment of intracranial dural arteriovenous fistulas with cortical venous drainage: new management using Onyx. AJNR Am J Neuroradiol. 2008; 29(2):235–241

[15] Torok CM, Nogueira RG, Yoo AJ, et al. Transarterial venous sinus occlusion of dural arteriovenous fistulas using ONYX. Interventional Neuroradiology. 2016; 22:711–716

[16] Tsai LK, Jeng JS, Liu HM, Wang HJ, Yip PK. Intracranial dural arteriovenous fistulas with or without cerebral sinus thrombosis: analysis of 69 patients. J Neurol Neurosurg Psychiatry. 2004; 75(11):1639–1641

[17] Piske RL, Campos CM, Chaves JB, et al. Dural sinus compartment in dural arteriovenous shunts: a new angioarchitectural feature allowing superselective transvenous dural sinus occlusion treatment. AJNR Am J Neuroradiol. 2005; 26(7):1715–1722

[18] Urtasun F, Biondi A, Casaco A, et al. Cerebral dural arteriovenous fistulas: percutaneous transvenous embolization. Radiology. 1996; 199(1):209–217

[19] Roy D, Raymond J. The role of transvenous embolization in the treatment of intracranial dural arteriovenous fistulas. Neurosurgery. 1997; 40(6):1133–1141, discussion 1141–1144

[20] Olteanu-Nerbe V, Uhl E, Steiger H-J, Yousry T, Reulen H-J. Dural arteriovenous fistulas including the transverse and sigmoid sinuses: results of treatment in 30 cases. Acta Neurochir (Wien). 1997; 139(4):307–318

[21] Cannizzaro D, Peschillo S, Cenzato M, et al. Endovascular and surgical approaches of ethmoidal dural fistulas: a multicenter experience and a literature review. Neurosurg Rev. 2018; 41(2):391–398

[22] Kakarla UK, Deshmukh VR, Zabramski JM, Albuquerque FC, McDougall CG, Spetzler RF. Surgical treatment of high-risk intracranial dural arteriovenous fistulae: clinical outcomes and avoidance of complications. Neurosurgery. 2007; 61(3):447–457, discussion 457–459

[23] Piippo A, Niemelä M, van Popta J, et al. Characteristics and long-term outcome of 251 patients with dural arteriovenous fistulas in a defined population. J Neurosurg. 2013; 118(5):923–934

[24] Quiñones D, Duckwiler G, Gobin PY, Goldberg RA, Viñuela F. Embolization of dural cavernous fistulas via superior ophthalmic vein approach. AJNR Am J Neuroradiol. 1997; 18(5):921–928

[25] Houdart E, Saint-Maurice JP, Chapot R, et al. Transcranial approach for venous embolization of dural arteriovenous fistulas. J Neurosurg. 2002; 97(2):280–286

[26] Starke RM, McCarthy DJ, Chen CJ, et al. Evaluation of stereotactic radiosurgery for cerebral dural arteriovenous fistulas in a multicenter international consortium. J Neurosurg. 2019 Jan 4; 132(1):114–121

[27] Ambekar S, Gaynor BG, Peterson EC, Elhammady MS. Long-term angiographic results of endovascularly "cured" intracran dural arteriovenous fistulas. J Neurosurg. 2016; 124(4):1123–1127

10

11 Vein of Galen Malformations

Lekhaj C. Daggubati, Jeffrey Watkins, and Kenneth C. Liu

Abstract

Vein of Galen aneurysmal malformations (VGAMs) are rare congenital intracranial vascular malformations with high mortality and morbidity, which have been a challenge to treat. They represent 30% of pediatric vascular lesions. Symptoms vary by severity and patient's age. In neonates, the primary presentation is high-output heart failure; in infants, neurological deficits and hydrocephalus are the presenting symptoms. In older children and adults, headache and mental delay are the typical symptoms. Treatment focuses on symptom management with reversal of vascular shunting to physiological equilibrium. The treatment paradigm has shifted from microsurgical to endovascular with the advancement of new technologies. This chapter recounts the natural history and advances in treatment for VGAMs.

Keywords: vein of Galen aneurysmal malformation, management, cardiac failure, endovascular treatment, median prosencephalic vein of Markowski, hydrocephalus

11.1 Goals

1. Describe the embryologic origin of vein of Galen aneurysmal malformations (VGAMs).
2. Detail the age-related presentations of symptomatic VGAMs.
3. Review the literature on the advancement of treatments in VGAM.
4. Review the management of VGAM based on age-related symptoms.

11.2 Case Example

11.2.1 History of Present Illness

A 5-month-old boy presented a recently discovered VGAM with a witnessed complex partial seizure. The patient was back to baseline after 2 minutes of unresponsiveness. He was being followed up earlier for increasing head circumference, and a nonurgent cranial ultrasound revealed a VGAM.

Past medical history: None.
Past surgical history: Previous circumcision.
Family history: Denies history of cerebrovascular pathology.
Social history: Lives with family.
Review of systems: As per the above.
Neurological examination: Head circumference 49 cm (90%), otherwise unremarkable.
Imaging studies: Cranial ultrasound. See ▶ Fig. 11.1.

11.2.2 Treatment Plan

With the patient's symptomatic VGAM, he was taken to have a transarterial diagnostic cerebral angiogram for VGAM classification. Subsequently, a staged approach for a transarterial Onyx embolization of the various anterior and posterior circulation feeders was planned. After successful embolization of the various arterial feeders, the venous enlargement was treated with coils and Onyx (▶ Fig. 11.2).

11.2.3 Follow-up

The patient performed well through the various stages of transarterial embolizations. During his last transvenous embolization,

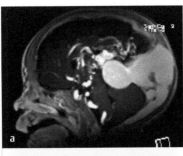
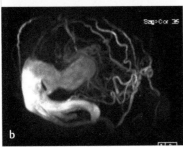
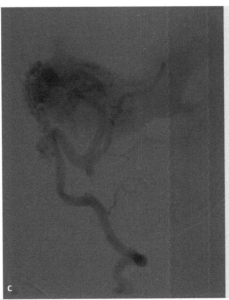

Fig. 11.1 Magnetic resonance angiography (MRA) of the brain (**a,b**) and angiogram (**c**) of the vein of Galen aneurysmal malformation (VGAM). VGAM is receiving supply from the pericallosal artery and bilateral posterior cerebral artery (PCA).

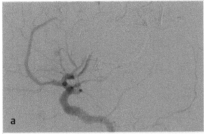
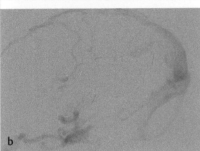
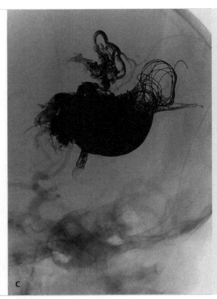

Fig. 11.2 Angiography **(a)** and magnetic resonance imaging (MRI) **(b)** after the endovascular transarterial and transvenous treatment of the vein of Galen aneurysmal malformation (VGAM) with Onyx and coils. The patient underwent six stepwise treatments ranging from age 10 to 15 months. **(c)** Unsubstracted angiogram demonstrating the coil mass and Onyx cast following treatment.

the patient suffered worsening seizures secondary to an intracranial hemorrhage post coiling of the venous enlargement. He did not require any surgical intervention and went home with his parents. Interval follow-up showed good adaptation and continued achievement of appropriate developmental milestones. At the 1-year follow-up, he had a successfully treated VGAM on repeat diagnostic cerebral angiogram.

11.3 Case Summary

1. *What is the embryological origin of VGAM?*
   a) VGAMs are congenital vascular malformations that form during the generation of primitive vasculature of the brain parenchyma. Though commonly called a vein of Galen malformation, it is actually a failed regression of the medial prosencephalic vein of Markowski (mProV of Markowski).[1] Between weeks 10 and 11 of development, the primary arterial flow shifts from the choroidal arteries to the cortical arteries; this results in the formation of the paired internal cerebral veins that connect to the posterior mProV of Markowski. With decreased flow, the anterior portion involutes. A residual arterial shunt, usually from the anterior choroidal, posterior choroidal, and anterior cerebral arteries, causes the failed involution of the anterior mProV of Markowski and the subsequent dilation into a VGAM.[2,3]

2. *What are the different symptomatic presentations of VGAM?*
   a) The symptoms for a VGAM patient are largely determined by age and the severity of the VGAM. The presentations are divided into neonates, infants, and older children/adults.
   b) Neonates
      1. Neonates already have a disproportionate distribution of blood flow to the brain, but the additional high-flow, low-resistance VGAM sequesters as much as 80% of the cardiac output.[4] Quiet and initially controlled by the presence of the placenta, another low-resistance system, the VGAM presents postpartum and is worsened by a patent ductus arteriosus and/or patent foramen ovale.[5] The increased venous return causes pulmonary hypertension, and arterial steal with increased cardiac demand causes myocardial infarctions.[6,7]
   c) Infants
      1. The presenting signs in an infant are hydrocephalus and macrocephaly. The robust deep cerebral venous drainage can keep primitive occipital and marginal sinuses patent and cause hypoplastic galenic veins.[8] This causes venous hypertension and subsequently intracranial hypertension. Though the dilated vein of Galen may cause communicating hydrocephalus, the hydrocephalus associated with VGAM is typically a noncommunicating hydrocephalus, secondary by the decreased hydrovenous equilibrium. The intracranial hypertension and venous hypertension can cause impaired cortical development, calcifications, and epilepsy.[1,9]
   d) Older children/Adults
      1. Quiescent VGAMs may present out of infancy with seizures, headaches, or intracranial hemorrhages.[8] These are usually smaller and less severe, but could be associated with flow-related microaneurysms.[5]

3. *What are the different classifications of VGAM? (▶ Fig. 11.3)*
   a) Lasjaunias grouped VGAMs in three forms. Mural and choroidal are the true VGAMs: Mural type has distinct direct arterial connections to the wall of the mProV of Markowski while choroidal type has many choroidal arteries forming a nidus that drains into the mProV of Markowski. The secondary VGAM is from high flow of a deep arteriovenous malformation (AVM).[10]
   b) Yasargil categorized VGAMs by the arterial feeder pattern. Type 1 are direct fistulas from the pericallosal or posterior cerebral arteries. Type 2 is supplied by the thalamoperforator arteries. Type 3 has multiple fistulas from Type 1 and 2 supplying the VGAM. Type 4 is a flow-related false VGAM formed by a deep AVM. Similar to Lasjaunias, Yasargil distinguishes Type 1 to 3 as the true VGAMs.[11]

4. *What is the gold standard for neuroimaging of the VGAM? What other tests should be ordered?*

11

Vein of Galen Aneurysmal Malformation (VGAM) Classification Systems			
Lasjaunias		**Yasargil**	
True VGAM		*True VGAM*	
Choroidal	Multiple feeders from thalamoperforating, chorodial and pericallosal arteries	1	Few direct Fistulas from the Pericallosal and Posterior Cerebral Artery
Mural	Single or few fistula(s) into the MProsV of Markowski	2	Few direct fistulas from the thalamoperforating arterial feeders to the MProsV of Markowski
		3	Multiple fistulous connection to the MProsV of Markowski with a nidus-like formation proximal to the vein
AVM related Secondary VGAM		*AVM related Secondary VGAM*	
Secondary	Vein of Galen dilation due to a Parenchymal deep arteriovenous malformation	4	Vein of Galen dilation due to a Parenchymal deep arteriovenous malformation

Fig. 11.3 The right side shows the four-group Yasargil classification, while the left side shows the three-group Lasjaunias classification.

a) The gold standard is a diagnostic cerebral angiogram. However, a transfontanelle ultrasound, computed tomography angiography (CTA), and magnetic resonance angiography/venography (MRA/MRV) are all part of the initial work-up to diagnose a VGAM.[12] In addition, an electroencephalogram, echocardiogram, and liver and renal function tests should be checked for seizures, myocardial infarction, and liver and renal perfusion injuries, respectively.[13]

5. *What is the current management algorithm for VGAMs?*
   a) Neonates—Symptomatic
      1. The goal of intervention is to stabilize high-output cardiac failure and other end-organ damage until infancy for more definitive intervention. Diuretics, inotropic agents, and vasodilators are used for symptomatic control.[1,5] If unsuccessful, emergent embolization is carried out just enough to control the cardiac failure and attain organ equilibrium.[12] Unfortunately, neonates with severe cardiogenic shock, end-organ damage, or significant brain damage are not offered intervention. The Bicêtre neonatal evaluation score is to direct management; a score of below 8 is deemed futile, 8 to 12 will get emergent embolization of physiological stability, and above 12 will get medical management until 4 to 5 months of age.[12]
   b) Infancy—Symptomatic
      1. The endovascular treatments are limited until 6 months of age, until the infant is old enough to withstand the endovascular procedure. The goal of intervention is to normalize the hydrovenous equilibrium to physiological levels. A combination of n-butyl cyanoacrylate and Onyx is used in a stepwise fashion. Zerah et al discovered that hydrocephalus is reversed in VGAMs once hydrovenous equilibrium is achieved. Sixty-six percent of nonshunt VGAMs as opposed to 33% of shunt VGAMs were neurologically normal.[9]

c) *Older children/Adults—Symptomatic*
   1. When discovered later in life, VGAMs can be treated immediately. Except for mild headaches, which could be asymptomatic, patients presenting with a hemorrhage or neurological deficits need treatment to minimize the vascular steal.
d) Asymptomatic
   1. Neurological delays can occur in asymptomatic and incidentally found VGAMs. Patients should be carefully monitored for deficits through neurocognitive assessments.

6. *What is the mortality and morbidity of the different treatment modalities?*
   a) Initially, treatment was done through microsurgery, which had poor outcomes, with Gold et al experiencing 100% mortality in nine neonates. Until endovascular techniques became available, mortality was commonly close to 100%. Early embolization treatment had 50% mortality, but with the advent of better embolic material and improved medical care, Lasjaunias et al's series in 2006 of 233 patients had a morality of 10.6% and normal neurological development in 74% of survivors.[12,14] Payne et al published an eight-patient series in 2000 for VGAMs treated with gamma knife radiosurgery. His treatment dosage ranged from 17 to 50 Gy, with a maximum size of 8.0 cm^3. Results showed 50% did not have filling, remainder had decreased filling, and none of the patients had nonreversible complications.[15]

11.4 Level of Evidence[16]

Microsurgical treatment: Microsurgical treatment of VGAMs is associated with excess of morbidity and mortality compared to endovascular treatment (Class III, Level of Evidence B—non-randomized).

Endovascular treatment: Endovascular treatment should be initiated at 5 months of age, unless deemed emergent in neonates, in a stepwise fashion to achieve hydrovenous equilibrium (Class I, Level of Evidence B—nonrandomized).

Hydrocephalus: Shunting of patients with hydrocephalus in VGAMs is potentially harmful unless it is a life-threatening situation (Class III, Level of Evidence C).

11.5 Landmark Papers

Boldrey E, Miller ER. Arteriovenous fistula (aneurysm) of the great cerebral vein (of Galen) and the circle of Willis: report of two treated patients. Trans Am Neurol Assoc 1948;73(73 Annual Meet.):122–124.

In 1948, Boldrey and Miller were the first to surgically treat two patients with aneurysms of the vein of Galen.[17] In case one, a 16-month-old patient with progressive head enlargement and papilledema was discovered to have a large vein of Galen aneurysm with enlarged right posterior communicating and posterior cerebral arteries. The patient was treated with right common carotid artery ligation. The result was resolution of papilledema and normalized head circumference. A postligation angiogram showed no filling of the fistula and once confirmed, the posterior cerebral artery was clipped. Three years postintervention, the patient's development was normal. In case two, a 15-year old presented with right eye exophthalmos and an audible bruit. Angiogram showed a fistulous connection between dilated posterior communicating and posterior cerebral arteries with a bulbous great vein. The right internal and external arteries were ligated, the venous engorgement disappeared, and bruit was reduced without neurological deficits.

Boldrey and Miller were the first to publish the diagnosis using carotid angiography and treatment of vein of Galen dilation. Prior to this, vein of Galen dilations were only described in cadavers and incidental intraoperative discovery. They attributed to the findings to cerebral AVMs and argued bruits, macrocephaly, and pineal gland calcification should be examined for AVMs. Recent reviews note that only one of the cases was likely a true VGAM; nonetheless, they were the first to intervene on VGAMs and more importantly, show restoration of normal cerebrovascular physiology with treatment.

Gold A, Ransohoff J, Carter S. Vein of Galen aneurysm malformation. Acta Neurol Scand Suppl 1964;40(Suppl 11):1.

In 1964, Gold et al presented a review of literature with 8 patients from the Columbia-Presbyterian Medical Center in New York and 35 previously published cases.[18] They defined that an AVM of the vein of Galen occurs when "one or more branches of the carotid or vertebral circulation communicates directly with this vein." The authors acknowledged it as a unique entity with congenital end-to-end anastomosis and a network of poorly differentiated noncapillary vessels between the artery and vein.

Reviewing the available literature, Gold et al found three major subsets of symptomatic VGAMs. Early neonates presented with marked deficits in cardiovascular function, often with cyanosis and respiratory distress. Gold and his colleagues suggested that in neonates, the shunt is of such severe magnitude that it

elicited peripheral congestion and congestive heart failure; none of the neonates survived. In contrast to neonates, infants presented primarily with hydrocephalus, convulsions, and distension of scalp veins. In infants, the shunt is of lesser magnitude than in neonates, such that it resulted in marked dilation of the vein of Galen and cerebral compression. Cerebral compression resulted in a diversity of clinical presentations, but included hydrocephalus, convulsions, psychomotor retardation, cardiomegaly, papilledema, and harsh intracranial bruits. In late childhood or adulthood, the patients typically presented with headaches and central nervous system (CNS) dysfunction. These include convulsions, paresis, ataxia, aphasia, cranial nerve palsies, ocular disturbances, and subarachnoid hemorrhage. Finally, X-rays of the skull in the oldest group showed concentric calcification in the wall of the VGAM.

Gold and his colleagues established a consistent definition for VGAMs and related their functional hemodynamics, rather than anatomic similarities, to the clinical presentations. In addition, these symptoms correlated with three major age groups and started invaluable evaluation of VGAMs through age-associated severity and clinical findings.

Hoffman HJ, Chuang S, Hendrick EB, Humphreys RP. Aneurysms of the vein of Galen. Experience at The Hospital for Sick Children, Toronto. J Neurosurg 1982;57(3):316–322.

Hoffman et al reviewed the clinical course and management of 128 patients from 1937 to 1981 with an aneurysm of the vein of Galen.[19] Utilizing Gold's findings, Hoffman's 128 patients were divided into 45 neonates, 36 infants, and 47 older children and adults; moreover, 43 of 45 neonates presented with heart failure, 33 of 36 infants with hydrocephalus, and 18 of 47 adults with subarachnoid hemorrhage. Fifty-four of these patients were treated surgically. More importantly, Hoffman et al published the largest series of patients with 29 from 1950 to 1980 at The Hospital for Sick Children. Of this series, 16 were neonates, 8 were infants, and 5 were older children.

Overall, untreated patients did very poorly and none were reported as normal. Of those treated, most were through carotid ligation; 26 of the 54 treated patients were considered normal. In the single site series, 5 of 16 treated patients were considered normal and only 10 of 29 total patients survived. Notably, treatment was morbid in the neonate population with only 1 of 16 surviving on follow-up.

In Hoffman et al's review, neonates had the worst prognosis. Therefore, the authors suggest they require early treatment to avoid aneurysmal stealing of blood and subsequent cerebral infarction. In addition, early treatment was crucial to eliminate the hemodynamic abnormalities contributing to myocardial ischemia and infarction. Hoffman claimed that, instead of excision, like in AVMS, simple occlusion was sufficient to convert a malformed vein of Galen into a physiologically normal vein. Hoffman et al were the first to suggest favorable outcomes from the treatment of VGAMs for a significant part of the population.

Lasjaunias P, Rodesch G, Pruvost P, Laroche FG, Landrieu P. Treatment of vein of Galen aneurysmal malformation. J Neurosurg 1989;70(5):746–750.

In 1989, Lasjaunias reported the treatment of a VGAM in a 1-year-old baby with macrocephaly and divergent strabismus with the first endovascular treatment for VGAMs.[10] Initially with normal birth and cardiovascular and neurological development, the infant was found to have an intracranial bruit. Plan

11

skull X-ray revealed craniofacial dysmorphism, without signs of intracranial hypertension, pathological calcification, or posterior fossa abnormalities. The VGAM was found on follow-up CT and magnetic resonance imaging (MRI) and confirmed on subsequent cerebral angiography.

One week after the diagnosis, the VGAM was completely embolized through a left femoral approach, with occlusion of the artery and a reduction of VGAM flow. At 4-month follow-up, angiography confirmed the resolution of the AV fistula and demonstrated shrinkage of the torcular dilation. Clinically, the patient was neurologically normal. The authors argue that VGAMs are a therapeutic challenge due to their deep location and severe symptoms and urged the clinicians to consider arterial embolization as the primary treatment choice.

Lasjaunias P, Rodesch G, Terbrugge K, et al. Vein of Galen aneurysmal malformations: report of 36 cases managed between 1982 and 1988. Acta Neurochir (Wien) 1989;99(1–2):26–37.

Lasjaunias et al reported a series of 36 VGAM patients managed between 1982 and 1988 at Bicêtre Hospital.[20] These VGAMs ranged a variety of symptoms including systemic manifestations (36%), neurological symptoms (22%), hydrocephaly (17%), and intracranial hemorrhage (11%). In addition, the authors evaluated the angioarchitecture and natural or posttherapeutic history of the VGAMs.

VGAM was more commonly symptomatic in the pediatric population. However, isolated neurological signs and hemorrhage correlate more closely with adult symptomatology as no patient older than 15 years presented with systemic symptoms. Of the 36 patients, 30 angioarchitectural analyses were obtained. The authors classified VGAMs into five different subtypes. Mural arteriovenous fistulas (AVFs) (20% of total) and choroidal fissure AVFs (30% of total) were more common in neonates and infants, whereas parenchymal (44% of total), dural AVFs (3% of total), and vein of Galen varices (7% of total) were usually associated with late childhood or even adulthood. Patients were treated surgically, endovascularly, or not at all. Among the 36 patients, 6 passed away; of these, two were treated surgically, two were treated endovascularly, and two were too futile for any treatment. This represents a 13% mortality rate for embolized patient, significantly better than historical surgical prognosis (91% mortality in neonates, 38% in infants).

In this landmark series, Lasjaunias et al concluded that endovascular treatment of VGAM results in superior outcomes. Also, they differentiated VGAMs into five subtypes and associated them with different age groups. Historically, VGAMs carried high morbidity and mortality; however, Lasjaunias et al claimed that certain subtypes (mural or choroidal AVF) can probably be cured with appropriate diagnosis and treatment. Contrary to the leading practice of the time, Lasjaunias et al found cerebral tissue damage or uncontrollable systemic failure to be contraindications to treatment. Therefore, they assert that treatment is only indicated when there is a possibility to compensate for systemic failure that previously responded to maximal medical treatment.

Zerah M, Garcia-Monaco R, Rodesch G, et al. Hydrodynamics in vein of Galen malformations. Childs Nerv Syst 1992;8(3):111–117.

In 1992, Zerah et al published a series of 43 patients with VGAM seen between 1985 and 1990 and reviewed an additional 335 cases in literature.[9] These cases were reviewed with particular attention paid to the hydrodynamics associated with shunting. Similar to other literature, the patients in this series were categorized by age (prenatal [12%], newborn [50%], infant [19%], and child [16%]), and presenting symptoms (heart failure [26%], hydrocephalus/macrocephaly [15%], hemorrhage [1%], and clinical deterioration [1%]).

In addition to reviewing the cases, the authors explored several theories that could explain the development of hydrocephalus in VGAM. Zerah et al supported the hypothesis that increased venous pressure is the primary cause of VGAM hydrocephalus. They hypothesized that increased venous pressure inhibits cerebrospinal fluid (CSF) flow from the subarachnoid space into the venous system. Fifty percent of VGAM patients presented with macrocrania. In their experience, ventricular drainage of CSF through shunting worsened the complications associated with increased venous pressure. After shrinking the ventricles, the venous malformation enlarges to fill the potential space. Zerah et al considered embolization to be the best method of reducing the venous pressure and restoring the hydrovenous equilibrium and that VP shunting be avoided in order to prevent clinical deterioration.

Lasjaunias PL, Chng SM, Sachet M, Alvarez H, Rodesch G, Garcia-Monaco R. The management of vein of Galen aneurysmal malformations. Neurosurgery 2006; 59(5, Suppl 3)S184–S194.

In 2006, Lasjaunias et al presented a 20-year review of 317 patients with VGAM at the Hôpital de Bicêtre.[12] Of these, 233 (74%) were treated with endovascular embolization, 67 (21%) were deferred for treatment for a variety of reasons, and 17 (5%) were lost to follow-up. As a first-line treatment, the authors chose transarterial embolization using n-butylcyanoacrylate glue as the embolic agent with a goal to preserving normal development and avoiding neurologic deficits. A total or near total (90–100%) occlusion of the VGAM was obtained in 55% of the patients; only 6.2% of patients had an obliteration rate of less than 50%. Patients were followed up with clinical examination every year and MRI every 2 years. In their series, 74% of surviving patients were neurologically normal. Only 2% experienced permanent neurological disability.

With the largest series of VGAMs, Lasjaunias was able to provide multiple important observations. First, the angioarchitecture of an individual patient should direct the treatment decision. Fistulas involving the choroidal arteries and an interposed vascular network before opening into the vein of Galen tend to be more severe and correlate with poorer outcomes, thus lending themselves to earlier treatment. On the contrary, mural fistulas are direct AV fistulas and tend to be better tolerated. Second, there exists a "therapeutic window" in which endovascular treatment is optimized based on the evolution of clinical manifestations as outlined in the literature. Third, treatment should be stratified based on age and specific medical complications. Treatment should focus on restoration of physiological flow. Finally, contrary to the previous thought, a majority of children treated endovascularly survive and maintain normal neurological development.

Lasjaunias was among the first to combine clinical, anatomical, and pathophysiological aspects of VGAM to predict disease evolution and guide management decisions. From the series, the Bicêtre Neonatal Evaluation Score (▶ Table 11.1) was created to lead best management of neonatal VGAMs. Their data showed

11

Table 11.1 Bicêtre neonatal evaluation score[†]

Points	Cardiac function	Cerebral function	Respiratory function	Hepatic function	Renal function
5	Normal	Normal	Normal		
4	Overload, no medical treatment	Subclinical, isolated EEG abnormalities	Tachypnea finishes bottle		
3	Failure, stable with medical treatment	Nonconvulsive intermittent neurologic signs	Tachypnea does not finish bottle	No hepatomegaly, normal hepatic function	Normal
2	Failure, not stable with medical treatment	Isolated convulsions	Assisted ventilation, normal saturation FiO2 <25%	Hepatomegaly, normal hepatic function	Transient anuria
1	Ventilation necessary	Seizures	Assisted ventilation, normal saturation FiO2 >25%	Moderate or transient hepatic insufficiency	Unstable diuresis with treatment
0	Resistant to medical therapy	Permanent neurological signs	Assisted ventilation, desaturation	Abnormal coagulation, elevated enzymes	Anuria

[†] Score: Cardiac (5) + Cerebral (5) + Respiratory (5) + Hepatic (3) + Renal Function (3) = Maximal Score (21).
Interpretation: <8 Futile for intervention; 8–12 Emergent Endovascular Therapy; >12 Medical Treatment with Endovascular intervention at 5 months of age.
*Reviewed using the 2014 ACC/AHA Clinical Practice Guideline.
Source: Adapted from Lasjaunias et al.[1,2]

that patient selection and therapeutic timing are keys to successful outcomes.

Li AH, Armstrong D, terBrugge KG. Endovascular treatment of vein of Galen aneurysmal malformation: management strategy and 21-year experience in Toronto. J Neurosurg Pediatr 2011;7 (1):3–10.

In this study, the investigators reviewed the 21-year history of VGAM outcomes and considered factors that potentially affect survival and neurocognitive development at the Toronto Sick Children Hospital.[21] From 1984 to 2005, 26 patients with VGAM were managed by their group. The survival rate in this series was 76.9%. Based on the guidelines proposed by the team at Hôpital de Bicêtre, 21 patients were treated with endovascular embolization. Five patients were excluded from the treatment for minimal symptoms or severe comorbidities. Fourteen of the 21 endovascularly treated patients showed normal development. Of those with developmental delay, the patient's age at treatment was significantly higher than those who did not develop deficits.

Three main factors were associated with a poor prognosis: major comorbidities, failure of the embolization procedure, and the lack of the procedure's long-term effect as determined by clinical deterioration. The findings supported the Bicêtre strategy, with particular focus on the health of the brain, heart, kidneys, and liver. In addition, compared to transvenous embolization, open operation, and radiosurgery, transarterial intervention provided higher efficacy and lower morbidity.

In this series, Li et al found that a strategic approach to VGAM management led to long-term survival rate of more than 90% in infants and children and further validated the Bicêtre results. The authors looked at "experience-year equivalent" to account for any learning curve in their management expertise. There was no significant difference in experience-year equivalent among patients who survived to those who did not.

11.6 Recommendations

Still a rare congenital pathology, VGAM treatment has been slowly evolving. Since its definition by Gold et al, the treatment of VGAM has shifted from open microsurgical to endovascular

embolization as first-line treatment. In addition, medical management, gamma knife radiosurgery, and microsurgery still have an adjuvant role.[12,15] Medical management is primarily used to stabilize cardiac, hepatic, and renal function and temporize system complications until the therapeutic window can be achieved. This is accomplished through diuretics, vasodilators, and inotropic agents and should be directed by a pediatric cardiologist or a pediatric intensivist.[22] The goal of treatment is restoration of hemodynamic balance to allow for normal neurocognitive growth. Many symptoms, such as hydrocephalus, resolve with restoration of normal hydrodynamic flow, and thus, shunting should be avoided.[9] When embolization attempts fail, microsurgery or, to a lesser degree, gamma knife radiosurgery remains as a potential option. Finally, the therapeutic window minimizes complications, promotes normal cerebral maturation, and maximizes therapeutic benefit. Lasjaunias and colleagues defined the therapeutic window as 4 to 5 months of age, except in emergent circumstance to stabilize neonates.

11.6.1 Management by Age

Clinical presentation and management guidelines have typically been categorized into four groups. Antepartum diagnosis of VGAM is becoming increasingly common through the widespread use of ultrasonography and fetal MRI.[23,24] Uncomplicated VGAM is not an indication for termination of pregnancy or early induction. However, VGAM with concurrent heart failure and/or cerebral damage has been associated with high mortality rates and therefore may be appropriate for termination.

Neonates often have the most severe clinical picture and present with heart failure, cyanosis, and respiratory distress. Consequently, this group of patients also has the worst outcomes. In an attempt to address this disparity, Lasjaunias and collaborators were the first to propose a score (Bicêtre Neonatal Evaluation Score) to guide neonatal management. This scoring system accounts for cardiac, cerebral, respiratory, hepatic, and renal function. In their experience, a score of less than 8 indicates extensive comorbid conditions and results in a decision to abstain from treatment. A score between 8 and 12 indicates that emergency endovascular treatment should be performed.

11

A score more than 12 indicates that a patient is relatively stable and should be managed medically until they reach 5 months of age.[12]

Infants typically present with neurological manifestations including hydrocephalus, seizures, psychomotor retardation, and developmental delay. Thus, therapeutic management of infants depends largely on their age of presentation and the degree of their symptoms. Typically, when symptoms are present, intervention is necessitated.

Older children and adults most commonly present with headaches or intracranial hemorrhage. Hemorrhage can result in more marked CNS disturbances including CN palsies, aphasia, and ataxia. Treatment should be done to prevent neurocognitive decline or rehemorrhage.

Treatment may be guided by these recommendations, observational studies, and the Bicêtre Neonatal Evaluation Score, but, as always, treatment decisions should be individualized to each patient's circumstances.

11.7 Summary

1. VGAMs are rare congenital vascular malformations that were initially high morbid but continue to have improved prognosis with endovascular treatment.
2. VGAMs commonly present at three age groups with three distinct clinical symptomologies based on VGAM severity.
3. Neonatal patients are managed medically until 5 months of age except in severe situations where temporization through endovascular treatment is undertaken in select patients. Some patients are deemed futile based on systemic organ failure.

References

[1] Gailloud P, O'Riordan DP, Burger I, et al. Diagnosis and management of vein of Galen aneurysmal malformations. J Perinatol. 2005; 25(8):542–551

[2] Raybaud CA, Strother CM, Hald JK. Aneurysms of the vein of Galen: embryonic considerations and anatomical features relating to the pathogenesis of the malformation. Neuroradiology. 1989; 31(2):109–128

[3] Horowitz MB, Jungreis CA, Quisling RG, Pollack I. Vein of Galen aneurysms: a review and current perspective. AJNR Am J Neuroradiol. 1994; 15(8):1486–1496

[4] King WA, Wackym PA, Viñuela F, Peacock WJ. Management of vein of Galen aneurysms: combined surgical and endovascular approach. Childs Nerv Syst. 1989; 5(4):208–211

[5] Hoang S, Choudhri O, Edwards M, Guzman R. Vein of Galen malformation. Neurosurg Focus. 2009; 27(5):E8

[6] Pellegrino PA, Milanesi O, Saia OS, Carollo C. Congestive heart failure secondary to cerebral arterio-venous fistula. Childs Nerv Syst. 1987; 3(3):141–144

[7] Chevret L, Durand P, Alvarez H, et al. Severe cardiac failure in newborns with VGAM: prognosis significance of hemodynamic parameters in neonates presenting with severe heart failure owing to vein of Galen arteriovenous malformation. Intensive Care Med. 2002; 28(8):1126–1130

[8] Krings T, Geibprasert S, Terbrugge K. Classification and endovascular management of pediatric cerebral vascular malformations. Neurosurg Clin N Am. 2010; 21(3):463–482

[9] Zerah M, Garcia-Monaco R, Rodesch G, et al. Hydrodynamics in vein of Galen malformations. Childs Nerv Syst. 1992; 8(3):111–117, discussion 117

[10] Lasjaunias P, Rodesch G, Pruvost P, Laroche FG, Landrieu P. Treatment of vein of Galen aneurysmal malformation. J Neurosurg. 1989; 70(5):746–750

[11] Yasargil MG, Antic J, Laciga R, Jain KK, Boone SC. Arteriovenous malformations of vein of Galen: microsurgical treatment. Surg Neurol. 1976(3):195–200

[12] Lasjaunias PL, Chng SM, Sachet M, Alvarez H, Rodesch G, Garcia-Monaco R. The management of vein of Galen aneurysmal malformations. Neurosurgery. 2006; 59(5) Suppl 3:S184–S194, discussion S3–S13

[13] Rodesch G, Hui F, Alvarez H, Tanaka A, Lasjaunias P. Prognosis of antenatally diagnosed vein of Galen aneurysmal malformations. Childs Nerv Syst. 1994; 10(2):79–83

[14] Friedman DM, Verma R, Madrid M, Wisoff JH, Berenstein A. Recent improvement in outcome using transcatheter embolization techniques for neonatal aneurysmal malformations of the vein of Galen. Pediatrics. 1993; 91(3):583–586

[15] Payne BR, Prasad D, Steiner M, Bunge H, Steiner L. Gamma surgery for vein of Galen malformations. J Neurosurg. 2000; 93(2):229–236

[16] Jacobs AK, Anderson JL, Halperin JL. The evolution and future of ACC/AHA clinical practice guidelines: a 30-year journey: a report of the American College of Cardiology/American Heart Association Task Force on Practice Guidelines. J Am Coll Cardiol. 2014; 64(13):1373–1384

[17] Boldrey E, Miller ER. Arteriovenous fistula (aneurysm) of the great cerebral vein of Galen and the circle of Willis: report of two treated patients. Trans Am Neurol Assoc. 1948; 73 73 Annual Meet.:122–124

[18] Gold A, Ransohoff J, Carter S. Vein of Galen aneurysm malformation. Acta Neurol Scand Suppl. 1964; 40 Suppl 11– 1–31

[19] Hoffman HJ, Chuang S, Hendrick EB, Humphreys RP. Aneurysms of the vein of Galen: experience at The Hospital for Sick Children, Toronto. J Neurosurg. 1982; 57(3):316–322

[20] Lasjaunias P, Rodesch G, Terbrugge K, et al. Vein of Galen aneurysmal malformations: report of 36 cases managed between 1982 and 1988. Acta Neurochir (Wien). 1989; 99(1–2):26–37

[21] Li AH, Armstrong D, terBrugge KG. Endovascular treatment of vein of Galen aneurysmal malformation: management strategy and 21-year experience in Toronto. J Neurosurg Pediatr. 2011; 7(1):3–10

[22] Recinos PF, Rahmathulla G, Pearl M, et al. Vein of Galen malformations: epidemiology, clinical presentations, management. Neurosurg Clin N Am. 2012; 23(1):165–177

[23] Nuutila M, Saisto T. Prenatal diagnosis of vein of Galen malformation: a multidisciplinary challenge. Am J Perinatol. 2008; 25(4):225–227

[24] Vintzileos AM, Eisenfeld LI, Campbell WA, Herson VC, DiLeo PE, Chameides L. Prenatal ultrasonic diagnosis of arteriovenous malformation of the vein of Galen. Am J Perinatol. 1986; 3(3):209–211

11

Section II

Ischemic Stroke

12 Mechanical Thrombectomy in Acute Ischemic Stroke

Matias Negrotto, Mithun Sattur, and Alejandro M. Spiotta

Abstract

Acute ischemic strokes are a devastating condition and represent 85% of all cerebrovascular accidents.[1] For every minute of delay in the treatment of ischemic stroke, 1.9 million cells die in the brain and 13.8 million synapses and 12 kilometers of axonal fibers are lost.[2]

Rapid advances in devices have propelled the evolution of mechanical thrombectomy over the past decade from rudimentary mechanical disruption and intra-arterial thrombolytic infusions to increasingly effective thrombectomy devices.

The initial thrombectomy trials[3,4,5,6] failed to demonstrate a benefit of mechanical thrombectomy over intravenous tissue plasminogen activator (tPA). More recently, multiple, large, multicenter trials validated the efficacy of mechanical thrombectomy with newer generations of thrombectomy devices.[7,8,9,10,11] These trials changed the paradigm of ischemic stroke treatment, clearly demonstrating the efficacy of endovascular treatment for stroke patients with large vessel occlusions.

Keywords: stroke, mechanical thrombectomy, landmark papers, evidence, large vessel occlusion

12.1 Goals

1. Review the literature that forms the basis of mechanical thrombectomy in acute ischemic stroke for large-vessel occlusion (LVO).
2. Critically analyze the steps to follow on stroke protocol and the decision for endovascular treatment.
3. Critically analyze the importance of imaging studies and its role in patient selection.

12.2 Case Example

12.2.1 History of Present Illness

A 63-year-old woman with a history of hypertension and hyperlipidemia presented with left-sided facial palsy, right gaze deviation, left-sided weakness, and a National Institutes of Health Stroke Scale (NIHSS) score of 12. The patient had a noncontrast computed tomography (NCCT), a CT angiogram (CTA), and CT perfusion of the brain. The NCCT demonstrated an Alberta Stroke Program Early CT score (ASPECTS) of 10. The CTA demonstrated a right M1 occlusion with poor collaterals (▶ Fig. 12.1) and the CT perfusion demonstrated a large area of ischemic penumbra with no infarct (▶ Fig. 12.2). Time from symptom onset was 90 minutes. The patient received intravenous (IV) recombinant tissue plasminogen activator (rTPA) and was transported to the angiography suite for mechanical thrombectomy.

12.2.2 Treatment Plan

Under conscious sedation, the right common femoral artery was accessed and a 9 F sheath was introduced. A right carotid arteriogram showed complete occlusion of the right M1 (▶ Fig. 12.3).

The thrombus was removed using a direct aspiration first pass technique (ADAPT). Control angiography demonstrated thrombolysis in cerebral infarction (TICI) 3, complete recanalization of the branch with normal anterograde flow (▶ Fig. 12.4).

12.2.3 Follow-up

The patient was transferred to the intensive care unit following the procedure. She made a complete recovery within 6 hours of the procedure and was subsequently discharged home following a short stay in the hospital.

12.3 Case Summary

1. *Which were the main objectives of NCCT?*

   The noncontrast CT Head is obtained to exclude other possible etiologies for the patient's symptoms. In addition, these initial scans may identify an LVO (hyperdense artery sign) and/or early signs of completed infarctions (loss of gray-white differentiation, gyrus effacement, etc.).

   Numerous studies have shown that the baseline central infarct size is a powerful predictor of ischemic stroke treatment outcomes. Although diffusion-weighted magnetic resonance imaging (MRI) is the most accurate method of

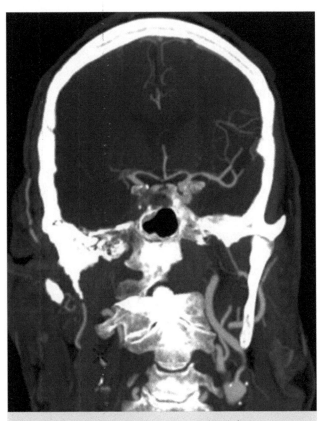

Fig. 12.1 Computed tomography angiogram (CTA) demonstrating right M1 occlusion.

12

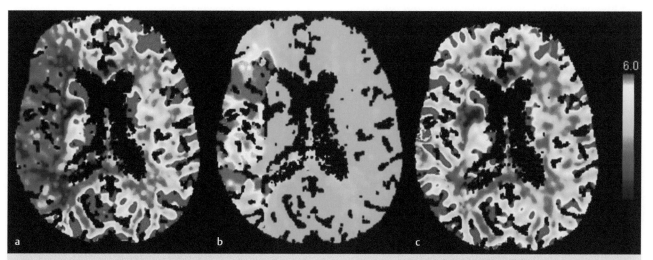

Fig. 12.2 Computed tomography (CT) perfusion cerebral blood flow (CBF) map demonstrating a region of decreased perfusion within the right middle cerebral artery (MCA) territory **(a)**. Mean transit time (MTT) map shows a corresponding prolongation within this region **(b)**. Cerebral blood volume (CBV) map demonstrates no abnormality **(c)**.

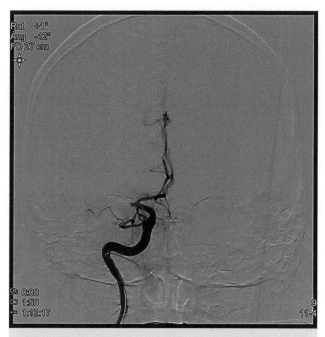

Fig. 12.3 Anteroposterior (AP) projections of the right internal carotid angiogram with occlusion of the right proximal M1 segment.

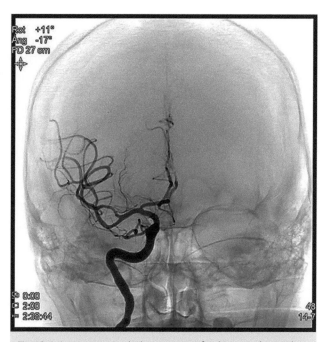

Fig. 12.4 Anteroposterior (AP) projections of right internal carotid angiogram demonstrating complete recanalization (thrombolysis in cerebral infarction [TICI] 3) with normal antegrade flow.

determining cerebral infarction, CT is still the most commonly used imaging modality due to its rapidity and availability.

ASPECTS is a favorable predictor of perfusion and is used for selection of candidates for thrombolytic and endovascular treatment.[12] This 10-point radiographic score is a semiquantitative classification system that improves the detection of ischemic changes. Elevated ASPECTS are significantly associated with improved functional outcomes, reduced mortality, and lower rates of symptomatic intracranial hemorrhage following thrombectomy, as well as a positive predictor of functional independence at 90 days.[13] The ASPECTS score is increasingly used due to its rapidity, simplicity, and reproducibility.[14]

ASPECTS segments the vascular territories of the middle cerebral artery and deducts one point for each affected territory.

- Caudate nucleus.
- Putamen.
- Internal capsule.
- Insular rim.
- M1: "anterior cortex of the middle cerebral artery (MCA)" corresponding to the frontal operculum.

12

- M2: "lateral cortex of MCA to the insular rim" corresponding to the anterior temporal lobe.
- M3: "posterior cortex of MCA" corresponding to posterior temporal lobe.
- M4: "territory of MCA immediately superior to M1."
- M5: "lateral territory immediately above M2."
- M6: "posterior territory immediately above M3."
  M1 to M3 are measured at the level of the basal ganglia, while the M4 to M6 territories are measured at the level of the lateral ventricles.[15]

2. *What are the main objectives of CTA?*
The CTA Head is obtained to determine the presence of an LVO and identify potential patients for mechanical thrombectomy.[16] In addition, it assesses the extent of the patient's collateral circulation, which plays an important role in maintaining the viability of tissues in the early hours of an ischemic stroke. CTA, rather than MRA, appears to be the most useful for the evaluation of cortical collaterals.[17] The prognostic impact of collaterals has been demonstrated on clinical outcome, initial NIHSS score, and infarct size.[18] In addition, cerebral blood volume (CBV), ASPECTS score, mean transit time (MTT), and time to max have all been found to correlate with the extent of collateral circulation.[19,20] Patient selection remains a critical area of further investigation for mechanical thrombectomy.[21]

3. *What is the role of CT perfusion in patient selection?*
The decrease in cerebral blood flow (CBF) is initially offset by the increase in collaterals manifested in local CBV. This maintains the viability of the tissue at risk (penumbra). This decrease in CBF is also demonstrated by an increase in the MTT. However, when both the CBF and CBV fall, the tissue is considered to be nonviable. Thus, the addition of perfusion techniques differentiates the hypoperfused territory (penumbra) from the infarcted territory (core).

4. *What other factors influence stroke outcome?*
In addition to the level of occlusion and NIHSS at presentation, several other factors (successful recanalization, established infarct core, ASPECTS, age, baseline functional status, and collateral status) also influence the outcome following stroke.[22]

5. *Is there a relation between NIHSS score and LVO?*
An NIHSS score of 8 was used to select candidates for intervention due to its high sensitivity and specificity in detecting LVOs.[17] However, patients with LVOs can also present with mild neurological deficits.[20] In addition, there is significant variability in outcomes of patients with LVOs and low-admission NIHSS.[23]
The presence of an underlying LVO in a patient with a low NIHSS can be a strong predictor of neurological deterioration.[24] These patients who underwent MT demonstrated a shift toward improved outcomes compared with the best medical management.[25]

6. *Should patients who do not meet the inclusion criteria of the published studies be considered for MT?*
While exceptions for use of MT in cases not meeting strict criteria are allowable, it remains unknown whether patients will be excluded from treatment.[26] Bhole et al[21] demonstrated that 33% of the cases in their series treated outside standard recommendations still attained a modified Rankin score (mRS) of ≤ 2 by 3 months. In addition, nearly half of their MT cases would have been denied MT if top-tier criteria were used to select patients.
In addition, basilar artery occlusions, which were not included in the initial or subsequent studies, are a particularly devastating event with uniformly poor outcomes if recanalization is not achieved early.[27]

7. *What would have happened if the patient experienced a wake-up stroke?*
Wake-up strokes represent up to 25% of acute ischemic strokes and largely fall outside of the traditional 6-hour window for MT.[28] However, studies suggest that the majority of these strokes occur closer to the time of awakening.[29,30,31,32,33,34] Additional imaging studies, such as CT and MR perfusion studies, can be employed to select these patients for treatment.[35,36,37]

12.4 Level of Evidence

An emergency NCCT is recommended prior to initiating any specific treatment for acute stroke (Class I, Level of Evidence A).

Noninvasive intracranial vascular study is strongly recommended during the initial imaging evaluation of the acute stroke patient but should not delay intravenous rTPA if indicated (Class I, Level of Evidence A).

Administration of intravenous rTPA is recommended for eligible patients who can be treated within 3 to 4.5 hours after stroke onset (Class I, Level of Evidence B).

Patients eligible for intravenous rTPA should receive intravenous rTPA even if endovascular treatments are being considered (Class I, Level of Evidence A).

Observing patients after intravenous rTPA to assess for clinical response before pursuing endovascular therapy is not recommended (Class III, Level of Evidence B-R).

Patients should receive MT if they meet the appropriate criteria (Class I, Level of Evidence A).

TICI 2b/3 recanalization following MT maximizes the probability of a good functional clinical outcome (Class I, Level of Evidence A).

Endovascular therapy should be carried out in an experienced stroke center with rapid access to qualified neurointerventionalists (Class I, Level of Evidence E).

12.5 Landmark Papers

Langhorne P, Williams BO, Gilchrist W, Howie K. Do stroke units save lives? Lancet. 1993 Aug 14;342(8868):395–398.[38]

This seminal paper initiated the fertile ground for stroke research and treatment. Using the newly introduced meta-analysis technique, the authors found that dedicated stroke units improved patient outcomes.

They performed a statistical overview of randomized controlled trials reported between 1962 and 1993 in which the management of stroke patients in a specialist unit was compared with that in general wards. They identified 10 trials, 8 of which used a strict randomization procedure. A total of 1,586 stroke patients were included: 766 were allocated to a stroke unit and 820 to general wards. The odds ratio (stroke unit vs. general wards) for mortality within the first 4 months (median follow-up 3 months) after a stroke was 0.72 (95% CI 0.56–0.92),

12

consistent with a reduction in mortality of 28% (2p < 0.01). This reduction persisted (odds ratio 0.79, 95% CI 0.63–0.99, 2p < 0.05) when calculated for mortality during the first 12 months. They concluded that management of stroke patients in a dedicated stroke unit was associated with a sustained reduction in mortality.

The National Institute of Neurological Disorders and Stroke rt-PA Stroke Study Group. Tissue plasminogen activator for acute ischemic stroke. N Engl J Med 1995; 333 (24): 1581–1587.[39]

In 1995, the first study with a positive impact for treatment of stroke patients was published demonstrating a statistically significant improvement in outcomes with administration of IV rTPA within 3 hours of symptom onset. Patients receiving the medication had at least a 30% better outcome in terms of disability at 3 months. Patients with IV rTPA also had a reduction in 3-month mortality of 17% versus 21% (*p* = 0.30). However, there was an increase in the percentage of hemorrhagic conversion of 6.4% versus only 0.6% in control (*p* < 0.001). The findings were statistically significant with a clear benefit of IV rTPA treatment with a required number needed to treat (NNT) of 8 to obtain favorable results.

Hacke W, Kaste M, Bluhmki E, et al; ECASS Investigators. Thrombolysis with alteplase 3 to 4.5 hours after acute ischemic stroke. N Engl J Med 2008;359(13):1317–1329.[40]

In 2008, the second statistically significant study was published that supported treatment with IV rTPA: ECASS III. This work increased the therapeutic window from 3 to 4.5 hours following symptom onset. There was no difference in mortality, but it demonstrated improved morbidity with an NNT of 14 for "favorable results." Based upon these two studies, for patients meeting national and international eligibility guidelines, IV rTPA improves functional outcomes at 3 and 6 months when given within the first 4.5 hours.

Endovascular treatment

Broderick JP, Palesch YY, Demchuk AM, et al; Interventional Management of Stroke (IMS) III Investigators. Endovascular therapy after intravenous t-PA versus t-PA alone for stroke. N Engl J Med 2013;368(10):893–903.[5]

Kidwell CS, Jahan R, Gornbein J, et al; MR RESCUE Investigators. A trial of imaging selection and endovascular treatment for ischemic stroke. N Engl J Med 2013;368(10):914–923.[3]

Ciccone A, Valvassori L, Nichelatti M, et al; SYNTHESIS Expansion Investigators. Endovascular treatment for acute ischemic stroke. N Engl J Med 2013;368(10):904–913.[4]

In March 2013, in a single issue the *New England Journal of Medicine* published three studies that evaluated the efficacy of endovascular treatment for ischemic stroke (IMS III, MR RESCUE, SYNTHESIS). In IMS III, a total of 656 participants underwent randomization (434 participants to endovascular therapy and 222 to intravenous tPA alone) at 58 study centers between August 25, 2006 and April 17, 2012 in the United States, Canada, Australia, and Europe. Eligibility criteria included receipt of intravenous tPA within 3 hours after symptom onset and a moderate-to-severe neurologic deficit (defined as an NIHSS score ≥ 10 or score of 8 to 9 with CT angiographic evidence of an occlusion of the first segment of the middle cerebral artery [M1], internal carotid artery, or basilar artery). Participants randomly assigned to the endovascular therapy group underwent angiography as soon as possible. Participants who had no angiographic evidence of a treatable occlusion received no addi-

tional treatment, while those with a treatable vascular occlusion received endovascular intervention. The angiographic procedure had to begin within 5 hours and be completed within 7 hours after the onset of stroke.

Reperfusion rates, as measured by a TICI score of 2b (partial reperfusion of half or more of the vascular distribution of the occluded artery) to 3, were 38% for an occlusion in the internal carotid artery, 44% for an occlusion in M1, 44% for a single M2 occlusion, and 23% for multiple M2 occlusions. The trial was terminated early due to futility as defined by the prespecified rules. There was no significant difference between the endovascular therapy and intravenous tPA groups in the overall proportion of participants with an mRS of 2 or less. It failed to show a benefit in functional outcome with the use of additional endovascular therapy, as compared with the standard therapy of intravenous tPA alone. The safety profiles were similar in the two treatment groups.

In MR RESCUE, 127 patients were randomized to embolectomy and studied clinical outcomes in subgroups with and without a "penumbral pattern" on MRI or CT of each treatment arm. There was no improvement in revascularization, tissue reperfusion, or clinical outcomes in the embolectomy group compared to the standard care group.

SYNTHESIS compared endovascular therapy versus IV tPA during the first 4.5 hours from symptom onset. The study included 362 patients (181 in each group). There were no significant differences with respect to prognosis (30.4% endovascular vs. 34.8% intravenous), hemorrhagic complications, or mortality.

Numerous concerns regarding various aspects of these trials were raised. First, only MR RESCUE routinely identified LVO with either CTA or MRA. In IMS III, CTA was performed in only 47% of patients and 20% of patients in the interventional arm either did not have an LVO or had an inaccessible, distally located thrombus. In SYNTHESIS expansion, approximately 10% of patients in the interventional arm did not have an LVO.

Moreover, modern thrombectomy devices, such as retrievable stents and aspiration catheters were used in only a minority of patients. The use of older, less effective endovascular technology resulted in significantly lower rates of successful recanalization. The rates of TICI 2b or 3 recanalization were 40% in IMS III and 27% in MR RESCUE. Recanalization rates were not reported in SYNTHESIS expansion. The use of first-generation thrombectomy devices and techniques could explain the low rates of recanalization seen in these studies.

Furthermore, patients with minor ischemic deficits were included. These patients may not have the same benefit as those with LVOs. SYNTHESIS expansion also compared thrombectomy versus IV tPA, rather than concomitant use. Despite the negative results, these studies pointed the way for new trials on mechanical thrombectomy in LVOs.

Bekhemer O, Beumer F, Berg V, Lingsma H, Schonewile Y, Nederkoom V. The randomized trial of intra-arterial treatment for acute ischemic stroke (Mr. CLEAN). N Engl J Med 2015;372.[7]

MR CLEAN was the first positive trial to be published in January 2015. Five hundred patients (233 intervention and 267 control group) were randomized to medical management versus mechanical thrombectomy. Inclusion criteria consisted of age > 18 years, NIHSS > 2, intervention < 6 hours since the onset of symptoms, proximal vascular occlusion by CTA, and an

12

ASPECTS > 7. IV rTPA was administered to 90% of the patients (87% intervention vs. 91% control). No significant changes were observed in terms of mortality; however, there was a statistically significant decrease in morbidity in the intervention arm with an mRS of 0–2 of 33% with endovascular treatment versus 19% in the control group. TICI 2b-3 reperfusion was achieved in 59% of the cases.

Despite the sample size, this study allowed for the estimation of the primary effect parameter with sufficient precision.

Goyal M, Demchuk A, Menon B, et al. Randomized assay of rapid endovascular treatment of ischemic stroke (ESCAPE). N Engl J Med 2015.[8]

The ESCAPE trial included a total of 315 patients (165 intervention vs. 150 control), with an NIHSS more than 12, ASPECTS more than 5, treatment within 12 hours, diagnosis of proximal occlusion by CTA, and perfusion imaging for evaluation of collateral circulation. IV rTPA was administered in 76% of the patients (72.7% intervention vs. 78.6% control group). This study was terminated early because of the clear benefit and efficacy of endovascular treatment in the control group. A TICI 2b-3 reperfusion rate of 72% was observed with a favorable outcome (mRS 0–2) in 53% with intervention versus 29% in the control group (NNT = 4) and a decrease in mortality of 10% versus 19%, respectively.

In the ESCAPE trial, a short imaging-to-reperfusion time significantly improved the chance of achieving a functionally independent outcome.

Campbell B, Mitchell P, Kleinig T, Dewey H, Churilov L, Yassi N. Endovascular therapy for ischemic stroke with perfusion-imaging selection (EXTEND-IA). N Engl J Med 2015;372(11):1009–1018.[9]

EXTEND-IA was the smallest trial with n = 70 (35 intervention vs. 35 control). The selection criteria were based on perfusion images of patients with LVO within 4.5 hours from onset of symptoms. There were no age limits or NIHSS limits. IV rTPA was administered in all patients. TICI 2b-3 reperfusion rate was 86% with a favorable outcome (mRS 0–2) in 71% with intervention versus 40% control group. Mortality was 9% in the thrombectomy arm and 20% in the control.

They concluded that early endovascular thrombectomy with stentrievers after IV rTPA resulted in greater reperfusion and early neurologic recovery than rTPA alone in a population with LVO and salvageable tissue on CT perfusion imaging.

In conclusion, the magnitude of the observed benefit in these trials, along with the SWIFT-PRIME[10] and REVASCAT[11] studies, was dramatic. The findings suggested a superior outcome following treatment with IV thrombolysis and thrombectomy using modern thrombectomy devices compared with best medical treatment alone. The successes from these trials compared with the earlier ones have been mostly attributed to improved thrombectomy devices with faster and higher rates of recanalization and improved study protocols.

Nogueira RG, Jadhav AP, Haussen DC, et al. Thrombectomy 6 to 24 hours after stroke with a mismatch between deficit and infarct. N Engl J Med. 2017 Nov 11.[41]

The DAWN trial was a multicenter, prospective, randomized, open-label trial with a Bayesian adaptive–enrichment design and with blinded assessment of end points. This study supported the use of a stent retriever beyond the 8-hour indicated time limit in late presenting ischemic stroke subjects.

The investigators selected patients arriving after 6 hours from symptom onset for inclusion in the trial by using perfusion imaging and clinical scores to identify those with "target mismatch"—a small core infarct volume with a large area of brain at risk for ischemia. From September 2014 through February 2017, a total of 206 patients were enrolled in the trial; 107 were randomly assigned to the thrombectomy group and 99 to the control group.

Patients with an LVO presenting between 6 and 24 hours (average 13 hours) underwent computed tomographic (CT) perfusion or magnetic resonance diffusion-weighted imaging. Patients were selected for randomization if they had a small infarct core in relation to their NIHSS score.

Results showed a two-point difference in the 90-day weighted mRS in favor of the thrombectomy group which translated into a 73% relative reduction of dependency in activities of daily living. In addition, there was a 35% absolute increase in the number of patients achieving functional independence (mRS 0–2), with an NNT of 2.8.

Albers GW, Marks MP, Kemp S, Christensen S, Tsai JP, Ortega-Gutierrez S, et al. Thrombectomy for stroke at 6 to16 hours with selection by perfusion imaging. The New England Journal of Medicine, 2018.[42]

DEFUSE 3 was a multicenter, randomized, open-label trial, with blinded outcome assessment, of thrombectomy in patients 6 to 16 hours after they were last known to be well and who had remaining ischemic brain tissue that was not yet infarcted. From May 2016 through May 2017, a total of 182 patients underwent randomization (92 to the endovascular-therapy group and 90 to the medical-therapy group) at 38 centers in the United States.

Patients with proximal middle-cerebral-artery or internal-carotid-artery occlusion, an initial infarct size of less than 70 mL, and a ratio of the volume of ischemic tissue on perfusion imaging to infarct volume of 1.8 or more were randomly assigned to endovascular therapy (thrombectomy) plus standard medical therapy (endovascular-therapy group) or standard medical therapy alone (medical-therapy group). RAPID software imaging was used for all the patients.

The primary outcome was the ordinal score on the modified Rankin scale (range, 0 to 6, with higher scores indicating greater disability) at day 90. Endovascular therapy plus standard medical therapy was associated with a more favorable distribution of disability scores on the modified Rankin scale at 90 days than standard medical therapy alone. Mortality at 90 days was 14% in the endovascular-therapy group and 26% in the medical-therapy group (p = 0.05). The rate of symptomatic intracranial hemorrhage did not differ significantly between the two groups.

The results of DAWN trial and the subsequent DEFUSE III trial expanded the population of patients who could benefit from mechanical thrombectomy for stroke, to significantly reduce functional impairment in the most severely affected patients.

The period, location, number of patients, and centers of the trials that demonstrated the benefit of endovascular stroke treatment are summarized in ▶ Table 12.1.

12.6 Recommendations

Prehospital stroke management: Stroke patients are dispatched at the highest level of care available in the shortest time

Table 12.1 Characteristics of trials

Trial	Trial period	Location	Total no. of patients	No. of centers
MR CLEAN	2010–2014	Europe	500	30
ESCAPE	2013–2014	North America, Europe, South Korea	315	22
EXTEND IA	2012–2014	Australia and New Zealand	70	14
SWIFT PRIME	2013–2014	North America, Europe	196	39
REVASCAT	2012–2014	Spain	206	4
DAWN	2014–2017	North America, Europe Australia	206	32
DEFUSE III	2016–2017	United States	182	38

possible. Travel time is equivalent to trauma or myocardial infarction calls.[43]

Emergency evaluation and diagnosis of acute ischemic stroke: The evaluation and initial treatment of patients with stroke should be performed expeditiously. A limited number of essential diagnostic tests are recommended.[43]

Early diagnosis, brain, and vascular imaging: An emergency brain imaging study is recommended prior to initiating any specific treatment for acute stroke (Class I, Level of Evidence A).[16] Noncontrast Head CT + CT angiography (CT perfusion can be added to protocol) or MRI.

Intravenous rTPA (0.9 mg/kg, maximum dose 90 mg) is recommended for administration to eligible patients who can be treated in the time period of 3 to 4.5 hours after stroke onset (Class I, Level of Evidence B). Patients eligible for intravenous rTPA should receive intravenous rTPA even if endovascular treatments are being considered (Class I, Level of Evidence A).[16]

Patients should receive endovascular therapy if they meet all the following criteria (Class I, Level of Evidence A)[16]:

- Prestroke mRS score 0 to 1.
- Acute ischemic stroke receiving intravenous rTPA within 4.5 hours of onset according to the published guidelines.
- LVO.
- Age ≥ 18 years.
- NIHSS score of ≥ 6.
- ASPECTS of ≥ 6.
- Treatment can be initiated (groin puncture) within 6 hours of symptom onset and a favorable CT Head or up to 24 hours with perfusion imaging.

A finding of intracranial LVOs during the initial diagnostic evaluation is strongly associated with worse functional outcome and higher mortality rate. Patients with emergent large-vessel occlusion (ELVO) are a heterogeneous group requiring rapid and effective revascularization with the likelihood of benefit decreasing over time elapsed from symptom onset.[44]

As already mentioned, endovascular treatment in cases not meeting strict criteria is allowable. Each patient should be discussed quickly, analyzing the level of occlusion, NIHSS at presentation, vascular anatomy, established infarct core, ASPECTS, age, baseline functional status, and collateral circulation.

The role of mechanical thrombectomy could be significantly expanded if patients are selected based on risk of severe disability and favorable parenchymal/collateral imaging findings, instead of time and occlusion location.[21]

Type of device: The use of retrievable stents is recommended with the highest level of evidence by American Heart Association (AHA), Canadian Stroke Best Practice (CSBP), and European Stroke Organization (ESO) guidelines with lower levels of

recommendations given to consider other devices based on local protocols. An analysis of the MR CLEAN data showed that choice of device did not influence outcomes in that data set. The majority were treated with the Trevo device 53%, Solitaire device 13%, and other device 17%.[45] The ASTER Trial concluded that among patients with ischemic stroke in the anterior circulation undergoing thrombectomy, first-line thrombectomy with direct aspiration compared with stent retriever were comparable with respect to revascularization, clinical efficacy, and adverse events.[46]

Type of anesthesia: Conscious sedation is preferred over general anesthesia (unless medically indicated) by both AHA and CSBP recommendations, albeit with reduced levels of evidence (Class IIb, Level C and Level B, respectively), whereas the ESO guideline leaves this as an individual patient decision. Several randomized controlled trials are under way to address this issue.[47]

12.7 Summary

1. The understanding of the natural history of ischemic stroke and its treatment relies on multiple landmark papers.
2. Endovascular thrombectomy is of benefit to patients with acute ischemic stroke caused by occlusion of the proximal anterior circulation, irrespective of patient characteristics.
3. Medical systems of care must be equipped to provide lifesaving treatment in a timely fashion to patients with acute ischemic stroke due to LVO.

References

[1] Fishser M, Aminoff M, Boller F, Swaab D. Handbook of clinical neurology. Vol. 92. 3rd ed. In: Fisher M, ed. Stroke. Part I. Elsevier B.V.;2009

[2] Casaubon L, Boulanger J, Blacquiere D, Boucher S, Brown K, Goddard T. Canadian stroke best practice recommendations: hyperacute stroke care guidelines. Update 2015

[3] Kidwell CS, Jahan R, Gornbein J, et al. MR RESCUE Investigators. A trial of imaging selection and endovascular treatment for ischemic stroke. N Engl J Med. 2013; 368(10):914–923–(MR RESCUE)

[4] Ciccone A, Valvassori L, Nichelatti M, et al. SYNTHESIS Expansion Investigators. Endovascular treatment for acute ischemic stroke. N Engl J Med. 2013; 368(10):904–913–(SYNTHESIS)

[5] Broderick JP, Palesch YY, Demchuk AM, et al. Interventional Management of Stroke (IMS) III Investigators. Endovascular therapy after intravenous t-PA versus t-PA alone for stroke. N Engl J Med. 2013; 368(10):893–903

[6] Przybylowski CJ, Ding D, Starke RM, Durst CR, Crowley RW, Liu KC. Evolution of endovascular mechanical thrombectomy for acute ischemic stroke. World J Clin Cases. 2014; 2(11):614–622

[7] Bekhemer O, Beumer F, Berg V, Lingsma H, Schonewile Y, Nederkoom V. The randomized trial of intra-arterial treatment for acute ischemic stroke (Mr. CLEAN). N Engl J Med. 2015; 372

12

[8] Goyal M, Demchuk A, Menon B, et al. Randomized assay of rapid endovascular treatment of ischemic stroke (ESCAPE). N Engl J Med. 2015

[9] Campbell B, Mitchell P, Kleinig T, Dewey H, Churilov L, Yassi N. Endovascular therapy for ischemic stroke with perfusion-imaging selection (EXTEND-IA). N Engl J Med. 2015; 372(11):1009:1018

[10] Saver J, Mayank M, Bonafe A, Diener M, Elad P, Levy I. Thrombectomy Stent-Retriever alter Intravenous t-PA vs. t-PA Alone in Stroke (SWIFT PRIME). N Engl J Med. 2015

[11] Jovin T, Chamorro A, Cobo E, Miquel M, Molina C, Rovira A. Thrombectomy within 8 hours after symptom onset in ischemic stroke (REVASCAT). N Engl J Med. 2015

[12] Yaghi S, Bianchi N, Amole A, Hinduja A. ASPECTS is a predictor of favorable CT perfusion in acute ischemic stroke. J Neuroradiol. 2014; 41(3):184–187

[13] Menon BK, Puetz V, Kochar P, Demchuk AM. ASPECTS and other neuroimaging scores in the triage and prediction of outcome in acute stroke patients. Neuroimaging Clin N Am. 2011; 21(2):407–423, xii

[14] Lassalle L, Turc G, Tisserand M, et al. ASPECTS (Alberta Stroke Program Early CT Score) assessment of the perfusion-diffusion mismatch. Stroke. 2016; 47(10):2553–2558

[15] Barber PA, Demchuk AM, Zhang J, Buchan AM. Validity and reliability of a quantitative computed tomography score in predicting outcome of hyper-acute stroke before thrombolytic therapy. ASPECTS Study Group. Alberta Stroke Programme Early CT Score. Lancet. 2000; 355(9216):1670–1674

[16] Powers WJ, Derdeyn CP. Guideline 2015 AHA/ASA focused update of the 2013 guidelines for the early management of patients with acute ischemic stroke regarding endovascular treatment: a guideline for healthcare professionals from the American Heart Association/American Stroke Association

[17] Fischer U, Arnold M, Nedeltchev K, et al. NIHSS score and arteriographic findings in acute ischemic stroke. Stroke 2005;36(10):2121–2125

[18] Attyé A, Boncoeur-Martel MP, Maubon A, et al. Diffusion-weighted imaging infarct volume and neurologic outcomes after ischemic stroke. J Neuroradiol. 2012; 39(2):97–103

[19] Lee JH, Kim YJ, Choi JW, et al. Multimodal CT: favorable outcome factors in acute middle cerebral artery stroke with large artery occlusion. Eur Neurol. 2013; 69(6):366–374

[20] Smith WS, Lev MH, English JD, et al. Significance of large vessel intracranial occlusion causing acute ischemic stroke and TIA. Stroke 2009;40(12):3834–384

[21] Bhole R, Goyal N, Nearing K, et al. Implications of limiting mechanical thrombectomy to patients with emergent large vessel occlusion meeting top tier evidence criteria. J Neurointerv Surg. 2017; 9(3):225–228

[22] Fields JD, Lutsep HL, Smith WS, MERCI Multi MERCI Investigators. Higher degrees of recanalization after mechanical thrombectomy for acute stroke are associated with improved outcome and decreased mortality: pooled analysis of the MERCI and Multi MERCI trials. AJNR Am J Neuroradiol. 2011; 32(11):2170–2174

[23] Mokin M, Masud MW, Dumont TM, et al. Outcomes in patients with acute ischemic stroke from proximal intracranial vessel occlusion and NIHSS score below 8. J Neurointerv Surg. 2014; 6(6):413–417

[24] Kim JT, Park MS, Chang J, Lee JS, Choi KH, Cho KH. Proximal arterial occlusion in acute ischemic stroke with low NIHSS scores should not be considered as mild stroke. PLoS One. 2013; 8(8):e70996

[25] Haussen DC, Bouslama M, Grossberg JA, et al. Too good to intervene? Thrombectomy for large vessel occlusion strokes with minimal symptoms: an intention-to-treat analysis. J Neurointerv Surg. 2017; 9(10):917–921

[26] Fiorella D, Mocco J, Arthur AS, et al. Too much guidance. J Neurointerv Surg. 2015; 7(9):626–627

[27] Kumar G, Shahripour RB, Alexandrov AV. Recanalization of acute basilar artery occlusion improves outcomes: a meta-analysis. J Neurointerv Surg. 2015; 7(12):868–874

[28] Mackey J, Kleindorfer D, Sucharew H, et al. Population-based study of wake-up strokes. Neurology. 2011; 76(19):1662–1667

[29] Fink JN, Kumar S, Horkan C, et al. The stroke patient who woke up: clinical and radiological features, including diffusion and perfusion MRI. Stroke. 2002; 33(4):988–993

[30] Thomalla G, Cheng B, Ebinger M, et al. STIR and VISTA Imaging Investigators. DWI-FLAIR mismatch for the identification of patients with acute ischaemic stroke within 4·5 h of symptom onset (PRE-FLAIR): a multicentre observational study. Lancet Neurol. 2011; 10(11):978–986

[31] Elliott WJ. Circadian variation in the timing of stroke onset: a meta-analysis. Stroke. 1998; 29(5):992–996– [PubMed: 9596248–]

[32] Casetta I, Granieri E, Fallica E, la Cecilia O, Paolino E, Manfredini R. Patient demographic and clinical features and circadian variation in onset of ischemic stroke. Arch Neurol. 2002; 59(1):48–53

[33] Marler JR, Price TR, Clark GL, et al. Morning increase in onset of ischemic stroke. Stroke. 1989; 20(4):473–476

[34] Huisa BN, Raman R, Ernstrom K, et al. Alberta Stroke Program Early CT Score (ASPECTS) in patients with wake-up stroke. J Stroke Cerebrovasc Dis. 2010; 19(6):475–479

[35] Thomalla G, Rossbach P, Rosenkranz M, et al. Negative fluid-attenuated inversion recovery imaging identifies acute ischemic stroke at 3 hours or less. Ann Neurol. 2009; 65(6):724–732

[36] Huisa BN, Liebeskind DS, Raman R, et al. University of California, Los Angeles Stroke Investigators. Diffusion-weighted imaging-fluid attenuated inversion recovery mismatch in nocturnal stroke patients with unknown time of onset. J Stroke Cerebrovasc Dis. 2013; 22(7):972–977

[37] Cho AH, Kim JS, Kim SJ, et al. Focal fluid-attenuated inversion recovery hyperintensity within acute diffusion-weighted imaging lesions is associated with symptomatic intracerebral hemorrhage after thrombolysis. Stroke. 2008; 39(12):3424–3426

[38] Langhorne P1, Williams BO, Gilchrist W, Howie K. Do stroke units save lives? Lancet. 1993 Aug 14; 342(8868):395–839

[39] The National Institute of Neurological Disorders and Stroke rt-PA Stroke Study Group. Tissue plasminogen activator for acute ischemic stroke. N Engl J Med. 1995; 333(24):1581–1587

[40] Hacke W, Kaste M, Bluhmki E, Brozman M, Dávalos A, Guidetti D, et al; ECASS Investigators. Thrombolysis with alteplase 3 to 4.5 hours after acute ischemic stroke. N Engl J Med 2008; 359 (13): 1317–1329

[41] Nogueira RG, Jadhav AP, Haussen DC, et al. Thrombectomy 6 to 24 hours after stroke with a mismatch between deficit and infarct. N Engl J Med. 2017 Nov 11

[42] Albers GW, Marks MP, Kemp S, Christensen S, Tsai JP, Ortega-Gutierrez S, et al. Thrombectomy for stroke at 6 to 16 hours with selection by perfusion imaging. The New England Journal of Medicine. 2018

[43] Jauch EC, Saver JL, Adams HP, Jr, et al. American Heart Association Stroke Council, Council on Cardiovascular Nursing, Council on Peripheral Vascular Disease, Council on Clinical Cardiology. Guidelines for the early management of patients with acute ischemic stroke: a guideline for healthcare professionals from the American Heart Association/American Stroke Association. Stroke. 2013; 44(3):870–947

[44] Khatri P, Yeatts SD, Mazighi M, et al. IMS III Trialists. Time to angiographic reperfusion and clinical outcome after acute ischaemic stroke: an analysis of data from the Interventional Management of Stroke (IMS III) phase 3 trial. Lancet Neurol. 2014; 13(6):567–574

[45] Dippel D, Majoie C, Roos Y, et al. Influence of device choice on the effect of intra-arterial treatment for acute ischemic stroke in MR CLEAN. Stroke. 2016; 47:2574–2581

[46] Lapergue B, Blanc R, Gory B, et al; ASTER Trial Investigators. Effect of endovascular contact aspiration vs stent retriever on revascularization in patients with acute ischemic stroke and large vessel occlusion: the ASTER randomized clinical trial. JAMA 2017; 318(5):443-452

[47] Sedation vs. intubation for endovascular stroke treatment (SIESTA). ClinicalTrials.gov NCT02126085. doi: 10.1111/ijs.12488

12

13 Intracranial Atherosclerosis

Wiebke Kurre and Hans Henkes

Abstract

Endovascular treatment of symptomatic atherosclerotic intracranial stenosis is a controversial issue. Two prospective randomized trials did not demonstrate any benefit of stent-angioplasty over medical management. Rather, endovascular therapy may even cause harm. Nevertheless, if stenosis-related cerebral ischemia recurs despite the best medical management, intracranial angioplasty—with or without stenting—can be considered a compassionate treatment. The decision on whether or not to perform endovascular therapy has to be taken on a case-to-case basis and requires a profound knowledge of the pathophysiology and prognosis of symptomatic intracranial atherosclerotic disease, medical treatment options, and the design and scope of the currently available randomized trials. Given this sensitive background, performing the procedure should be confined to operators with high individual expertise in this field.

Keywords: intracranial atherosclerosis, intracranial stenosis, best medical treatment, (stent-)angioplasty

13.1 Goals

1. Critically analyze the literature on medical management of symptomatic intracranial atherosclerotic disease.
2. Review relevant trials on endovascular treatment of symptomatic intracranial atherosclerotic disease.
3. Highlight key issues in endovascular therapy, periprocedural management, and follow-up after intracranial angioplasty and stenting.

13.2 Case Example

13.2.1 History of Present Illness

A 75-year-old patient complained of recurrent episodes of left-sided weakness and speech disturbance. Magnetic resonance (MR) imaging showed acute infarcts in the left cerebellar hemisphere, right pons, and left occipital lobe (▶ Fig. 13.1a, b). A basilar artery stenosis was detected on MR angiography (▶ Fig. 13.1c). Best medical treatment was initiated including dual antiplatelet treatment with acetylsalicylic acid (ASA) and clopidogrel, atorvastatin at 80 mg daily, and an optimization of antihypertensive medication. One month later, the patient experienced palpitations and was diagnosed with atrial fibrillation. The treating cardiologist performed cardioversion and replaced the dual antiplatelet treatment with rivaroxaban without any other change of medication.

Another month later, episodes of speech disturbance and perioral paresthesia occurred. These episodes were interpreted as brainstem transient ischemic attack (TIA), but MR imaging did not show any new infarcts or stenosis progression. ASA was added to rivaroxaban. A few weeks later, atrial fibrillation relapsed. The patient was readmitted and treated with amiodarone. During the course of the hospital stay, the patient experienced two more episodes of speech disturbance. This time MR imaging revealed a new pontine infarction. Since all infarcts and the TIA were in the territory of the basilar artery, it was assumed that a large artery atherosclerosis was the cause rather than atrial fibrillation. After interdisciplinary discussion with the neurologist, neuroradiologist, and cardiologist, endovascular therapy was regarded as the only treatment option left and the patient gave informed consent after careful consideration. During preprocedural medical work-up, a slight drop in hemoglobin was recognized. In view of the extensive postprocedural anticoagulation required, an endoscopy was performed. An angiodysplasia was found in the colon and coagulated.

Past Medical History: hypertension, hyperlipidemia, heterozygous factor-V-Leiden mutation with previous deep vein thrombosis, impaired glucose tolerance, atrial fibrillation (CHA2DS2-VASc 5).

Past surgical history: Previous bilateral cataract surgery.

Family history: Answered negative to family history of stroke.

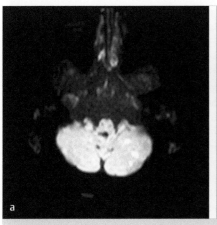 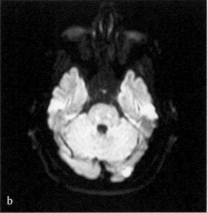 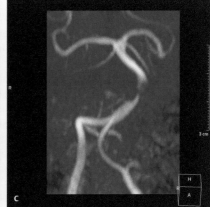

Fig. 13.1 The patient presented with recurrent episodes of left-sided weakness and speech disturbance. Diffusion-weighted magnetic resonance (MR) imaging revealed infarcts in the left cerebellar hemisphere (a), pons and left occipital lobe (b). A high-grade basilar stenosis was found in MR angiography (c).

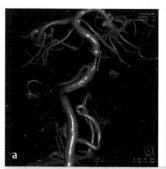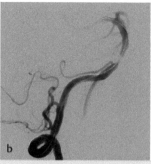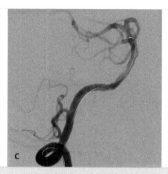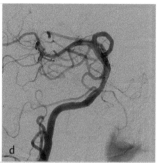

Fig. 13.2 Treatment and follow-up of a high-grade basilar artery stenosis. **(a)** A 3D rotational angiography was acquired to precisely measure the dimensions of the basilar artery and the stenosis. **(b)** After catheterization of the right posterior cerebral artery with a 0.014″ microwire, a 3.5- to 8-mm balloon-expandable stent was placed at the site of the stenosis (*arrows* indicate the proximal and distal balloon marker). **(c)** After stent deployment, the stenosis resolved completely. **(d)** Twelve-month control angiography revealed patency of the stent and no restenosis.

Social history: Answered negative to being a former or current smoker.
Review of systems: As per the above.
Neurological examination: Unremarkable.
Imaging studies: As described above.

13.2.2 Treatment Plan

The patient was scheduled for intracranial stenting under general anesthesia. A balloon-expandable stent was uneventfully implanted (▶ Fig. 13.2a–c). After the procedure, the anticoagulation medication was changed to dabigatran at 110 mg twice daily with ASA and clopidogrel for 4 weeks. Then, the medication was changed to rivaroxaban and clopidogrel.

13.2.3 Follow-up

Clinical, MRI, and angiographic follow-up was scheduled at 6 and 12 months. The patient did not experience any new ischemic symptoms. There was no evidence of new infarcts in imaging studies and no restenosis occurred (▶ Fig. 13.2d). At 12 months, the antithrombotic medication was changed to rivaroxaban and ASA.

13.3 Case Summary

1. *What is the recommended anticoagulation/antithrombotic treatment in patients with symptomatic intracranial atherosclerosis?*
   The first attempt to clarify the uncertainty about the optimal antithrombotic therapy in patients with symptomatic intracranial atherosclerosis was the "Warfarin and Aspirin for Symptomatic Intracranial Stenosis (WASID)" trial.[1] The trial was terminated early since the use of warfarin was associated with an increased mortality and major bleeding risk without any benefit in terms of stroke prevention. The increased risk of major hemorrhage was largely triggered by excess international normalized ratio (INR) values and low values were associated with an increased risk of stroke. Out of range INR was not infrequent within the trial. Novel anticoagulants (NOACs) are more suitable in this aspect and have proven to be superior to warfarin in terms of safety and efficacy in patients with cardioembolic stroke. Therefore, they might play a future role in the treatment of patients with symptomatic intracranial atherosclerosis.
   The "Stenting versus Aggressive Medical Therapy for Intracranial Arterial Stenosis (SAMMPRIS)" trial compared stenting with aggressive medical management to aggressive medical management alone for the treatment of high-grade symptomatic intracranial stenosis.[2,3] The likelihood of a primary end-point event in the noninterventional arm of the trial was only 5.8% at 30 days and much lower than expected. Dual antiplatelet treatment with ASA and clopidogrel during the first 3 months after randomization was an essential component of medical therapy.
   The superiority of dual antiplatelet treatment compared to ASA alone to prevent recurrence of cerebral ischemia without an increased risk of hemorrhage was demonstrated in the "Clopidogrel with Aspirin in Acute Minor Stroke or Transient Ischemic Attack (CHANCE)" trial.[4] A CHANCE subgroup analysis focusing on patients with intracranial atherosclerosis showed only a trend for improved outcome with dual antiplatelet therapy.[5] This may be attributable to the very common phenomenon of "clopidogrel resistance," which is caused by the inability to convert the prodrug clopidogrel into the active form via the CYP2C19 enzyme. An additional subgroup analysis showed that the benefit of dual antiplatelet therapy was not present in carriers of CYP2C19 loss-of-function alleles but was highly significant in noncarriers.[6] Ticagrelor has the same mode of action as clopidogrel but does not require enzymatic conversion. Therefore, it will likely overcome the issue of clopidogrel resistance. The safety and efficacy of ticagrelor in patients with intracranial large artery atherosclerosis has not been investigated yet.

2. *What are the most important adjunctive components of medical therapy in symptomatic intracranial atherosclerosis?*
   The medical treatment arm of the SAMMPRIS trial showed the most favorable clinical results in patients with symptomatic intracranial atherosclerosis so far.[3] Therefore, medical therapy in the real-world setting should ideally be aligned to the trial guidelines. Specific risk factor targets were as follows[7]: systolic blood pressure < 140 mm Hg (< 130 mm Hg if diabetic), LDL cholesterol < 70 mg/dL, non-HDL lipoprotein < 100 mg/dL, HbA1c < 7%, smoking cessation, weight management (for initial BMI of 25–27 kg/m²: target BMI < 25 kg/m²;

for initial BMI > 27 kg/m^2: target 10% weight loss), physical activity: ≥ 30 min of moderate exercise ≥ 3 times per week. The effectiveness of the components of risk factor management in the medical arm of SAMMPRIS was validated in a subgroup analysis. Interestingly, physical activity was the strongest predictor for favorable outcome.[8]

3. *What is the risk of endovascular therapy compared to medical management in intracranial atherosclerotic disease?*

Endovascular therapy was compared to best medical management in two prospective randomized trials. The leading trial was SAMMPRIS, which compared the clinical outcomes of patients with high-grade (≥ 70% degree of stenosis), symptomatic intracranial stenosis receiving stent-angioplasty with the self-expanding Wingspan device in conjunction with aggressive medical management versus aggressive medical management alone.[2,3] The "Vitesse Stent Ischemic Therapy (VISSIT)" trial followed using the balloon-expandable Pharos Vitesse stent as the study device in the endovascular treatment arm.[9] SAMMPRIS was halted after randomization of 451 patients due to safety concerns and VISSIT was stopped after the publication of the initial results from SAMMPRIS.

In both trials, the probability of a primary end-point event was higher in the endovascular treatment arm as compared to medical treatment alone. The primary end point in SAMMPRIS was any of the following: stroke or death within 30 days after enrollment, ischemic stroke in the territory of the qualifying artery beyond 30 days of enrollment, or stroke or death within 30 days after a revascularization procedure of the qualifying lesion during follow-up. During a median follow-up of 32.4 months, 34 (15%) of 227 patients in the medical group and 52 (23%) of 224 patients in the stenting group had a primary end-point event ($p = 0.0252$).

The primary end point of VISSIT was a composite of stroke in the same territory within 12 months of randomization or a TIA in the same territory from day 2 through month 12 postrandomization. The 1-year primary outcome occurred in more patients in the stent group 21 (36.2%) of 58 versus the medical group 8 (15.1%) of 53 ($p = 0.02$). Under the premises of these studies stent-angioplasty was inferior compared to medical management alone in the treatment of symptomatic intracranial large artery disease. The negative trial results were mainly driven by high procedure-related event rates. In SAMMPRIS, two-thirds of procedure-related events were ischemic and one-third were hemorrhagic.[10] Basilar artery stenosis, diabetes, and old age were predictors of procedural ischemic events and perforator stroke was the most critical issue. A higher grade of stenosis, a lower modified Rankin score, and a clopidogrel load associated with an activated clotting time above the target range predicted procedural hemorrhage. Delayed hemorrhage turned out to be the major contributor.

It is worth noting that patients with unstable clinical symptoms were excluded in both trials. Therefore, the results cannot be transferred to acute stroke treatment.

4. *What is the rationale for endovascular treatment of symptomatic intracranial atherosclerotic disease?*

Extensive subgroup analyses have been performed from the SAMMPRIS data to identify subgroups which would potentially benefit from endovascular therapy. Subgroup analyses have included the following (underlined representing prespecified subgroups): patients on and off antithrombotic therapy at the time of the qualifying event (QE), age < 60 versus ≥ 60, gender, black or white racial background, vascular risk factors (hypertension, lipid disorder, diabetes, smoking), location of the stenosis (internal carotid artery, middle cerebral artery, vertebral artery, basilar artery), anterior versus posterior circulation, percent stenosis (< 80% vs. ≥ 80%), type of QE (stroke vs. TIA), days to enrollment (≤ 7 days vs. > 7 days), old infarcts in the territory, proton pump inhibitors at QE, and hypoperfusion symptoms.[11,12] None of the above revealed an advantage of stent-angioplasty over medical treatment.

Both SAMMPRIS and VISSIT have been criticized in many ways, including the treatment being confined to a specific device, the development of devices for this purpose still being at an early stage, inadequate operator experience, patient selection issues, and a low enrollment rate. Nevertheless, from an evidence-based perspective, stent-angioplasty of intracranial atherosclerotic disease is a compassionate treatment and must be confined to a small patient group with recurrent cerebral ischemia despite having optimized medical management.

New prospective randomized trials with more advanced devices and techniques demonstrating a clinical benefit of intracranial stent-angioplasty are required to establish the stenting of intracranial stenosis as a standard treatment. For balloon angioplasty alone, scientific data are sparse and no meaningful prospective randomized trials exist. An early meta-analysis dated 2009 suggested that rates of recurrent stroke and restenosis are higher following balloon angioplasty compared to stent-assisted treatment.[13] Two more recent case series suggest that angioplasty alone may carry a lower procedural risk compared to stent-angioplasty.[14,15] From a practical point of view, balloon angioplasty alone is frequently associated with dissection and/or elastic recoil and does not result in reliable treatment results.

5. *What is the ideal endovascular treatment strategy?*

Intracranial stenting can be performed with either self-expanding or balloon-expandable stents. Since SAMMPRIS was conducted with a self-expanding stent and VISSIT with a balloon-expandable stent and both failed to prove superiority of endovascular therapy, no general recommendation can be given. The choice of the device must be made individually and is triggered by vascular anatomy, location of stenosis, and operator preference. In general, balloon-expandable stents are stiffer and lesion access may be hampered in tortuous anatomy. This may be the reason for the relatively low technical success rate in the VISSIT trial (54%). If vessel anatomy is appropriate, using balloon-expandable stents is more convenient as it is generally a one-step procedure. With a self-expanding stent, while nearly every lesion of a major intracranial artery is accessible, this is at the expense of it being a multiple step procedure and requiring at least one exchange maneuver. High rates of restenosis are described for both types of stents.[9,16] Drug-eluting devices may overcome this issue, but currently none have been approved for intracranial stenting.[17]

13

6. *What is the recommended postprocedural management and follow-up after endovascular treatment of intracranial atherosclerotic disease?*

Delayed hemorrhage was a major issue in SAMMPRIS, and therefore, postprocedural intensive care is recommended to ensure optimal blood pressure management and clinical observation. There is no general rule for how long dual antiplatelet medication should be taken. In SAMMPRIS and VISSIT, clopidogrel was added to ASA for 3 months, which appears reasonable but may vary with other devices and the morphological result of the procedure. With bare metal stents, the rate of restenosis generally exceeds 20% and restenosis is associated with new ischemic symptoms.[18] Therefore, a systematic follow-up regimen should be established.

13.4 Level of Evidence

Medical management is the first-line of treatment for patients with symptomatic intracranial stenosis (Class I, Level of Evidence A).

Dual antiplatelet treatment during the first 3 months after the ischemic event is most likely superior to ASA alone during the first 3 months of an event (Class IIa, Level of Evidence A).

Endovascular therapy of high-grade symptomatic intracranial stenosis can be offered as a compassionate treatment to patients with recurrent strokes despite being under optimal medical management, and who lack therapeutic alternatives as a compassionate treatment (Class IIb, Level of Evidence C).

13.5 Landmark Papers

Chimowitz MI, Lynn MJ, Howlett-Smith H, et al. Comparison of Warfarin and Aspirin for Symptomatic Intracranial Arterial Stenosis. New Engl J Med 2005; 352:1305–1316.

The study objective was to compare ASA (1300 mg/day) versus warfarin (INR 2.0–3.0) for the treatment of intracranial, symptomatic stenosis. The study population included patients with a 50–99% symptomatic stenosis of a major intracranial artery. Primary endpoint was a composite of stroke, brain hemorrhage and vascular death from other causes than stroke. A total of 569 patients were enrolled and the median follow-up was 1.8 years.

There was no difference in primary endpoint events (22.1% with ASA, 21.8% with warfarin, $p = 0.83$), but death of any cause (4.3% vs. 9.7%, $p = 0.02$), non-vascular death (1.1% vs. 3.9%, $p = 0.05$) and major hemorrhage (3.2% vs. 8.3%, $p = 0.01$) was less likely under ASA compared to warfarin. The trial was terminated early due to safety concerns.

The risk of stroke in the territory of the symptomatic artery was high at 1 year (12% under ASA, 11% under warfarin) with most events occurring during the first weeks of randomization. A subgroup analysis revealed the degree of stenosis as the most important predictor of recurrent stroke. In high-grade stenosis ($\geq 70\%$) the risk of stroke at 1 year nearly hit 20%. These patients served as the target population for endovascular therapy as an alternative treatment in future trials.

Chimowitz MI, Lynn MJ, Derdeyn CP, et al; SAMMPRIS Trial Investigators. Stenting versus aggressive medical therapy for intracranial arterial stenosis. N Engl J Med 2011;365(11):993–1003.

In SAMMPRIS trial 451 patients with a 70 to 99% symptomatic intracranial stenosis were randomized to receive either aggressive medical management plus endovascular treatment with the Wingspan self-expanding stent or aggressive medical management alone. The primary end point was stroke or death within 30 days after enrollment or after a revascularization procedure for the qualifying lesion during the follow-up period or stroke in the territory of the qualifying artery beyond 30 days. The trial was stopped early because the rate of stroke or death within 30 days in the endovascular treatment group was 14.7% compared to 5.8% with aggressive medical management alone ($p = 0.002$). In the final analysis after a median of 32.4 months 23% in the endovascular group and 15% in the medical group had an end-point event ($p = 0.0252$). Apart from the primary end point, any stroke (26% vs. 19%, $p = 0.0468$) and any major hemorrhage (13% vs. 4%, $p = 0.0009$) were more frequent in the endovascular treatment group. The disadvantage of the endovascular treatment group was mainly driven by periprocedural events. Multiple subgroup analyses were performed but no population that benefitted from endovascular treatment was identified.

Zaidat OO, Fitzsimmons BF, Woodward BK, et al. Effect of a balloon-expandable intracranial stent vs medical therapy on risk of stroke in patients with symptomatic intracranial stenosis. The VISSIT Randomized Clinical Trial. JAMA 2015; 313:1240–1248.

VISSIT also compared intracranial stenting with medical management and best medical management alone for the treatment of symptomatic intracranial stenosis. The Pharos Vitesse balloon-expandable stent was used as a study device. The primary outcome measure was a composite of stroke in the same territory within 12 months of randomization or hard TIA in the same territory day 2 through month 12 postrandomization. The trial was halted after the publication of the initial SAMMPRIS results. One hundred and twelve of the intended 210 patients were enrolled. Primary end-point events occurred more frequently in the endovascular treatment group (36.2% vs. 15.1%, $p = 0.02$), and most of the end-point events were strokes. Interestingly, the predefined criteria for stent placement success (across the lesion, residual stenosis $\leq 20\%$) were only met in 54% of the patients receiving endovascular therapy.

Alexander MJ, Zauner A, Chaloupka JC, et al; WEAVE Trial Sites and Interventionalists. WEAVE trial: final results in 152 on-label patients. Stroke 2019;50(4):889–894.

The WEAVE trial re-explored the role of the Wingspan stent system in patients presenting with symptomatic intracranial atherosclerosis.[19] However, in contrast to the SAMMPRIS trial, only the on-label use of the Wingspan stent was allowed. This postmarket surveillance trial assessed the risk of stroke and death within 72 hours of the procedure. While the goal of the trial was to enroll 389 on-label patients, the study was terminated early when a predetermined interim analysis demonstrated a lower than expected periprocedural stroke and death rate of 2.6%. The authors attributed their results to experienced operators and the strict inclusion criteria. However, this study does not consider the long-term results of patients following their treatment, and the authors recommend further investigations to properly establish the role of intracranial stenting in the treatment of symptomatic intracranial atherosclerotic disease.

13.6 Recommendations

According to the current evidence, medical management is the first line of treatment for patients with symptomatic intracranial atherosclerosis. Aggressive medical therapy should include dual antiplatelet treatment for 3 months followed by ASA alone. Clopidogrel may be replaced by ticagrelor if there is a resistance, but data on the use of ticagrelor in large artery atherosclerosis do not exist. The role of NOACs is unclear so far. Other well-known vascular risk factors need to be treated and monitored closely. Patients should be advised to increase physical activity.

In cases of recurrent stroke under aggressive medical therapy, endovascular repair could be offered as a compassionate treatment. No definite recommendation can be given regarding the type of device in terms of periprocedural outcome. Balloon-expandable stents may ease the procedure but are limited to cases with favorable anatomy. Drug-eluting stents have the potential to improve long-term patency, but no devices approved for intracranial use exist yet.

13.7 Summary

1. From an evidence-based perspective, the liberal use of intracranial stenting in patients with symptomatic high-grade intracranial stenosis cannot be recommended given the two negative prospective randomized trials. Balloon angioplasty may be an alternative but data on this are sparse and clinical experience often shows insufficient results.

2. Best medical treatment has to be regarded as a first-line therapy and endovascular repair should be reserved for patients with recurrent stroke despite optimized medical therapy. Even with aggressive medical management, the risk of stroke recurrence exceeds 10% in the first year. Therefore, developing new devices and techniques which would allow more promising studies would be valuable. Progress in this field is currently hampered by the limitations of existing treatment indications.

References

[1] Chimowitz MI, Lynn MJ, Howlett-Smith H, et al. Warfarin-Aspirin Symptomatic Intracranial Disease Trial Investigators. Comparison of warfarin and aspirin for symptomatic intracranial arterial stenosis. N Engl J Med. 2005; 352(13):1305–1316

[2] Chimowitz MI, Lynn MJ, Derdeyn CP, et al. SAMMPRIS Trial Investigators. Stenting versus aggressive medical therapy for intracranial arterial stenosis. N Engl J Med. 2011; 365(11):993–1003

[3] Derdeyn CP, Chimowitz MI, Lynn MJ, et al. Stenting and Aggressive Medical Management for Preventing Recurrent Stroke in Intracranial Stenosis Trial Investigators. Aggressive medical treatment with or without stenting in high-risk patients with intracranial artery stenosis (SAMMPRIS): the final results of a randomised trial. Lancet. 2014; 383(9914):333–341

[4] Wang Y, Wang Y, Zhao X, et al. CHANCE Investigators. Clopidogrel with aspirin in acute minor stroke or transient ischemic attack. N Engl J Med. 2013; 369(1):11–19

[5] Liu L, Wong KS, Leng X, et al. CHANCE Investigators. Dual antiplatelet therapy in stroke and ICAS: subgroup analysis of CHANCE. Neurology. 2015; 85 (13):1154–1162

[6] Wang Y, Zhao X, Lin J, et al. CHANCE Investigators. Association between cyp2c19 loss-of-function allele status and efficacy of clopidogrel for risk reduction among patients with minor stroke or transient ischemic attack. JAMA. 2016; 316(1):70–78

[7] Turan, TN, Lynn, MJ, Nizam, A. Rationale, design, and implementation of aggressive risk factor management in the SAMMPRIS Trial. Circ Cardiovasc Qual Outcomes. 2012; 5:e51–e60

[8] Turan TN, Nizam A, Lynn MJ, et al. Relationship between risk factor control and vascular events in the SAMMPRIS trial. Neurology. 2017; 88(4):379–385

[9] Zaidat, OO, Fitzsimmons, BF, Woodward, BK, et al. Effect of a balloon-expandable intracranial stent vs medical therapy on risk of stroke in patients with symptomatic intracranial stenosis. The VISSIT Randomized Clinical Trial. JAMA. 2015; 313:1240–1248

[10] Fiorella D, Derdeyn CP, Lynn MJ, et al. SAMMPRIS Trial Investigators. Detailed analysis of periprocedural strokes in patients undergoing intracranial stenting in Stenting and Aggressive Medical Management for Preventing Recurrent Stroke in Intracranial Stenosis (SAMMPRIS). Stroke. 2012; 43(10):2682–2688

[11] Lutsep HL, Barnwell SL, Larsen DT, et al. SAMMPRIS Investigators. Outcome in patients previously on antithrombotic therapy in the SAMMPRIS trial: subgroup analysis. Stroke. 2015; 46(3):775–779

[12] Lutsep HL. Does stenting versus aggressive medical therapy for intracranial arterial stenosis support stenting during medical therapy for subpopulations of patients with intracranial arterial stenosis? Stroke. 2015; 46:3282–3284

[13] Siddiq F, Memon MZ, Vazquez G, Safdar A, Qureshi AI. Comparison between primary angioplasty and stent placement for symptomatic intracranial atherosclerotic disease: meta-analysis of case series. Neurosurgery. 2009; 65 (6):1024–1033, discussion 1033–1034

[14] Siddiq F, Chaudhry SA, Khatri R, et al. Rate of postprocedural stroke and death in SAMMPRIS trial: eligible patients treated with intracranial angioplasty and/or stent placement in practice. Neurosurgery. 2012; 71(1):68–73

[15] Al-Ali F, Cree T, Duan L, et al. How effective is endovascular intracranial revascularization in stroke prevention? Results from Borgess Medical Center Intracranial Revascularization Registry. AJNR Am J Neuroradiol. 2011; 32 (7):1227–1231

[16] Levy EI, Turk AS, Albuquerque FC, et al. Wingspan in-stent restenosis and thrombosis: incidence, clinical presentation, and management. Neurosurgery. 2007; 61(3):644–650, discussion 650–651

[17] Kurre W, Aguilar-Pérez M, Fischer S, et al. Solving the issue of restenosis after stenting of intracranial stenoses: experience with Two Thin-Strut Drug-Eluting Stents (DES)-Taxus Element™ and Resolute Integrity™. Cardiovasc Intervent Radiol. 2015; 38(3):583–591

[18] Jin M, Fu X, Wei Y, Du B, Xu XT, Jiang WJ. Higher risk of recurrent ischemic events in patients with intracranial in-stent restenosis. Stroke. 2013; 44 (11):2990–2994

[19] Alexander MJ, Zauner A, Chaloupka JC, et al. WEAVE Trial Sites and Interventionalists. WEAVE trial: final results in 152 on-label patients. Stroke. 2019; 50 (4):889–894

13

14 Symptomatic Carotid Stenosis

Chesney S. Oravec, Ahmed Cheema, and Adam S. Arthur

Abstract

Symptomatic carotid stenosis carries significant risk of stroke and disability. Management is aimed at reducing the lifetime risk of disabling stroke and death. Carotid endarterectomy (CEA) is usually our first choice for patients without contraindications, but carotid angioplasty and stenting is another excellent choice for a subset of patients who may not be eligible for CEA. Selection of one or the other depends on several factors, necessitating a thorough understanding of the individual patient's health status and risks. Treatment should be selected and carried out in order to dramatically lower the risk of recurrent stroke without incurring treatment-related complications.

Keywords: carotid stenosis, symptomatic, stroke, TIA, CEA, CAS

14.1 Goals

1. Review the natural history of symptomatic carotid stenosis.
2. Review and analyze the evidence supporting the indications for treatment of symptomatic carotid stenosis.
3. Review and analyze risk factors favoring endovascular versus open treatment.
4. Discuss the literature related to outcomes following treatment of symptomatic carotid stenosis.

14.2 Case Example

14.2.1 History of Present Illness

The patient is a 63-year-old male who presents immediately after an episode of acute onset vision loss in his right eye, which occurred while reading. He described it as a "black spot" in his right visual field that appeared suddenly. Full vision returned after approximately 2 minutes. The patient denied any associated pain, headache, nausea/vomiting, photophobia, recent trauma, illness, or cough, as well as any history of ocular disease or stroke.

Past medical history: Hypertension, hyperlipidemia, myocardial infarction (MI), chronic obstructive pulmonary disease.
Past surgical history: Cardiac stents.
Family history: Hypertension in parents.
Social history: Tobacco—two packs per day for 20 years; denies alcohol and illicit drugs.
Medications: Metoprolol, aspirin, plavix, atorvastatin.
Allergies: Penicillin (causes rash).
Review of systems: As per the above.
Neurological examination: Unremarkable.
Imaging studies: See figures. In ▶ Fig. 14.1, ▶ Fig. 14.2, and ▶ Fig. 14.3, digital subtraction angiography (DSA) shows severe stenosis of right common carotid artery.

14.2.2 Treatment Plan

The patient was admitted to the hospital and underwent a right-sided carotid endarterectomy (CEA) without complication.

14.2.3 Follow-up

The patient did well following the CEA and had no further issues with stroke or stroke-like symptoms. He was seen for a follow-up in clinic at 3 weeks postoperatively and was symptom free.

14.3 Case Summary

1. *What factors influence the decision to offer a revascularization procedure to this patient?*

   The major factors that support surgical treatment of the stenosis are the presence of symptoms, severity of the stenosis, the type of symptoms, and timing of presentation after symptom onset. Symptoms consistent with carotid stenosis should initiate imaging such as CT angiogram or four-vessel angiogram to evaluate severity of the stenosis, as well as studies to rule out other potential etiologies, such as isolated ophthalmologic issues, seizures, or multiple sclerosis.

   Based on the North American Symptomatic Carotid Endarterectomy Trial (NASCET), patients presenting with symptomatic stenosis measuring 70 to 99% and treated with medical

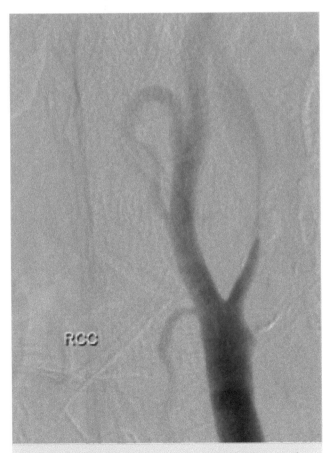

Fig. 14.1 Right common carotid artery injection, lateral view, early arterial phase.

14

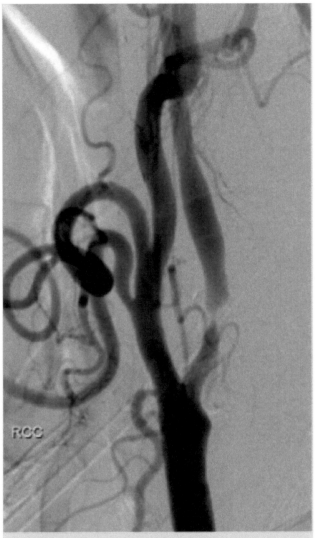

Fig. 14.2 Right common carotid artery injection, lateral view, showing severe stenosis of the right internal carotid artery stenosis.

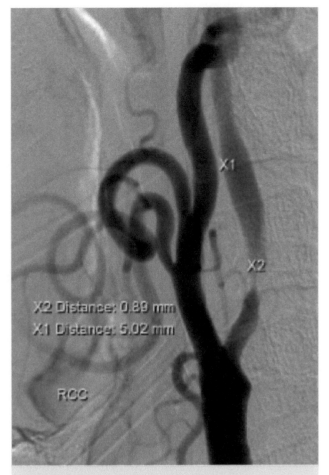

Fig. 14.3 Right common carotid artery injection, lateral view, with measurements of right internal carotid artery stenosis.

therapy had a 26% risk of any stroke at 2 years and a 13.1% risk of a major stroke or death at 2 years.[1] The NASCET study data also showed a reduced risk of any stroke, major stroke, and fatal stroke when patients were treated with CEA over medical therapy alone in a center that routinely performs carotid interventions.[1] Therefore, to avoid subsequent stroke, the patient with symptomatic carotid stenosis should be counseled to undergo treatment.

The type of presenting symptoms can stratify high-risk and low-risk patients and help determine the type and timing of intervention. For a recent transient ischemic attack (TIA), some symptoms have been shown to confer a higher short-term risk of stroke. As determined by a secondary analysis of the NASCET trial data, patients who had a hemispheric TIA—defined as distinct neurological dysfunction lasting less than 24 hours—as the qualifying event experienced a higher risk of short-term stroke than those with hemispheric stroke.[2] For these patients, the risk of stroke following the hemispheric TIA was 5.5% at 48 hours and 20.1% at 90 days. Comparatively, patients who presented after experiencing a

hemispheric stroke (defined as stroke symptoms persisting beyond 24 hours) had only a 2.3% risk of stroke at 90 days. Of note, this 90-day stroke risk was not independently predicted by degree of stenosis.

2. *What patient factors would influence the decision to recommend CEA versus carotid angioplasty and stenting (CAS)?*

a) Age—Patient's age is an important consideration for determining the type of revascularization procedure. There are data showing that patients undergoing stenting over the age of 70 and endarterectomy over the age of 80 are considered high risk due to the risk of periprocedural stroke and risks of general anesthesia, respectively. To minimize the risks of general anesthesia, carotid stenting offers an alternative to patients who, due to age or other risk factors, are not candidates for general anesthesia. Some centers offer CEA without general anesthesia for this reason.

1. Patients aged 70 or older treated with CAS had a 12% risk of stroke or death within 120 days, compared to a 6% risk in those patients treated with CEA.[3] In addition, compared to the patients below the age of 60, patients above the age of 70 have a four times greater periprocedural risk following CAS.[4]

2. Patients with greatly advanced age, defined as greater than or equal to 85 years, are at an especially increased risk of morbidity and mortality when

14

undergoing general anesthesia.[5] In addition, patients aged 80 and older had higher rates of postoperative complications, and there were higher 30-day mortality rates among those who experienced complications.[6]

b) Sex—Male patients with atherosclerotic stenosis have a fourfold greater risk for future stroke than similar female patients and therefore are more likely to benefit from CEA.[7]

c) Ability to take antiplatelet drugs—Patients who are unable or unwilling to take antiplatelet drugs are better served with CEA because stent placement requires dual antiplatelet therapy to reduce the risk of perioperative complications, including stroke and in-stent thrombosis.[8,9,10] Patients can undergo CEA while taking either aspirin alone or dual antiplatelet medications.

d) Cardiovascular/Renal risk—As predicted by the Revised Cardiac Index for vascular surgery (which includes multiple risk factors such as hypertension, congestive heart failure, ischemic heart disease, cerebrovascular disease, insulin-dependent diabetes, renal failure, or age > 75), patients with three or more risk factors are at an increased risk of perioperative MI when undergoing vascular surgery; therefore, patients deemed to be high risk for vascular surgery may benefit more from CAS.[11] On the other hand, stenting in patients with renal disease is an unfavorable option due to the need for contrast administration.

3. *What technical factors would influence the decision to pursue CEA versus CAS?*

a) Surgical accessibility—Patients with a high carotid bifurcation (i.e., at the level of C2 or higher) may be better candidates for endovascular therapy; however, a high carotid lesion has not been associated with increased risk of cranial nerve injury with open surgery.[12]

b) Prior CEA—Prior surgery to the region may make it more difficult to separate structures without incurring injury, especially nerve injury, due to the presence of scar tissue.[12]

c) Other—Other features that may increase surgical difficulty include radiation to the head/neck region as well as prior neck surgery of any sort, both of which can lead to scarring and increase the risk of nerve injury as discussed above.

4. *What treatment, if any, should be pursued for the contralateral carotid artery?*

A staged CEA may be pursued for the contralateral carotid artery, to be performed following successful recovery from surgery on the symptomatic side first, if needed.

5. *What is the follow-up regimen?*

The first follow-up should occur around 2 weeks postoperatively to ensure proper wound healing and check for postoperative complications, including any further stroke-like symptoms or to check for the evolution of any nerve injuries that may have occurred during surgery. At 3 months postoperatively, a carotid ultrasound should be done to evaluate the artery for any new stenosis or restenosis. If there is no evidence of stenosis on ultrasound, follow-up should proceed with an annual surveillance ultrasound. If restenosis has occurred, further evaluation should be undertaken with either CT angiography or catheter-based angiography.

14.4 Level of Evidence

Presence of symptoms: For symptomatic stenosis, treatment should be performed (Class I, Level of Evidence A).

Severity of the stenosis: For stenosis 70 to 99%, treatment should be performed (Class I, Level of Evidence B).

Timing: Treatment performed within 2 weeks of the last symptomatic event may be beneficial in reducing the risk of recurrent stroke (Class IIb, Level of Evidence C).

Age: For patients over the age of 70, performing CEA instead of CAS may be beneficial in decreasing the risk of periprocedural stroke (Class IIa, Level of Evidence B).

Sex: For male patients, CEA should be performed (Class I, Level of Evidence A).

Ability to take antiplatelet drugs: Because stenting requires adherence to an antiplatelet regimen, patients who are unable or unwilling to follow such a regimen should undergo CEA (Class I, Level of Evidence B).

Cardiovascular risk: In patients with multiple vascular risk factors, CAS may be more beneficial than CEA (Class IIa, Level of Evidence B).

Renal risk: In patients with renal disease, it is reasonable to choose CEA over CAS due to the renal risks of contrast administration (Class IIa, Level of Evidence C).

Surgical accessibility: It may be reasonable to treat stenosis in patients with high carotid bifurcations with CAS over CEA (Class IIb, Level of Evidence C).

Prior CEA: It is reasonable to treat stenosis in patients with prior CEA with CAS to avoid the risk of nerve injury with repeat CEA (Class IIa, Level of Evidence C).

14.5 Landmark Papers

Barnett HJM, Taylor DW, Haynes RB, et al; North American Symptomatic Carotid Endarterectomy Trial Collaborators. Beneficial effect of carotid endarterectomy in symptomatic patients with high-grade carotid stenosis. N Engl J Med 1991;325(7):445–453.[13]

The NASCET trial was among the first of its kind in investigating the effect of CEA on the risk of stroke for patients with symptomatic carotid stenosis. Patients with a recent hemispheric or retinal TIA, and 70 to 99% stenosis of the ipsilateral carotid artery, were randomized to receive either optimal medical care alone or optimal medical care plus CEA. A total of 659 patients with stenosis of 70 to 99% were randomized; 331 were assigned to the medical therapy group and 328 were assigned to undergo CEA. Patients were followed at multiple intervals for a total of 2 years, with an average completed follow-up of 18 months. In the assigned medical group, 6.3% of patients crossed-over to receive surgery, and in the CEA group, only one patient crossed over to medical therapy after refusing the operation.

The rate of perioperative (within 30 days after surgery) stroke and death was 5.8% in the CEA group but was 3.3% in a comparable time period for the medical therapy group. At the 2-year follow-up, the rate of ipsilateral stroke was 26% in the medical therapy group and 9% in the CEA group. This represented an absolute risk reduction of 17%. The short-term risk of any ipsilateral stroke in the CEA group was slightly higher than the medical group until 3 months, after which point the risk of

14

ipsilateral stroke was persistently higher in the medical therapy group. This trend was similarly observed for the risk of any stroke, any major stroke, and death. Furthermore, the protective effect of CEA on the risk of stroke appeared to last for at least 30 months.

Overall the NASCET trial determined that for patients with symptomatic 70 to 99% stenosis, perioperative risk of CEA was outweighed by the reduced risk of major stroke or death for at least 24 to 30 months postoperatively. Based on this information, the authors recommended that patients with TIAs or recent minor stroke, along with arteriography-confirmed high-grade carotid stenosis, should be referred to medical centers with low rates of perioperative morbidity and mortality when performing CEAs.

ECSTC Group. Randomised trial of endarterectomy for recently symptomatic carotid stenosis: final results of the MRC European Carotid Surgery Trial (ECST). Lancet 1998;351:1379–1387.[14]

This landmark paper was a randomized trial following 3,024 patients between 1981 and 1994 who had recently symptomatic carotid stenosis. Patients were assigned to either the treatment or control group. Treatment was CEA and control was to avoid surgery as long as possible; there were 1,811 and 1,213 patients in each respective group. Mean follow-up was 6.1 years, and the primary end point studied was major stroke or death. Surgery was to be performed within 1 year of randomization for the CEA group, and this was done for 96% of those assigned to CEA (95% received surgery within 70 days). Surgery was also performed within 1 year of randomization for 3.5% of those assigned to the control group and were thus classified as crossovers. A total of 11.5% of those assigned to the control group underwent surgery during the trial period which was most often done to treat recurrent symptoms.

Major stroke or death was seen in 37% of the CEA group and 36.5% of the control group. Major stroke or death within 30 days of surgery was seen in 7% of patients in the treatment group. At 3 years' follow-up, major stroke or death was seen in 14.9% of the CEA group and 26.5% of the control group.

Outcomes were examined according to the degree of severity of carotid stenosis. In the control group the risk of stroke in the first 3 years following randomization positively correlated with stenosis severity, but after 3 years it did not. However, when considering the risk of major ipsilateral stroke in the 3 years following a successful CEA, there was an absolute risk reduction of 18.6% over the control group for stenosis above 80%.

Overall, ECST demonstrated that the operative risk of major stroke or death associated with CEA was not insignificant. However, for patients with ≥ 80% stenosis, the rate of stroke-free survival at 3 years was significantly lower after CEA. The authors concluded that the evidence indicates the short-term operative risk of CEA is outweighed by the significant risk reduction over the long term in patients with severe stenosis.

Eckstein HH, Ringleb P, Allenberg JR, et al; Results of the Stent-Protected Angioplasty versus Carotid Endarterectomy (SPACE) study to treat symptomatic stenoses at 2 years: a multinational, prospective, randomised trial. Lancet Neurol 2008;7(10):893–902.[15]

This study aimed to compare carotid artery stenting (CAS) and CEA for symptomatic carotid stenosis. A total of 1,214 patients were randomized to receive 1 of these 2 treatments. Patients were required to have had TIA or moderate stroke

(defined as modified Rankin scale score of 0–3) in the previous 6 months. Carotid stenting was assigned to 613 patients and CEA to 601 patients. Eighteen patients were excluded from the analysis due to withdrawal of consent prior to treatment. The primary end point of the study was the rate of stroke or death within 30 days postoperatively. At the 2-year follow-up, additional end points included any stroke, death, and recurrent stenosis of at least 70%.

The primary end point showed a similar rate of death or ipsilateral stroke within 30 days of either procedure, with a rate of 6.92% in patients treated with CAS and 6.45% in patients treated with CEA. At 2 years, the overall mortality was 6.3% versus 5.0% in the CAS and CEA groups, respectively, and the rate of ipsilateral stroke was 9.5% versus 8.8% in the CAS and CEA groups, respectively. When analyzed by intention-to-treat, the rate of recurrent stenosis > 70% at 2 years was 10.7% in the CAS group and 11.1% in the CEA group, with most cases occurring within 6 months of initial treatment (51.9% in the CAS group and 52.2% in the CEA group). In subgroup analyses, a few trends were noted. The rate of outcome events within 30 days was found to increase with increasing age for those in the CAS group. Examining this trend out to 2 years, it was found that patients > 68 years tended to have more events when treated with CAS compared to CEA, suggesting a benefit for patients over 68 to be treated with CEA.

In conclusion, this study failed to show noninferiority for CAS with regard to 30-day event rates, but at 2 years, there was no difference seen between CEA and CAS with regard to rates of clinical outcomes or recurrent events.

Mantese VA, Timaran CH, Chiu D, Begg RJ, Brott TG. CREST Investigators. The Carotid Revascularization Endarterectomy versus Stenting Trial (CREST): stenting versus carotid endarterectomy for carotid disease. Stroke 2010; 41(10, Suppl)S31–S34.[16]

In this major randomized trial comparing CEA to CAS, 2,502 symptomatic and asymptomatic patients were enrolled with 1,240 assigned to receive CEA and 1,262 assigned to receive CAS. Patients were required to have symptoms within the preceding 6 months and/or have severe stenosis at randomization. The primary end point was any stroke, MI, or death within the periprocedural period (a defined period following the procedure); any ipsilateral stroke within 4 years after the procedure was also considered part of the primary end point.

When the primary end point was considered as a whole, there was no significant difference between the two groups. However, when broken down by the individual component of primary end point, there were some differences that proved significant. CAS had a higher incidence of stroke (4.1% vs. 2.3%) and death (0.7% vs. 0.3%) in the periprocedural period, but CEA had a higher incidence of MI (2.3% vs. 1.1%) in this period. For symptomatic patients, the risk of stroke and death was higher with CAS (6.0%) than CEA (3.2%). There was no difference in ipsilateral stroke out to 4 years follow-up.

The authors included a discussion of follow-up data at 1 year. This tended to suggest that despite being lower in the short term, the rate of MI following CAS approached that of CEA. On the other hand, the lower risk of stroke following CEA appeared to persist out to 1 year. Age may also play a role as patients > 70 years tended to do better with CEA and patients < 70 years did better with CAS.

14

Mas JL, Trinquart L, Leys D, et al; EVA-3S investigators. Endarterectomy versus angioplasty in patients with symptomatic severe carotid stenosis (EVA-3S) trial: results up to 4 years from a randomised, multicentre trial. Lancet Neurol 2008;7(10):885–892.[17]

In this study conducted at 30 centers in France, investigators compared outcomes after carotid stenting and CEA. The authors sought to determine the long-term patient outcomes and prevention of stroke and death. Patients with carotid stenosis of at least 60% and who were recently symptomatic (defined as hemispheric or retinal TIA, or nondisabling stroke within the past 4 months) were randomized to receive either CAS or CEA. Patients were followed for 30 days postprocedure to determine the primary end point of rate of stroke or death. Patients were also followed out to 4 years to determine the secondary end point of any stroke or death in the follow-up period. A total of 527 patients were randomized, with 262 assigned to CEA and 265 to CAS.

The analysis included 520 patients as 7 of the 527 randomized did not undergo treatment. Median follow-up was 43 months in the CEA group and 42 months in the CAS group. At 30 days, the rate of stroke or death in the CEA group was 3.9% and in the CAS group, it was 9.6%. In the 4-year follow-up analysis, the rate of any stroke was similar in both groups: 4.94% among CEA and 4.49% among CAS patients. A subgroup analysis found that the excess risk of ipsilateral stroke among CAS patients was higher in patients who were male, were ≥ 70 years of age, had prior stroke, and those who had stroke as their qualifying event as opposed to TIA.

In conclusion, the authors describe a 4-year cumulative risk of stroke or death that is higher after stenting than CEA. This difference is attributed to the higher short-term (within 30 days) risk of event after stenting because the risk was relatively low and similar in both groups in the follow-up period between 31 days and 4 years. Therefore, the authors conclude that CAS is as effective as CEA for medium-term prevention of stroke.

Bonati LH, Dobson J, Featherstone RL, et al; International Carotid Stenting Study investigators. Long-term outcomes after stenting versus endarterectomy for treatment of symptomatic carotid stenosis: the International Carotid Stenting Study (ICSS) randomised trial. Lancet 2015;385(9967):529–538.[18]

Symptomatic patients with carotid stenosis of at least 50% were randomized to receive either carotid stenting or endarterectomy. The primary end point was rate of fatal or disabling stroke within the follow-up period. In total, 1,713 patients were randomized, with 855 assigned to the CAS group and 858 to the CEA group. Patients were followed for at least 5 years, with a median follow-up time of 4.2 years, and some patients continued follow-up out to 10 years.

The CAS group experienced a cumulative risk of fatal or disabling stroke of 6.4% over 5 years, while the CEA group experienced a rate of 6.5%. Thus, there was no significant difference in the primary end point. The rate of any stroke was higher in the CAS group (15.2%) compared with the CEA group (9.4%); however, this did not lead to significant differences in functional outcomes as measured by the modified Rankin Scale score. The rate of all-cause mortality was not different between the groups, nor was the rate of severe recurrent carotid stenosis.

Overall, the authors conclude that both procedures are equally effective in preventing fatal or disabling stroke as well as in achieving similar functional outcomes. There is currently a CREST2 study underway to investigate the benefits of intervention for asymptomatic high-grade stenosis.

14.6 Recommendations

Patients with symptomatic moderate- to high-grade stenosis should undergo a revascularization procedure. CEA remains the mainstay of treatment for revascularization; however, carotid stenting, in select patients, based upon their overall clinical picture, may be an excellent option. Medical management and risk factor reduction should still be maximized in addition to revascularization.

14.7 Summary

1. The natural history of symptomatic carotid stenosis includes a high risk of stroke; therefore, these patients should be treated.
2. Multiple factors related to the patient and/or the stenosis should be taken into account when evaluating a patient to determine a treatment course.
3. CEA has been shown to be more effective than CAS in some cases.[3,4] However, if there is a reason to avoid CEA as discussed above, CAS is a reasonable alternative treatment option.

References

[1] Ferguson GG, Eliasziw M, Barr HW, et al. The North American Symptomatic Carotid Endarterectomy Trial: surgical results in 1415 patients. Stroke. 1999; 30(9):1751–1758

[2] Eliasziw M, Kennedy J, Hill MD, Buchan AM, Barnett HJ, North American Symptomatic Carotid Endarterectomy Trial Group. Early risk of stroke after a transient ischemic attack in patients with internal carotid artery disease. CMAJ. 2004; 170(7):1105–1109

[3] Bonati LH, Fraedrich G, Carotid Stenting Trialists' Collaboration. Age modifies the relative risk of stenting versus endarterectomy for symptomatic carotid stenosis: a pooled analysis of EVA-3S, SPACE and ICSS. Eur J Vasc Endovasc Surg. 2011; 41(2):153–158

[4] Howard G, Roubin GS, Jansen O, et al. Carotid Stenting Trialists' Collaboration. Association between age and risk of stroke or death from carotid endarterectomy and carotid stenting: a meta-analysis of pooled patient data from four randomised trials. Lancet. 2016; 387(10025):1305–1311

[5] Fleisher LA, Pasternak LR, Herbert R, Anderson GF. Inpatient hospital admission and death after outpatient surgery in elderly patients: importance of patient and system characteristics and location of care. Arch Surg. 2004; 139 (1):67–72

[6] Hamel MB, Henderson WG, Khuri SF, Daley J. Surgical outcomes for patients aged 80 and older: morbidity and mortality from major noncardiac surgery. J Am Geriatr Soc. 2005; 53(3):424–429

[7] Petty GW, Brown RD, Jr, Whisnant JP, Sicks JD, O'Fallon WM, Wiebers DO. Ischemic stroke subtypes: a population-based study of incidence and risk factors. Stroke. 1999; 30(12):2513–2516

[8] Dalainas I, Nano G, Bianchi P, Stegher S, Malacrida G, Tealdi DG. Dual antiplatelet regime versus acetyl-acetic acid for carotid artery stenting. Cardiovasc Intervent Radiol. 2006; 29(4):519–521

[9] Enomoto Y, Yoshimura S. Antiplatelet therapy for carotid artery stenting. Intervent Neurol. 2013; 1(3–4):151–163

[10] McKevitt FM, Randall MS, Cleveland TJ, Gaines PA, Tan KT, Venables GS. The benefits of combined anti-platelet treatment in carotid artery stenting. Eur J Vasc Endovasc Surg. 2005; 29(5):522–527

[11] Bauer SM, Cayne NS, Veith FJ. New developments in the preoperative evaluation and perioperative management of coronary artery disease in patients undergoing vascular surgery. J Vasc Surg. 2010; 51(1):242–251

14

[12] Tsantilas P, Kuehnl A, Brenner E, Eckstein HH. Anatomic criteria determining high-risk carotid surgery patients. J Cardiovasc Surg (Torino). 2017; 58 (2):152–160

[13] Barnett HJM, Taylor DW, Haynes RB, et al. North American Symptomatic Carotid Endarterectomy Trial Collaborators. Beneficial effect of carotid endarterectomy in symptomatic patients with high-grade carotid stenosis. N Engl J Med. 1991; 325(7):445–453

[14] ECSTC Group. Randomised trial of endarterectomy for recently symptomatic carotid stenosis: final results of the MRC European Carotid Surgery Trial (ECST). Lancet. 1998; 351:1379–1387

[15] Eckstein HH, Ringleb P, Allenberg JR, et al. Results of the Stent-Protected Angioplasty versus Carotid Endarterectomy (SPACE) study to treat symptomatic stenoses at 2 years: a multinational, prospective, randomised trial. Lancet Neurol. 2008; 7(10):893–902

[16] Mantese VA, Timaran CH, Chiu D, Begg RJ, Brott TG, CREST Investigators. The Carotid Revascularization Endarterectomy versus Stenting Trial (CREST): stenting versus carotid endarterectomy for carotid disease. Stroke. 2010; 41 (10) Suppl:S31–S34

[17] Mas JL, Trinquart L, Leys D, et al. EVA-3S investigators. Endarterectomy versus angioplasty in patients with symptomatic severe carotid stenosis (EVA-3S) trial: results up to 4 years from a randomised, multicentre trial. Lancet Neurol. 2008; 7(10):885–892

[18] Bonati LH, Dobson J, Featherstone RL, et al. International Carotid Stenting Study investigators. Long-term outcomes after stenting versus endarterectomy for treatment of symptomatic carotid stenosis: the International Carotid Stenting Study (ICSS) randomised trial. Lancet. 2015; 385(9967):529–538

14

15 Asymptomatic Carotid Stenosis

Philip G. R. Schmalz, Paul M. Foreman, and Mark R. Harrigan

Abstract

The management of carotid stenosis is a fundamental component of the neurointerventionalist's practice. Decision making for these patients weighs the risk of future stroke with the procedural risks. Though historical studies have shown benefit for revascularization procedures, newer medical therapies have narrowed the therapeutic index for these procedures. Careful patient selection, based on established evidence, is necessary to ensure revascularization will provide benefit.

Keywords: endarterectomy, carotid, stroke, cardiovascular diseases, atherosclerosis, cerebrovascular disorders, carotid stenosis

15.1 Goals

1. Understand the risk profile of a patient with asymptomatic carotid stenosis. Review medical and anatomical risk factors for stroke in patients with asymptomatic carotid stenosis and understand how medical, surgical, or interventional management can alter this risk profile.
2. Review the literature on medical, surgical, and interventional treatment of patients with asymptomatic carotid stenosis.
3. Understand the risks and benefits of all the three management strategies.

15.2 Case Example

15.2.1 History of Present Illness

An 80-year-old female presented to her primary care physician with complaints of right-sided intermittent headache. She had a history of cigarette smoking and both coronary and peripheral arterial disease. Examination revealed a bruit over the left carotid artery. Duplex carotid ultrasonography and computed tomography (CT) angiography of the head and neck were obtained demonstrating left-sided extracranial internal carotid artery (ICA) stenosis. She was referred for neurosurgical consultation. Other than intermittent headaches, she had no neurological complaints or symptoms attributable to cerebral ischemia, including motor or sensory change or language dysfunction.

Past medical history: Notable for hyperlipidemia, coronary artery disease, and peripheral arterial disease. There was no history of stroke or transient ischemic attack (TIA).
Past surgical history: Bilateral iliac artery stenting 2 years prior.
Social history: More than 50 pack-year smoker with several recent attempts at smoking cessation.
Examination: There were no neurological abnormalities on examination. A bruit was heard over the left carotid artery.
Imaging studies: See ▶ Fig. 15.1 and ▶ Fig. 15.2.

15.2.2 Treatment Plan

The importance of smoking cessation was stressed and the patient agreed to additional efforts to stop smoking. Medical treatment for smoking cessation was offered but declined. The patient was taking 81 mg of aspirin daily but had stopped taking her prescribed statin medication. Plans were made to coordinate with the patient's primary physician to facilitate smoking cessation and achieve cholesterol goals with use of a statin. In addition, the patient was counseled on symptoms of cerebral ischemia and encouraged to report these immediately. Plans were made for follow-up in 1 year with an additional carotid duplex ultrasound.

15.2.3 Follow-up

Working with her primary physician, the patient was able to successfully stop smoking. Cholesterol goals were targeted initially with simvastatin, and ultimately the patient achieved her cholesterol goals with the addition of ezetemibe. Aspirin therapy was continued. No symptoms of ischemia developed. A repeat carotid ultrasound study showed decreased velocities in the ICA.

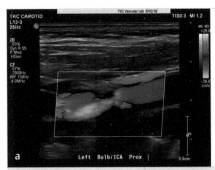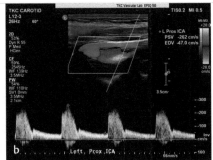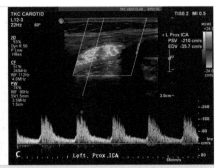

Fig. 15.1 **(a)** Carotid duplex ultrasound of the left carotid bifurcation demonstrating atherosclerotic stenosis and increased velocities. **(b)** More distal view of the left internal carotid artery (ICA) with Doppler peak systolic velocities (PSV) of 262 cm/s, which was interpreted to represent > 80% stenosis. Note the shadowing (absence of soft-tissue signal deep to the plaque) of the heavily calcified plaque at the right of the image. **(c)** Follow-up carotid duplex ultrasound after 1 year of medical management demonstrates mild reduction in PSV.

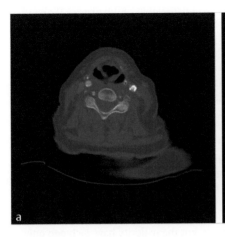
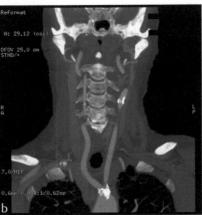

Fig. 15.2 Computed tomography (CT) angiogram of the neck **(a)** axial and **(b)** coronal views demonstrating a heavily calcified plaque at the left carotid bifurcation. There is no enhancement at the region of stenosis. Note the heavily calcified origin of the common carotid artery at the aortic arch.

15.3 Case Summary

1. *What is the risk of stroke in a patient with asymptomatic carotid stenosis without surgical or endovascular treatment? How have changes in the medical treatment changed the clinical course of patients with asymptomatic carotid stenosis treated with medical therapy alone?*

   Atherosclerotic stenosis of the extracranial carotid arteries is a relatively common disease of older adults, affecting approximately 7% of women and > 12% of men aged 70 years or above.[1] Our knowledge of the risk posed by asymptomatic carotid stenosis has evolved considerably in the last 20 years, largely due to the advances in medical therapies. Several landmark papers, reviewed in greater detail later in this chapter, have contributed to this progression in understanding. The two largest trials that have addressed the issue of asymptomatic carotid stenosis are the Asymptomatic Carotid Atherosclerosis Study (ACAS) and the Asymptomatic Carotid Surgery Trial (ACST).[2,3] These studies, both performed in the 1990s, were two randomized trials of carotid endarterectomy (CEA) versus medical therapy. In both studies, the annual risk of stroke from asymptomatic stenosis greater than 60% was found to be approximately 2% in the nonsurgical arms.

   While these studies are important as a foundation for our understanding of this disease process, it is important to bear in mind that they were performed over 20 years ago, prior to widespread use of aggressive medical management including statins and newer antiplatelet agents. Newer studies suggest that the risk of stroke from asymptomatic stenosis treated medically has fallen in the last 30 years.[4] Several recent studies suggest that the annual stroke risk of nonsurgical treatment of asymptomatic carotid stenosis ranges from 0.3 to 1.3%.[5,6,7,8] Thus, while ACAS and ACST remain important studies in the history of the disease, they have largely been eclipsed by contemporary data which show a very low risk in asymptomatic patients treated with medical therapy alone. Despite this overall low risk, certain patients may benefit from intervention if properly selected on the basis of certain anatomical and medical factors.

2. *What clinical or radiological variables can aid in risk stratification and decision making for intervention?*

   Our understanding of the risk of asymptomatic carotid stenosis has become more nuanced in recent years. Several clinical

and radiological features have been identified as risk factors for stroke in these patients. These risk factors provide a means for risk stratification and may allow clinicians to select patients for which an alteration in medical therapy or an intervention may be beneficial. The simplest means of risk stratification which is widely available is the percentage of stenosis. Though this method is simple and available, it demonstrates a lack of understanding of the pathogenesis of stroke due to carotid disease, which is overwhelmingly thromboembolic rather than related to hemodynamic failure. Accordingly, study data on the degree of stenosis as an accurate predictor of ipsilateral stroke risk are mixed.[9,10] Thus, more specific risk factors are likely to prove helpful for decision making. These include progression of stenosis on serial carotid ultrasound, plaque features, and findings on additional cranial studies including transcranial Doppler (TCD) ultrasound and standard axial imaging.

The overall plaque burden (which includes the cross-sectional area of plaque from the clavicle to the mandible) has been shown to predict ipsilateral stroke significantly better than the degree of stenosis.[10] In addition, approximately 25% of patients will show progression of stenosis on annual carotid ultrasound studies. This progression has been shown to increase the risk of stroke to as high as 27% over a mean follow-up period of 42 months.[11] Other features of the plaque itself have been shown to increase the risk of stroke. A systematic review showed that plaque echolucency on ultrasound, which is suggestive of lipid-rich necrotic core, raised stroke risk to approximately 10%, a roughly 2.5 relative risk increase, over a follow-up period of 30 months.[12] In addition to echolucency, motion within the plaque is suggestive of plaque instability. This finding has also been shown to increase the risk of stroke in one study (hazard ratio ~5).[13] Other findings suggestive of plaque instability that are thought to increase the risk of stroke include the volume of plaque ulceration on three-dimensional ultrasonography, as well as enhancement of the carotid bulb on CT angiography.[14,15]

In addition to features of the carotid plaque itself, TCD can be used to stratify stroke risk.[16] Approximately 10% of patients with asymptomatic carotid stenosis have evidence of emboli on TCD.[17] TCD recording showing two or more embolic signals over 1 hour has been shown to elevate the absolute annual risk of stroke to 7%.[18] In this study, the hazard ratio

15

for ipsilateral stroke in patients who had emboli detected on TCD was > 6.[18] Finally, as might be expected, evidence of previous silent stroke on CT or magnetic resonance imaging (MRI) predicts ischemia, raising the annual event rate of stroke or TIA to 4.6%.[19]

In this particular patient's case, though the degree of stenosis was severe, the plaque was heavily calcified, dense, and though somewhat heterogeneous in appearance, did not have evidence of ulceration (▶ Fig. 15.1 and ▶ Fig. 15.2). Thus, the patient's risk of stroke was deemed relatively low. TCD studies were not performed.

3. *What are the key aspects of maximal medical management for patients with asymptomatic carotid stenosis? What is the optimal antiplatelet strategy in these patients?*

The medical management of asymptomatic carotid stenosis focuses on modifiable risk factors for stroke including cholesterol reduction, treatment of hypertension, and antiplatelet medication. Hypertension is the most prevalent risk factor for stroke and is increasing with increasing age and obesity.[20,21] More than two-thirds of the U.S. population above 65 years of age is hypertensive.[22] The treatment of hypertension has been shown to decrease the risk of stroke and is recommended for primary stroke prevention.[23] With the advent of multiple antihypertensive medications and sophisticated risk stratification, the treatment of hypertension has become complex and algorithm based with recommendations often in flux.[22,24] Patients with high-grade stenosis and longstanding untreated hypertension are at risk for hemodynamic failure if hypertension is overcorrected or corrected too rapidly. It is recommended that neurointerventional specialists coordinate antihypertensive care for prevention of stroke with involvement of the primary care physician.

Smoking has been clearly established in numerous longitudinal studies to increase stroke risk. A systematic review assessing the risk for ischemic stroke in smokers showed a nearly twofold relative risk increase compared to nonsmokers.[25] Furthermore, it has been shown that smoking cessation rapidly decreases stroke and other cardiovascular risk to a level that approaches but does not quite reach that of the nonsmoking population.[26,27,28] Numerous strategies are available to assist patients in smoking cessation including FDA-approved medications. These treatments should be offered to smokers with asymptomatic carotid stenosis.[23,29,30] In this case, the patient had attempted smoking cessation but was initially unsuccessful. Working with the primary physician, this patient was able to stop smoking without the use of adjunctive medications.

Elevated total cholesterol, as well as elevation of low-density lipoprotein (LDL) relative to high-density lipoprotein (HDL) have been established as risk factors both for atherosclerosis and ischemic stroke.[31,32] More specifically, hyperlipidemia has been established as a risk factor for both carotid atherosclerosis and stenosis with lipid-rich plaque.[33,34] Treatment of these conditions with statin drugs has been shown to both slow the progression of carotid atherosclerosis and reduce the relative risk for ischemic stroke by 21%.[35,36] Research on other lipid-lowering agents is nascent; however, a clinical trial demonstrated a reduction in the risk of ischemic stroke in patients with diabetes with the addition of ezetimibe to statin therapy (as used in this patient).[37] Specific guidelines

for the management of hypercholesterolemia are regularly updated by the National Institutes of Health through the National Cholesterol Education Program Adult Treatment Panel (NCEP-ATP).

The benefit of antiplatelet therapy for patients with carotid atherosclerotic disease is well established. The Mayo Asymptomatic Carotid Endarterectomy Study, which did not use aspirin in the surgical arm, was terminated early due to the higher number of coronary and cerebral ischemic events in the surgical arm.[38] This underscores the importance of antiplatelet therapy in this disease. Aspirin is the mainstay of antiplatelet therapy for asymptomatic carotid stenosis; however, the optimal dose of aspirin in this setting is not well established.[39] Several large trials have examined dual antiplatelet therapy or alternative antiplatelet agents for patients with carotid stenosis, but the majority have included only those patients with prior stroke or TIA.[40,41] At present, there is a lack of clinical trial data to support the use of dual antiplatelet therapy, or antiplatelet therapy other than aspirin for the prevention of a first stroke in asymptomatic patients.[39] In this case, the patient was treated with aspirin 81 mg daily.

4. *What are the benefits of CEA? What is the risk of surgery in patients with asymptomatic carotid stenosis? What factors serve to alter this risk?*

The largest studies of the surgical management of asymptomatic carotid stenosis, ACAS and ACST, found an approximately 50% risk reduction with CEA as compared to medical therapy. These studies showed perioperative stroke and death rates of 2.3 and 3.1%, respectively.[2,3] More recently, the Carotid Revascularization Endarterectomy versus Stent Trial (CREST) found 30-day perioperative stroke and death rates in asymptomatic patients undergoing CEA of 1.4%, much lower than the aforementioned trials. However, CREST was notable for the rigorous credentialing and lead-in period for operators and thus may underestimate procedural risk.[42]

A recent study using data on Medicare beneficiaries in New York State undergoing CEA for asymptomatic stenosis used a multivariate logistic regression analysis to identify clinical features predictive of perioperative stroke and death. These findings were then developed and validated as the CEA-8 Risk Score (▶ Table 15.1), which ranges from 0.6 to 9.6%.[43] Current guidelines recommend CEA only in those patients with a perioperative risk of stroke and death less than 3%; thus, this tool may prove helpful in selecting patients who may benefit from CEA.[39]

5. *What are the benefits of carotid angioplasty and stenting (CAS) for asymptomatic stenosis? What is the risk? In which patients might this therapy be offered?*

Most major noninferiority trials comparing CAS to CEA, including the Stent Supported Percutaneous Angioplasty of the Carotid versus Endarterectomy (SPACE), Endarterectomy versus Angioplasty in Patients with Symptomatic Severe Carotid Stenosis (EVA-3S), and the International Carotid Stenting Study (ICSS) trials, enrolled patients with symptomatic carotid stenosis.[44,45,46] One major study to date, the Stenting and Angioplasty with Protection in Patients at High Risk for Endarterectomy (SAPPHIRE) trial included asymptomatic patients with at least 80% stenosis deemed high risk for surgery. Though this study was stopped prematurely, stenting was found to be noninferior to endarterectomy and

15

a trend toward benefit for stenting was noted at 1 year.[47] The perioperative complication rate was 4.8% in the stenting group, but it should be noted that patients in SAPPHIRE were selected to have high-risk comorbidities. The benefits of stenting as demonstrated in the CREST study are similar to that demonstrated with CEA in ACAS.[48] The perioperative risk for CAS in asymptomatic patients in CREST was 2.5%. Interestingly, the risk of CAS was slightly higher in older patients (see below). Relative indications for CAS are provided in ► Table 15.2.

15.4 Level of Evidence[39]

Medical treatment: Patients with asymptomatic carotid stenosis, whether treated medically or surgically, should receive treatment with both aspirin and a statin and receive counseling on lifestyle modification to include smoking cessation (Class I, Level of Evidence C).

Carotid endarterectomy: Offering CEA for patients with > 70% stenosis is reasonable if the risk of perioperative stroke and death is < 3%. The effectiveness of CEA versus medical therapy is not yet well established (Class IIa, Level of Evidence A).

Carotid angioplasty and stenting: Performing CAS in highly selected patients with > 70% stenosis and contraindications to CEA may be considered; however, the effectiveness of this procedure versus current medical therapy is not yet established (Class IIb, Level of Evidence B).

Selection of revascularization technique: Although many patients with carotid stenosis are suitable candidates for CEA

and CAS, a number of factors may favor one technique over the other for any given patient.

- The risk of procedural stroke is slightly higher with CAS than CEA, while the risk of myocardial infarction (MI) is slightly higher with CEA than CAS.[48]
- Patients > 70 years have a slightly greater risk of stroke with CAS.[48]
- After the periprocedural period, the two techniques are equivalent in their efficacy to prevent stroke, and there is no significant difference in the risk of restenosis.[49]
- Current FDA approval for stenting in asymptomatic patients is limited to patients with at least 80% stenosis, while Medicare reimbursement requires patients with high-risk comorbidities such as heart failure or unstable angina.[50,51]

Detailed patient selection criteria for both CAS and CEA are presented in ► Table 15.2 and ► Table 15.3, respectively. Centers for Medicare and Medicaid Services (CMS) high-risk criteria are provided in ► Table 15.4.

15.5 Landmark Papers

15.5.1 Natural History

Marquardt L, Geraghty OC, Mehta Z, Rothwell PM. Low risk of ipsilateral stroke in patients with asymptomatic carotid stenosis on best medical treatment: a prospective, population-based study. Stroke 2010;41(1):e11–e17.

The Oxford Vascular Study is the most recent study to address asymptomatic carotid stenosis treated medically. This population-based study enrolled 1,153 patients with a history of either TIA or ischemic stroke in 1 hemisphere and > 50% stenosis of the contralateral (asymptomatic) carotid artery. All patients were treated with antiplatelet agents (aspirin and clopidogrel for the first 30 days after stroke/TIA, then aspirin-dipyridamole thereafter) and a statin (most commonly simvastatin 40 mg). In addition, all patients with blood pressure > 130/80 mm Hg were treated with one or more antihypertensive agents. Lifestyle modification was also discussed with each patient. Over a mean follow-up period of 3 years (range 1–84 mo), the authors reported an annual risk of 0.34% for ischemic stroke and 1.78% for TIA. Though this study focused on patients with asymptomatic stenosis, all patients had a prior stroke or TIA of the contralateral hemisphere. Thus, patients without a prior history of contralateral stroke or TIA might have an even lower risk than is reported in this study. The remarkably low annual stroke/TIA

Table 15.1 CEA-8 risk score predicting 30-day risk of stroke or death[43]

Risk factor	CEA-8 risk score points
Female sex	1
Nonwhite race	1
Contralateral stenosis ≥ 50%	1
Congestive heart failure	1
Coronary artery disease	1
Valvular heart disease	1
Severe disability	2
Quantitative risk category (percent risk)	**Total risk score points**
Low risk (0.6–2.2%)	0–2
Medium risk (4.7%)	3
High risk (≥ 6.6%)	≥ 4

Table 15.2 Patient selection for carotid angioplasty and stenting

Carotid angioplasty and stenting	
Relative indications	**Relative contraindications**
• Age < 70 y	• Age > 70 y
• Poor surgical candidate	• Elongated aortic arch or otherwise difficult vascular access
• Accessible vascular anatomy	• High-grade carotid stenosis
• Focal stenosis	• Long region of stenosis
• Tandem stenoses	• Aortic or femoral artery occlusion
• Previous neck surgery	• Intolerance to antiplatelet agents
• Radiation-induced stenosis	• Intolerance to iodinated contrast
• High risk for anesthesia complications	• Intraluminal thrombus

15

Table 15.3 Patient selection for carotid endarterectomy

Carotid endarterectomy	
Relative indications	**Relative contraindications**
• Age > 70 y	• Contralateral laryngeal palsy
• Few medical conditions	• Multiple medical conditions
• No previous neck surgery or radiation	• Previous neck surgery or radiation
• Thin, supple neck	• Short, thick neck
• Patent, nonstenotic contralateral carotid artery	• Contralateral carotid occlusion
• Low carotid bifurcation	• High carotid bifurcation

Table 15.4 CMS high-risk conditions

CMS "High risk for endarterectomy" conditions[51]
• Congestive heart failure class III or IV
• Left ventricular ejection fraction < 30%
• Unstable angina
• Contralateral carotid occlusion
• Recent myocardial infarction
• Previous CEA with recurrent stenosis
• Prior radiation treatment of the neck
• Other conditions that were used to determine patients at high risk for CEA in prior stenting trials and studies

Abbreviations: CEA, carotid endarterectomy; CMS, Centers for Medicare and Medicaid Services.

rates demonstrated in this study emphasizes the efficacy of medical management of this disease.

15.5.2 Endarterectomy versus Medical Therapy

Walker MD, Marler JR, Goldstein M, et al; Executive Committee for the Asymptomatic Carotid Atherosclerosis Study. Endarterectomy for asymptomatic carotid artery stenosis. JAMA 1995;273 (18):1421–1428.

The ACAS was a prospective, multicenter randomized controlled trial that enrolled 1,662 patients with at least 60% stenosis. The study was conducted at 39 clinical sites across the United States and Canada between 1987 and 1993. All patients were treated with 325-mg aspirin daily and counseled on lifestyle modification. Patients were randomized to either medical therapy alone or medical therapy plus CEA. The primary end point of the study was 5-year ipsilateral stroke rate and the perioperative stroke and death rate. This study was stopped prematurely when a significant benefit for surgery was identified. The combined risk of stroke over 5 years and perioperative stroke and death were 11% in the medical arm and 5.1% in the surgical arm for a 53% risk reduction for surgery. In the surgical group, the risk of perioperative stroke and death was 2.3%. This study demonstrated that CEA in patients with asymptomatic carotid stenosis roughly halves stroke risk over 5 years. It should be noted that this study was performed over 30 years ago and predated significant advancements in medical therapy. Thus, clinicians should be familiar with its findings; however, it may be better viewed in a historical context.

Halliday A, Mansfield A, Marro J, et al; MRC Asymptomatic Carotid Surgery Trial (ACST) Collaborative Group. Prevention of disabling and fatal strokes by successful carotid endarterectomy in patients without recent neurological symptoms: randomised controlled trial. Lancet 2004;363(9420):1491–1502.

ACST, the largest multicenter prospective randomized trial to evaluate CEA for asymptomatic carotid stenosis, enrolled 3,120 patients at 126 centers in 30 countries from 1993 to 2003. Eligible patients had 60 to 99% stenosis identified by ultrasound. Patients were randomized to either immediate CEA or indefinite deferral of CEA. Patients in both arms were treated medically with antiplatelet agents, antihypertensives when indicated, and in the latter years of the trial, statins. The primary outcomes included the perioperative stroke and death rate in patients undergoing CEA and the 5-year risk of stroke. This study found a perioperative risk of 3.1% in all patients undergoing CEA, including crossovers. Patients assigned to the immediate CEA group had a 5-year stroke rate of 6.4% compared to 11.8% in the deferred group. Unlike ACAS, ACST was able to show a benefit for CEA in women with a 5-year stroke rate of 3.8% in the immediate group versus 7.48% in the deferral group. This trial demonstrated an approximate 50% reduction in 5-year stroke risk for patients receiving CEA, which is a similar finding to ACAS. This lends support to the findings, but again, this trial should be viewed with an eye to more recent data addressing medical management of asymptomatic stenosis.

15.5.3 Endarterectomy versus Angioplasty and Stenting

Brott TG, Hobson RW II, Howard G, et al; CREST Investigators. Stenting versus endarterectomy for treatment of carotid-artery stenosis. N Engl J Med 2010;363(1):11–23.

The Carotid Revascularization Endarterectomy versus Stent Trial (CREST) was a multicenter randomized controlled trial comparing CEA versus CAS in patients with atherosclerotic carotid stenosis. The trial enrolled 2,502 patients with both asymptomatic and symptomatic carotid stenoses treated at 117 centers in the United States and Canada. The trial initially focused on symptomatic patients, but asymptomatic patients were allowed in the latter years of the trial. Asymptomatic patients were required to have slightly greater stenosis than symptomatic patients. Patients were randomized to either CEA or CAS with a single stent and embolic protection system permitted. All patients were treated medically both with antiplatelet agents (dual antiplatelet agents in the case of stenting), statins and antihypertensive medications when indicated. Surgeons underwent a selection process that required a minimum of 12 procedures per year and a complication rate of < 3% in asymptomatic patients. Similar requirements were made for interventionists. Unlike prior stenting trials, embolic protection devices were used in 96% of patients. The primary end point was a composite of perioperative stroke, MI, or death, and any ipsilateral stroke within 4 years. For asymptomatic patients, the primary end point was met in 3.5% of patients stented and 3.6% of patients treated with CEA. The risk of stroke, MI, and death was 2.5% in those stented and 1.4% in the surgical arm in the peri-procedural period, both of which were significantly lower than perioperative risk seen in symptomatic patients. The data from this study suggest that the perioperative risk of stroke is slightly higher for CAS than CEA, while the risk of MI was slightly higher for CEA. Interestingly, CAS showed slightly greater efficacy for those below 70 years of age, while CEA was more beneficial in older patients. This difference has been attributed to the greater tortuosity of older vessels. Long-term results of CREST have recently been published. Over a follow-up period of 10 years, patients who were assigned to stenting had a higher risk of stroke than those assigned to CEA; however, the postprocedural rate of stroke was equivalent between the two arms. Thus, the increased risk was attributable to procedural differences.[49]

A follow-up study to CREST, CREST-2 is currently enrolling patients. CREST-2 combines two randomized controlled trials comparing aggressive medical therapy alone to medical therapy with either CEA or CAS for asymptomatic carotid stenosis.[52]

15.6 Recommendations

Asymptomatic carotid stenosis is likely benign in many patients and medical management may be superior to surgery or endovascular treatment. Medical management versus intervention with either CEA or CAS is currently undergoing evaluation in the CREST 2 Trial. A certain subset of patients with asymptomatic carotid stenosis may benefit from surgery or endovascular treatment. These include patients with rapid progression of stenosis, ultrasound evidence suggestive of plaque instability or thrombogenicity, evidence of prior silent infarction on cranial imaging, and predicted surgical risk of stroke and death of < 3%.

15.7 Summary

1. Asymptomatic carotid stenosis is a risk factor for stroke. This risk can be decreased with medical therapy as well as revascularization procedures.
2. Medical treatment of carotid stenosis has advanced since initial trials which showed benefit to revascularization, thus narrowing the benefit margin for asymptomatic patients.
3. Clinical features and decision tools may help identify patients in whom revascularization could be of benefit; however, complication rates must be exceedingly low to achieve this result.

References

[1] de Weerd M, Greving JP, de Jong AWF, Buskens E, Bots ML. Prevalence of asymptomatic carotid artery stenosis according to age and sex: systematic review and metaregression analysis. Stroke. 2009; 40(4):1105–1113

[2] Walker MD, Marler JR, Goldstein M, et al. Executive Committee for the Asymptomatic Carotid Atherosclerosis Study. Endarterectomy for asymptomatic carotid artery stenosis. JAMA. 1995; 273(18):1421–1428

[3] Halliday A, Mansfield A, Marro J, et al. MRC Asymptomatic Carotid Surgery Trial (ACST) Collaborative Group. Prevention of disabling and fatal strokes by successful carotid endarterectomy in patients without recent neurological symptoms: randomised controlled trial. Lancet. 2004; 363(9420):1491–1502

[4] Abbott AL. Medical (nonsurgical) intervention alone is now best for prevention of stroke associated with asymptomatic severe carotid stenosis: results of a systematic review and analysis. Stroke. 2009; 40(10):e573–e583

[5] Nicolaides AN, Kakkos SK, Griffin M, et al. Asymptomatic Carotid Stenosis and Risk of Stroke (ACSRS) Study Group. Severity of asymptomatic carotid stenosis and risk of ipsilateral hemispheric ischaemic events: results from the ACSRS study. Eur J Vasc Endovasc Surg. 2005; 30(3):275–284

[6] Abbott AL, Chambers BR, Stork JL, Levi CR, Bladin CF, Donnan GA. Embolic signals and prediction of ipsilateral stroke or transient ischemic attack in asymptomatic carotid stenosis: a multicenter prospective cohort study. Stroke. 2005; 36(6):1128–1133

[7] Goessens BMB, Visseren FLJ, Kappelle LJ, Algra A, van der Graaf Y, for the, SMART Study Group. Asymptomatic carotid artery stenosis and the risk of new vascular events in patients with manifest arterial disease: the SMART study. Stroke. 2007; 38(5):1470–1475

[8] Marquardt L, Geraghty OC, Mehta Z, Rothwell PM. Low risk of ipsilateral stroke in patients with asymptomatic carotid stenosis on best medical treatment: a prospective, population-based study. Stroke. 2010; 41(1): e11–e17

[9] Norris JW, Zhu CZ, Bornstein NM, Chambers BR. Vascular risks of asymptomatic carotid stenosis. Stroke. 1991; 22(12):1485–1490

[10] Yang C, Bogiatzi C, Spence JD. Risk of stroke at the time of carotid occlusion. JAMA Neurol. 2015; 72(11):1261–1267

[11] Balestrini S, Lupidi F, Balucani C, et al. One-year progression of moderate asymptomatic carotid stenosis predicts the risk of vascular events. Stroke. 2013; 44(3):792–794

[12] Gupta A, Kesavabhotla K, Baradaran H, et al. Plaque echolucency and stroke risk in asymptomatic carotid stenosis: a systematic review and meta-analysis. Stroke. 2015; 46(1):91–97

[13] Kashiwazaki D, Yoshimoto T, Mikami T, et al. Identification of high-risk carotid artery stenosis: motion of intraplaque contents detected using B-mode ultrasonography. J Neurosurg. 2012; 117(3):574–578

[14] Kuk M, Wannarong T, Beletsky V, Parraga G, Fenster A, Spence JD. Volume of carotid artery ulceration as a predictor of cardiovascular events. Stroke. 2014; 45(5):1437–1441

[15] Romero JM, Pizzolato R, Atkinson W, et al. Vasa vasorum enhancement on computerized tomographic angiography correlates with symptomatic patients with 50% to 70% carotid artery stenosis. Stroke. 2013; 44(12):3344–3349

[16] King A, Markus HS. Doppler embolic signals in cerebrovascular disease and prediction of stroke risk: a systematic review and meta-analysis. Stroke. 2009; 40(12):3711–3717

[17] Spence JD, Tamayo A, Lownie SP, Ng WP, Ferguson GG. Absence of microemboli on transcranial Doppler identifies low-risk patients with asymptomatic carotid stenosis. Stroke. 2005; 36(11):2373–2378

[18] Markus HS, King A, Shipley M, et al. Asymptomatic embolisation for prediction of stroke in the Asymptomatic Carotid Emboli Study (ACES): a prospective observational study. Lancet Neurol. 2010; 9(7):663–671

[19] Kakkos SK, Sabetai M, Tegos T, et al. Asymptomatic Carotid Stenosis and Risk of Stroke (ACSRS) Study Group. Silent embolic infarcts on computed tomography brain scans and risk of ipsilateral hemispheric events in patients with asymptomatic internal carotid artery stenosis. J Vasc Surg. 2009; 49(4): 902–909

[20] Sacco RL, Wolf PA, Gorelick PB. Risk factors and their management for stroke prevention: outlook for 1999 and beyond. Neurology. 1999; 53(7) Suppl 4: S15–S24

[21] Cutler JA, Sorlie PD, Wolz M, Thom T, Fields LE, Roccella EJ. Trends in hypertension prevalence, awareness, treatment, and control rates in United States adults between 1988–1994 and 1999–2004. Hypertension. 2008; 52(5): 818–827

[22] Chobanian AV, Bakris GL, Black HR, et al. National Heart, Lung, and Blood Institute Joint National Committee on Prevention, Detection, Evaluation, and Treatment of High Blood Pressure, National High Blood Pressure Education Program Coordinating Committee. The Seventh Report of the Joint National Committee on Prevention, Detection, Evaluation, and Treatment of High Blood Pressure: the JNC 7 report. JAMA. 2003; 289(19):2560–2572

[23] Goldstein LB, Bushnell CD, Adams RJ, et al. American Heart Association Stroke Council, Council on Cardiovascular Nursing, Council on Epidemiology and Prevention, Council for High Blood Pressure Research, Council on Peripheral Vascular Disease, and Interdisciplinary Council on Quality of Care and Outcomes Research. Guidelines for the primary prevention of stroke: a guideline for healthcare professionals from the American Heart Association/American Stroke Association. Stroke. 2011; 42(2):517–584

15

[24] James PA, Oparil S, Carter BL, et al. 2014 evidence-based guideline for the management of high blood pressure in adults: report from the panel members appointed to the Eighth Joint National Committee (JNC 8). JAMA. 2014; 311(5):507–520

[25] Shinton R, Beevers G. Meta-analysis of relation between cigarette smoking and stroke. BMJ. 1989; 298(6676):789–794

[26] Burns DM. Epidemiology of smoking-induced cardiovascular disease. Prog Cardiovasc Dis. 2003; 46(1):11–29

[27] Fagerström K. The epidemiology of smoking: health consequences and benefits of cessation. Drugs. 2002; 62 Suppl 2:1–9

[28] Robbins AS, Manson JE, Lee IM, Satterfield S, Hennekens CH. Cigarette smoking and stroke in a cohort of U.S. male physicians. Ann Intern Med. 1994; 120 (6):458–462

[29] Anczak JD, Nogler RA, II. Tobacco cessation in primary care: maximizing intervention strategies. Clin Med Res. 2003; 1(3):201–216

[30] Fiore MC, Baker TB. Clinical practice: treating smokers in the health care setting. N Engl J Med. 2011; 365(13):1222–1231

[31] Iso H, Jacobs DRJ, Jr, Wentworth D, Neaton JD, Cohen JD. Serum cholesterol levels and six-year mortality from stroke in 350,977 men screened for the multiple risk factor intervention trial. N Engl J Med. 1989; 320(14):904–910

[32] Leppälä JM, Virtamo J, Fogelholm R, Albanes D, Heinonen OP. Different risk factors for different stroke subtypes: association of blood pressure, cholesterol, and antioxidants. Stroke. 1999; 30(12):2535–2540

[33] Sacco RL, Roberts JK, Boden-Albala B, et al. Race-ethnicity and determinants of carotid atherosclerosis in a multiethnic population. The Northern Manhattan Stroke Study. Stroke. 1997; 28(5):929–935

[34] Wasserman BA, Sharrett AR, Lai S, et al. Risk factor associations with the presence of a lipid core in carotid plaque of asymptomatic individuals using high-resolution MRI: the multi-ethnic study of atherosclerosis (MESA). Stroke. 2008; 39(2):329–335

[35] Baldassarre D, Veglia F, Gobbi C, et al. Intima-media thickness after pravastatin stabilizes also in patients with moderate to no reduction in LDL-cholesterol levels: the carotid atherosclerosis Italian ultrasound study. Atherosclerosis. 2000; 151(2):575–583

[36] Amarenco P, Labreuche J, Lavallée P, Touboul P-J. Statins in stroke prevention and carotid atherosclerosis: systematic review and up-to-date meta-analysis. Stroke. 2004; 35(12):2902–2909

[37] Giugliano RP, Cannon CP, Blazing MA, et al. IMPROVE-IT (Improved Reduction of Outcomes: Vytorin Efficacy International Trial) Investigators. Benefit of adding ezetimibe to statin therapy on cardiovascular outcomes and safety in patients with versus without diabetes mellitus: results from IMPROVE-IT (Improved Reduction of Outcomes: Vytorin Efficacy International Trial). Circulation. 2018; 137(15):1571–1582

[38] Mayo Asymptomatic Carotid Endarterectomy Study Group. Results of a randomized controlled trial of carotid endarterectomy for asymptomatic carotid stenosis. Mayo Clin Proc. 1992; 67(6):513–518

[39] Meschia JF, Bushnell C, Boden-Albala B, et al. American Heart Association Stroke Council, Council on Cardiovascular and Stroke Nursing, Council on Clinical Cardiology, Council on Functional Genomics and Translational Biology, Council on Hypertension. Guidelines for the primary prevention of stroke: a statement for healthcare professionals from the American Heart Association/ American Stroke Association. Stroke. 2014; 45(12):3754–3832

[40] Diener H-C, Bogousslavsky J, Brass LM, et al. MATCH Investigators. Aspirin and clopidogrel compared with clopidogrel alone after recent ischaemic stroke or transient ischaemic attack in high-risk patients (MATCH): randomised, double-blind, placebo-controlled trial. Lancet. 2004; 364(9431):331–337

[41] CAPRIE Steering Committee. A randomised, blinded, trial of clopidogrel versus aspirin in patients at risk of ischaemic events (CAPRIE). Lancet. 1996; 348 (9038):1329–1339

[42] Hopkins LN, Roubin GS, Chakhtoura EY, et al. The Carotid Revascularization Endarterectomy versus Stenting Trial: credentialing of interventionalists and final results of lead-in phase. J Stroke Cerebrovasc Dis. 2010; 19(2):153–162

[43] Calvillo-King L, Xuan L, Zhang S, Tuhrim S, Halm EA. Predicting risk of perioperative death and stroke after carotid endarterectomy in asymptomatic patients: derivation and validation of a clinical risk score. Stroke. 2010; 41 (12):2786–2794

[44] Ringleb PA, Allenberg J, Brückmann H, et al. SPACE Collaborative Group. 30 day results from the SPACE trial of stent-protected angioplasty versus carotid endarterectomy in symptomatic patients: a randomised non-inferiority trial. Lancet. 2006; 368(9543):1239–1247

[45] Mas J-L, Trinquart L, Leys D, et al. EVA-3S investigators. Endarterectomy versus angioplasty in patients with Symptomatic Severe Carotid Stenosis (EVA-3S) trial: results up to 4 years from a randomised, multicentre trial. Lancet Neurol. 2008; 7(10):885–892

[46] Ederle J, Dobson J, Featherstone RL, et al. International Carotid Stenting Study Investigators. Carotid artery stenting compared with endarterectomy in patients with symptomatic carotid stenosis (International Carotid Stenting Study): an interim analysis of a randomised controlled trial. Lancet. 2010; 375(9719):985–997

[47] Yadav JS, Wholey MH, Kuntz RE, et al. Stenting and Angioplasty with Protection in Patients at High Risk for Endarterectomy Investigators. Protected carotid-artery stenting versus endarterectomy in high-risk patients. N Engl J Med. 2004; 351(15):1493–1501

[48] Brott TG, Hobson RW, II, Howard G, et al. CREST Investigators. Stenting versus endarterectomy for treatment of carotid-artery stenosis. N Engl J Med. 2010; 363(1):11–23

[49] Brott TG, Howard G, Roubin GS, et al. CREST Investigators. Long-term results of stenting versus endarterectomy for carotid-artery stenosis. N Engl J Med. 2016; 374(11):1021–1031

[50] Tillman D-B. FDA approval of the ACCULINK Carotid Stent System and RX ACCULINK Carotid Stent System. In: Services HH, ed. Rockville, MD; 2004

[51] Medicare National Coverage Determinations Manual. Chapter 1, Part 1 (Sections 10–80.12) Coverage Determinations. 2007

[52] Howard VJ, Meschia JF, Lal BK, et al. CREST-2 study investigators. Carotid revascularization and medical management for asymptomatic carotid stenosis: Protocol of the CREST-2 clinical trials. Int J Stroke. 2017; 12(7):770–778

15

16 Carotid Dissection

John D. Nerva, Brian M. Corliss, and W. Christopher Fox

Abstract

Carotid artery dissection (CAD) can develop spontaneously or from trauma. Dissections occur in both the carotid and vertebral arteries with the majority of literature combining the two entities despite different natural histories. The main risk of CAD is stroke, which typically happens either with the initial arterial injury or during the early postdissection period. The severity of CADs and corresponding risk of stroke are graded based on the degree of luminal narrowing and pseudoaneurysm formation. The first-line treatment is medical therapy with antiplatelet or anticoagulant medication for prevention of thromboembolic stroke, with endovascular or open surgical therapy being reserved for patients with progressive ischemia and/or symptomatic luminal stenosis despite adequate medical therapy.

Keywords: dissection, carotid artery, vertebral artery, blunt cerebrovascular injury, antiplatelet therapy, anticoagulant therapy, endovascular therapy, transcranial Doppler ultrasonography

16.1 Goals

1. Describe the pathophysiology and natural history of carotid artery dissection (CAD).
2. Review the screening, diagnosis, and grading of blunt cerebrovascular injury (BCVI).
3. Review medical and endovascular therapy (EVT) for cervical artery dissection, both spontaneous and traumatic.

16.2 Case Examples

16.2.1 Case 1

A 46-year-old right-handed female with no past medical history presented to the emergency department with acute onset aphasia and right hemibody numbness. Over the prior month, she had intermittent blurry vision including the day of presentation.

Past medical history: No history of trauma.

Past surgical history: Noncontributory.

Social history: No history of tobacco or drug use.

Family history: No history of familial stroke or connective tissue disorders.

Examination: The patient was alert and following commands appropriately. She was unable to answer the questions due to word-finding difficulty and dysarthria. Visual field testing demonstrated right lower quadrantanopia. There was no pronator drift or lower extremity weakness. Right-sided touch was diminished. The National Institutes of Health Stroke Scale (NIHSS) score was 8.

Computed tomography angiography (CTA) of the brain revealed no evidence of hemorrhage or intracranial arterial thrombus, or dissection. CTA of the neck showed near occlusive luminal narrowing, 1.5 cm in length, consistent with the "string

sign" of a dissection in the cervical segment of the left internal carotid artery (ICA) proximal to the skull base (▶ Fig. 16.1).

CT perfusion revealed prolonged time-to-peak (TTP) and mean transit time (MTT) with preserved cerebral blood volume (CBV), indicating at-risk perfusion, of the entire left hemisphere (▶ Fig. 16.2).

Magnetic resonance imaging (MRI) demonstrated punctate foci of subacute infarction in the left hemisphere deep white matter.

Hospital course: The patient was admitted to the neuroscience ICU and administered an Aspirin bolus. During the course of hospital day (HD) 1, neurological examination fluctuated with intermittent global aphasia and mild right pronator drift

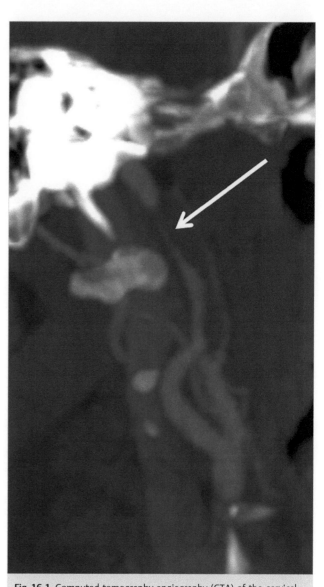

Fig. 16.1 Computed tomography angiography (CTA) of the cervical spine (sagittal view) demonstrates high-grade stenosis of the distal cervical internal carotid artery (ICA) consistent with arterial dissection (*white arrow*).

16

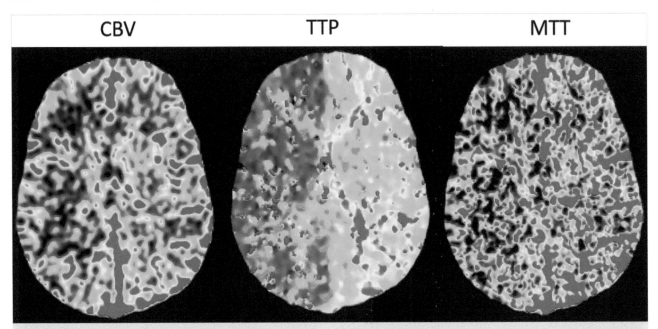

Fig. 16.2 Computed tomography (CT) perfusion demonstrates relatively preserved cerebral blood volume and prolonged time-to-peak (TTP) and mean transit time (MTT) consistent with delayed blood flow and reduced perfusion from the high-grade cervical internal carotid artery (ICA) dissection.

and full-dose heparin drip was initiated. These fluctuations persisted on HD 2. The decision was made to proceed with urgent carotid artery stent placement, and the patient was loaded with clopidogrel.

Under monitored anesthesia care with conscious sedation, the patient underwent diagnostic angiography followed by left ICA stenting and angioplasty. Left ICA angiography confirmed near-occlusive dissection with delayed intracranial ICA flow (▶ Fig. 16.3a). Given the high degree of stenosis, luminal irregularity, and lack of atherosclerotic plaque, a .017 microcatheter/ .014 microwire combination was used to navigate the dissection. We elected not to use distal embolic protection as, with the high degree of stenosis and the lack of atherosclerotic disease, we prefer the greater ability to torque and steer the .014 microwire compared to the wire of a distal protection device. Microcatheter angiography was also performed to confirm that the catheter remained in the true lumen. Carotid artery stent placement was performed with poststent balloon angioplasty to improve stent expansion (▶ Fig. 16.3b,c). Post-angioplasty angiography demonstrated excellent filling of the left ICA and distal branches.

Postoperatively, systolic blood pressure (SBP) was maintained less than 140 to avoid reperfusion injury and the heparin drip was weaned. The patient's examination improved dramatically, and she was discharged home on HD 5 with mild aphasia (NIHSS score 1). She was maintained on dual antiplatelet therapy. At 3-month follow-up, she had returned to her neurologic baseline.

Case 1 review: Spontaneous carotid artery dissection

Spontaneous cervical artery dissection (SCAD) is a leading cause of stroke in patients less than 40 years of age. It occurs at an annual incidence of 3 per 1,00,000 for the ICA and 1 per 1,00,000 for the vertebral artery (VA).[1] Fisher et al provided one of the early descriptions of SCAD including definition of the "string sign," distal pouch formation (i.e., pseudoaneurysm), and occlusion.[2] SCAD arise from a tear in one or more of the three arterial layers (i.e., tunica intima, media, and adventitia). Tears allow blood to enter the arterial wall and create an intramural hematoma, that is, false lumen.[3] Subintimal dissection can result in stenosis of the arterial lumen, and more extensive subadventitial dissection can create an aneurysmal dilation (commonly referred to as a pseudoaneurysm) that may also compromise the arterial lumen.[3] SCAD occurs in the absence of major trauma but can result from arteriopathies such as fibromuscular dysplasia, Marfan syndrome, and Ehler-Danlos type IV. Comorbidities associated with SCAD include infection, radiation and cervical tumors, and repeated microtrauma including chiropractic cervical manipulation, coughing, and abrupt head turns.[3,4] Headache, neck pain, oculosympathetic palsy with miosis and ptosis, and lower cranial neuropathy as well as ischemic manifestations from hypoperfusion and thromboembolic phenomena are common presentations of SCAD.[3,5,6] ICA stenosis or occlusion is associated with a 0.3% annual risk of transient neurologic deficit and 0.7% annual risk of stroke.[7] A prospective study of 970 patients with SCAD of the ICA ($n = 668$) and VA ($n = 302$) revealed that ischemic presentations were more common in the VA (84% vs. 70%, $p < 0.001$), but stroke severity was worse with ICA dissection (10 +/– 7.1 vs. 5 +/– 5.9, $p < 0.001$).[8] As well, VA dissections had more favorable outcomes at 3 months but also had more recurrent ischemic symptoms.[8] In a recent study of patients who present without ischemia, the absolute risk of stroke was 1.25% over the first 2 weeks with no significant increase in stroke over the subsequent 10 weeks.[9] Both antiplatelet and antithrombotic agents are used to treat SCADs to decrease the risk of stroke and have

16

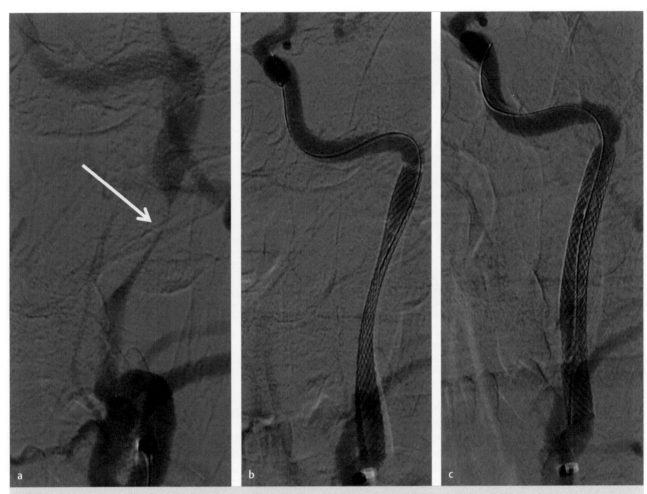

Fig. 16.3 Angiography confirms the high-grade flow limiting stenosis (**a**, *white arrow*). After carotid artery stent placement (**b**) and post-stenting balloon angioplasty (**c**), the stenosis had significantly improved and blood flow patterns normalized.

recently been shown to provide similar benefit in the Cervical Artery Dissection in Stroke Study (CADISS) trial.[10,11] The indications for endovascular intervention are uncertain with no randomized trials to demonstrate efficacy.[4,12,13,14,15]

This case demonstrates the presentation of a patient with recurrent transient symptoms followed by cerebral ischemia from SCAD resulting in near occlusion of the left cervical ICA. Initial therapy with aspirin for SCAD is supported by Class IIb recommendation, Level B-Randomized evidence in the 2018 Guidelines for Management of Acute Ischemic Stroke, which is reviewed in a subsequent section.[15] Despite medical therapy, the patient had a worsening neurological examination and severe perfusion deficit on CT with the entire left hemisphere at risk of stroke from the high-grade dissection. The decision to proceed with EVT is supported by multiple retrospective studies demonstrating effectiveness in patients who have failed medical management.[16,17,18,19,20] EVT is supported by Class IIb recommendation, Level C-Limited Data evidence in the 2018 Guidelines, which state that "consideration of EVT should be reserved for patients with definite recurrent cerebral ischemic events despite medical therapy."[15]

16.2.2 Case 2

A 19-year-old male was in an automobile struck by a semi-trailer truck at high speed and was brought to an outside institution after stabilization at the scene. His traumatic injuries included pulmonary contusions, liver and splenic lacerations, and right radial/femur/ankle fractures. Initial CT brain imaging was negative. The orthopaedic injuries were stabilized. On HD 2, the patient developed left upper extremity weakness. CT head revealed multiple hypodensities in the right hemisphere confirmed by MRI (▶ Fig. 16.4a, b). MRA revealed distal cervical ICA dissection with pseudoaneurysm formation (▶ Fig. 16.4c). The patient was subsequently transferred to a tertiary center for a higher level of care.

On examination upon arrival, the patient was intubated but obeying commands off sedation. The right upper extremity was casted and right lower extremity was in an immobilizer. He was able to follow simple commands on the left but weaker than on the right. CTA with perfusion on arrival confirmed the right distal cervical ICA pseudoaneurysm and identified a left distal cervical ICA dissection with mild luminal narrowing with intact

16

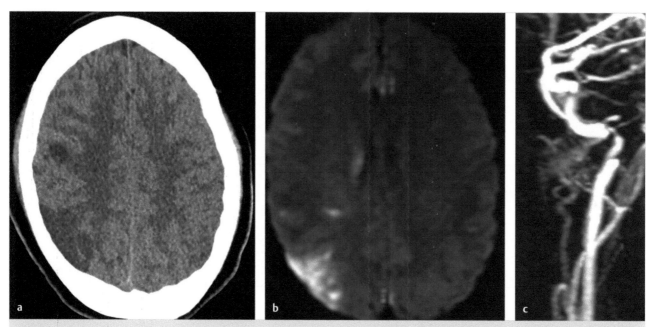

Fig. 16.4 Computed tomography (CT) demonstrates multiple areas of hypodensity in separate arterial distributions consistent with thromboembolic phenomena **(a)**, which is confirmed on magnetic resonance imaging (MRI) **(b)**. Magnetic resonance angiography (MRA) demonstrates dissection and pseudoaneurysm formation in the petrous/cervical segment of the right internal carotid artery (ICA) **(c)**.

perfusion of both hemispheres except areas of reduced blood volume associated with prior thromboembolic events. Full-dose heparin drip was initiated after embolization of the splenic and hepatic lacerations and stabilization of hematocrit. We recommended cerebral angiography to determine the severity and type of the dissections and assess blood flow and collateral circulation. Angiography on HD 2 confirmed the dissections and demonstrated delayed right hemispheric flow through the right ICA but adequate collateral flow from the left ICA and vertebrobasilar system (▶ Fig. 16.5). The right cervical ICA dissection had 50 to 60% luminal narrowing and endovascular intervention was not performed due to the risk of dual antiplatelet therapy with multiple traumatic injuries and adequate cerebrovascular reserve.

The patient was maintained on heparin drip and followed with daily transcranial Doppler ultrasonography with microembolic monitoring of bilateral middle cerebral artery (MCA) territories (TCDe). Microembolic signals (MES, 9 per hour) were detected on HD 3, and daily aspirin was started after a loading dose due to ongoing emboli from the dissection. Over the next several days, MES were intermittently detected but declining in number in the right MCA and the patient remained neurologically stable after extubation on HD 4. Once MES were absent for 3 consecutive days and the patient was neurologically unchanged, repeat CTA was performed which demonstrated stable appearance of the dissections. Therapeutic heparin was discontinued and aspirin was continued with no evidence of MES. After a prolonged hospitalization and repair of other injuries, he was discharged home on HD 25. At 3 months, the patient returned to clinic continuing to rehab from his orthopaedic injuries but otherwise neurologically intact. CTA head and neck demonstrated stable appearance of the bilateral ICA dissections, and the patient was maintained on aspirin monotherapy.

Case 2 review: Blunt cerebrovascular injury

BCVI is a type of traumatic cervical arterial dissection. The incidence of BCVI has increased over the past two decades with improved CTA screening protocols for asymptomatic patients with traumatic presentations and is present in 0.5 to 1.0% of admissions for trauma.[21,22,23] CTA as opposed to diagnostic cerebral angiography and MRA is generally used for screening patients presenting with trauma because it is less invasive than angiography, part of overall trauma screening with CT and quicker than MRA.[24,25,26,27,28] Typical screening protocols for BCVI include patients with cervical soft tissue hematoma, carotid bruit, cerebral infarction, Horner syndrome, lateralizing neurological deficit, intracranial hemorrhage, and transient ischemic attack (TIA) as well as high-energy trauma resulting in LeFort fractures and cervical spine fractures.[24,25]

BCVI involves the ICA more commonly than the VA (62% vs. 38% cases).[22,29] The most commonly used BCVI grading scale is the Denver (also known as the Biffl) criteria, which has five grades of decreasing incidence and increasing stroke risk (<10% for Grade I and 100% for Grade V).[22,24,29] Grade I (54% of BCVI) is luminal irregularity or dissection with < 25% luminal narrowing; Grade II (20%) is dissection or intramural hematoma with ≥ 25% luminal narrowing; Grade III (13%) involves any dissection with pseudoaneurysm formation; Grade IV (10%) is traumatic occlusion; and Grade V (3%) is transection with free extravasation.[29]

Treatment of BCVI typically involves antiplatelet or anticoagulant medication. There have not been direct randomized trials comparing antiplatelet or anticoagulation for stroke prevention, but in retrospective analysis, antiplatelet and anticoagulant agents have similar effectiveness in preventing stroke and injury healing rates.[30] Low-dose heparin (i.e., PTT 40–50 s) is the typical anticoagulant used during the acute phase with

16

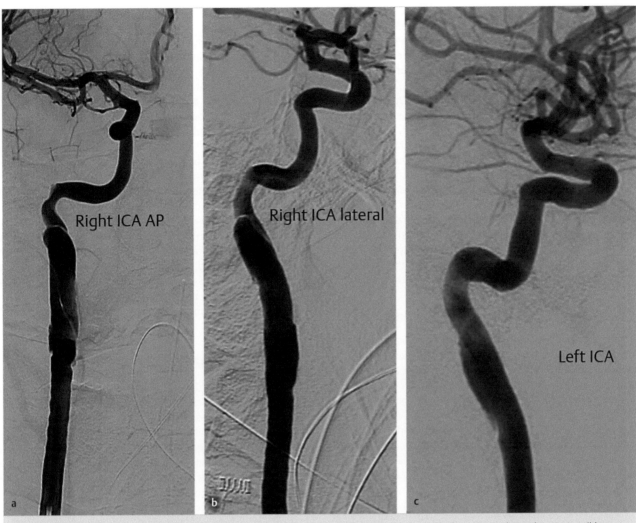

Fig. 16.5 (a) Right internal carotid artery (ICA) angiography (anteroposterior [AP], lateral) confirms the dissection and pseudoaneurysm (blunt cerebrovascular injury [BCVI] grade III). **(b)** Flow limitation is not observed. **(c)** The patient also sustained a grade I BCVI of the left distal cervical ICA.

aspirin or other antiplatelet agents reserved for patients with contraindications to anticoagulation or for long-term therapy. TCDe has been used to help monitor and guide medical therapy with the presence of continued emboli requiring additional antiplatelet or anticoagulant agents or potentially EVT.[31,32,33,34] Serial imaging with CTA or angiography can be used to monitor low-grade lesions due to risk of progression and pseudoaneurysm development (8% risk with Grade I and 43% with Grade II at 7–10 postinjury); however, more recent studies have questioned the utility of early follow-up injury, especially for high-grade injuries.[29,35] Endovascular stenting or arterial sacrifice may be warranted for patients with progressive stenosis, enlarging pseudoaneurysms, persistent microemboli, and progressive neurological deficits despite adequate medical therapy.[24,29,31,36,37,38] Routine EVT for low-grade lesions has not been shown to provide additional benefit compared to anticoagulant therapy.[39] However, EVT reserved for symptomatic patients and major dissections may reduce the risk of stroke.[38] Grade V injury (transection) warrants immediate endovascular intervention, either arterial sacrifice or covered stenting or open surgical repair/sacrifice due to acute and active arterial extravasation.

This case demonstrates the presentation of a patient with multiple traumatic injuries who sustained a stroke from a right cervical ICA Grade III BCVI and also sustained a left cervical ICA Grade I BCVI. Initial therapy with heparin drip with plan to transition to aspirin therapy in the absence of a contraindication is supported by Level B-Non Randomized evidence and recommended by trauma surgery guidelines.[24,40] Medical therapy was tailored based on TCDe and aspirin was initiated when emboli were present, which may signify that therapy with heparin alone was insufficient. Early repeat imaging was also used to monitor response to therapy and progression of the dissections, which is also supported by guidelines for BCVI.[24,40]

16.3 Level of Evidence and Recommendations

16.3.1 Spontaneous Cervical Artery Dissection

Based on the 2018 Guidelines for the Early Management of Patients with Acute Ischemic Stroke, a Class IIb recommendation

16

(i.e., Weak, Benefit ≥ Risk) based on Level B-R evidence (i.e., moderate-quality evidence from one or more randomized controlled trials [RCTs] or meta-analysis of moderate-quality RCTs), "For patients with AIS and extracranial carotid or vertebral arterial dissection, treatment with either antiplatelet or anticoagulant therapy for 3 to 6 months may be reasonable."[11] This recommendation is largely based on data from the CADISS trial. The patients in CADISS trial presented with spontaneous dissections and as such, may not apply to patients with BCVI.

Based on the 2018 Guidelines for the Early Management of Patients with Acute Ischemic Stroke, a Class IIb recommendation (i.e., Weak, Benefit ≥ Risk) based on Level C-LD evidence (i.e., randomized or nonrandomized observational or registry studies with limitations of design or execution or meta-analyses of such studies), "for patients with AIS and extracranial carotid or vertebral arterial dissection who have definite recurrent cerebral ischemic events despite medical therapy, the value of EVT (stenting) is not well established."[11] Again this recommendation may not apply for patients presenting with BCVI.

16.3.2 Blunt Cerebrovascular Injury

The data on BCVI management is based on nonrandomized data from prospective cohorts and retrospective review largely from single institutions. A system for BCVI registries, a clinical trials network, and observational studies followed by randomized trials has been proposed.[41] A peer-reviewed online database maintained by authors highly published in BCVI updates recommendations for BCVI management and provides similar recommendations to previously published guidelines and recommendations from the Western Trauma Associations and the Eastern Association for the Surgery of Trauma (EAST) as well as other single institution guidelines.[40,42,43]

Aggressive screening for patients presenting with risk factors and signs/symptoms of BCVI has proven cost-effective for preventing stroke.[24,44,45,46] The risk factors include: LeFort fracture, mandible fracture, skull base fracture, occipital condyle fracture, severe traumatic brain injury, cervical spine fracture or subluxation, hanging injury, clothesline-type injury, scalp degloving, and major thoracic injuries.[24,43] Signs/symptoms of BCVI include cervical/nasal/oral hemorrhage, cervical bruit in patients less than 50 year of age, focal neurological deficits including TIA, hemiparesis, Horner syndrome, vertebrobasilar insufficiency, stroke on CT/MRI, or neurological deficit inconsistent with CT findings.[24,43] Asymptomatic patients with significant blunt head trauma are at a significantly increased risk for BCVI and screening should be considered. Risk factors include: Glasgow Coma Scale score ≤ 8, petrous bone fracture, diffuse axonal injury, cervical spine fracture particularly those with (i) fracture of C1 to C3 and (ii) fracture through the foramen transversarium, cervical spine fracture with subluxation or rotational component, Lefort II or III facial fractures.[40]

Imaging for screening according to the EAST trauma guidelines says with Level 2 evidence, diagnostic four-vessel cerebral angiography (FVCA) remains the gold standard for the diagnosis of BCVI. Duplex ultrasound and CTA with a four (or less)-slice multidetector array is not adequate for screening for BCVI. There is Level III evidence that multislice (eight or greater) multidetector CTA has a similar rate of detection for BCVI when compared with historic control rates of diagnosis with FVCA

and may be considered as a screening modality in place of FVCA.

For patients with BCVI without neurological deficit and no contraindications to antiplatelets or anticoagulation (heparin infusion), treatment is recommended over no therapy for prevention and treatment of stroke.[24,43] This is a Grade 1B recommendation, which "is a strong recommendation, and applies to most patients. Clinicians should follow a strong recommendation unless a clear and compelling rationale for an alternative approach is present."[43] The duration of therapy is unknown, but aspirin therapy could be used indefinitely in patients with persistent BCVI on follow-up imaging. However, this recommendation did not receive a formal grade.[24,43] Surgical exploration can be considered for accessible BCVI lesions in symptomatic patients with EVT reserved for surgically inaccessible lesions near the skull base with BCVI grades II (flow-limiting stenosis), III (pseudoaneurysm formation), or V (transection), although no studies have directly compared surgical and endovascular modalities.[24,43] Follow-up imaging at 7 to 10 days for nonocclusive BCVI is recommended as well as imaging at 3 months if long-term anticoagulant or antiplatelet therapy is needed.[24,43]

16.4 Landmark Papers

Fisher CM, Ojemann RG, Roberson GH. Spontaneous dissection of cervico-cerebral arteries. Can J Neurol Sci 1978;5(1):9–19.

This manuscript was one of the early series describing spontaneous CAD in six patients with verified lesions. Clinical presentations included headache, facial pain, bruit, transient monocular blindness, oculosympathetic palsy, TIA, hemiplegia, and aphasia. The authors described four angiographic profiles including long dissection (i.e., "string sign"), tell-tale pouch, postsinus tapering occlusion, and distal pouch (i.e., pseudoaneurysm with luminal narrowing). The decision to treat with antiplatelet or anticoagulant therapy was a question that "cannot be answered reliably." Surgical exploration was considered in patients with complete occlusion and neurological deficit of < 12-hour duration. The authors concluded that proper management was largely unknown.

Srinivasan J, Newell DW, Sturzenegger M, Mayberg MR, Winn HR. Transcranial Doppler in the evaluation of internal carotid artery dissection. Stroke 1996;27(7):1226–1230.

This manuscript described the use of transcranial Doppler (TCD) with emboli monitoring in an attempt to identify a subset of patients with CAD at risk for stroke. Emboli monitoring was performed of the MCA ipsilateral to the dissection. Ten patients presented with trauma, and seven patients presented with spontaneous CAD. Patients with microemboli detected by TCD presented with stroke more commonly than patients without microemboli (70% vs. 14%). The authors suggested that TCD could be an adjunctive tool to evaluate and monitor response to medical therapy.

Fabian TC, Patton JH, Jr., Croce MA, Minard G, Kudsk KA, Pritchard FE. Blunt carotid injury: importance of early diagnosis and anticoagulant therapy. Ann Surg 1996;223(5):513–522; discussion 522–515.

Prior to this study, blunt ICA injury was considered uncommon. The authors hypothesized that it was underdiagnosed, and early treatment could improve outcome. Sixty-seven patients were identified from a prospective registry. The overall incidence was 0.33% and 0.67% after motor vehicle accidents during the 11-year study period compared to previous reports of < 0.1%. Screening with diagnostic cerebral angiography was performed for patients with soft tissue neck swelling, neurological examination incongruent with head CT, and development of neurological deficit and Horner syndrome. Patients were treated with heparin, and routine follow-up angiography was performed. Heparin therapy was independently associated with survival ($p < 0.02$) and improvement in neurological outcome ($p < 0.01$). The authors concluded that liberal screening could improve outcome in patients with blunt ICA injury by allowing early diagnosis and initiation of heparin therapy prior to neurological decline.

Biffl WL, Moore EE, Offner PJ, Brega KE, Franciose RJ, Burch JM. Blunt carotid arterial injuries: implications of a new grading scale. J Trauma 1999;47(5):845–853.

This manuscript defined a grading scale based on 109 blunt ICA injuries in 79 patients that has since been used throughout the BCVI literature:

- Grade I: Luminal irregularity or dissection with < 25% luminal narrowing.
- Grade II: Dissection or intramural hematoma with ≥ 25% luminal narrowing.
- Grade III: Any dissection with pseudoaneurysm formation.
- Grade IV: Traumatic occlusion.
- Grade V: Transection with free extravasation.

Stroke risk increased with injury grade. Majority of grade I injuries healed; grade II injuries were at a risk of progression; grade III injuries were more likely to heal with EVT; grade IV injuries did not recanalize; and grade V injuries were often lethal. The authors advocated for early surgical/endovascular repair for accessible lesions; a recommendation which has since been changed by this group.[24,39] An important limitation of this manuscript was the high incidence of head injury (Glasgow Coma Scale score ≤ 6, 46% patients), which confounded results. Nonetheless, this grading scale has helped define the BCVI literature.

Biffl WL, Cothren CC, Moore EE, et al. Western Trauma Association critical decisions in trauma: screening for and treatment of blunt cerebrovascular injuries. J Trauma 2009;67(6):1150–1153.

This manuscript described an algorithm for the diagnosis and management of BCVI based on the institution's extensive experience and literature review. Screening criteria, imaging requirements at initial diagnosis and follow-up, and indications for angiography, heparin therapy, and EVT were defined. The group has since amended recommendations for early imaging follow-up and EVT based on nonrandomized data and retrospective review; however, these issues remain controversial within the BCVI literature and management remains institution-dependent.[20,27,30,31,35,38,39,40,42,47,48]

Markus HS, Hayter E, Levi C, et al. Antiplatelet treatment compared with anticoagulation treatment for cervical artery dissection (CADISS): a randomized trial. Lancet Neurol 2015;14(4):361–367.

CADISS was a multicenter, prospective, randomized trial comparing antiplatelet and anticoagulant therapy for extracranial carotid and VA dissection. Two hundred and fifty patients were enrolled. The majority of patients presented with stroke or TIA (90% patients). The risk of stroke after randomization was rare in both groups at 2% (four patients), and there was no difference

between therapies. After randomization, the exact therapy was left to the discretion of the treating clinician. The mean time to randomization was 3.65 days due to delays in obtaining imaging to diagnosis of cervical artery dissection. Importantly, the diagnosis of dissection was not confirmed on central review of the imaging in 52 (21%) patients. In addition, the results of carotid and VA injury were combined, and these injuries have been shown to have different presentations, stroke risk, and natural histories.[8] Despite these limitations, the trial demonstrates that with treatment the risk of stroke with antiplatelet or anticoagulant therapy is low.

16.5 Summary

1. Cervical artery dissection can occur spontaneously or from trauma and may affect either the carotid or VA.
2. Patients may present with ischemic symptoms, local symptoms such as neck pain or cranial nerve deficit, or asymptomatically.
3. Screening for BCVI has proven cost-effective for prevention and treatment of stroke in the setting of trauma.
4. The five-tier Denver grading system for BCVI correlates with prognosis and has implications for therapy.
5. Antiplatelet and anticoagulant therapy both provide benefit for stroke prevention and treatment in patients with spontaneous dissection and BCVI.
6. TCD with emboli monitoring may provide benefit for following response to medical therapy.
7. EVT is generally reserved for patients with persistent neurological symptoms or progression of cervical artery dissection despite adequate medical therapy.

References

[1] Pelkonen O, Tikkakoski T, Leinonen S, Pyhtinen J, Lepojärvi M, Sotaniemi K. Extracranial internal carotid and vertebral artery dissections: angiographic spectrum, course and prognosis. Neuroradiology. 2003; 45(2):71–77

[2] Fisher CM, Ojemann RG, Roberson GH. Spontaneous dissection of cervicocerebral arteries. Can J Neurol Sci. 1978; 5(1):9–19

[3] Schievink WI. Spontaneous dissection of the carotid and vertebral arteries. N Engl J Med. 2001; 344(12):898–906

[4] Fusco MR, Harrigan MR. Cerebrovascular dissections: a review part I: spontaneous dissections. Neurosurgery. 2011; 68(1):242–257, discussion 257

[5] Mokri B, Silbert PL, Schievink WI, Piepgras DG. Cranial nerve palsy in spontaneous dissection of the extracranial internal carotid artery. Neurology. 1996; 46(2):356–359

[6] Silbert PL, Mokri B, Schievink WI. Headache and neck pain in spontaneous internal carotid and vertebral artery dissections. Neurology. 1995; 45 (8):1517–1522

[7] Kremer C, Mosso M, Georgiadis D, et al. Carotid dissection with permanent and transient occlusion or severe stenosis: long-term outcome. Neurology. 2003; 60(2):271–275

[8] von Babo M, De Marchis GM, Sarikaya H, et al. Differences and similarities between spontaneous dissections of the internal carotid artery and the vertebral artery. Stroke. 2013; 44(6):1537–1542

[9] Morris NA, Merkler AE, Gialdini G, Kamel H. Timing of incident stroke risk after cervical artery dissection presenting without ischemia. Stroke. 2017; 48 (3):551–555

[10] Kennedy F, Lanfranconi S, Hicks C, et al. CADISS Investigators. Antiplatelets vs anticoagulation for dissection: CADISS nonrandomized arm and meta-analysis. Neurology. 2012; 79(7):686–689

[11] Markus HS, Hayter E, Levi C, Feldman A, Venables G, Norris J, CADISS trial investigators. Antiplatelet treatment compared with anticoagulation treatment for cervical artery dissection (CADISS): a randomised trial. Lancet Neurol. 2015; 14(4):361–367

16

[12] Touzé E, Randoux B, Méary E, Arquizan C, Meder JF, Mas JL. Aneurysmal forms of cervical artery dissection: associated factors and outcome. Stroke. 2001; 32 (2):418–423

[13] Menon R, Kerry S, Norris JW, Markus HS. Treatment of cervical artery dissection: a systematic review and meta-analysis. J Neurol Neurosurg Psychiatry. 2008; 79(10):1122–1127

[14] Brott TG, Halperin JL, Abbara S, et al. 2011 ASA/ACCF/AHA/AANN/AANS/ACR/ASNR/CNS/SAIP/SCAI/SIR/SNIS/SVM/SVS guideline on the management of patients with extracranial carotid and vertebral artery disease: executive summary: a report of the American College of Cardiology Foundation/American Heart Association Task Force on Practice Guidelines, and the American Stroke Association, American Association of Neuroscience Nurses, American Association of Neurological Surgeons, American College of Radiology, American Society of Neuroradiology, Congress of Neurological Surgeons, Society of Atherosclerosis Imaging and Prevention, Society for Cardiovascular Angiography and Interventions, Society of Interventional Radiology, Society of Neuro-Interventional Surgery, Society for Vascular Medicine, and Society for Vascular Surgery. J Am Coll Cardiol. 2011; 57(8):1002–1044

[15] Powers WJ, Rabinstein AA, Ackerson T, et al. American Heart Association Stroke Council. 2018 Guidelines for the early management of patients with acute ischemic stroke: a guideline for healthcare professionals from the American Heart Association/American Stroke Association. Stroke. 2018; 49 (3):e46–e110

[16] Kadkhodayan Y, Jeck DT, Moran CJ, Derdeyn CP, Cross DT, III. Angioplasty and stenting in carotid dissection with or without associated pseudoaneurysm. AJNR Am J Neuroradiol. 2005; 26(9):2328–2335

[17] Jeon P, Kim BM, Kim DI, et al. Emergent self-expanding stent placement for acute intracranial or extracranial internal carotid artery dissection with significant hemodynamic insufficiency. AJNR Am J Neuroradiol. 2010; 31 (8):1529–1532

[18] Masahira N, Ohta T, Fukui N, et al. A direct aspiration first pass technique for retrieval of a detached coil. J Neurointerv Surg. 2015

[19] Hauck EF, Natarajan SK, Ohta H, et al. Emergent endovascular recanalization for cervical internal carotid artery occlusion in patients presenting with acute stroke. Neurosurgery. 2011; 69(4):899–907, discussion 907

[20] Ohta H, Natarajan SK, Hauck EF, et al. Endovascular stent therapy for extracranial and intracranial carotid artery dissection: single-center experience. J Neurosurg. 2011; 115(1):91–100

[21] Berne JD, Norwood SH, McAuley CE, Vallina VL, Creath RG, McLarty J. The high morbidity of blunt cerebrovascular injury in an unscreened population: more evidence of the need for mandatory screening protocols. J Am Coll Surg. 2001; 192(3):314–321

[22] Biffl WL, Moore EE, Offner PJ, Brega KE, Franciose RJ, Burch JM. Blunt carotid arterial injuries: implications of a new grading scale. J Trauma. 1999; 47 (5):845–853

[23] Fabian TC, Patton JH, Jr, Croce MA, Minard G, Kudsk KA, Pritchard FE. Blunt carotid injury: importance of early diagnosis and anticoagulant therapy. Ann Surg. 1996; 223(5):513–522, discussion 522–525

[24] Biffl WL, Cothren CC, Moore EE, et al. Western Trauma Association critical decisions in trauma: screening for and treatment of blunt cerebrovascular injuries. J Trauma. 2009; 67(6):1150–1153

[25] Burlew CC, Biffl WL, Moore EE, Barnett CC, Johnson JL, Bensard DD. Blunt cerebrovascular injuries: redefining screening criteria in the era of noninvasive diagnosis. J Trauma Acute Care Surg. 2012; 72(2):330–335, discussion 336–337, quiz 539

[26] DuBose J, Recinos G, Teixeira PG, Inaba K, Demetriades D. Endovascular stenting for the treatment of traumatic internal carotid injuries: expanding experience. J Trauma. 2008; 65(6):1561–1566

[27] Emmett KP, Fabian TC, DiCocco JM, Zarzaur BL, Croce MA. Improving the screening criteria for blunt cerebrovascular injury: the appropriate role for computed tomography angiography. J Trauma. 2011; 70(5):1058–1063, discussion 1063–1065

[28] Wang AC, Charters MA, Thawani JP, Than KD, Sullivan SE, Graziano GP. Evaluating the use and utility of noninvasive angiography in diagnosing traumatic blunt cerebrovascular injury. J Trauma Acute Care Surg. 2012; 72(6):1601–1610

[29] Biffl WL, Ray CE, Jr, Moore EE, et al. Treatment-related outcomes from blunt cerebrovascular injuries: importance of routine follow-up arteriography. Ann Surg. 2002; 235(5):699–706, discussion 706–707

[30] Cothren CC, Biffl WL, Moore EE, Kashuk JL, Johnson JL. Treatment for blunt cerebrovascular injuries: equivalence of anticoagulation and antiplatelet agents. Arch Surg. 2009; 144(7):685–690

[31] Morton RP, Levitt MR, Emerson S, et al. Natural history and management of blunt traumatic pseudoaneurysms of the internal carotid artery: the Harborview Algorithm based off a 10-year experience. Ann Surg. 2016; 263(4):821–826

[32] Morton RP, Hanak BW, Levitt MR, et al. Blunt traumatic occlusion of the internal carotid and vertebral arteries. J Neurosurg. 2014; 120(6):1446–1450

[33] Bonow RH, Witt CE, Mosher BP, et al. Transcranial Doppler microemboli monitoring for stroke risk stratification in blunt cerebrovascular injury. Crit Care Med. 2017; 45(10):e1011–e1017

[34] Srinivasan J, Newell DW, Sturzenegger M, Mayberg MR, Winn HR. Transcranial Doppler in the evaluation of internal carotid artery dissection. Stroke. 1996; 27(7):1226–1230

[35] Wagenaar AE, Burlew CC, Biffl WL, et al. Early repeat imaging is not warranted for high-grade blunt cerebrovascular injuries. J Trauma Acute Care Surg. 2014; 77(4):540–545, quiz 650

[36] Seth R, Obuchowski AM, Zoarski GH. Endovascular repair of traumatic cervical internal carotid artery injuries: a safe and effective treatment option. AJNR Am J Neuroradiol. 2013; 34(6):1219–1226

[37] Coldwell DM, Novak Z, Ryu RK, et al. Treatment of posttraumatic internal carotid arterial pseudoaneurysms with endovascular stents. J Trauma. 2000; 48(3):470–472

[38] DiCocco JM, Fabian TC, Emmett KP, et al. Optimal outcomes for patients with blunt cerebrovascular injury (BCVI): tailoring treatment to the lesion. J Am Coll Surg. 2011; 212(4):549–557, discussion 557–559

[39] Burlew CC, Biffl WL, Moore EE, et al. Endovascular stenting is rarely necessary for the management of blunt cerebrovascular injuries. J Am Coll Surg. 2014; 218(5):1012–1017

[40] Bromberg WJ, Collier BC, Diebel LN, et al. Blunt cerebrovascular injury practice management guidelines: the Eastern Association for the Surgery of Trauma. J Trauma. 2010; 68(2):471–477

[41] Fabian TC. Blunt cerebrovascular injuries: anatomic and pathologic heterogeneity create management enigmas. J Am Coll Surg. 2013; 216(5):873–885

[42] Shahan CP, Magnotti LJ, Stickley SM, et al. A safe and effective management strategy for blunt cerebrovascular injury: avoiding unnecessary anticoagulation and eliminating stroke. J Trauma Acute Care Surg. 2016; 80(6):915–922

[43] Biffl WL, Burlew CC, Monroe EE. Blunt cerebrovascular injury: treatment and Outcomes. In: Collins KA, ed. UpToDate. Waltham MA

[44] Biffl WL, Moore EE, Offner PJ, et al. Optimizing screening for blunt cerebrovascular injuries. Am J Surg. 1999; 178(6):517–522

[45] Biffl WL, Ray CE, Jr, Moore EE, Mestek M, Johnson JL, Burch JM. Noninvasive diagnosis of blunt cerebrovascular injuries: a preliminary report. J Trauma. 2002; 53(5):850–856

[46] Cothren CC, Moore EE, Biffl WL, et al. Anticoagulation is the gold standard therapy for blunt carotid injuries to reduce stroke rate. Arch Surg. 2004; 139 (5):540–545, discussion 545–546

[47] Scott WW, Sharp S, Figueroa SA, et al. Clinical and radiographic outcomes following traumatic Grade 1 and 2 carotid artery injuries: a 10-year retrospective analysis from a Level I trauma center. The Parkland Carotid and Vertebral Artery Injury Survey. J Neurosurg. 2015; 122(5):1196–1201

[48] Scott WW, Sharp S, Figueroa SA, et al. Clinical and radiographic outcomes following traumatic Grade 3 and 4 carotid artery injuries: a 10-year retrospective analysis from a Level 1 trauma center. The Parkland Carotid and Vertebral Artery Injury Survey. J Neurosurg. 2015; 122(3):610–615

16

17 Vertebral Artery Origin Stenosis

Andre Monteiro, Victor Hugo Da Costa, Roberta Santos, Ricardo Hanel, Eric Sauvageau, and Amin Nima Aghaebrahim

Abstract

Stroke is the leading cause of severe disability in the United States. Ischemic stroke accounts for 80% of all strokes and, of these, 20% affect the posterior circulation. Posterior circulation strokes can be especially devastating due to the high concentration of motor tracts in this territory and are associated with higher mortality rates than strokes in the anterior circulation. Etiologies include small vessel disease, cardioembolism, intra- and extracranial atherosclerotic disease, including vertebral artery origin stenosis (VAOS) and other segments. Stenosis of the origin of the vertebral artery has been found in 20% of posterior circulation ischemic stroke patients (up to 30,000 patients per year) and is likely underdiagnosed. Noninvasive imaging, such as computed tomography (CT) and magnetic resonance (MR) angiograms, does not always provide good visualization of the vertebral ostium due to artifact. Doppler ultrasonography is also not adequate to evaluate the vertebral arteries, notably their origins. Optimized treatment of VAOS is unclear. Unfortunately, there has not been a large-scale prospective study or randomized trial of VAOS management. Therefore, we do not have any good evidence regarding potential benefit of stents in reducing the recurrent stroke risk. While little is known about the natural history of medically treated VAOS, we have accumulated significant evidence from retrospective studies to state that stenting of VAOS is a low-risk procedure with periprocedural complications (stroke, transient ischemic attack [TIA], and death) occurring in 1 to 3% of patients. Restenosis rates may be reduced by use of drug-eluting stents.

Keywords: vertebral artery, stenosis, stenting, angioplasty, vertebrobasilar insufficiency, stroke

17.1 Goals

1. Review the literature that forms the basis of our understanding of the natural history of vertebral artery stenosis.
2. Review the literature that supports treatment of vertebral artery origin stenosis.
3. Critically analyze the literature on the natural history of vertebral origin stenosis and evidence-based decisions regarding management.

17.2 Case Example

17.2.1 History of Present Illness

A 66-year-old male presented to the emergency department with dizziness which he described as balance issues and a spinning sensation with exertion. He denied any other complaints and his physical examination was unremarkable. The patient was on daily aspirin (ASA) and clopidogrel due to previous cardiovascular history and risk factors. Imaging assessment with noncontrast computed tomography of the head was negative for ischemic and hemorrhagic stroke. Magnetic resonance imaging showed subacute cerebellar infarction. Computed tomography angiogram (CTA) of the head and neck revealed severe stenosis of the right vertebral artery ostium. The left vertebral artery was occluded at the origin. Both carotid arteries were patent. He was then transferred to a comprehensive stroke center for further management.

Past medical history: Coronary and peripheral artery disease, hypertension, diabetes type II, hyperlipidemia, and atrial fibrillation (treated with cardioversion, denied use of anticoagulation).

Past surgical history: Coronary and peripheral artery stenting, bilateral carotid endarterectomies.

Family history: Denies cardiovascular events in the family.

Social history: Denies tobacco smoking, alcohol abuse, or illicit drugs.

Neurological examination: Unremarkable.

Imaging studies: See ▶ Fig. 17.1 and ▶ Fig. 17.2.

17.2.2 Treatment Plan

After arrival at the comprehensive stroke center, the patient was started on a low-dose heparin drip and underwent digital subtraction angiography (DSA) for further evaluation of vessel stenosis. The left vertebral artery was found to be occluded, and there was 90% stenosis of the right vertebral artery origin. He then underwent successful angioplasty and stenting of the vertebral artery origin on the right using a balloon mounted stent. There was no complication related to the procedure.

17.2.3 Follow-up

The patient's symptoms improved after the procedure. Magnetic resonance imaging of the head was negative for ischemic stroke and he was discharged home 2 days after the intervention. At the 2-month follow-up visit, he reported no recurrence of symptoms and was doing well. At the 6-month follow-up visit, the patient remained asymptomatic and imaging demonstrated patency of the stent.

17.3 Case Summary

1. *What are the indications for vertebral artery stenting?*
   In patients with vertebrobasilar insufficiency, revascularization of the vertebral artery origin can be considered if degree of stenosis is significant. Even though vertebral artery origin stenting is a relatively safe procedure, the evidence of its superiority over medical management is lacking. When reviewing literature, VAOS stenting should also be separated from intracranial vertebral artery stenting as intracranial stenting has been shown to have higher rate of preprocedural risks likely due to its anatomy, location, and presence of perforators. A recent meta-analysis of the stenting versus medical management for vertebral artery stenosis showed high risks of periprocedural stroke or death for intracranial stenting and did not demonstrate any evidence of benefit for stenting over medical management in

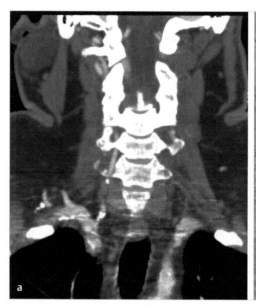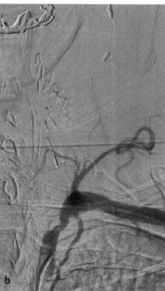

Fig. 17.1 Computed tomography angiogram demonstrates severe stenosis of the right vertebral artery origin **(a)**. Digital subtraction angiogram shows occlusion of the left vertebral artery **(b)** at the origin.

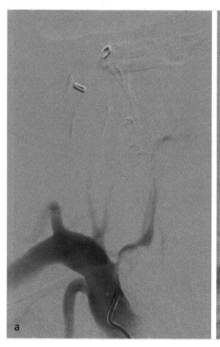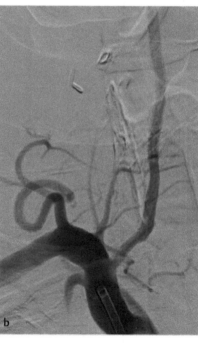

Fig. 17.2 Severe stenosis (90%) at the right vertebral artery ostium **(a)**. Right vertebral artery after angioplasty and stenting **(b)** demonstrates restoration of flow.

extracranial stenosis. It should be noted that the number of extracranial stenosis were small, and no randomized study, as of today, has looked exclusively at the vertebral artery origin stenosis (VAOS).[1]

Previous retrospective studies, however, have shown that VAOS stenting is feasible and relatively safe. Selection of appropriate patients with vertebrobasilar disease due to VAOS and no other causes is also very important. A detail history, clinical examination, and imaging are key. Patients with unilateral vertebral artery disease and contralateral vertebral artery hypoplasia or bilateral vertebral artery disease may be at higher risk of thromboembolic events. Advanced imaging, such as large-vessel quantitative magnetic resonance angiography (QMRA), can be used to select patients with poor posterior circulation flow.

2. *What are the symptoms of vertebrobasilar insufficiency?*
   Ischemia in the vertebrobasilar circulation can result in a wide variety of symptoms often occurring simultaneously. Symptoms include perioral numbness, vertigo, unilateral weakness, and visual disturbances. Other potential manifestations include syncopal episodes, nausea, vomiting, tinnitus, headache, dysarthria, ataxia, motor and sensory disturbances, and cranial nerves deficits.

3. *What are the risks of vertebral artery stenting?*
   Periprocedural risks associated with vertebral artery stenting is low (1–3%) when performed by skilled operators.[2] Inherent complications associated with endovascular manipulation of vessels are further embolization of atherosclerotic material causing strokes/transient ischemic attacks (TIAs), potential myocardial infarction, and death. The most

17

frequent complication after stenting the vertebral artery is in-stent restenosis, which can be reduced by the use of drug-eluting stents. Fractures of the stent due to elastic recoil at the ostium may also occur.[3]

4. *What patient factors were considered in the decision of revascularization versus medical treatment in this case?*

Even though the optimized management of the VAOS remains unclear, our patient in this case was thought to be a good candidate for revascularization. He had evidence of a prior cerebellar stroke. His contralateral vertebral artery was occluded and he did not have well-developed posterior communicating arteries or other evidence of collateral circulation. Therefore, he relied on the stenotic right vertebral artery to provide blood to the posterior circulation. Therefore, he underwent stent revascularization to reestablish blood supply to the vertebrobasilar system.

5. *What are the technical factors to consider for vertebral artery stenting?*

There are several technical aspects to consider when VAOS stenting is planned. Importantly, medical management should be optimized with dual antiplatelet therapy and statin, if indicated. Dual antiplatelet regimen is typically continued for at least 6 months poststenting. Access is also important, as these lesions lend themselves particularly well to the transradial approach. A balloon-mounted stent is typically used, and drug-eluting stents may decrease risk of in-stent stenosis. While placing the stent, it is important to cover the entire vertebral artery origin as the diseased area is typically at the ostium.

17.4 Level of Evidence

Natural history of VAOS: The natural history of VAOS is derived from studies examining the natural history of both intra- and extracranial stenosis. Specific information regarding the VAOS is gleaned from multiple large-scale studies (Class IIB, Level of Evidence B).

Endovascular treatment: Multiple, randomized controlled trials have been performed which included patients with vertebral artery ostium stenosis. However, these studies included patients with stenosis in other segments including intracranial stenosis (Class IIB, Level of Evidence B).

Choice of stent: Bare metal and drug-eluting stents have both been used in the treatment of VAOS (Class IIB, Level of Evidence C).

Follow-up of vertebral artery origin stents: The rates of restenosis have been examined with regard to stents in the vertebral artery ostium in large, multicenter trials. However, the restenosis rate of bare metal and drug-eluting stents has been examined in retrospective series only (Class IIB, Level of Evidence B).

17.5 Landmark Papers

Amin-Hanjani S, Pandey DK, Rose-Finnell L, et al; Vertebrobasilar Flow Evaluation and Risk of Transient Ischemic Attack and Stroke Study Group. Effect of hemodynamics on stroke risk in symptomatic atherosclerotic vertebrobasilar occlusive disease. JAMA Neurol 2016;73(2):178–185.[3]

This was a prospective, observational, blinded, multicenter (U.S. and Canada) study. It included patients with previous recent TIAs or stroke and ≥ 50% atherosclerotic stenosis in the vertebrobasilar system during a 5-year period. The 82 patients enrolled were subsequently studied with large-vessel QMRA. Follow-up was performed with monthly phone calls and biannual clinical consultation with physicians blinded to the status of QMRA. After central review of angiograms, 72 patients remained eligible, of which 69 completed 12 months follow-up. All patients received similar management of risk factors at 6 months interval. One quarter of the patients (18) had low distal-flow status. This group had significantly higher risk of stroke in the posterior circulation ($p = 0.4$) and lower 12- and 24-months event-free survival rates (78% and 70%) than the normal flow group (96% and 87%). After adjustment for age and risk factors, the low flow group remained significantly associated with a higher risk of subsequent stroke (Hazard Ratio 11.55, 95% CI 1.88–71.00; $p = 0.008$).

Considering the study results, it was concluded that noninvasive imaging methods, such as QMRA, are emerging useful tools in the assessment of patients with vertebrobasilar ischemia, and those with low flow status are particularly at risk of subsequent strokes.

Markus HS, Harshfield EL, Compter A, et al; Vertebral Stenosis Trialists' Collaboration. Stenting for symptomatic vertebral artery stenosis: a preplanned pooled individual patient data analysis. Lancet Neurol 2019;18(7):666–673.[4]

This was a meta-analysis to analyze the results of three trials and other reviews about vertebral artery stenosis. The major trials included Vertebral Artery Stenting Trial (VAST), Vertebral Artery Ischemia Stenting Trial (VIST), and stenting versus aggressive medical management for preventing recurrent stroke in intracranial stenosis (SAMMPRIS). The analysis was done using the intention-to-treat in each trial result and estimated hazard ratios, separating the patients in extracranial and intracranial stenosis, which were randomly assigned to medical management versus stenting. One hundred and twenty-two patients with extracranial stenosis were enrolled in each treatment modality. In the stenting group, the analysis showed higher risk of periprocedural major vascular events (stroke or death) in patients with intracranial stenosis than those with extracranial stenosis (16% vs. 1%, $p < 0.0001$). However, they did not identify evidence of benefit for stroke prevention in either treatment group. Further, large-scale trials should be performed to determine the benefit of stenting in vertebral artery extracranial stenosis.

SSYLVIA Study Investigators. Stenting of Symptomatic Atherosclerotic Lesions in the Vertebral or Intracranial Arteries (SSYLVIA): study results. Stroke 2004;35(6):1388–1392.[2]

The Stenting of Symptomatic Atherosclerotic Lesions in the Vertebral or Intracranial Arteries (SSYLVIA) study was a multicenter, nonrandomized, prospective study and was aimed at evaluating the safety and procedural feasibility of the NEUROLINK System (Guidant Corporation) for treatment of vertebral or intracranial artery stenosis. The patients enrolled were between 18 and 80 years old with TIA or stroke attributed to a single target lesion of ≥ 50% stenosis by angiography. The primary end points were rate of (1) death or stroke in the first 30 days postprocedure and (2) successful placement of stent resulting in < 50% stenosis covering an area no longer than the original lesion. Secondary end points included follow-up angiography at 6 months, stroke in the distribution of the target lesion at 12 months, and access site events requiring treatment.

17

The SSYLVIA study included a total of 61 patients from November 9, 2000 through November 19, 2001. Thirty-seven (60.7%) patients suffered a stroke, while 24 (39.3%) patients had a TIA. The treated vessels were intracranial in 43 (70.5%) patients and extracranial in 18 (29.5%), 6 (9.8%) of which were in the vertebral ostium. No deaths occurred within 30 days postprocedure, but 4 (6.6%) patients had strokes, 3 of them major and ipsilateral. Successful stent placement was achieved in 58/61 (95%) cases. At 6 months, stenosis > 50% was seen in 12/37 (32.4%) intracranial stents and 6 of 14 (42.9%) extracranial vertebral stents. Of these extracranial vertebral stents, 67% (4/6) occurred in the vertebral ostium.

An exploratory analysis was performed which determined that certain factors such as diabetes, greater postprocedure stenosis, smaller pretreatment vessel size, and vertebral ostium lesions contributed significantly to the prediction of restenosis at 6 months. According to the trial, restenosis occurred in 67% of vertebral ostium lesions, compared with only 25% of pre-posterior inferior cerebellar artery (PICA) vertebral lesions, suggesting that ostial recoil may require a more robust stent.

Coward LJ, McCabe DJ, Ederle J, Featherstone RL, Clifton A, Brown MM; CAVATAS Investigators. Long-term outcome after angioplasty and stenting for symptomatic vertebral artery stenosis compared with medical treatment in the Carotid And Vertebral Artery Transluminal Angioplasty Study (CAVATAS): a randomized trial. Stroke 2007;38(5):1526–1530.[5]

The Carotid and Vertebral Artery Transluminal Angioplasty Study (CAVATAS) was a multicenter clinical trial that incorporated three separate randomized clinical trials: (1) endovascular versus surgical treatment in patients with carotid stenosis, (2) endovascular treatment versus medical management alone in patients with carotid stenosis, and (3) endovascular treatment versus medical management alone in patients with vertebral artery stenosis. The natural history of vertebral artery stenosis is not completely understood, and there is not a clear consensus on the optimal therapeutic approach in symptomatic patients. CAVATAS is the first clinical trial that sought to address this uncertainty. Coward et al[5] reported on the long-term outcome of endovascular intervention compared with medical management alone in patients with symptomatic vertebral artery stenosis.

A total of 16 patients with symptomatic vertebral stenosis were randomly split into equal proportions to receive endovascular therapy (balloon angioplasty or stenting) or best medical management alone from March 1992 through July 1997. There were no significant differences in baseline clinical characteristics or medical therapy used between groups. Fifteen of the 16 (94%) patients had VAOS. There were no 30-day strokes or deaths in either group, although two of the eight patients who underwent endovascular treatment experienced TIAs. No posterior circulation infarct was recorded in either arm during follow-up, but three patients in each treatment arm died of myocardial infarction or carotid territory stroke. One patient, in the endovascular treatment arm, had a nonfatal carotid territory stroke.

The trial failed to show benefit of endovascular therapy of vertebral artery stenosis over medical management alone. Three of the six patients treated with balloon angioplasty alone developed restenosis of the treated artery on follow-up imaging. The limitations of this study were that six of the eight patients in the endovascular treatment arm were only treated with angioplasty, possibly due to the unavailability of stents for use in the vertebral artery prior to 1994, and the small number of patients included in the study.

Compter A, van der Worp HB, Schonewille WJ, et al; VAST investigators. Stenting versus medical treatment in patients with symptomatic vertebral artery stenosis: a randomised open-label phase 2 trial. Lancet Neurol 2015;14(6):606–614.[1]

Another trial comparing percutaneous vertebral intervention with medical therapy is VAST. VAST was an open-label, phase 2 clinical trial that randomly assigned 115 patients with a recent TIA or minor stroke associated with an intracranial or extracranial vertebral artery stenosis of at least 50% to either stenting plus best medical treatment or best medical treatment alone between January 22, 2008 and April 8, 2013. The primary outcome was the composite of vascular death, myocardial infarction, or any stroke within the 30 days after the start of treatment. The secondary outcomes included stroke in the territory of the symptomatic vertebral artery during follow-up, the composite outcome during follow-up, and the degree of stenosis in the symptomatic vertebral artery at 12 months.

Fifty-seven patients were assigned to the stenting plus best medical treatment group and 58 to the best medical treatment alone. Forty-seven (82%) patients in the stenting group and 46 (79%) patients in the medical treatment group had a VAOS. Although the medical treatment group had more patients with a modified Rankin score of greater than 1 at inclusion (9 vs. 20), the remaining baseline characteristics between both groups were similar. Three patients (5%) in the stenting group had vascular death, myocardial infarction, or any stroke within 30 days after the start of treatment compared with one (2%) patient in the medical treatment group. During a median follow-up of 3 years, 7 (12%) of the patients in the stenting and 4 (7%) in the medical treatment group had a stroke in the territory of the symptomatic vertebral artery, questioning the need for a phase 3 trial to assess the benefit of stenting in a comparable patient population.

Markus HS, Larsson SC, Kuker W, et al; VIST Investigators. Stenting for symptomatic vertebral artery stenosis: The Vertebral Artery Ischaemia Stenting Trial. Neurology 2017;89(12):1229–1236.[6]

VIST was a randomized, open-blinded end point clinical trial which aimed to compare treatment options for patients with symptomatic vertebral artery (VA) stenosis. The prospective study placed patients in two groups: (1) VA stenting or angioplasty with best medical therapy (BMT) and (2) BMT only. Follow-ups with patients occurred periodically, and any outcomes were recorded. The primary outcomes included fatal or nonfatal stroke in any arterial area. Secondary outcomes were stroke or TIA, fatal or nonfatal stroke in any arterial area within 90 days after randomization, or death.

Patients were recruited between October 23, 2008 and February 4, 2015 from 14 hospitals in the United Kingdom. Only 182 patients were enrolled out of the initial goal of 540 patients due to lack of funding. An additional three patients later withdrew from the study. The remaining 179 patients were randomly assigned, with stratification based on the VA stenosis site, to the 2 groups. Ninety-one were assigned to the stenting group and 88 were assigned to the BMT-only group. Most patients had an extracranial stenosis, with 81% in the stenting group

17

and 84% in the BMT-only group. Baseline characteristics for the two groups were comparable, and the median follow-up was 3.5 years with data available for all 179 patients until March 2016.

In the stenting group, a few complications arose. One intracranial stenosis patient died of hemorrhage and another had a nonfatal stroke. An extracranial stenosis patient had a nonfatal stroke within 30 days of treatment. A primary outcome occurred in 5 of the stent group patients and in 12 of the BMT-only group patients. The absolute risk was reduced by 25 strokes per 1,000 person-years. For both groups overall, the secondary outcome of a fatal or nonfatal stroke or TIA had a hazard ratio of 0.50 (95% CI 0.25–1.01). There was no statistical difference between the two groups for the remaining secondary outcomes.

17.6 Recommendations

In patients with vertebrobasilar insufficiency, revascularization of the vertebral artery origin can be considered if the degree of stenosis is significant. However, evidence of superiority of stenting over medical therapy is lacking. A recent meta-analysis of the stenting versus medical management for vertebral artery stenosis showed high risk of periprocedural stroke or death for intracranial stenting and did not show any evidence of a benefit for stenting over medical management in extracranial stenosis.[4] Stenting was safe for patients with extracranial stenosis with a low procedural risk, although there was no significant difference in stroke risk between the medical and interventional cohorts. Sample size, time between randomization and treatment, and the location of the stenosis were the main limitations for this study. The stenting group also had a shorter average waiting time between randomization and treatment. When compared to the BMT group, stenting also resulted in a nonsignificant reduced risk of recurrent stroke.

Further, current retrospective and prospective evidence concerning extracranial vertebral artery stenosis are pooled data involving all segments of the extracranial vertebral artery, and no separate analysis of the VAOS has been performed. In the experience of many operators, as reported in retrospective studies, VAOS stenting is feasible and safe when patients are carefully selected, taking into consideration the clinical details, extension of the disease (i.e., unilateral, bilateral), anatomical characteristics of the posterior circulation (i.e., presence of contralateral hypoplasia), and use of proper imaging tools, such as QMRA. This information must be combined to delineate a subset of eligible patients who are truly symptomatic from VAOS and would benefit from stenting without a high risk of periprocedural complications.[3]

17.7 Summary

1. The natural history of vertebral artery stenosis can be better understood using the evidence provided by multiple prospective and retrospective studies. However, most studies do not differentiate between stenosis involving varying segments of the vertebral artery.
2. Since there is not enough evidence to suggest benefit of stenting over medical management, it is crucial to take into account the lesion's and patient's characteristics (i.e., recurrent symptoms despite best medical management, degree of stenosis, status of the contralateral vertebral artery) before considering endovascular intervention.
3. The VAOS has not been studied separately. Recommendations regarding this specific segment are still to be formulated in future studies.

References

[1] Compter A, van der Worp HB, Schonewille WJ, et al. VAST investigators. Stenting versus medical treatment in patients with symptomatic vertebral artery stenosis: a randomised open-label phase 2 trial. Lancet Neurol. 2015; 14 (6):606–614

[2] SSYLVIA Study Investigators. Stenting of Symptomatic Atherosclerotic Lesions in the Vertebral or Intracranial Arteries (SSYLVIA): study results. Stroke. 2004; 35(6):1388–1392

[3] Amin-Hanjani S, Pandey DK, Rose-Finnell L, et al. Vertebrobasilar Flow Evaluation and Risk of Transient Ischemic Attack and Stroke Study Group. Effect of hemodynamics on stroke risk in symptomatic atherosclerotic vertebrobasilar occlusive disease. JAMA Neurol. 2016; 73(2):178–185

[4] Markus HS, Harshfield EL, Compter A, et al. Vertebral Stenosis Trialists' Collaboration. Stenting for symptomatic vertebral artery stenosis: a preplanned pooled individual patient data analysis. Lancet Neurol. 2019; 18(7):666–673

[5] Coward LJ, McCabe DJ, Ederle J, Featherstone RL, Clifton A, Brown MM, CAVATAS Investigators. Long-term outcome after angioplasty and stenting for symptomatic vertebral artery stenosis compared with medical treatment in the Carotid And Vertebral Artery Transluminal Angioplasty Study (CAVATAS): a randomized trial. Stroke. 2007; 38(5):1526–1530

[6] Markus HS, Larsson SC, Kuker W, et al. VIST Investigators. Stenting for symptomatic vertebral artery stenosis: the Vertebral Artery Ischaemia Stenting Trial. Neurology. 2017; 89(12):1229–1236

17

18 Cerebral Venous Sinus Thrombosis

Michael G. Brandel, Christian Lopez Ramos, Robert C. Rennert, Peter Abraham, Kevin Porras, Arvin R. Wali, Jeffrey A. Steinberg, David R. Santiago-Dieppa, J. Scott Pannell, and Alexander A. Khalessi

Abstract

Cerebral venous sinus thrombosis (CVST) is the acute occlusion of the brain's dural venous sinuses by a thrombus. CVST is a rare cause of stroke that primarily affects children and young adults. Diagnosis of CVST is often delayed due to variable clinical manifestations, and mortality ranges from 5 to 30%. While systemic anticoagulation is the primary initial treatment for CVST, endovascular therapies including local thrombolysis or mechanical thrombectomy can be considered in refractory cases, although efficacy data remain mixed. Decompressive hemicraniectomy may be performed in patients presenting with severely increased intracranial pressures and impending herniation, despite an increased risk for poor outcomes that is independent of endovascular recanalization. Understanding the scope and quality of evidence regarding neurosurgical and neurointerventional procedures for refractory cases of CVST is critical.

Keywords: cerebral venous sinus thrombosis, anticoagulation, thrombolysis, mechanical thrombectomy

18.1 Goals

1. Review the literature that describes the risk factors and prognosis for cerebral venous sinus thrombosis.
2. Review the diagnostic methods used to distinguish cerebral venous sinus thrombosis from other neurological conditions.
3. Review the literature that describes the traditional treatments for cerebral venous sinus thrombosis.
4. Critically analyze endovascular treatments for cerebral venous sinus thrombosis.

18.2 Case Example

18.2.1 History of Present Illness

A 25-year-old woman presented to the emergency room with altered mental status. As per her family, she had been complaining of a progressively worsening headache and nausea for 3 days. On the morning of presentation, she was found to be poorly responsive with slurred speech. She had no sick contacts, fever, or neck stiffness, and no recent trauma or travel.

Past medical history: Ovarian cysts managed with oral contraceptives (OCPs) started 3 months prior to presentation.
Past surgical history: None.
Family history: Maternal history of migraines.
Social history: No tobacco, alcohol, or substance use.
Review of systems: As per the above.
Neurological examination: On examination, the patient attempted to vocalize with moaning but was unable to answer any questions. She opened her eyes to noxious stimuli, flexor postured to pain in the upper extremities bilaterally, and triple flexed in the lower extremities bilaterally.

She had no spontaneous movement of the extremities. Pupils were equal in size and reactive to light. Ophthalmological examination was notable for mild papilledema.
Imaging studies: See ▶ Fig. 18.1.

18.2.2 Treatment Plan

The patient was started on anticoagulation with intravenous heparin for treatment of a cerebral venous thrombosis of the straight and transverse sinuses. Despite therapeutic anticoagulation, the patient's clinical status continued to deteriorate, and she was taken to the neurointerventional suite for a diagnostic angiogram and embolectomy.

During the procedure, a 4-Fr diagnostic catheter and guidewire were introduced into a right common femoral artery sheath for catheterization of the right internal carotid artery. Angiograms of the anterior circulation demonstrated no opacification of the straight and left transverse sinus and a large thrombus in the right transverse sinus (▶ Fig. 18.2a). An aspiration catheter and guidewire were then advanced through a right internal jugular vein guide sheath to catheterize the straight and transverse sinuses. Venograms demonstrated a large thrombus burden of the straight sinus (▶ Fig. 18.2b). Mechanical aspiration of thrombus resulted in adequate recanalization of the straight and transverse sinuses.

18.2.3 Follow-up

The patient responded well to the treatment and was transitioned to oral anticoagulation with warfarin for 6 months. OCPs were discontinued and thrombophilia work-up was negative. Subsequent imaging demonstrated recanalization of the straight and transverse sinuses. At follow-up, the patient denied any complaints and had an unremarkable neurological examination.

18.3 Case Summary

1. *When is intervention indicated for a patient with cerebral venous sinus thrombosis (CVST)?*
   Anticoagulation therapy with either dose-adjusted unfractionated heparin or weight-based low-molecular-weight heparin (LMWH) is recommended for patients with CVST even in the presence of hemorrhagic lesions.[1] This recommendation is based on limited evidence from randomized controlled trials (RCTs)[2,3,4,5] and several observational studies,[3,6,7,8,9,10,11,12,13,14,15] the largest of which was the International Study on Cerebral Vein and Dural Sinus Thrombosis (ISCVT).[6] While limited nonrandomized studies suggest that LMWH is more effective compared to unfractionated heparin, no definitive evidence exists.[16]
   Endovascular intervention for CVST is generally indicated for patients with progressive neurological deterioration or poor prognosis despite adequate anticoagulation therapy.[1] Endovascular methods include direct catheter chemical

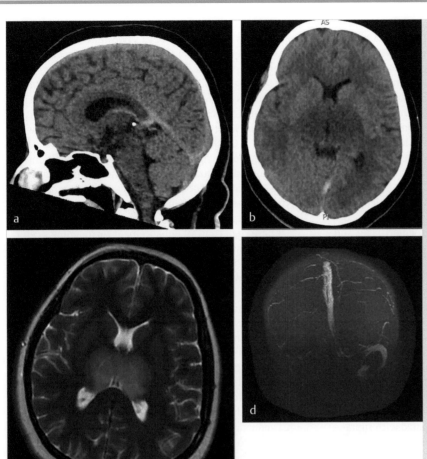

Fig. 18.1 Diagnostic imaging studies. Preoperative noncontrast computed tomography (CT) scan and magnetic resonance imaging and venography (MRI/MRV). **(a)** Noncontrast sagittal CT scan revealed a hyperdense cord sign indicating a thrombosed straight sinus. Hyperdensities within the deep cerebral veins, vein of Galen, and transverse sinuses were also noted. **(b)** Noncontrast axial CT scan revealed hypodense bilateral thalami indicative of edema and concerning for infarction. There was no evidence of intracranial hemorrhage. **(c)** MRI showed symmetric bilateral edema of the thalamus, internal capsule, and basal ganglia. **(d)** MRV showed thrombosis of the straight sinus, right transverse sinus, and internal cerebral veins.

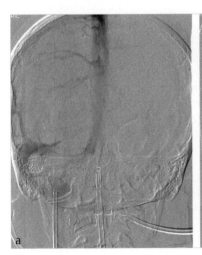
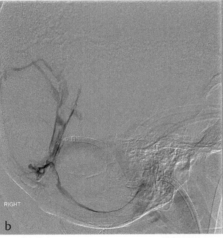

Fig. 18.2 Intraprocedural imaging. **(a)** Diagnostic angiogram of anterior circulation (delayed venous phase) demonstrated occlusion of the left transverse sinus and severe stenosis of the right transverse sinus due to large thrombus in the transverse sinus. **(b)** Diagnostic angiogram (lateral view) revealed positioning of aspiration catheter in the straight sinus with contrast-filling defect due to a thrombosed straight sinus.

thrombolysis or direct mechanical thrombectomy (balloon-assisted or aspiration catheter) with or without thrombolysis. In a systematic review of 169 patients who received local thrombolysis, more than 80% were independent at follow-up.[17] Another systematic review of 185 patients treated with mechanical thrombectomy demonstrated that 84% and 74% of patients had a good outcome and near-to-complete or complete recanalization after the procedure, respectively.[18] However, no RCTs have evaluated the efficacy and safety of endovascular intervention for the treatment of CVST. A decompressive craniectomy is considered for critically ill CVST patients with impending herniation secondary to a large venous hemorrhage and parenchymal infarctions. In a review of 69 patients with ischemic or hemorrhagic parenchymal lesions that underwent decompressive surgery, only 17% had unfavorable outcomes (modified Rankin scale [mRS] score of 5–6), whereas 59% were independent (mRS 0–2) at the end of follow-up.[19]

18

2. *What is the long-term management of CVST?*

Patients are transitioned to oral anticoagulation for 3 to 12 months with an international normalized ratio (INR) goal of 2–3.[1] Treatment duration depends on the presence of risk factors for recurrent CVST or other venous thromboembolisms (VTE). Patients with idiopathic CVST and a mild thrombophilia may be treated for 6 to 12 months, compared to 3 to 6 months in patients with provoked CVST.[1] Long-term or indefinite anticoagulation may be considered for patients with a severe inherited thrombophilia, recurrent CVST, or VTE after CVST.

3. *What is the clinical presentation of CVST?*

Clinical presentation of CVST is highly variable and dependent on acuity, site, number of occluded vessels, presence of cerebral lesions (edema, venous infarction, hemorrhage), and patient age. The mean age for women and men is 34 and 42 years, respectively.[20] Patients may present with an isolated intracranial hypertension (ICH) syndrome (headache, papilledema), neurological deficits (motor weakness, aphasias, focal or generalized seizures), or signs of encephalopathy (mental status changes).[1,21]

The most common symptom of CVST is severe headache, occurring in 90% of patients.[21] Headaches are typically slow in onset, with increasing severity over multiple days. Patients with parenchymal lesions are more likely to have diminished mental status or neurological deficits such as motor weakness, aphasia, and seizures.[21] In the ISCVT, 39% of patients presented with seizures, which were associated with supratentorial lesions, motor deficits, and sagittal sinus and cortical vein thrombosis.[22]

4. *What are the most commonly involved sites in CVST and their associated clinical characteristics?*

In the ISCVT cohort, the most common cerebral venous sites involved were the transverse (86%), superior sagittal (62%), and straight sinuses (18%).[6] Sagittal sinus thrombosis commonly manifests with motor deficits and seizures. Transverse sinus thromboses may present with isolated signs and symptoms of ICH. Aphasia is generally associated with thrombus in the left transverse sinus. Involvement of the straight sinus results in more severe signs and symptoms, including coma or altered mental status, and is typically associated with bilateral thalamic lesions, as in the case example patient.[23]

5. *What risk factors should you consider for the development of cerebral venous sinus thrombosis (CVST)?*

A genetic or acquired prothrombotic state is the most common risk factor for the development of CVST, identified in 85% of patients.[6] Genetic hypercoagulable states include deficiencies in antithrombin, protein C, and protein S, or mutations in factor V Leiden and prothrombin genes.[24] Acquired prothrombotic conditions include antiphospholid syndrome, polycythemia, homocysteinemia, inflammatory diseases, malignancies, and severe systemic infections.[1,21] Patients with CVST should be evaluated for underlying hypercoagulable states. Head trauma, pregnancy, obstetric delivery, and surgery may precipitate CVST in patients with risk factors for a hypercoagulable state.

CVST commonly affects people in their third decade of life. Of note, 80% of newly diagnosed cases occur in women of childbearing age.[6] Increased incidence of CVST among women is likely related to the prothrombotic effects of OCPs.

In the prospective International Study on Cerebral Vein and Dural Sinuses Thrombosis (ISCVT), two-thirds of women with CVST were either on OCPs, hormone replacement therapy, or were pregnant.[20]

6. *What imaging modalities are used for diagnosing CVST and what findings are suggestive of the diagnosis?*

a) Computed tomography (CT) and CT venography

Given the wide variability in clinical presentation, the diagnosis of CVST is often challenging. A head CT is the first investigation to rule out other neurological conditions, yet it is normal in about 70% of CVST cases.[25] Direct signs of CVST include the "dense triangle sign," characterized by a triangular-shaped hyperdensity caused by the thrombus.[26] On contrast CT, the "empty delta sign" is a triangular pattern of contrast enhancement surrounding a central region lacking contrast enhancement in the sinus due to the thrombus.[26] Another is the "cord sign," typically observed with a contrast CT as a linear patchy hyperdensity of the occluded vein.[27] Dilated or tortuous cerebral veins, edema, and hemorrhagic venous infarctions can also be seen. About 30 to 40% of patients with CVST present with an intracerebral hemorrhage.[6]

Per AHA/ASA guidelines, venography (either CT venography or magnetic resonance [MR] venography) should be performed in suspected CVST following a negative CT or magnetic resonance imaging (MRI), or to characterize the extent of thrombosis after a suggestive CT or MRI.[1] CT venography increases the accuracy of diagnosis of CVST to 90 to 100%.[25] CT venography provides visualization of the major dural sinuses and may demonstrate filling defects, sinus wall enhancement, and increased collateral venous drainage secondary to the presence of a thrombus.[25]

b) MRI and MR venography

MR venography in combination with MRI (particularly T2 susceptibility weighted sequences) is also highly sensitive for diagnosing CVST.[26] In the acute phase, thrombosed sinuses appear isointense and hypointense on T1-weighted and T2-weighted images, respectively.[25] Subacutely, the signal increases on both T1- and T2-weighted MRI images. Other lesions, including edema or venous infarction, appear hypointense or isointense on T1-weighted MRI and hyperintense on T2-weighted images. Hemorrhagic venous infarcts can also be seen on MRI, and appear as hyperintense lesions on both T1 and T2 sequences. It is nonetheless important to be aware of normal anatomic variants that may mimic findings of CVST, such as sinus hypoplasia or atresia and asymmetric sinus drainage.[25]

c) Angiography

In the event of inconclusive results from CT or MRI, catheter angiography may be used to diagnose CVST.[25] Findings on angiography include lack of or delayed opacification of the affected vein or sinus, indicative of a thrombus. Similar to MRI, normal asymmetric angiographic venous anatomy may potentially result in a misdiagnosis of CVST.[27]

7. *What is the prognosis of patients with CVST?*

The overall ISCVT cohort mortality rate was 8.3% (approximately half of which occurred acutely), with other studies reporting mortality rates up to 21%.[6,28] Nonetheless, nearly

25% of patients experience neurologic deterioration after admission, and acute herniation secondary to hemorrhage is the most common cause of death in the acute period.[1] Thirty-day mortality predictors include mental status changes, hemorrhage of the right hemisphere, and thrombosis of deep venous structures.[6,7] Patients with ICH as their only presentation of CVST have favorable outcomes. Poor long-term prognosis is associated with infection, hemorrhage, Glasgow Coma Scale (GCS) < 9 on admission, mental status abnormalities, and male sex.[6,7] Complete recovery at the end of follow-up (mean 18.6 months) was observed in 80% of patients in the ISCVT cohort.[6] Risk of recurrent CVST and VTE in other sites is 2 to 4% and 4 to 7%, respectively.[6] Male patients and those with severe thrombophilias are at higher risk for developing thromboembolic events.[6]

18.4 Level of Evidence

18.4.1 Patient Characteristics

Age: Mean age 34 in women, 42 in men (Level of Evidence B).[6]
  Symptoms:
- Headache is the most frequent symptom of CVST (Level of Evidence B).[6]
- CVST can present similarly to idiopathic ICH (vomiting, papilledema, visual disturbances) (Level of Evidence B).[6,29]
- Symptoms of encephalopathy (altered mental status, stupor, coma) are common (Level of Evidence B).[6]
  Past medical history: OCPs are a risk factor for CVST (Level of Evidence A).[30]
  Family history (maternal history of migraines): Headaches of CVST may resemble migraine with aura (Level of Evidence C).[31]
  Neurological examination: Aphasia, papilledema, decreased consciousness.

18.4.2 Work-up

- Imaging of the cerebral venous system to rule out CVST in patients presenting with symptoms of idiopathic ICH (Class I, Level of Evidence C).[1]

18.4.3 Treatment

- Acute antithrombotic treatment with subcutaneous LMWH or intravenous heparin (Class II, Level of Evidence B).[1]
- Endovascular intervention for patients with progressive neurological deterioration or poor prognosis despite adequate anticoagulation therapy (Class II, Level of Evidence C).[1]
- Decompressive craniectomy for patients with mass effect or hemorrhage causing ICH and neurological deterioration (Class II, Level of Evidence C).[1]

18.4.4 Follow-up

- Oral anticoagulation for 3 to 12 months (Class II, Level of Evidence C).[1]
- Thrombophilia work-up after completion of anticoagulation (Class II, Level of Evidence B).[1]

18.5 Landmark Papers

Bousser MG, Chiras J, Bories J, Castaigne P. Cerebral venous thrombosis: a review of 38 cases. Stroke 1985;16(2):199–213.

Prior to the landmark paper by Professor Marie-Germaine Bousser and colleagues in 1985, most reports on CVST were based on autopsy findings.[32] However, the advent of angiographic techniques enabled the authors to report a series of 38 living patients (17 women, 21 men) between 1975 and 1982 with angiographically proven CVST. All patients underwent unilateral or bilateral carotid angiography, either by percutaneous direct puncture or right-sided brachial/femoral arteries, which showed partial or complete lack of sinus filling.

Etiology was identified as infective for 4 patients, local causes including head trauma for 5, general (autoimmune disease, malignancy, or OCP use) for 19, and idiopathic (no identifiable cause) for 10 patients. Sixteen patients had a well-defined ICH syndrome, whereas 22 patients had focal symptoms with or without ICH symptoms. Frequent neurological signs among patients included headache (74%), papilledema (45%), hemiplegia (34%), and seizures (29%). Other focal and multifocal signs such as dysphagia and multiple cranial nerve palsies were also observed.

CT scans with and without contrast were performed for 25 patients, with normal findings in 20% and abnormal findings in 80% of patients. Observed abnormalities included small ventricles (52%), enlarged ventricles (12%), focal parenchymal lesions (40%), tentorial enhancement (16%), and an empty delta sign (12%). Treatments varied, including anticoagulants (61%), steroids (45%), anticonvulsants (26%), antibiotics (21%), and no treatment (11%). Immediate outcomes were mostly favorable, with 71% of patients recovering completely, 18% with residual deficits, and 11% dead. The authors observed that patients presenting with focal deficits were more likely to experience sequelae (31%) or die (19%), whereas those presenting with ICH syndrome had mostly favorable outcomes.

Despite the importance of this study, its generalizability is limited. A case series does not provide information on CVST incidence, and there was selection bias due to the exclusion of autopsy-identified patients. Modern diagnostic and treatment guidelines and technologies were also not yet available in the time period (pre-1982).

de Brujin SF, Stam J. Randomized, placebo-controlled trial of anticoagulant treatment with low-molecular-weight heparin for cerebral sinus thrombosis. Stroke 1999;30(3):484–488.

In 1999, de Brujin et al compared LMWH to placebo in imaging-confirmed CVST patients.[2] In a randomized, partially double-blinded, placebo control trial, patients were randomized to either nadroparin 180 anti-factor Xa units/kg per 24 hours (30 patients) or placebo (30 patients). Primary outcomes were death or poor outcome, defined as a Barthel Index (BI) of activities of daily living < 15 3 weeks after randomization. Secondary outcome was death or dependence, defined as the Oxford Handicap Scale grade 3–5 (partial dependence), at 12 weeks.

Unlike prior studies that showed a statistically significant benefit for heparin in CVST patients,[3] the treatment and placebo groups in this study did not statistically differ in the rate of poor outcomes at 3 weeks (20% vs. 24%, respectively). Similarly, death or dependence at 12 weeks also did not statistically differ (13% vs. 21%, respectively). Nadroparin was not associated

18

with new symptomatic cerebral hemorrhages, even in patients initially presenting with hemorrhage. Although heparin was not shown to have significant benefit, this study helped demonstrate its safety.

Study limitations include potential unblinding of trial patients to their treatment allocation due to treatment side effects (e.g., injection-site hemorrhages from nadroparin), potential bias from the open design after the 3-week mark, and a small sample size that was not powered to detect small or moderate treatment effects.

Canhao P, Falcao F, Ferro JM. Thrombolytics for cerebral sinus thrombosis: a systematic review. Cerebrovasc Dis 2003;15:159–166.

In 2003, Canhao et al published a systematic review of papers between 1966 and 2001 on the use of thrombolytics for CVST.[17] In the absence of RCT data, this study was a landmark in its aggregation of data for a rare treatment of CVST with unknown efficacy or safety. One hundred and sixty-nine patients from 72 studies were included. Patients had an average age of 34 years (37% male, 63% female) and most were in poor clinical condition (78% with encephalopathy or coma, 15% with the ICH syndrome).

Most patients received urokinase only (75%) or recombinant tissue plasminogen activator (rtPA) only (22%), with a few others receiving streptokinase or multiple agents. Administration was local in 88% of cases. Duration of local thrombolytic therapy averaged 41 hours (range < 1–244 h). Fifty-six percent of cases were single administration and 44% involved repeated administration or prolonged infusion (> 24 h). Nearly all (97%) patients were anticoagulated, and 10% also underwent mechanical thrombus disruption.

Complications included intracranial hemorrhage (17%), extracranial hemorrhage (21%), infections (4%), pulmonary embolism (2%), and groin pseudoaneurysm (1%). Discharge disposition for study patients was 86% independent, 7% dependent, and 9% deceased. Average patient follow-up was 8.4 months (range 0.3–37 mo).

Recanalization was observed in most patients and was statistically more likely in those who received local, rather than systemic, thrombolytic therapy. Complete recovery was statistically more likely in patients who did not present with a coma, were treated within 7 days of symptoms onset, and received urokinase. Serious hemorrhages were more common among patients treated with tPA than with other thrombolytics.

Limitations of this study include acquisition of data from case reports or case series, which represents level 5 evidence, and the absence of randomization, control group, or blinding. There was substantial variation in baseline patient characteristics, in addition to treatment characteristics such as thrombolytic dose, duration, and route of administration. Furthermore, several patients had concurrent or subsequent therapies that may confound the associations identified. However, this study established that thrombolytic therapy is relatively safe for CVST treatment as only 5% of patients experienced intracranial hemorrhages associated with clinical deterioration and only 5% of patients died.

Ferro JM, Canhão P, Stam J, Bousser MG, Barinagarrementeria F; ISCVT Investigators. Prognosis of cerebral vein and dural sinus thrombosis: results of the International Study on Cerebral Vein and Dural Sinus Thrombosis (ISCVT). Stroke 2004;35(3):664–670.

The International Study on Cerebral Vein and Dural Sinus Thrombosis (ISCVT) was a prospective observational study of 624 consecutive symptomatic CVST patients from 89 centers in 21 countries.[6] To date, the ISCVT is the largest longitudinal study of CVST patients, and its 16-month median follow-up enabled analysis of long-term functional status and mortality.

Acuity of onset was classified as either acute (37%), subacute (56%), or chronic (7%). An isolated ICH syndrome was present in 23% of patients. Before treatment, 14% of patients had moderate brain injury (GCS 9–13) and 5% were comatose. Most patients (83%) were therapeutically anticoagulated with IV heparin or subcutaneous LMWH in the acute phase. A minority of patients underwent local endovascular thrombolysis (2.1%) or decompressive craniotomy (1.6%). Other treatments used included antiepileptic drugs (44%), osmotherapy (13%), steroids (24%), acetazolamide 10%, and diuretics (6%).

At the time of discharge, 66% of patients had complete recovery, 15% were dependent, and 4% were dead. At 6 months, 78% were completely recovered, 7% were dependent, and 7% were dead. Nearly half (44%) of deaths following the acute phase were due to underlying conditions other than CVST. Outcomes at last follow-up were 79% completely recovered, 5% dependent, and 8% dead.

Ferro et al identified increased age (> 37 years), male sex, GCS < 9, intracranial hemorrhage, mental status disorders, deep vein thrombosis (DVT), central nervous system (CNS) infection, and cancer as significant predictors of death or dependency. They also observed better outcomes for patients presenting with isolated ICH syndrome than for those who presented differently (7% vs. 14% dead/dependent). Interestingly, there was no significant difference in outcome for patients who were therapeutically anticoagulated in the acute phase compared to those who were not.

This landmark paper was the first multicenter, multinational prospective study on CVST and is likely more generalizable than prior prospective studies. Its methods adhered to established consensus criteria and diagnostic techniques. In addition, there was minimal (1%) loss to follow-up. Drawbacks of the study include lack of generalizability to children, as patients less than 15 years of age were excluded, and possible selection bias, as study site participants were primarily neurologists rather than intensive care providers or neurosurgeons who may treat more severe cases of CVST. Finally, some bias in this longitudinal study may be due to incomplete case ascertainment, although investigators were reminded to continuously search for cases at their institutions.

Ferro JM, Crassard I, Coutinho JM, et al; Second International Study on Cerebral Vein and Dural Sinus Thrombosis (ISCVT 2) Investigators. Decompressive surgery in cerebrovenous thrombosis: a multicenter registry and a systematic review of individual patient data. Stroke 2011;42(10):2825–2831.

Given the rarity of CVST, no formal trials have compared surgical and medical interventions. However, multiple case studies have documented the benefit of surgical intervention for CVST. Ferro et al completed a retrospective analysis of decompressive surgery for CVST.[19] Data were derived from a multicenter registry of 69 patients and published case studies of patients receiving decompressive craniectomy, hematoma evacuation, or both. End points included neurologic outcome and level of patient dependence at last follow-up as described by the mRS.

Of 69 total patients, 82.6% had a favorable outcome (mRS 0–4) and only 12.4% had an unfavorable outcome (mRS 5 or death).

Twenty-six patients (37.7%) had complete recovery (mRS 0–1). At the last follow-up, 56.5% of patients were independent (mRS 0–2), 5.8% were severely dependent (mRS 4–5), and 15.9% were dead.

The authors concluded that decompressive surgery for patients with CVST is beneficial in most cases. Moreover, even in patients with the most severe symptom of brain herniation, bilateral fixed pupils, a third had complete recovery (three of nine patients). Similarly, about a third of comatose patients recovered completely. A prospective study to assess the safety and efficacy of decompressive surgery for CVST is needed.

Siddiqui FM, Dandapat S, Banerjee C, et al. Mechanical thrombectomy in cerebral venous thrombosis: systematic review of 185 cases. Stroke 2015;46(5):1263–1268.

Although mechanical thrombectomy has been used for many CVST patients unresponsive to anticoagulation since its first published use by Gurley et al in 1996,[33] indications have been unclear. To address this, Siddiqui et al completed a systematic review of papers published between 1995 and 2014 on mechanical thrombectomy for CVST.[18] One hundred and eighty-five cases from 42 studies were identified, which included only 1 prospective study and no RCTs. Overall, patients presented in severe clinical condition, with 64% having pretreatment ICH and 47% stuporous or comatose. Eighty-two percent of patients had at least two thrombosed venous sinuses and 70% received pretreatment therapeutic anticoagulation.

Nearly all procedures were completed under general anesthesia (98%), with intraprocedural heparin (90%), and via a transjugular or transfemoral approach. Seventy-one percent received concurrent intrasinus thrombolysis.

Overall, 84% of patients had a good outcome (mRS 0–2), 4% had a poor outcome (mRS 3–5), and 12% died. Main causes of death were worsening of hemorrhage and herniation (45%) and lack of clinical improvement, with eventual withdrawal of care (27%). Recanalization rates were 74% complete, 21% partial, and 5% none. The complication rate was 26%, including new or worsening ICH, which occurred in 10% of patients. Significant risk factors for poor outcome or death included pretreatment stupor/coma and baseline ICH. Patients with stupor/coma were also less likely to have complete recanalization and more likely to experience a complication. Complete recanalization was associated with good outcome and inversely associated with complications.

The authors noted that their findings of poor outcome or death in 16% of thrombectomy patients exceeded the results of the ISCVT, which had a 13% death or dependence rate. However, patients in this study more commonly presented in a stuporous/comatose state (47%) than those of the ISCVT (19%). They also observed an 11% rate of postprocedure hemorrhage in patients who received concurrent intrasinus thrombolysis, compared to 7% in those who did not, although this difference was not statistically significant. Despite low levels of evidence for source data and the absence of a comparison group, this study suggests that mechanical thrombectomy is relatively safe with unclear efficacy for CVST.

18.6 Recommendations

Although anticoagulation is the core treatment strategy for CVST in both adults and children, acute phase mortality is nearly 5%, and approximately 10% of patients may die in the long term. Rapidly deteriorating patients refractory to anticoagulation may benefit from endovascular therapy. Local thrombolytic therapy with urokinase or tPA has been shown to achieve higher rates of recanalization than systemic thrombolytic therapy, and is relatively safe for these patients despite an increased risk of hemorrhage.[17] Mechanical thrombectomy has been shown to effectively recanalize thrombosed venous sinuses.[18] Patients with impending herniation before treatment may present too late for effective endovascular therapy,[18,34] but still may benefit from decompressive craniectomy.[19] The Thrombolysis or Anticoagulation for Cerebral Venous Thrombosis (TO-ACT) RCT, which compared endovascular thrombolysis (with or without mechanical thrombectomy) to heparin, sought to elucidate the optimal role of endovascular therapy for CVST (ClinicalTrials.gov *NCT01204333*).[35] However, this trial was ended early for futility in 2017, as endovascular therapy did not improve the clinical outcome for patients with severe CVST. Future publications describing the results of this trial in detail may provide more insight into the clinical role of endovascular therapy in CVST patients.

18.7 Summary

1. The safety and efficacy of various CVST treatments is described by multiple landmark papers, including systematic reviews of endovascular therapies.
2. While anticoagulation remains the primary initial and long-term therapy for CVST, severe cases of CVST may benefit from endovascular treatments or decompressive hemicraniectomy.
3. Local thrombolysis and mechanical thrombectomy have been shown to be relatively safe for CVST, but their efficacy is unclear. Preliminary data from the TO-ACT trial failed to demonstrate an improvement in clinical outcome for severe CVST patients getting endovascular therapy. Future reports may nonetheless better define the role for endovascular therapy in these patients.

References

[1] Saposnik G, Barinagarrementeria F, Brown RD, Jr, et al. American Heart Association Stroke Council and the Council on Epidemiology and Prevention. Diagnosis and management of cerebral venous thrombosis: a statement for healthcare professionals from the American Heart Association/American Stroke Association. Stroke. 2011; 42(4):1158–1192

[2] de Bruijn SF, Stam J. Randomized, placebo-controlled trial of anticoagulant treatment with low-molecular-weight heparin for cerebral sinus thrombosis. Stroke. 1999; 30(3):484–488

[3] Einhäupl KM, Villringer A, Meister W, et al. Heparin treatment in sinus venous thrombosis. Lancet. 1991; 338(8767):597–600

[4] Stam J, De Bruijn SF, DeVeber G. Anticoagulation for cerebral sinus thrombosis. Cochrane Database Syst Rev. 2002(4):CD002005

[5] de Bruijn SF, Budde M, Teunisse S, de Haan RJ, Stam J. Long-term outcome of cognition and functional health after cerebral venous sinus thrombosis. Neurology. 2000; 54(8):1687–1689

[6] Ferro JM, Canhão P, Stam J, Bousser MG, Barinagarrementeria F, ISCVT Investigators. Prognosis of cerebral vein and dural sinus thrombosis: results of the International Study on Cerebral Vein and Dural Sinus Thrombosis (ISCVT). Stroke. 2004; 35(3):664–670

[7] Girot M, Ferro JM, Canhão P, et al. ISCVT Investigators. Predictors of outcome in patients with cerebral venous thrombosis and intracerebral hemorrhage. Stroke. 2007; 38(2):337–342

[8] Ferro JM, Correia M, Pontes C, Baptista MV, Pita F, Cerebral Venous Thrombosis Portuguese Collaborative Study Group (Venoport). Cerebral vein and dural sinus thrombosis in Portugal: 1980–1998. Cerebrovasc Dis. 2001; 11(3):177–182

18

[9] Daif A, Awada A, al-Rajeh S, et al. Cerebral venous thrombosis in adults: a study of 40 cases from Saudi Arabia. Stroke. 1995; 26(7):1193–1195

[10] Preter M, Tzourio C, Ameri A, Bousser MG. Long-term prognosis in cerebral venous thrombosis: follow-up of 77 patients. Stroke. 1996; 27(2):243–246

[11] Maqueda VM, Thijs V. Risk of thromboembolism after cerebral venous thrombosis. Eur J Neurol. 2006; 13(3):302–305

[12] Breteau G, Mounier-Vehier F, Godefroy O, et al. Cerebral venous thrombosis 3-year clinical outcome in 55 consecutive patients. J Neurol. 2003; 250 (1):29–35

[13] Cakmak S, Derex L, Berruyer M, et al. Cerebral venous thrombosis: clinical outcome and systematic screening of prothrombotic factors. Neurology. 2003; 60(7):1175–1178

[14] Stolz E, Rahimi A, Gerriets T, Kraus J, Kaps M. Cerebral venous thrombosis: an all or nothing disease? Prognostic factors and long-term outcome. Clin Neurol Neurosurg. 2005; 107(2):99–107

[15] Brucker AB, Vollert-Rogenhofer H, Wagner M, et al. Heparin treatment in acute cerebral sinus venous thrombosis: a retrospective clinical and MR analysis of 42 cases. Cerebrovasc Dis. 1998; 8(6):331–337

[16] Coutinho JM, Ferro JM, Canhão P, Barinagarrementeria F, Bousser MG, Stam J, ISCVT Investigators. Unfractionated or low-molecular weight heparin for the treatment of cerebral venous thrombosis. Stroke. 2010; 41(11):2575–2580

[17] Canhão P, Falcão F, Ferro JM. Thrombolytics for cerebral sinus thrombosis: a systematic review. Cerebrovasc Dis. 2003; 15(3):159–166

[18] Siddiqui FM, Dandapat S, Banerjee C, et al. Mechanical thrombectomy in cerebral venous thrombosis: systematic review of 185 cases. Stroke. 2015; 46 (5):1263–1268

[19] Ferro JM, Crassard I, Coutinho JM, et al. Second International Study on Cerebral Vein and Dural Sinus Thrombosis (ISCVT 2) Investigators. Decompressive surgery in cerebrovenous thrombosis: a multicenter registry and a systematic review of individual patient data. Stroke. 2011; 42(10):2825–2831

[20] Coutinho JM, Ferro JM, Canhão P, et al. Cerebral venous and sinus thrombosis in women. Stroke. 2009; 40(7):2356–2361

[21] Stam J. Thrombosis of the cerebral veins and sinuses. N Engl J Med. 2005; 352 (17):1791–1798

[22] Ferro JM, Canhão P, Bousser MG, Stam J, Barinagarrementeria F, ISCVT Investigators. Early seizures in cerebral vein and dural sinus thrombosis: risk factors and role of antiepileptics. Stroke. 2008; 39(4):1152–1158

[23] Kothare SV, Ebb DH, Rosenberger PB, Buonanno F, Schaefer PW, Krishnamoorthy KS. Acute confusion and mutism as a presentation of thalamic strokes secondary to deep cerebral venous thrombosis. J Child Neurol. 1998; 13(6):300–303

[24] Marjot T, Yadav S, Hasan N, Bentley P, Sharma P. Genes associated with adult cerebral venous thrombosis. Stroke. 2011; 42(4):913–918

[25] Leach JL, Fortuna RB, Jones BV, Gaskill-Shipley MF. Imaging of cerebral venous thrombosis: current techniques, spectrum of findings, and diagnostic pitfalls. Radiographics. 2006; 26 Suppl 1:S19–S41, discussion S42–S43

[26] Rizzo L, Crasto SG, Rudà R, et al. Cerebral venous thrombosis: role of CT, MRI and MRA in the emergency setting. Radiol Med (Torino). 2010; 115(2):313–325

[27] Linn J, Ertl-Wagner B, Seelos KC, et al. Diagnostic value of multidetector-row CT angiography in the evaluation of thrombosis of the cerebral venous sinuses. AJNR Am J Neuroradiol. 2007; 28(5):946–952

[28] Borhani Haghighi A, Edgell RC, Cruz-Flores S, et al. Mortality of cerebral venous-sinus thrombosis in a large national sample. Stroke. 2012; 43(1):262–264

[29] Biousse V, Ameri A, Bousser MG. Isolated intracranial hypertension as the only sign of cerebral venous thrombosis. Neurology. 1999; 53(7):1537–1542

[30] Roach ES, Golomb MR, Adams R, et al. American Heart Association Stroke Council, Council on Cardiovascular Disease in the Young. Management of stroke in infants and children: a scientific statement from a Special Writing Group of the American Heart Association Stroke Council and the Council on Cardiovascular Disease in the Young. Stroke. 2008; 39(9):2644–2691

[31] Agostoni E. Headache in cerebral venous thrombosis. Neurol Sci. 2004; 25 Suppl 3:S206–S210

[32] Bousser MG, Chiras J, Bories J, Castaigne P. Cerebral venous thrombosis: a review of 38 cases. Stroke. 1985; 16(2):199–213

[33] Gurley MB, King TS, Tsai FY. Sigmoid sinus thrombosis associated with internal jugular venous occlusion: direct thrombolytic treatment. J Endovasc Surg. 1996; 3(3):306–314

[34] Stam J, Majoie CB, van Delden OM, van Lienden KP, Reekers JA. Endovascular thrombectomy and thrombolysis for severe cerebral sinus thrombosis: a prospective study. Stroke. 2008; 39(5):1487–1490

[35] Coutinho JM, Ferro JM, Zuurbier SM, et al. Thrombolysis or anticoagulation for cerebral venous thrombosis: rationale and design of the TO-ACT trial. Int J Stroke. 2013; 8(2):135–140

18

Section III

Neurointerventional Oncology

III

19 Meningioma Embolization

Joshua S. Catapano, Rami O. Almefty, Nader Sanai, Felipe Albuquerque, and Andrew F. Ducruet

Abstract

Preoperative embolization of meningiomas remains controversial and is often dependent on surgeon preference. Endovascular techniques have advanced significantly over the past several decades, making embolization of meningiomas safer and more effective. However, the medical literature regarding the safety and efficacy of preoperative embolization of meningiomas is scarce. It is therefore imperative to examine the landmark papers in the field to acquire a thorough understanding of the subject and to form an evidence-based opinion to facilitate decision-making on the use of embolization in the treatment of meningiomas.

Keywords: embolization, meningiomas, neurointerventional procedures, Onyx, tumor

19.1 Goals

1. Review the medical literature on preoperative embolization of meningiomas.
2. Critically analyze the medical literature on the preoperative embolization of meningiomas.
3. Provide recommendations for preoperative embolization of meningiomas.

19.2 Case Example

19.2.1 History of Present Illness

A 46-year-old woman presented to the emergency room with a new onset of a generalized tonic-clonic seizure and was found on magnetic resonance imaging (MRI) to have a right frontal operculum extra-axial mass consistent with a large meningioma with extensive surrounding edema and brain compression (▶ Fig. 19.1a–e). She denied any other neurological complaints, including loss of consciousness, numbness, weakness, and speech/vision difficulty.
   Medical history: Denied a history of cancer or any other pertinent history.
   Surgical history: Previous tonsillectomy.
   Family history: Denied a history of previous central nervous system tumors.
   Social history: Denied tobacco, alcohol, and illicit drug use.
   Review of systems: As per the above.
   Neurological examination: Unremarkable.
   Imaging studies: See ▶ Fig. 19.1 and ▶ Fig. 19.2.

19.2.2 Treatment Plan

The patient consented to a preoperative embolization followed by surgical resection the next morning. A distal branch of the right middle meningeal artery (MMA) was the primary vascular supply to the lesion (▶ Fig. 19.1d, e). Successful transcatheter, transarterial embolization with Onyx (Medtronic plc) within the right MMA was performed, without any evidence of residual tumor vascularity or nontarget embolization (▶ Fig. 19.2a, b). The patient experienced no complications after embolization and subsequently underwent a right-sided craniotomy for complete resection of the tumor (▶ Fig. 19.2c, d).

19.2.3 Follow-up

The patient initially woke from surgery with word-finding difficulties, which resolved on postoperative day 1. The patient was discharged home on postoperative day 2 without neurological deficits and was doing well on follow-up.

19.3 Case Summary

1. *What factors would you consider when deciding on preoperative embolization of meningiomas?*
   Preoperative embolization of meningiomas may facilitate surgical resection.[1,2,3,4] Several studies have described reduced blood loss, shorter length of operative time, and a greater capability of achieving gross total resections of skull base and large meningiomas.[1,2,3,4,5,6] However, preoperative embolization of such lesions does pose the risk of severe complications, including stroke and hemorrhage.[1,7] The risks and benefits of preoperative embolization must be carefully weighed. Preoperative embolization has been beneficial in patients with anterior skull base and large supratentorial lesions.[1,8,9] In these patients, preoperative embolization causes central softening and necrosis, which creates a plane between the adjacent brain and tumor, making removal simpler and safer for adjacent vital structures.[1,8,9] Furthermore, highly vascular giant convexity tumors with a complex blood supply may benefit the most from preoperative embolization because of a decrease in vascularity and a reduction of intraoperative blood loss.[1] The majority of skull base meningiomas are supplied by branches from the external carotid artery (ECA), which allows for safer catheterization and embolization with a low risk of neurological morbidity. However, careful attention is necessary to avoid common extracranial-intracranial anastomoses and ECA branches with distal cranial nerve supply.[10,11] Cases where the internal carotid artery supplies the majority of the vascular supply of a meningioma are generally poor cases for preoperative embolization, as the majority of the supply generally arises either from the ophthalmic or ethmoidal vessels, which are largely accessible early in surgery, or from the meningohypophyseal trunk, which can be challenging to catheterize safely.[10] Preoperative embolization is thought to be valuable in rare complex meningiomas that are associated with a vascular lesion or aneurysm, where the vascular lesion or aneurysm can be dealt with before surgery, making resection safer.[1,12,13,14] Another example where preoperative embolization is useful is in orbital lesions, where embolization theoretically reduces intraoperative blood loss, which improves visualization and allows for safer resection.[1,7]

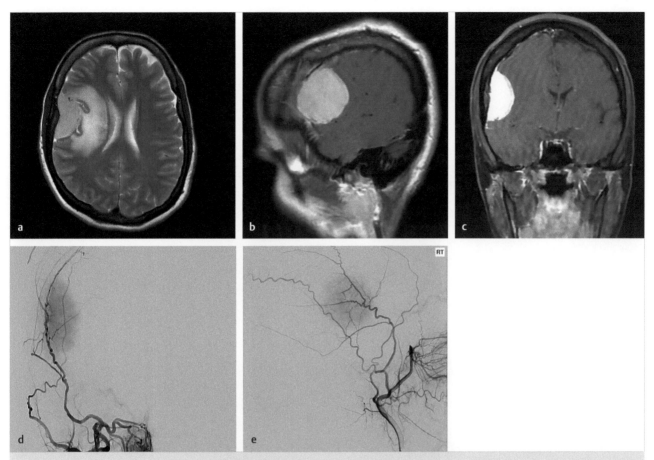

Fig. 19.1 (a) Axial T2 magnetic resonance imaging (MRI) showing an avidly enhancing, T2 isointense extra-axial mass overlying the right frontal operculum, with a dural tail. The mass has imaging characteristics of a large meningioma, measuring 4.2 × 4.3 × 2.3 cm (anteroposterior × craniocaudal × transverse). There is a large arterial feeder overlying the superior, anterior, and inferior aspects of the meningioma. **(b)** Sagittal T1 MRI with contrast. **(c)** Coronal T1 MRI with contrast. **(d)** Pre-embolization right external carotid angiogram (RECA) injection, posteroanterior view, showing highly vascular tumor with main supply from the right middle meningeal artery. **(e)** Pre-embolization lateral view of RECA injection. (Used with permission from Barrow Neurological Institute, Phoenix, Arizona.)

2. *What technical considerations were important for embolization of this patient's lesion?*

In the case described, the meningioma was a large, highly vascular, operculum lesion, with a blood supply from the MMA of the ECA. Because of the size and vascularity of the lesion, preoperative embolization was deemed beneficial to reduce intraoperative blood loss and create a necrotic core, thus facilitating a safer gross total resection. Although catheterization and embolization of the MMA is technically feasible and carries a low risk of neurological morbidity, careful attention was paid to avoiding occlusion of the petrosal branch of the MMA, which supplies the facial nerve.[11] Embolization was performed with ethylene vinyl alcohol copolymer Onyx, which is a liquid agent that is dissolved in dimethyl sulfoxide to create a low precipitation in the blood at the site of injection, allowing for deep intratumoral vessel penetration.[6,15,16] Hence, Onyx is thought to aid in devascularization of larger lesions, as in the case described. Furthermore, Onyx is less adhesive than other liquid embolizing agents such as n-butyl cyanoacrylate (NBCA), reduces the risk of microcatheter entrapment or fracture, and allows for longer injections with more control angiograms.[16,17]

19.4 Level of Evidence

Given the patient's lesion location, size, and vascular pedicle, preoperative embolization of the tumor was deemed beneficial (Class III, Level of Evidence C).

19.5 Landmark Papers

Manelfe C, Guiraud B, David J, et al. Embolization by catheterization of intracranial meningiomas [In French]. Rev Neurol (Paris) 1973;128:339–351.

In 1973, Manelfe et al[18] first reported the use of preoperative embolization by catheterization of intracranial meningiomas. The authors reported a series of five meningiomas treated via embolization with fragments of Spongel (Magic srl). This series included three convexity and two skull base lesions embolized, each with primary feeders from the ECA. Four of the patients were subsequently operated on within 3 to 13 days. One patient did not undergo resection because the tumor was deemed highly malignant; however, that patient was described as making enough progress to resume daily activities 6 months postembolization. The authors described a practically bloodless

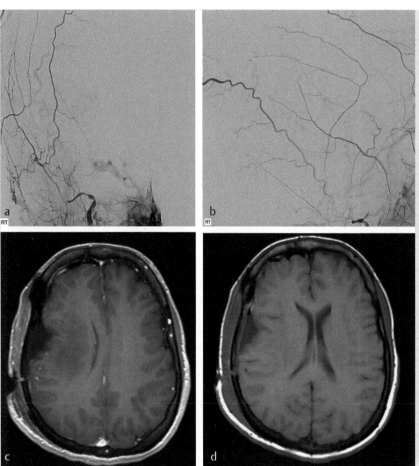

Fig. 19.2 **(a)** Postembolization Towne's view of right external carotid angiogram (RECA) injection showing complete occlusion of tumor vessels with 100% devascularization of the lesion. **(b)** Postembolization lateral view of RECA injection showing complete devascularization of the lesion. **(c)** Axial T1 (with contrast) magnetic resonance image (MRI) after complete resection of the tumor. **(d)** Axial T1 (without contrast) MRI after complete resection of the tumor. (Used with permission from Barrow Neurological Institute, Phoenix, Arizona.)

operation, which greatly facilitated the resection of the lesions, in the four patients with resection. In pathological specimens, each lesion was confirmed to have been embolized, with fragments of Spongel visible in intratumoral capillaries. The authors concluded that percutaneous catheter embolization is beneficial for large meningiomas, particularly lesions located in the skull base with feeders from the ECA because this practice greatly decreased the risk of operative hemorrhage.

Oka H, Kurata A, Kawano N, et al. Preoperative superselective embolization of skull-base meningiomas: indications and limitations. J Neurooncol 1998;40:67–71.

In 1998, Oka et al[4] retrospectively analyzed all skull base meningiomas in Kitasato University Hospital in Japan from 1980 to the early 1990s. Of the 324 patients, 20 patients fit their selection criteria of a skull base meningioma with ECA feeders, tumor size > 4 cm, patients without coagulopathy or anemia, and total or subtotal tumor resection. Twelve patients underwent preoperative embolization, and eight patients did not. In all patients treated with embolization, a superselective catheterization was performed and polyvinyl alcohol was used as the embosylate.

The authors found a statistically significantly lower volume of blood transfusion needed during resection in patients with 4- to 6-cm tumors treated with preoperative embolization. For tumors > 6 cm, fewer units of blood were transfused to the embolized patients than to the nonembolized patients (11.5 vs.

14 units); however, this difference was not statistically significant. The authors also did not find a difference in operative time between the embolized and the nonembolized patients.

As mentioned by the authors, all nonembolized patients were treated from 1980 to 1989, and embolized patients were treated from 1980 to the early 1990s. Hence, minor improvements in surgical techniques for the later cases present a limitation to this study. Another major limitation was the small sample size.

Rosen CL, Ammerman JM, Sekhar LN, Bank WO. Outcome analysis of preoperative embolization in cranial base surgery. Acta Neurochir (Wien) 2002;144:1157–1164.

In 2002, Rosen et al[5] reported the largest retrospective review in the medical literature on preoperative embolization of meningiomas. However, their study specifically analyzed only skull base meningiomas. A total of 167 patients with skull base meningiomas who had undergone a preoperative angiogram or embolization were analyzed. Twenty patients (12%) did not undergo embolization because of the lack of a suitable feeding artery. A total of 36 patients (21.6%) were reported to experience a neurological complication. These complications ranged from minor neurological deficits (e.g., temporary paresthesias) in 21 patients to severe neurological deficits (e.g., cranial nerve deficit, hemorrhage, and retinal artery thrombosis) in 15 patients. Another five patients experienced non-neurological complications, including groin hematomas, puncture site infection, and arrhythmias.

The most common vessel embolized was the MMA (60% of patients), followed by the meningohypophyseal trunk (41% of patients). In their study, the authors did not identify a specific vessel that carried a significantly greater risk of complication when embolized.

The authors compared skull base meningiomas that were preoperatively embolized to 157 other meningiomas that were not embolized before resection. The authors strongly favored embolization of skull base lesions. As a result, most of the lesions in the comparison cohort were convexity and falcine tumors, which introduced a significant selection bias into the analysis. Although tumor diameter was greater in the embolized patients than in the nonembolized patients (3.6 vs. 2.9 cm), there was no statistically significant difference in operative time, tumor consistency, gross total resection, or the need for intraoperative transfusion. Furthermore, the length of stay (19 vs. 12 days) and ICU days (5.1 vs. 1.8 days) were longer for the preoperatively embolized patients. The authors hypothesized that these findings were likely due to tumor locations and not due to whether the tumors were embolized. The authors concluded that the indiscriminate use of embolization is not warranted, that institutions must have policies for emergency surgery after embolization if necessary, and that close monitoring of patients after embolization is essential.

Kai Y, Hamada JI, Morioka M, et al. Clinical evaluation of cellulose porous beads for the therapeutic embolization of meningiomas. AJNR Am J Neuroradiol 2006;27:1146–1150.

In 2006, Kai et al[8] described the use of porous cellulose beads for embolization of 128 patients with meningiomas. They performed a retrospective cohort study of 203 patients with meningiomas. They selected 141 patients with tumors that were > 4 cm in diameter and that had at least 50% of their blood supply from the ECA. These patients presented with a great variety of lesion locations, including the sphenoid ridge, frontal base, convexity, cavernous sinus, cerebellopontine angle, middle fossa, parasagittal, petroclival, and occipital. The authors found that 50 of the 141 patients had lesions with blood supplied entirely from the ECA. Thirteen patients did not undergo embolization because of either a positive provocation test or vasospasm during angiography. Of the remaining 128 patients, the authors reported complete devascularization of the tumor in 29 patients (23%), significant devascularization in 63 patients (49%), and partial devascularization in 36 patients (28%). On postembolization MRI, 125 patients were found to have nonenhancing portions within the tumor. Importantly, the degree of nonenhancement was not correlated with the percentage of devascularization on the angiogram.

The authors compared two groups. Group 1 had resection before 1996, with surgery occurring 1 to 7 days after embolization. Group 2 had resection after 1996, with surgery that was delayed from 8 to 26 days after embolization. The delayed group was found to have a greater percentage of tumors that were deemed soft during surgery (17% vs. 6.7%) and a significantly lower Simpson Grade after resection (1.91 vs. 2.6). The authors concluded that delayed resection (>7 days) after embolization provided the greatest tumor softening, which facilitated a safer and simpler resection. These conclusions are limited by the fact that tumors with improved Simpson grades were also resected more recently, leading to potential bias of improved surgeon skills resulting from greater surgical experience.

Quiñones-Hinojosa A, Kaprealian T, Chaichana KL, et al. Preoperative factors affecting resectability of giant intracranial meningiomas. Can J Neurol Sci 2009;36:623–630.

In 2009, Quiñones-Hinojosa et al[6] performed a retrospective analysis at the University of California San Francisco on 67 patients who underwent resection for a large intracranial meningioma (> 5 cm) between 1998 and 2004. The authors set out to establish preoperative factors that affected the resectability of giant intracranial meningiomas. Thirty-nine patients (58%) were found to have a gross total resection. Preoperative embolization was found to be positively correlated with gross total resection in all large meningiomas that were studied (odds ratio: 8.1). A separate analysis examining only supratentorial meningiomas found similar results, with preoperative embolization predicting gross total resection (odds ratio: 10.5). These findings support other previous studies that suggest safer gross total resection in patients with meningiomas after embolization.

Shah AH, Patel N, Raper DM, et al. The role of preoperative embolization for intracranial meningiomas. J Neurosurg 2013;119:364–372.

Shah et al[1] reviewed the role of preoperative embolization for intracranial meningiomas. In their review, they analyzed a total of 36 studies over an 18-year period that included a total of 459 patients. They reported a complication rate of 4.6%, although most complications were transient. Nonetheless, two deaths were observed, and one patient sustained a permanent complication after embolization. Given the limited quality of the evidence, they were unable to provide specific guidelines for the use of preoperative embolization of meningiomas. However, they did suggest that giant convexity tumors with complex blood supplies may benefit the most from preoperative embolization. Furthermore, they found that preoperative embolization was practically essential in lesions with associated vascular lesions and aneurysms. In addition, they noted that preoperative embolization may be of value in anterior skull base lesions with most of their vascular supply from ECA feeders. Although some medical literature has shown that delayed resection after embolization provides a softer core and facilitates resection, Shah et al and others have found that delayed resection may cause severe edema with elevated intracranial pressures that necessitate emergency surgical resection.[1,19]

19.6 Recommendations

Significant controversy remains regarding the utility of preoperative embolization of intracranial meningiomas. The medical literature on the topic is scarce, and there have been no randomized control trials, making either argument onerous. Some investigators of case series have suggested that preoperative embolization is associated with decreased surgical blood loss, decreased operative time, improved neurological outcomes, and softening of the tumor, thus facilitating a safer gross total resection.[1,2,3,4,6,20,21] However, it remains uncertain whether these potential benefits outweigh the risks of embolization. Nonetheless, with the advent of more sophisticated and safer instruments for neurointerventionalists over the past decade, preoperative embolization of lesions has become more frequent.

As previously stated, a 4.6% complication rate from preoperative embolization has been reported in a large review.[1] The same review suggested that preoperative embolization for cranial meningiomas may be of most benefit for giant lesions with complex vascularity.[1] However, no formal recommendations were made because of the poor level of evidence.

There remains no consensus on the appropriate embolysate for the embolization of these lesions. Currently, either particles or liquid embolic agents are frequently used. Particle embolization is typically accomplished via polyvinyl alcohol and trisacryl gelatin microspheres. The mechanism of action of such particles is the occlusion of the vessel after slow injection into the target vessel.[16] In addition, these particles mediate an inflammatory reaction, leading to fibrosis of the vessel.[16] When larger feeding vessels are encountered, coil embolization may be of value for greater devascularization after embolization via particles.[10] When the distal vasculature is difficult to catheterize, particle embolization may be used for occlusion of the vessel. Another potential benefit of these embosylates is that the size of the particles (300–500 μm) is larger than the vasa nervosum vessels, making them safer for distal branches supplying cranial nerves.[16]

The primary liquid embosylate agents used are Onyx and NBCA. As mentioned earlier, Onyx possesses several advantages, including deeper intratumoral penetration and more controlled embolization.[6,15,16,17] However, because of its low precipitation in blood, Onyx has the potential to occlude off-target vessels and cause severe neurological deficits. Unlike Onyx, which is dissolved in dimethyl sulfoxide for low precipitation in blood, NBCA is a free-flowing monomer that polymerizes upon contact with blood.[22] However, NBCA does not need a high infusion pressure, which possibly reduces the risk of postembolization hemorrhage.[23] This reduced risk of postembolization hemorrhage must be weighed against a major shortcoming of NBCA, which is its adhesive nature. The adhesive nature of NBCA requires the microcatheter to be retracted after injection and necessitates a rapid and potentially less controlled embolization.[16]

As mentioned previously, ECA feeders are often catheterized more safely, with a low risk of neurological complication. However, ECA branches such as the petrosal branch of the MMA provide much of the blood supply to the facial nerve and extracranial-intracranial anastomoses with other critical vessels such as the stylomastoid branch of the posterior auricular artery may lead to severe neurological deficits if exceptional caution is not exercised during embolization.[10] In addition, internal carotid artery contributions are typically poor indications for embolization, as the majority of feeders are from either the ophthalmic or ethmoidal vessels, and there is a risk of blindness after embolization.[10]

Future research in preoperative embolization of intracranial meningiomas is of great importance. No guidelines for embolization have been made, and the risk-to-benefit profile remains elusive. Although a randomized control trial would potentially provide the requisite information needed, it is highly unlikely that such a trial would be conducted given the heterogeneity of tumors and surgeon preferences. The creation of larger prospective databases with high-quality longitudinal outcome data is necessary. Future studies should focus on the clinical benefit of preoperative embolization of meningiomas and whether they outweigh the inherent risk.

19.7 Summary

1. The risks and benefits of preoperative embolization of meningiomas are largely undecided. The available medical literature has too low level of evidence for recommending meaningful guidelines.
2. Although specific guidelines for preoperative embolization cannot be made, giant lesions with complex vascularity, anterior skull base lesions, and tumors associated with vascular lesions and aneurysms are likely to benefit from embolization.
3. Currently, there is no consensus regarding the best embolysate for the embolization of meningiomas. Onyx may provide greater devascularization of larger tumors, with a risk profile that is comparable to that of other agents.

References

[1] Shah AH, Patel N, Raper DM, et al. The role of preoperative embolization for intracranial meningiomas. J Neurosurg. 2013; 119(2):364–372
[2] Chun JY, McDermott MW, Lamborn KR, Wilson CB, Higashida R, Berger MS. Delayed surgical resection reduces intraoperative blood loss for embolized meningiomas. Neurosurgery. 2002; 50(6):1231–1235, discussion 1235–1237
[3] Dean BL, Flom RA, Wallace RC, et al. Efficacy of endovascular treatment of meningiomas: evaluation with matched samples. AJNR Am J Neuroradiol. 1994; 15(9):1675–1680
[4] Oka H, Kurata A, Kawano N, et al. Preoperative superselective embolization of skull-base meningiomas: indications and limitations. J Neurooncol. 1998; 40(1):67–71
[5] Rosen CL, Ammerman JM, Sekhar LN, Bank WO. Outcome analysis of preoperative embolization in cranial base surgery. Acta Neurochir (Wien). 2002; 144(11):1157–1164
[6] Quiñones-Hinojosa A, Kaprealian T, Chaichana KL, et al. Pre-operative factors affecting resectability of giant intracranial meningiomas. Can J Neurol Sci. 2009; 36(5):623–630
[7] Boulos PT, Dumont AS, Mandell JW, Jane JA, Sr. Meningiomas of the orbit: contemporary considerations. Neurosurg Focus. 2001; 10(5):E5
[8] Kai Y, Hamada JI, Morioka M, et al. Clinical evaluation of cellulose porous beads for the therapeutic embolization of meningiomas. AJNR Am J Neuroradiol. 2006; 27(5):1146–1150
[9] Manelfe C, Lasjaunias P, Ruscalleda J. Preoperative embolization of intracranial meningiomas. AJNR Am J Neuroradiol. 1986; 7(5):963–972
[10] Waldron JS, Sughrue ME, Hetts SW, et al. Embolization of skull base meningiomas and feeding vessels arising from the internal carotid circulation. Neurosurgery. 2011; 68(1):162–169, discussion 169
[11] Geibprasert S, Pongpech S, Armstrong D, Krings T. Dangerous extracranial-intracranial anastomoses and supply to the cranial nerves: vessels the neurointerventionalist needs to know. AJNR Am J Neuroradiol. 2009; 30(8):1459–1468
[12] Javadpour M, Khan AD, Jenkinson MD, Foy PM, Nahser HC. Cerebral aneurysm associated with an intracranial tumour: staged endovascular and surgical treatment in two cases. Br J Neurosurg. 2004; 18(3):280–284
[13] Maekawa H, Tanaka M, Hadeishi H. Middle meningeal artery aneurysm associated with meningioma. Acta Neurochir (Wien). 2009; 151(9):1167–1168
[14] O'Neill OR, Barnwell SL, Silver DJ. Middle meningeal artery aneurysm associated with meningioma: case report. Neurosurgery. 1995; 36(2):396–398
[15] Trivelatto F, Nakiri GS, Manisor M, et al. Preoperative onyx embolization of meningiomas fed by the ophthalmic artery: a case series. AJNR Am J Neuroradiol. 2011; 32(9):1762–1766
[16] Vaidya S, Tozer KR, Chen J. An overview of embolic agents. Semin Intervent Radiol. 2008; 25(3):204–215
[17] Crowley RW, Ducruet AF, McDougall CG, Albuquerque FC. Endovascular advances for brain arteriovenous malformations. Neurosurgery. 2014; 74 Suppl 1:S74–S82
[18] Manelfe C, Guiraud B, David J, et al. Embolization by catheterization of intracranial meningiomas [In French]. Rev Neurol (Paris). 1973; 128:339–351
[19] Przybylowski CJ, Baranoski JF, See AP, et al. Preoperative embolization of skull base meningiomas: outcomes in the Onyx Era. World Neurosurg. 2018; 116:e371–e379

[20] Bendszus M, Rao G, Burger R, et al. Is there a benefit of preoperative meningioma embolization? Neurosurgery. 2000; 47(6):1306–1311, discussion 1311–1312

[21] Raper DM, Starke RM, Henderson F, Jr, et al. Preoperative embolization of intracranial meningiomas: efficacy, technical considerations, and complications. AJNR Am J Neuroradiol. 2014; 35(9):1798–1804

[22] Pollak JS, White RI, Jr. The use of cyanoacrylate adhesives in peripheral embolization. J Vasc Interv Radiol. 2001; 12(8):907–913

[23] Kominami S, Watanabe A, Suzuki M, Mizunari T, Kobayashi S, Teramoto A. Preoperative embolization of meningiomas with N-butyl cyanoacrylate. Interv Neuroradiol. 2012; 18(2):133–139

20 Paraganglioma Embolization

Justin Schwarz, Ibrahim Hussain, Alejandro Santillan, David Kutler, and Jared Knopman

Abstract

Head-and-neck paragangliomas are a relatively rare disease entity, but one that is encountered occasionally in clinical practice, particularly in tertiary care centers. Due to their highly vascular nature, location, and natural history, these tumors are most aptly treated with a multidisciplinary approach involving neurointerventionalists, head-and-neck surgeons, vascular neurosurgeons, and vascular surgeons. The decision to proceed with preoperative embolization of these tumors is controversial, with many conflicting studies supporting surgical resection with or without preoperative embolization. Due to their relatively rare incidence, it has been difficult to study the role of preoperative embolization with rigor, but a close analysis of the available literature is important for the appropriate neurointerventional management of these tumors.

Keywords: carotid body tumor, paraganglioma, embolization

20.1 Goals

1. Review and understand the literature that describes the symptomatology and natural history of head-and-neck paragangliomas, specifically carotid body tumors (CBTs).
2. Review the classification scheme of CBTs and how it applies to the treatment decision for these tumors.
3. Critically analyze the literature that evaluates the utility of preoperative embolization of these tumors.

20.2 Case Example

20.2.1 History of Present Illness

A 47-year-old female presents for a painless and progressively enlarging swelling of the right side of her neck. An ultrasound ordered by her general internist revealed an approximately 5-cm mass situated at the right carotid bifurcation. The patient initially noticed this swelling 16 months ago, but it has noticeably enlarged since that time, albeit slowly. She also complains of hoarseness of her voice that started approximately 1 year ago. She denies any difficulty swallowing, or other significant neurologic complaints.

Past medical history: Chronic headaches, basal cell carcinoma, asthma.

Past surgical history: Excision of a basal cell carcinoma of the right face, open reduction and internal fixation of a left humerus fracture.

Family history: Denies any familial history of cancer or masses.

Social history: Two to three glasses of red wine per week, no smoking or other illicit substance use.

Review of systems: As per the above.

Examination: There is a firm, nontender, and pulsatile mass of the right neck at the anterior border of the right sternocleidomastoid, mobile in the medial-lateral direction but immobile in the rostral-caudal dimension (Fontaine sign). Firm

compression of the mass leads to a slight decrease in its size, with re-expansion on release of pressure in a series of pulsations (sign of Recluse and Chevassu).[1] Her voice is slightly hoarse, but otherwise her physical and neurologic examination is unremarkable.

Imaging studies: See figures.

Carotid Doppler: A 5-cm heterogeneously hypoechoic circumscribed mass in the right neck, lateral to the right submandibular gland, with the medial aspect of the mass inseparable from the adjacent carotid vasculature and carotid bifurcation, which remains widely patent.

Computed tomography (CT) neck with contrast in ▶ Fig. 20.1 shows an avidly enhancing mass in the right carotid space that splays the proximal right internal and external carotid arteries. It is intimately associated with the carotid bulb, measuring 5.0 × 4.2 × 4.0 cm, most consistent with a carotid body tumor. The tumor partially encases both the right external and internal carotid arteries, consistent with a Shamblin 2 carotid body tumor.

Diagnostic cerebral angiogram in ▶ Fig. 20.2a, b demonstrates a hypervascular lesion at the right carotid bifurcation that splays the internal and external carotid arteries apart. The tumor receives vascular supply primarily from robust branches from the ascending pharyngeal artery, the superior thyroid artery, and occipital artery. There is no significant tumor blush identified from selective injections of the right internal carotid artery. There was no vessel wall abnormality to suggest significant invasion of the internal or external carotid arteries. The patient had a widely patent anterior communicating artery with brisk collateralization from left common carotid artery injections.

▶ Fig. 20.2c, d: Diagnostic cerebral angiogram postselective catheterization and embolization. The ascending pharyngeal, superior thyroid, and occipital arteries were selectively catheterized and embolized with a combination of polyvinyl alcohol (PVA) particles and Onyx, with overall a 95% reduction in tumor blush.

20.2.2 Treatment Plan

The patient agreed to definitive treatment of her right-sided CBT, which included preoperative embolization followed by surgical resection with an interdisciplinary team including an experienced neurointerventionalist, vascular neurosurgeon, and otorhinolaryngologist.

20.2.3 Follow-up

The patient did very well after definitive treatment of her right CBT, including preoperative embolization followed by surgical resection by an interdisciplinary team involving a neurointerventionalist, vascular neurosurgeon, and otorhinolaryngologist. Total operative time for surgical resection was 189 minutes with an estimated blood loss of 100 mL. The patient was discharged home on postoperative day 2, with 1 additional day of hospital stay preceding surgical resection

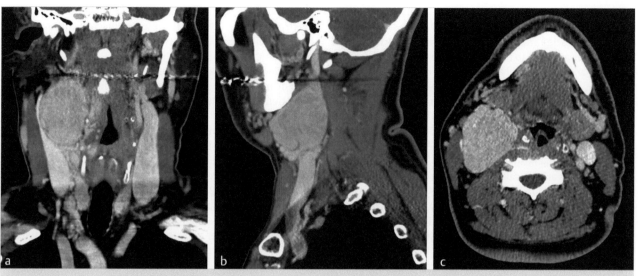

Fig. 20.1 Computed tomography (CT) neck with contrast showing a right-sided Shamblin 2 carotid body tumor in the (a) coronal, (b) sagittal, and (c) axial planes.

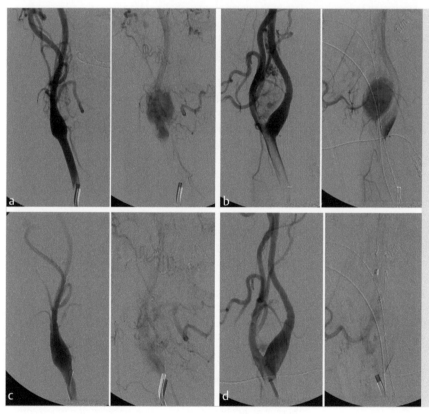

Fig. 20.2 Angiogram of right-sided carotid body tumor in the (a) anteroposterior, and (b) lateral projections prior to embolization. Postembolization angiogram of the same carotid body tumor in the (c) anteroposterior and (d) lateral projections.

for her embolization. The patient remained at her neurologic baseline following surgery, with slight hoarseness. At her 6-month follow-up appointment, she had persistent mild hoarseness of voice, but otherwise had no complaints.

20.3 Case Summary

1. *What are the general characteristics, symptomatology, and natural history of carotid body paragangliomas?*
Paragangliomas are highly vascular, slow growing, and relatively rare tumors of neural crest cell origin with an incidence of approximately 1:30,000.[2,3] CBTs are the most common paraganglioma of the head and neck and account for roughly 70% of head-and-neck paragangliomas.[3] They originate from the carotid body, as their namesake implies, and they are generally nonsecretory, although 10% can be.[4] Historically they have been called by many names including chemodectoma, glomus caroticum, in addition to carotid body paraganglioma. They derive their blood supply from branches of the external carotid artery, with the most common arterial supply coming from branches of the ascending pharyngeal artery.[5]

A majority of CBTs are diagnosed due to an insidious neck swelling, typically at the anterior border of the sternocleido-mastoid muscle.[6] The mass tends to be firm and painless and can be pulsatile due to their high degree of vascularity. These tumors are usually highly mobile in the medial-lateral direction but resist manipulation in the rostral-caudal dimension due to the tumor's attachment to the carotid body and carotid bifurcation (Fontaine's sign).[1] CBTs also may be found due to progressive cranial nerve dysfunction, including hoarse voice or difficulty swallowing.[7,8] A minority of these masses are found incidentally.

These lesions are typically slow growing and their symptomatology is explained by direct compression of nearby neurovascular structures, with an average rate of growth of 0.5 cm per year.[9] While mostly benign, there is a small but definite risk of malignancy that is approximately 2 to 5%.[10,11,12] The treatment modality of choice for these lesions is surgical resection with or without preoperative embolization, given their predictable growth and small, but definite, risk of malignancy.

2. *What patient factors would you consider when deciding on your recommendation for treatment versus observation?*

As with all candidates for surgery, the age and medical comorbidities of the patient need to be carefully considered in the context of the patient's symptoms. A young, relatively healthy patient should have definitive treatment of their paraganglioma regardless of symptomatology as the natural history dictates that the tumor will invariably enlarge and eventually become symptomatic.[7,8,9,10,11,12] However, an elderly patient with multiple medical comorbidities and an asymptomatic or mildly symptomatic CBT may be better served by either close observation or radiation therapy, as opposed to undergoing a relatively higher risk surgery.

3. *What tumor factors would you consider when deciding on your recommendations for observation or treatment of carotid body paragangliomas?*

Classification of carotid body paragangliomas based on operative risk was first proposed by Shamblin in 1970 based on retrospective review of 90 patients who underwent CBT resection.[5] He identified three groups in his classification scheme, with group 1 including CBTs that were not associated with the carotid vessels and were easily dissected from the vessel adventitia. Group 2 includes those tumors that partially encase the carotid vessels, while group 3 includes tumors that completely encase the carotid artery. Group 1 tumors are the easiest to surgically resect, while the group 3 tumors are much more difficult, sometimes requiring external carotid artery sacrifice or internal carotid artery repair.

The Shamblin grade alone does not inform a decision regarding the need for surgical resection as these lesions should be surgically resected if the patient is medically able to tolerate surgery. It does, however, inform the surgeon of the potential difficulty of surgical resection and potential benefit of adjuvant treatments, such as preoperative embolization. Group 2 and 3 patients' tumors are more difficult to dissect and resect due to their proximity to and involvement of the carotid vasculature, making vessel injury requiring repair or bypass more likely. This potentially could increase intraoperative blood loss,

operative time, and potential for ischemic events or strokes.[13,14,15] Given that these tumors will continue to grow without definitive treatment, these tumors should be resected despite their Shamblin classification. However, the Shamblin classification does provide important information for the physician in managing the patient's expectations and informing them about the potential risks of the surgical resection. It also provides information regarding the utility of preoperative angiography, including balloon-test occlusion and preoperative tumor embolization.

4. *What preoperative imaging should be performed for adequate work-up of a CBT?*

Appropriate preoperative imaging is essential for proper diagnosis and treatment planning for CBTs. All patients should have either a CT neck with contrast or an MRI with contrast, and a preoperative angiogram. The preoperative angiogram helps elucidate the vascular anatomy of the tumor, which may aid in appropriate diagnosis (differentiating between a schwannoma vs. a paraganglioma) and also gives information that is useful for surgical resection, regardless of the decision to embolize.[14] It allows the surgeon to have a working map of important vascular feeders and helps identify possible tumor invasion of the carotid vasculature, thereby alerting the surgeon to the possibility of having to perform a vessel sacrifice, repair, or bypass during resection. In addition, the angiogram provides critical information about the intracranial circulation, such as whether there is a patent anterior or posterior communicating artery with adequate collateral flow. These details are essential to know if there is a possibility of temporary or permanent occlusion of the internal carotid artery during surgery. In patients where carotid injury, repair, or bypass may be unavoidable, the patient should undergo provocative testing at the time of angiogram to determine whether the patient would be able to tolerate vessel sacrifice or temporary occlusion without ischemic consequences.

5. *When is preoperative embolization appropriate?*

Surgical resection is the definitive treatment of carotid body paragangliomas. Given their highly vascular nature, preoperative embolization can provide a significant benefit by decreasing operative time and blood loss and making surgical resection of the tumor easier and safer, especially for Shamblin 2 and 3 tumors.[12,13,15,16,17,18,19,20,21,22,23] However, the exact role of preoperative embolization in CBTs remains controversial owing to several contradicting case series. The relative rarity of these tumors makes them difficult to study in a more rigorous way. Several groups have proposed that there is no benefit of preoperative embolization when compared to surgical resection alone without embolization.[24,25,26,27,28]

When analyzing the series that shows no difference, the number of patients included is small and the complication rate from embolization is higher than expected for the majority of these cases. Many of these studies have cited the stroke rate associated with embolization to be as high as 10%, an unacceptably high rate for an appropriately trained interventionalist, especially with the safe technology now available for embolization.[12,19,26] Not surprisingly, studies citing such a high rate of stroke from embolization were published more than 15 years ago. Most of the studies showing no benefit from preoperative embolization are not stratified based on Shamblin classification of these tumors. Shamblin group 1 tumors are typically small and can be easily dissected off the carotid vasculature, so preoperative embolization should not affect overall operative time, estimated blood loss, or neurologic outcomes. Shamblin group 2 and 3 tumors are larger, more complex, and more intimately related with the carotid vasculature, allowing for greater potential for benefit from preoperative embolization.

Transarterial embolization is the standard method for tumor embolization, consisting of superselective catheterization and embolization using a combination of PVA particles, N-butyl cyanoacrylate (NBCA) glue, and Onyx. As with all head-and-neck tumor embolization, it is imperative to understand potential external to internal carotid artery anastomoses to ensure that embolization is performed safely. The proximity of tumor supplying arterial branches to the internal carotid artery is also important, as reflux of embolic material can lead to ischemic events. Percutaneous embolization using Onyx has more recently been described and has been shown to be effective in significantly reducing tumor blush.[29,30] However, some interventionalists remain wary of percutaneous embolization with tumors intimately related to the internal carotid artery, as reflux could result in embolic stroke.

6. *What treatment would you recommend for this patient's CBT?*
The patient was recommended preoperative embolization followed by surgical resection of her paraganglioma. The patient is young and healthy with a symptomatic Shamblin 2 right CBT paraganglioma. The natural history of the tumor dictates that it will continue to enlarge, albeit slowly. The patient already has developed hoarseness, but is otherwise asymptomatic. As the tumor continues to grow the patient's hoarseness will undoubtedly worsen and she will likely develop additional symptoms from local compression of vital structures in the region of the carotid body. As the tumor continues to enlarge, it may eventually fully encase the external and internal carotid arteries (Shamblin group 3), which has been shown to carry a significantly higher operative risk than Shamblin grade 1 and 2 tumors. The Shamblin grade 3 tumors have more morbidity associated with resection, including a greater risk of cranial nerve injury, vessel injury, and stroke.[31] All of these factors favor early surgical resection for this patient.

A CT or MRI neck with contrast is necessary to characterize the location of the tumor and delineate its anatomic relation with other important neurovascular structures. Catheter angiogram is an exceptionally useful modality to characterize the vascularity of the tumor, delineate the vascular supply to the tumor for intraoperative planning, and to ensure the appropriate preoperative diagnosis. The angiogram also allows for better characterization of the intracranial circulation, including the presence of patent anterior or posterior communicating arteries. It can also identify invasion of the external or internal carotid arteries and allow for further provocative testing, such as balloon-test occlusion, in case vessel sacrifice or temporary occlusion is needed intraoperatively. Lastly, preoperative embolization of Shamblin group 2 and 3 CBTs has been shown to decrease operative time and estimated blood loss, and allows for less burdensome tumor resection.

A multidisciplinary team, including a head-and-neck surgeon, vascular surgeon or vascular neurosurgeon, and experienced neurointerventionalist, is recommended when treating paragangliomas. This patient underwent preoperative CT neck with contrast indicating a highly vascular tumor partially encasing the internal and external carotid arteries, consistent with a Shamblin group 2 CBT. A preoperative angiogram was performed which redemonstrated the tumor's size and hypervascularity with multiple direct arterial feeders arising from the right superior thyroid artery, right occipital, and right ascending pharyngeal arteries. Each of these feeding arteries was successfully selectively catheterized and embolized utilizing a combination of PVA particles and Onyx to reduce tumor blush by 95% (▶ Fig. 20.1 and ▶ Fig. 20.2).

20.4 Level of Evidence

Preoperative embolization: There is a significant reduction on operative time and estimated blood loss that is consistently seen with preoperative embolization in Shamblin 2 and 3 group tumors, when embolization is performed by a qualified neuro-interventionalist (Class 2A, Level of Evidence B). There is not a consistent significant reduction in rate of cranial nerve injury with paragangliomas treated with resection alone versus embolization followed by resection.

20.5 Landmark Papers

Shamblin WR, ReMine WH, Sheps SG, Harrison EG. Carotid body tumor (chemodectoma): clinicopathologic analysis of ninety cases. Am J Surg 1971;122:732–739.

This represents the first, and still most widely used, classification system for CBTs to this date. Shamblin et al retrospectively analyzed the experience with CBT resection at the Mayo Clinic from 1931 to 1967. This study identified 58 patients who underwent partial or complete resections of pathology-confirmed CBTs. Through careful study of gross pathology and operative reports, the authors were able to propose a classification scheme composed of three different groups that was related to the relationship of the tumor to the carotid vessels. Group 1 was comprised of relatively small tumors that were easily dissected from the carotid vessels whereas Group 2 tumors partially surrounded the carotid vessels and were more difficult to dissect away due to vessel adherence. Group 3 was comprised of tumors that had circumferential growth around carotid bifurcation and could only be resected by entering the vessel lumen, requiring a patch or graft. This study established a framework with which surgeons could stratify patients in terms of extent of surgical resection required (including vessel replacement or bypass) and has been important as a basis for comparison, particularly for studies evaluating the utility of preoperative embolization.

Shick PM, Hieshima AB, White RA. Arterial catheter embolization followed by surgery for large chemodectoma. Surgery 1980;87:459–464.

This paper describes the first successful preoperative transarterial embolization of a CBT in 1980.[32] The tumor was Shamblin group 3 and large, measuring 10 × 12 cm, and had a 2-week staged course of preoperative embolization with an overall reduction of 90% tumor blush on angiography following embolization. The authors supported the routine use of preoperative transarterial embolization in treatment of large CBTs, and recommended consideration for preoperative embolization with smaller tumors as well.

Power AH, Bower TC, Kasperbauer J, et al. Impact of preoperative embolization on outcomes of carotid body tumor resections. J Vasc Surg 2012;56:979–989.

This retrospective study analyzed all surgically resected CBTs at Mayo Clinic from January 1985 to December 2010, including 144 resected tumors. The authors compared patients who underwent preoperative embolization followed by surgical resection to surgical resection alone, particularly comparing both groups based on the tumor's Shamblin group. For Shamblin 2 and 3 tumors, the authors concluded that the embolized group required significantly less extensive resection (simple excision in 97% vs. 82%, $p = 0.03$) and had less blood loss (EBL 263 vs. 599 mL, $p = 0.02$). There was no significant difference in operative time, but importantly there was no difference in intraoperative events or stroke between the embolized and non-embolized groups. While most other studies on CBTs lack the power to find significance, this study had enough patients to make comparisons between Shamblin groups for preoperative embolization. In total, 21 of 71 Shamblin 2 tumors and 8 of 33 Shamblin 3 tumors underwent embolization. The quality of preoperative embolization was also very high with an average devascularization of 76% without postembolization strokes, transient ischemic attacks, or access-site hematomas. Other studies that have found no advantage with preoperative embolization did not achieve an adequate tumor embolization and have a complication rate that is unacceptably high.

Li J, Wang S, Zee C, et al. Preoperative angiography and transarterial embolization in the management of carotid body tumor: a single-center, 10-year experience. Neurosurgery 2010;67:941–948.

The authors retrospectively identified 66 CBTs that were surgically removed between 1997 and 2007 and compared the CBTs that were preoperatively embolized (33 patients) to those that were treated with surgery alone (29 patients). The authors concluded that estimated blood loss (354 vs. 656 mL, $p = 0.008$), operative time (170 vs. 225 min, $p = 0.034$), and mean hospital stay (8.0 vs. 9.5 days, $p = 0.042$) was significantly lower in the embolized group. The authors achieved high-quality embolization with complete tumor vascularization in 76% of patients with no strokes, demonstrating the benefit and safety of preoperative tumor embolization when performed by qualified physicians.

20.6 Recommendations

Head-and-neck paragangliomas are slow growing tumors with a small, but definite, risk of malignancy that should be treated definitively with surgical resection. Adjunctive embolization is a somewhat controversial topic in the management of these tumors. There is evidence to support the use of preoperative embolization of CBTs, with embolization resulting in a significant reduction in overall operative time and estimated blood loss in patients with Shamblin group 2 and 3 tumors. Many experts also argue that the preoperative embolization allows for a more bloodless and simpler resection, but this has not resulted in a significant decrease in overall postoperative cranial

nerve deficits. Preoperative embolization of Shamblin group 1 tumors does not appear to confer the same benefit as with Shamblin group 2 and 3 tumors.

One of the criticisms of preoperative embolization of CBTs has been an unacceptably high rate of stroke described in earlier studies, which has been quoted as high as 5 to 10%.[12,19,26] Given advancements in technology, more recent studies show the incidence of stroke with CBT embolization to be considerably lower, especially in the hands of qualified and experienced neurointerventionalists.[15,16,17,18,19,20,21,22,23] Treatment of head-and-neck paragangliomas requires a multidisciplinary team including qualified neurointerventionalists, head-and-neck surgeons, and vascular surgeons or neurosurgeons. Ultimately, the decision to perform preoperative embolization is left to the best judgment of the treating physicians, but it has been shown to confer a significant benefit in Shamblin group 2 and 3 tumors by decreasing estimated blood loss and operative time, while anecdotally allowing for greater ease of resection.[15,16,17,18,19,20,21,22,23]

Regardless of the decision to embolization preoperatively, these head-and-neck tumors should have a diagnostic catheter angiogram preoperatively to ensure proper diagnosis and to characterize the arterial supply of the tumor to aid with surgical planning. Angiography can also identify vessel wall invasion by tumor, allowing for accurate characterization of the intracranial circulation and provocative testing (balloon-test occlusion) to better assess the risk of ischemia if the internal carotid artery requires temporary clamping, repair, bypass, or sacrifice.

20.7 Summary

1. Head-and-neck paragangliomas should be definitively treated with surgical resection with or without embolization. These tumors continually enlarge causing worsening symptoms due to direct compression of neurovascular structures and have a small, but definite, risk of malignancy. Those patients who cannot undergo surgical resection due to severe medical comorbidities can be managed expectantly or treated with radiation therapy.

2. Preoperative embolization remains somewhat controversial for treatment of head-and-neck paragangliomas, and specifically CBTs. There is evidence to suggest that it is effective in reducing blood loss and operative time in patients with Shamblin group 2 and 3 tumors, and anecdotal evidence that allows for easier surgical resection.

3. Head-and-neck paragangliomas should be treated by an interdisciplinary team including head-and-neck surgeons, vascular surgeons or vascular neurosurgeons, and adequately trained neurointerventionalists.

References

[1] Monro RS. The natural history of carotid body tumours and their diagnosis and treatment; with a report of five cases. Br J Surg. 1950; 37(148):445–453

[2] Sajid MS, Hamilton G, Baker DM, Joint Vascular Research Group. A multicenter review of carotid body tumour management. Eur J Vasc Endovasc Surg. 2007; 34(2):127–130

[3] Pellitteri PK, Rinaldo A, Myssiorek D, et al. Paragangliomas of the head and neck. Oral Oncol. 2004; 40(6):563–575

[4] Kruger AJ, Walker PJ, Foster WJ, Jenkins JS, Boyne NS, Jenkins J. Important observations made managing carotid body tumors during a 25-year experience. J Vasc Surg. 2010; 52(6):1518–1523

[5] Shamblin WR, ReMine WH, Sheps SG, Harrison EG, Jr. Carotid body tumor (chemodectoma). Clinicopathologic analysis of ninety cases. Am J Surg. 1971; 122(6):732–739

[6] Martinelli O, Irace L, Massa R, et al. Carotid body tumors: radioguided surgical approach. J Exp Clin Cancer Res. 2009; 28:148

[7] Bernard RP. Carotid body tumors. Am J Surg. 1992; 163(5):494–496

[8] Boedeker CC, Ridder GJ, Schipper J. Paragangliomas of the head and neck: diagnosis and treatment. Fam Cancer. 2005; 4(1):55–59

[9] Abu-Ghanem S, Yehuda M, Carmel NN, Abergel A, Fliss DM. Impact of preoperative embolization on the outcomes of carotid body tumor surgery: a meta-analysis and review of the literature. Head Neck. 2016; 38 Suppl 1:E2386–E2394

[10] Hallett JW, Jr, Nora JD, Hollier LH, Cherry KJ, Jr, Pairolero PC. Trends in neurovascular complications of surgical management for carotid body and cervical paragangliomas: a fifty-year experience with 153 tumors. J Vasc Surg. 1988; 7(2):284–291

[11] Nora JD, Hallett JW, Jr, O'Brien PC, Naessens JM, Cherry KJ, Jr, Pairolero PC. Surgical resection of carotid body tumors: long-term survival, recurrence, and metastasis. Mayo Clin Proc. 1988; 63(4):348–352

[12] Persky MS, Setton A, Niimi Y, Hartman J, Frank D, Berenstein A. Combined endovascular and surgical treatment of head and neck paragangliomas: a team approach. Head Neck. 2002; 24(5):423–431

[13] Power AH, Bower TC, Kasperbauer J, et al. Impact of preoperative embolization on outcomes of carotid body tumor resections. J Vasc Surg. 2012; 56 (4):979–989

[14] Li J, Wang S, Zee C, et al. Preoperative angiography and transarterial embolization in the management of carotid body tumor: a single-center, 10-year experience. Neurosurgery. 2010; 67(4):941–948, discussion 948

[15] Economopoulos KP, Tzani A, Reifsnyder T. Adjunct endovascular interventions in carotid body tumors. J Vasc Surg. 2015; 61(4):1081–91.e2

[16] Vogel TR, Mousa AY, Dombrovskiy VY, Haser PB, Graham AM. Carotid body tumor surgery: management and outcomes in the nation. Vasc Endovascular Surg. 2009; 43(5):457–461

[17] Ward PH, Liu C, Vinuela F, Bentson JR. Embolization: an adjunctive measure for removal of carotid body tumors. Laryngoscope. 1988; 98(12):1287–1291

[18] Muhm M, Polterauer P, Gstöttner W, et al. Diagnostic and therapeutic approaches to carotid body tumors: review of 24 patients. Arch Surg. 1997; 132(3):279–284

[19] Kafie FE, Freischlag JA. Carotid body tumors: the role of preoperative embolization. Ann Vasc Surg. 2001; 15(2):237–242

[20] Liapis CD, Evangelidakis EL, Papavassiliou VG, et al. Role of malignancy and preoperative embolization in the management of carotid body tumors. World J Surg. 2000; 24(12):1526–1530

[21] Wang SJ, Wang MB, Barauskas TM, Calcaterra TC. Surgical management of carotid body tumors. Otolaryngol Head Neck Surg. 2000; 123(3):202–206

[22] Kalani MYS, Ducruet AF, Crowley RW, Spetzler RF, McDougall CG, Albuquerque FC. Transfemoral transarterial onyx embolization of carotid body paragangliomas: technical considerations, results, and strategies for complication avoidance. Neurosurgery. 2013; 72(1):9–15, discussion 15

[23] Duffis EJ, Gandhi CD, Prestigiacomo CJ, et al. Society for Neurointerventional Surgery. Head, neck, and brain tumor embolization guidelines. J Neurointerv Surg. 2012; 4(4):251–255

[24] Ozay B, Kurc E, Orhan G, et al. Surgery of carotid body tumour: 14 cases in 7 years. Acta Chir Belg. 2008; 108(1):107–111

[25] Litle VR, Reilly LM, Ramos TK. Preoperative embolization of carotid body tumors: when is it appropriate? Ann Vasc Surg. 1996; 10(5):464–468

[26] Zeitler DM, Glick J, Har-El G. Preoperative embolization in carotid body tumor surgery: is it required? Ann Otol Rhinol Laryngol. 2010; 119(5): 279–283

[27] Bercin S, Muderris T, Sevil E, Gul F, Kılıcarslan A, Kiris M. Efficiency of preoperative embolization of carotid body tumor. Auris Nasus Larynx. 2015; 42(3): 226–230

[28] Cobb AN, Barkat A, Daungjaiboon W, et al. Carotid body tumor resection: just as safe without preoperative embolization. Ann Vasc Surg. 2018; 46: 54–59

[29] Elhammady MS, Peterson EC, Johnson JN, Aziz-Sultan MA. Preoperative onyx embolization of vascular head and neck tumors by direct puncture. World Neurosurg. 2012; 77(5–6):725–730

[30] Wanke I, Jäckel MC, Goericke S, Panagiotopoulos V, Dietrich U, Forsting M. Percutaneous embolization of carotid paragangliomas using solely Onyx. AJNR Am J Neuroradiol. 2009; 30(8):1594–1597

[31] Pacheco-Ojeda LA. Carotid body tumors: surgical experience in 215 cases. J Craniomaxillofac Surg. 2017; 45(9):1472–1477

[32] Shick PM, Hieshima AB, White RA. Arterial catheter embolization followed by surgery for large chemodectoma. Surgery. 1980;87:459–464

21 Retinoblastoma

Elias Atallah and Pascal Jabbour

Abstract

Intra-arterial delivery of chemotherapy for retinoblastoma is a safe, feasible, and efficacious adjuvant route for this disease process. Although cannulation of the ophthalmic artery can be challenging, especially in very young children, the local delivery of chemotherapy allows for minimization of systemic side effects in this vulnerable population. In this chapter, we summarize the advances in local delivery of chemotherapy using endovascular techniques for this disease.

Keywords: retinoblastoma, intra-arterial, chemotherapy

21.1 Goals

1. Review the indications for the use of intra-arterial chemotherapy (IAC) for retinoblastoma.
2. Summarize the literature on the use of intra-arterial delivery of chemotherapy for retinoblastoma.

21.2 Case Example

21.2.1 History

A 9-month-old boy was found to have a white right eye on photographs and diagnosed with a unilateral retinoblastoma of the right orbit on ocular ultrasound and magnetic resonance imaging (MRI) scans. After an initial evaluation by an ophthalmologist and a pediatric oncology team, it was found that the tumor was not a candidate for more conservative methods of control (i.e., cryotherapy, thermotherapy, or plaque radiotherapy). The family elected to defer enucleation as an initial treatment.

Past medical history: Noncontributory.
Past surgical history: Noncontributory.
Family history: No history of retinoblastoma or other cancers within the family.
Social history: Noncontributory.
Examination: Well-developed, well-nourished child in no acute distress. Unremarkable neurological examination. Ocular examination demonstrates a large macular retinoblastoma (▶ Fig. 21.1).

21.2.2 Clinical Course

After a thorough discussion with the multidisciplinary team and the patient's family, the plan was made to proceed with IAC with melphalan (▶ Fig. 21.2). Follow-up ophthalmological examinations after the first treatment demonstrated complete regression of the retinoblastoma (▶ Fig. 21.3).

21.3 Case Summary

1. *What are the genetic mutations involved with retinoblastoma development?*
   a) Retinoblastoma development has been associated with mutations in the *RB1* tumor suppressor gene. In hereditary retinoblastomas, patients will frequently have bilateral retinoblastomas developed. Approximately one-third of all retinoblastoma patients will have the hereditary form which is passed along in an autosomal-dominant pattern. There is often a family history of retinoblastomas.
   b) In this specific case example, there was no history of retinoblastomas in the family and the patient presented with unilateral disease.
2. *What treatment options are available for retinoblastoma patients?*
   a) There are multiple treatment options for retinoblastoma depending on the presentation. Focal therapies include cryotherapy or laser therapy for smaller isolated tumors or recurrent tumors. Enucleation can be used for more aggressive cases. Chemotherapy can be administered locally via intravitreous injections or via IAC. Systemic chemotherapy in conjunction with focal therapies can also be employed depending on the extent of involvement.
3. *What are the routes of delivery of IAC for retinoblastomas?*
   a) The most direct route for delivery of IAC involves the ophthalmic artery (▶ Fig. 21.2). While this is the preferred vessel, there are several other variations to the arterial

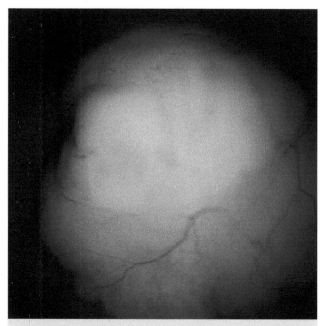

Fig. 21.1 Large macular retinoblastoma of the right orbit.

21

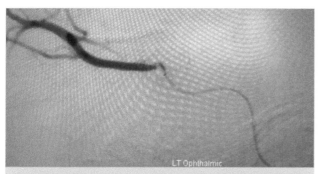

Fig. 21.2 Superselective injection of the right ophthalmic artery with the microcatheter engaged in the ophthalmic artery.

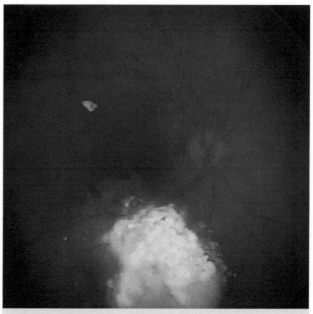

Fig. 21.3 Complete response after one dose of intra-arterial chemotherapy.

supply to the eye. In addition, vasospasm, vessel tortuosity, or small size may preclude successful canalization of the ophthalmic artery. In approximately 3 to 5% of cases, the ophthalmic artery arises from the middle meningeal artery. IAC can be delivered via catheterization through the middle meningeal artery.

b) The Japanese technique of temporary distal occlusion of the internal carotid artery with infusion of diluted drug into the internal carotid artery can be used in cases with difficult direct catheterization of the ophthalmic artery.

4. *What chemotherapeutic agents are available for IAC?*

a) Melphalan is an alkylating agent that is a nitrogen mustard derivative. The typical dose is 5 mg (< 0.5 mg/kg) with a range from 3 to 7.5 mg.

b) Topotecan is a semisynthetic camptothecin derivative and a topoisomerase 1 inhibitor with a dose range of 1 to 2 mg for IAC (standard dose 1 mg).

c) Carboplatin is a platinum-based derivative and is routinely used in multiagent intravenous protocols. Recommended doses are 15 to 30 mg.

21.4 Recommendations

21.4.1 Endovascular Technique

Currently, this treatment is employed for retinoblastoma patients as primary treatment for unilateral or bilateral retinoblastoma, and as secondary treatment following failure from other treatments. Under general anesthesia, the site of cannulation in the femoral artery is prepped in a sterile fashion avoiding the use of cotton material in order to prevent foreign body microembolization.

A pediatric arterial sheath is placed at the femoral artery. Anticoagulation with heparin is utilized with activated clotting time (ACT), being 2 to 2.5 times the normal at all times. No guidewire is used in this procedure. Selectively, the internal carotid artery is catheterized with a greatly flexible Marathon Flow Directed MicroCatheter (Medtronic, Minneapolis, Minnesota, ev3, Covidien, USA). An internal carotid artery injection is then performed to visualize the cerebral vasculature and to select the best approach showing the takeoff of the ophthalmic artery from the internal carotid artery. Then, the same microcatheter is guided all the way toward the origin of the ophthalmic artery. The ophthalmic artery is the first intracranial branch of the internal carotid artery. Using fluoroscopic guid-

ance, the ostium of the ophthalmic artery of the affected eye is subsequently superselectively catheterized. Due to the angle of origin of the ophthalmic artery, this turn of the catheter tip is technically challenging and requires proficiency and expertise.[1] Once the microcatheter is in stable position at the ostium of the ophthalmic artery, a superselective injection is formed to confirm the catheter positioning, to make sure that there is no reflux of contrast in the carotid artery and, if there is, to gauge the pressure of injection to avoid such a reflux.

Once the catheter positioning is confirmed, chemotherapy is delivered. The drugs are diluted in 30 mL of normal saline and are injected very slowly over 30 minutes at the rate 1 mL/min. The chemotherapy injection is pulsatile to avoid drug streaming (varying drug concentration due to laminar flow in arteries) and to deliver drug homogeneously. After the injection of each chemotherapeutic agent, an angiogram of the globe and brain is performed to rule out an embolic or hemorrhagic complication. The contrast is flushed with saline, and the microcatheter is then slowly withdrawn from the ophthalmic artery, the guide is removed, protamine is administered to reverse the heparin effect, and hemostasis is achieved at the femoral puncture site with 30 minutes of manual compression. The entire procedure (including time of injection of chemotherapy) takes 1 to 5 hours depending on the vascular anatomy of the patient. The child has to be on complete bed rest for 6 hours with a temporary cast in the leg to avoid bleeding from the femoral site. Oral aspirin is usually given in the dose of 1 to 3 mg/kg for 2 weeks to prevent vascular thrombosis, and topical atropine is given for 1 week.

Alternative catheterization technique in the event of failure to selectively catheterize ophthalmic artery includes[2]:

• Utilization of a 4 French (F-1.3-mm diameter) pediatric arterial sheath. Catheterization of the internal carotid artery with 4 French Berenstein II pediatric guide (Cordis Neurovascular, Miami Lakes, Florida). Then, the ophthalmic artery is superselectively catheterized with a microcatheter (Prowler 10) (Cordis Neurovascular, Miami Lakes, Florida) and a microwire (Synchro 10) (Boston Scientific, Natick, Massachusetts).

- Catheterization of the ipsilateral middle meningeal artery, in 3 to 5% of the patients, the ophthalmic artery arises from the middle meningeal artery instead of the internal carotid artery.[3]
- Utilization of the Japanese technique which involves placement of a temporary balloon to occlude the internal carotid artery prior to delivery of chemotherapy. With this technique, the chemotherapy is infused much more rapidly because of the limitation of occlusion of the internal carotid artery. This technique likely results in more widespread delivery of the chemotherapy.

For bilateral cases, both eyes have been treated in the same session. After infusing chemotherapy in one eye, the catheter is retracted to the aorta and then advanced to the contralateral internal carotid artery and ophthalmic artery. Caution is advised to dose the chemotherapy to avoid cumulative toxicity.[4] Munier and coworkers cautioned against the use of this technique of bilateral IAC as there is risk of causing sight threatening vaso-occlusive complications, potentially in both eyes.[5]

21.4.2 Medications

The pharmacological advantage of IAC is the first pass of the drug through the tumor circulation prior to reaching systemic circulation. Certain characteristics of medications that are advantageous for intra-arterial administration are high extraction fraction within target organ, high capillary permeability, and rapid systemic metabolism.[1] The drug dosage is determined by the ocular size and not by the body weight.[6]

- Melphalan is a nitrogen mustard alkylating agent. In experimental studies, retinoblastoma cell lines were very sensitive to this drug, but it was not used systematically due to severe adverse effect profile.[7] In the IAC technique, the systemic absorption is minimal, and melphalan has become the primary chemotherapeutic agent. Melphalan is ideally suited for this technique because of its short half-life of 1.5 hours.[2]
- Topotecan belongs to the group of topoisomerases I inhibitor. Topotecan has shown effective activity against retinoblastoma in mouse models[8] and has been used systematically for metastatic retinoblastoma with other chemotherapeutic agents.[9]
- Carboplatin is an alkylating agent, is the primary drug of choice for systemic chemotherapy, and is also used as a periocular chemotherapeutic agent.
- Methotrexate is an antimetabolite and has been used for the treatment of systemic retinoblastoma and pinealoblastoma.
- Digoxin belongs to the class of cardenolides and has been in use for many years to treat congestive heart failure. Antczak and associates studied the effect of cardenolide ouabain in a xenograft model of retinoblastoma. In their experimental model, they found complete regression of the tumor in 14 days with no evidence of toxicity even at high doses.[10] Based on the preclinical study, Patel and coworkers reported the use of systemic and intra-arterial digoxin, but documented measurable, although incomplete, tumor regression with intra-arterial digoxin. They suggested further clinical trials to evaluate the dosage and utility of digoxin in the management of retinoblastoma.[11]

21.4.3 Advantages

The intra-arterial technique allows selective delivery of chemotherapy to the eye with minimal systemic absorption. Approximately 11% of patients develop transient neutropenia that does not require transfusion.[2][6] Severe drug toxic effects have not been witnessed with the intra-arterial injection. As toxicity and infection rates are low, there is little need for hospitalization. In our experience, systemic chemotherapy (chemoreduction) was remarkably effective for retinoblastoma but carried the potential risk for serious systemic side effects like secondary leukemia, nephrotoxicity, and ototoxicity. In our experience with more than 300 children treated with chemoreduction for retinoblastoma, only 1 developed leukemia[12] and none developed nephrotoxicity.[7] In an analysis of 248 children with retinoblastoma treated with systemic chemotherapy, 5.6% had abnormal audiograms prior to treatment, but no new auditory impairment was noted after chemotherapy.[13] The lack of toxicities in our cases is likely due to strict use of only six cycles of chemotherapy with careful dosing and monitoring.

With the localized delivery of chemotherapy, these long-term complications could be minimized. However, there are ocular toxicities that are encountered after IAC therapy that were never seen with systemic chemotherapy (chemoreduction), and these include ophthalmic artery stenosis, retinal vascular obstruction, and retinal and choroidal ischemia which are elaborated later in this chapter.[5]

The dose delivered to the eye is 10 times that achieved with systemic chemotherapy. This high dose of chemotherapy delivered to the eye accelerates regression of tumor and seeds. The long-term outcome of these patients and recurrence rates after IAC are still not completely understood.

IAC is an effective treatment for recurrences occurring after systemic chemotherapy. Melphalan is not routinely used in systemic chemotherapy and is the primary agent used in intra-arterial therapy and hence development of resistance is unlikely (▶ Fig. 21.1).

21.4.4 Limitations

There are many considerations when deciding on IAC. The chemotherapy infusion has to be repeated every 3 to 4 weeks for up to three to six injections for complete regression of the tumor. There is concern that in the pediatric population with repeated vascular interventions, the complication rate would be higher.

The cannulation of ophthalmic artery is difficult in children particularly in infants less than 6 months and requires surgical expertise and precision. Anomalous ophthalmic artery origin is seen in 5% of the patients, and, in these instances, it is not possible to cannulate the ophthalmic artery and the procedure has to be abandoned. Gobin et al reported 98.5% successful catheterization in their report of 289 chemotherapy infusions.[6] Structural brain anomalies can impose significant risk with the procedure and hence preoperative MRI is performed. The technique may not be accessible to all centers especially in developing countries as neuroendovascular skill is needed.

A benefit of IAC is the focal infusion of medication to a site of visible malignancy, but this can also be a limitation as the dose to potentially subclinical metastasis would be inadequate. Chemotherapy delivered in this technique is localized to the eye with little systemic effects and hence might not offer protective effects for high-risk retinoblastoma that carries potential for metastatic disease. In particularly advanced cases of retinoblastoma, such as International Classification of Retinoblastoma (ICRB) Group E, this lack of systemic chemotherapeutic benefit could be detrimental. Enucleation had been the treatment of choice for advanced retinoblastoma for many decades, and in the presence of histopathologic high-risk features, systemic intravenous chemotherapy was delivered. In a retrospective analysis of 297 eyes treated for retinoblastoma with enucleation, 18.5% has high-risk features requiring systemic chemotherapy.[14]

The inability to detect high-risk features with intra-arterial therapy has raised significant concerns among ocular oncologists and pediatric oncologists. Some reported three clinicopathologic descriptions after IAC for advanced retinoblastoma. In their case series, all three patients had viable tumor on pathologic examination and two of them had high-risk characteristics necessitating systemic chemotherapy. Eagle and coworkers evaluated the histopathological changes after IAC in eight enucleated eyes. They found viable vitreous seeds in four eyes, optic nerve invasion in three eyes with laminar invasion in one eye and choroidal invasion in one eye. The viable tumor noted on histopathology correlated with clinical suspicion of nonregression, and all patients who appeared clinically regressed had no viable tumor on histopathology.[14] Also, as the IAC has little systemic circulation, the protective effect against pinealoblastoma and second cancers is nonexistent.

21.4.5 Adverse Effects

Local Side Effects

The intra-arterial procedure requires catheterization of the femoral artery, and this has to be repeated with every session of chemotherapy. Gobin et al reported one patient who developed transient occlusion of the superficial femoral artery that recanalized after aspirin therapy,[6] and Peterson et al reported one episode of groin hematoma that was self-limiting.[2] There is a theoretical risk of limb ischemia, although it has not been reported to date. Cerebral angiography with IAC has been used for many years for brain tumors. In the pediatric and adult literature for brain tumors, the local complications include groin hematoma (2.6%), carotid arterial dissections (0.5%), and popliteal embolism (0.3%). Catheter-induced vessel spasm and dissection are most commonly encountered in the internal carotid artery and are reported in around 1% of cases based on literature for cerebral aneurysms. Other studies reported higher complication rate with larger catheter diameter, longer procedure time with exchange of catheter during the procedure.

Ocular Side Effects

Minor ocular side effects include periorbital edema, ciliary madarosis, cutaneous hyperemia, and mechanical ptosis, most of which are self-limited.[15] Vascular orbitopathy with extraocular dysmotility is frequently encountered, but it usually resolves in 2 to 3 months.[16] Vitreous hemorrhage has also been reported with intra-arterial injections, and in persistent cases enucleation is performed.[2] [16] The hemorrhage is probably related to the

fragile tumor vascularization with rapid necrosis but could also reflect a toxicity of melphalan.[13] Shields and coworkers in their series of 16 eyes treated with IAC, reported eyelid edema (81%), blepharoptosis (63%), and eyelash loss (75%).[16]

The more serious and vision-threatening complication involves insult to the ophthalmic, choroidal, and retinal artery vasculature. Ophthalmic artery obstruction manifests with pale optic nerve, reduced retinal blood flow, and patchy reduction in choroidal blood flow, which may resolve spontaneously in some cases.[16] Retinal vascular toxicity manifests as central artery or branch retinal artery occlusion, and usually is an early manifestation. Choroidal ischemia, in contrast, is a delayed process and manifests as subtle retinal pigment epithelium changes over many months following IAC.[16]

The group from Wills Eye Institute evaluated the fluorescein angiographic changes after IAC therapy in 24 eyes after 55 catheterizations. They found varying degrees of intraocular vascular alterations in 20% of eyes, including branch and central retinal artery obstruction, ophthalmic artery obstruction, and choroidal vascular obstruction. Importantly, some of these vascular manifestations were subclinical and would have been undetectable without fluorescein angiography.[17] This suggests that there could be subclinical ischemic changes in the eye. The pathogenesis of the vascular insult is either related to endothelial damage, chemotherapy toxicity, or embolic phenomenon due to foreign body reaction.

In a histopathologic study of eight eyes treated with IAC, Eagle and coworkers found evidence of ischemic atrophy in the outer retina and choroid in four eyes (50%). In five eyes, they found evidence of vascular thrombosis involving the orbital ciliary arteries, the scleral emissary vessels, small choroidal vessels, and the central retinal artery. Surprisingly, they found intravascular birefringent foreign material inciting a granulomatous reaction within some thrombosed vessels. The foreign material was considered and was postulated to be introduced at the time of the IAC procedure via the catheter or room air suspended pariculates.[10] Foreign body embolization have been reported with angiography of other organs, but the ensuing vascular thrombosis are probably functionally inconsequential in large solid organs. This sight threatening complication emphasizes the need to attempt intra-arterial injection only in one eye to avoid bilateral vision loss.

The toxicity to the retina could also be an effect of the chemotherapeutic agent. Brodie and coworkers evaluated nine patients with electroretinogram following intra-arterial therapy and reported persistence or recovering of retinal function suggesting tolerable drug toxicity.[18] The toxicity of IAC, when used for brain tumors, was higher when used after or concomitant with brain radiation therapy. This has not been clearly documented in the ophthalmic literature, probably due to low numbers but needs to be considered.

21.5 Landmark Papers

Gobin YP, Dunkel IJ, Marr BP, Brodie SE, Abramson DH. Intra-arterial chemotherapy for the management of retinoblastoma: four-year experience. Arch Ophthalmol 2011;129(6):732–737.

Abramson DH, Dunkel IJ, Brodie SE, Marr B, Gobin YP. Bilateral superselective ophthalmic artery chemotherapy for bilateral reti-

21

noblastoma: tandem therapy. Arch Ophthalmol 2010;128 (3):370–372.

Abramson DH, Dunkel IJ, Brodie SE, Kim JW, Gobin YP. A phase I/II study of direct intraarterial (ophthalmic artery) chemotherapy with melphalan for intraocular retinoblastoma initial results. Ophthalmology 2008;115(8):1398–1404, 1404.e1.[19]

Gobin and coworkers reported a series of 95 eyes but did not stratify the results based on group of diseases. In their series, 43 eyes were primary treatments (success rate: 82%) and 52 were secondary treatments (success rate: 58%). In their series, two patients developed metastatic disease that was successfully treated with systemic chemotherapy. The other major systemic complications included significant neutropenia in 11.4% and 24 occurrences of bronchospasm during the procedure. Major ophthalmic side effects included avascular retinopathy in four eyes and phthisis in two eyes.

Shields CL, Shields JA. Intra-arterial chemotherapy for retinoblastoma: the beginning of a long journey. Clin Exp Ophthalmol 2010;38(6):638–643.

Shields CL, Bianciotto CG, Jabbour P, et al. Intra-arterial chemotherapy for retinoblastoma: report No. 2, treatment complications. Arch Ophthalmol 2011;129(11):1407–1415.

Shields CL, Ramasubramanian A, Rosenwasser R, Shields JA. Superselective catheterization of the ophthalmic artery for intra-arterial chemotherapy for retinoblastoma. Retina 2009;29 (8):1207–1209.

Shields and coworkers found that IAC provides tumor control with globe salvage in 100% of Group C and 100% of Group D eyes. Group E eyes with extensive vitreous seeds were the most resistant to therapy and globe salvage rate was 33%. In their series of 16 eyes, IAC was the primary treatment in 12 eyes (success rate: 58%) and for 4 eyes (success rate: 50%).[20] In their series, there was no reported metastasis and no serious systemic side effects. Major ocular complications included ophthalmic artery stenosis (25%), vitreous hemorrhage (6%), and choroidal atrophy (31%). In a subsequent study, Shields and coworkers evaluated the effect of minimal exposure IAC defined as one to two cycles of chemotherapy. They reported eight eyes treated with either one cycle of IAC ($n = 3$) or two cycles of IAC ($n = 5$). Globe salvage was achieved in 100% of Group C eyes, 100% of Group D eyes, 0% of Group E eyes, and 50% of salvage treatments. They made an important point that one to two cycles of IAC could be sufficient in achieving tumor control in Group C or Group D eyes.[21] There were no cases of brain complications or systemic metastases in any patient from this collaborative group.

Peterson EC, Elhammady MS, Quintero-Wolfe S, Murray TG, Aziz-Sultan MA. Selective ophthalmic artery infusion of chemotherapy for advanced intraocular retinoblastoma: initial experience with 17 tumors. J Neurosurg 2011;114(6):1603–1608.

Peterson and coworkers reported 17 eyes treated with IAC and all eyes were classified as Group D. Only in one patient, IAC was used as primary treatment with complete tumor regression. In the remaining 16 eyes, IAC was used as a salvage treatment and the reported globe salvage rate was 75%. None of their patients developed metastasis, but 11.5% developed neutropenia. Ocular complications included ischemic retinopathy in one patient and vitreous hemorrhage in 15% of eyes.

Munier FL, Beck-Popovic M, Balmer A, Gaillard MC, Bovey E, Binaghi S. Occurrence of sectoral choroidal occlusive vasculop-

athy and retinal arteriolar embolization after superselective ophthalmic artery chemotherapy for advanced intraocular retinoblastoma. Retina 2011;31(3):566–573.

Munier and coworkers reported 13 eyes treated with IAC of which one eye was staged as Group B (success rate: 100%) and the remaining were staged as Group D (success rate: 92%). The IAC was used as primary treatment in nine eyes (success rate: 100%) and as secondary treatment in four eyes (success rate: 75%). The only documented major systemic adverse effect was transient perioperative.

21.6 Summary

The era of cancer chemotherapy began in the 1940s with the use of nitrogen mustards and folic acid antagonist medications. These medications were delivered via the intravenous route for effective control of malignancy. Much later, a unique method of chemotherapy delivery was explored, the intra-arterial technique, whereby the medication was delivered directly to the affected organ by an intra-arterial catheter. This concept was popularized in the 1990s and was used to treat tumors of the head and neck, pancreas, liver, and others. The technique allowed for a concentrated high-dose administration of chemotherapy to a focal site with limited systematic side effects.[22]

There was initial enthusiasm for IAC with satisfactory tumor control, but later adverse effects limited its use for some cancers. For example, intra-arterial cisplatin was used for pediatric osteosarcomas, but later reports showed minimal benefit over systemic chemotherapy and also intolerable ischemic (often painful) limb complications; hence, the intra-arterial approach was abandoned.[23] For advanced inoperable head and neck tumors, IAC has been explored over many years with direct catheterization, into the central nervous system vascular tree, but the overall benefit has not been found to be superior to systemic chemotherapy.[24]

Based on these experiences, Shields and Shields have cautioned that the lessons learned from IAC use for other organs should be kept in mind while pursuing this novel treatment for retinoblastomas.[25] For retinoblastomas, the intra-arterial technique was first described by Reese and coworkers in 1957 with direct catheterization and infusion into the internal carotid artery. Later, in 1966, Kiribuchia showed favorable tumor response with frontal or supraorbital artery infusion with 5-fluorouracil.[26] Most recently, in the early 1990s, the Japanese group with Yamane carried out catheterization of the internal carotid artery with distal balloon occlusion for delivery of chemotherapy.[27] Unlike the description of direct carotid artery instillation of chemotherapy by Reese, the Japanese collaborators used remote femoral artery access to cannulate the internal carotid artery.[27] Gobin and coworkers in the United States modified the Japanese technique to directly enter the proximal portion of the ophthalmic artery without the need of a balloon occlusion.[6]

21.7 Conclusion

In summary, intra-arterial delivery of chemotherapy for retinoblastoma has seen an evolution toward focal delivery with minimization of side effects for this at-risk population. The endovascular techniques have matured to provide a robust, safe route for delivery. The advent of newer catheters has solved some of the issues around access to the ophthalmic artery, especially among the very young. This route of delivery has distinct advantages and may be broadly applied to many other cancer types, especially in the deep reaches of the brain.

References

[1] Newton HB. Intra-arterial chemotherapy of primary brain tumors. Curr Treat Options Oncol. 2005; 6(6):519–530– [published Online First: 2005/10/26]

[2] Peterson EC, Elhammady MS, Quintero-Wolfe S, Murray TG, Aziz-Sultan MA. Selective ophthalmic artery infusion of chemotherapy for advanced intraocular retinoblastoma: initial experience with 17 tumors. J Neurosurg. 2011; 114 (6):1603–1608– [published Online First: 2011/02/08]

[3] Hayreh SS, Dass R. The ophthalmic artery: II. Intra-orbital course. Br J Ophthalmol. 1962; 46(3):165–185– [published Online First: 1962/03/01]

[4] Abramson DH, Dunkel IJ, Brodie SE, Marr B, Gobin YP. Bilateral superselective ophthalmic artery chemotherapy for bilateral retinoblastoma: tandem therapy. Arch Ophthalmol. 2010; 128(3):370–372– [published Online First: 2010/03/10]

[5] Munier FL, Beck-Popovic M, Balmer A, Gaillard MC, Bovey E, Binaghi S. Occurrence of sectoral choroidal occlusive vasculopathy and retinal arteriolar embolization after superselective ophthalmic artery chemotherapy for advanced intraocular retinoblastoma. Retina. 2011; 31(3):566–573– [published Online First: 2011/01/29]

[6] Gobin YP, Dunkel IJ, Marr BP, Brodie SE, Abramson DH. Intra-arterial chemotherapy for the management of retinoblastoma: four-year experience. Arch Ophthalmol. 2011; 129(6):732–737– [published Online First: 2011/02/16]

[7] Friedman DL, Himelstein B, Shields CL, et al. Chemoreduction and local ophthalmic therapy for intraocular retinoblastoma. J Clin Oncol. 2000; 18(1):12–17– [published Online First: 2000/01/07]

[8] Laurie NA, Gray JK, Zhang J, et al. Topotecan combination chemotherapy in two new rodent models of retinoblastoma. Clin Cancer Res. 2005; 11 (20):7569–7578– [published Online First: 2005/10/26]

[9] Dunkel IJ, Khakoo Y, Kernan NA, et al. Intensive multimodality therapy for patients with stage 4a metastatic retinoblastoma. Pediatr Blood Cancer. 2010; 55(1):55–59– [published Online First: 2010/05/21]

[10] Gelman M, Chakeres DW, Newton HB. Brain tumors: complications of cerebral angiography accompanied by intraarterial chemotherapy. Radiology. 1999; 213(1):135–140– [published Online First: 1999/11/30]

[11] Patel M, Paulus YM, Gobin YP, et al. Intra-arterial and oral digoxin therapy for retinoblastoma. Ophthalmic Genet. 2011; 32(3):147–150– [published Online First: 2011/03/31]

[12] Turaka K, Shields CL, Meadows AT, Leahey A. Second malignant neoplasms following chemoreduction with carboplatin, etoposide, and vincristine in 245 patients with intraocular retinoblastoma. Pediatr Blood Cancer. 2012; 59 (1):121–125– [published Online First: 2011/08/10]

[13] Lambert MP, Shields C, Meadows AT. A retrospective review of hearing in children with retinoblastoma treated with carboplatin-based chemotherapy. Pediatr Blood Cancer. 2008; 50(2):223–226– [published Online First: 2007/02/06]

[14] Eagle RC, Jr. High-risk features and tumor differentiation in retinoblastoma: a retrospective histopathologic study. Arch Pathol Lab Med. 2009; 133 (8):1203–1209– [published Online First: 2009/08/06]

[15] Marr B, Gobin PY, Dunkel IJ, Brodie SE, Abramson DH. Spontaneously resolving periocular erythema and ciliary madarosis following intra-arterial chemotherapy for retinoblastoma. Middle East Afr J Ophthalmol. 2010; 17 (3):207–209– [published Online First: 2010/09/17]

[16] Shields CL, Bianciotto CG, Jabbour P, et al. Intra-arterial chemotherapy for retinoblastoma: report No. 2, treatment complications. Arch Ophthalmol. 2011; 129(11):1407–1415– [published Online First: 2011/06/15]

[17] Bianciotto C, Shields CL, Iturralde JC, Sarici A, Jabbour P, Shields JA. Fluorescein angiographic findings after intra-arterial chemotherapy for retinoblastoma. Ophthalmology. 2012; 119(4):843–849– [published Online First:–2011/12/06]

[18] Brodie SE, Pierre Gobin Y, Dunkel IJ, Kim JW, Abramson DH. Persistence of retinal function after selective ophthalmic artery chemotherapy infusion for retinoblastoma. Doc Ophthalmol. 2009; 119(1):13–22– [published Online First: 2009/01/27]

[19] Abramson DH, Dunkel IJ, Brodie SE, Kim JW, Gobin YP. A phase I/II study of direct intraarterial (ophthalmic artery) chemotherapy with melphalan for intraocular retinoblastoma initial results. Ophthalmology. 2008; 115 (8):1398–1404, 1404.e1– [published Online First: 2008/03/18]

[20] Shields CL, Ramasubramanian A, Rosenwasser R, Shields JA. Superselective catheterization of the ophthalmic artery for intraarterial chemotherapy for retinoblastoma. Retina. 2009; 29(8):1207–1209– [published Online First: 2009/09/08]

[21] Shields CL, Kaliki S, Shah SU, et al. Minimal exposure (one or two cycles) of intra-arterial chemotherapy in the management of retinoblastoma. Ophthalmology. 2012; 119(1):188–192– [published Online First: 2011/10/07]

[22] Higgins KM, Wang JR. State of head and neck surgical oncology research–a review and critical appraisal of landmark studies. Head Neck. 2008; 30 (12):1636–1642– [published Online First: 2008/07/22]

[23] Bielack SS, Bieling P, Erttmann R, Winkler K. Intraarterial chemotherapy for osteosarcoma: does the result really justify the effort? Cancer Treat Res. 1993; 62:85–92– [published Online First: 1993/01/01]

[24] Rasch CR, Hauptmann M, Balm AJ. Intra-arterial chemotherapy for head and neck cancer: is there a verdict? Cancer. 2011; 117(4):874–, 874–875

[25] Shields CL, Shields JA. Intra-arterial chemotherapy for retinoblastoma: the beginning of a long journey. Clin Exp Ophthalmol. 2010; 38(6):638–643– [published Online First: 2010/06/30]

[26] Reese AB, Hyman GA, Merrian CR, Jr, Forrest AW. The treatment of retinoblastoma by radiation and triethylene melamine. Trans Am Acad Ophthalmol Otolaryngol. 1957; 61(4):439–446– [published Online First: 1957/07/01]

[27] Yamane T, Kaneko A, Mohri M. The technique of ophthalmic arterial infusion therapy for patients with intraocular retinoblastoma. Int J Clin Oncol. 2004; 9 (2):69–73– [published Online First: 2004/04/27]

21

22 Intra-arterial Chemotherapy

Karen S. Chen and Ali Aziz-Sultan

Abstract

Intra-arterial chemotherapy (IAC) for malignant gliomas is an attractive treatment strategy that utilizes the selective nature of arterial catheterization to minimize nontarget drug toxicity allowing for higher local drug concentration. However, early case reports and randomized controlled trials (RCTs) failed to show discernable survival benefit. The interval development of more navigable catheters, fine-tuning of tumor-specific chemotherapy agents, and innovative blood–brain barrier disruption techniques have enabled increased selectivity for treatment. Early reports are showing modest but persistent survival benefits of adjunct IAC for malignancies of the intracranial compartment, as well as the head and neck. Reviewed here is the evidence of IAC in the treatment of recurrent malignant gliomas, primary central nervous system (CNS) lymphoma, lacrimal gland malignancies, and squamous cell carcinoma of the head and neck. RCTs have evaluated a select few chemotherapy agents for malignant gliomas and squamous cell carcinomas of the head and neck and the remainder of the evidence rests on case series and case reports. However, many phase III trials for IAC are open and recruiting.

Keywords: intra-arterial chemotherapy, malignant gliomas, squamous cell carcinoma, primary CNS lymphoma, intracranial metastases

22.1 Goals

1. Review the current clinical applications of intra-arterial chemotherapy (IAC) beyond retinoblastoma.
2. Critically analyze the literature on IAC on gliomas, squamous cell carcinomas of the head and neck, primary central nervous system (CNS) lymphoma, intracranial metastases, and adenoid cystic carcinoma (ACC) of the lacrimal gland.
3. Briefly review the variety of applications of IAC in the treatment of uncommon intracranial tumors and experimental efforts to expand the use of IAC.

22.2 Case Example

22.2.1 History of Present Illness

A 43-year-old woman who initially presented approximately 1 year after noticing a small nodule over the right superolateral globe which eventually was associated with mild right temporal discomfort. The condition was initially treated as a prolapsed lacrimal gland that was repositioned surgically. Biopsy at the time demonstrated mild chronic inflammation. Follow-up imaging performed a year later showed progressive enlargement. Excisional biopsy of the nodule demonstrated ACC. Follow-up imaging noted persistent asymmetry of the right lacrimal gland but no abnormally enhancing lesion.

Past medical history: Left arm and ankle fracture after car accident.

Past surgical history: Laparoscopic cholecystectomy 2011, nasal septum repair 1988.

Family history: Father died of stomach cancer; mother alive at age 66 with chronic obstructive pulmonary disease (COPD). Brother and sister in their 40 s are in good health.

Social history: University professor. Denies smoking or other chemical exposures. Social drinker.

Review of systems: Some blurry vision and eye pain.

Neurological examination: CN II-IX, XI, XII intact, PERRL, EOMI, 5/5 motor strength and sensation.

Imaging studies: See ▸ Fig. 22.1 and ▸ Fig. 22.2.

22.2.2 Treatment Plan

There is a significant reduction in cause-specific mortality at 5 years with intra-arterial cytoreductive chemotherapy (IACC).

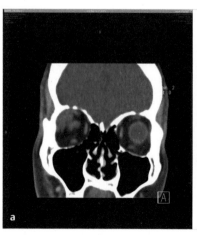 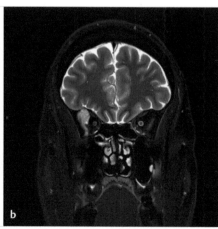

Fig. 22.1 Coronal noncontrast computed tomography (CT) of the orbits **(a)** demonstrates asymmetrically enlarged soft tissue density of the right lacrimal gland. Corresponding coronal T2 image of the orbits **(b)** demonstrates heterogenous T2 hypertense asymmetric soft tissue abnormality of the right lacrimal gland. (Photo credit: Priyank Khandelwal, MD.)

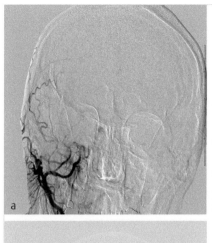
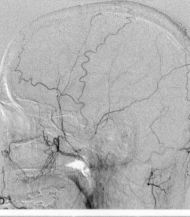
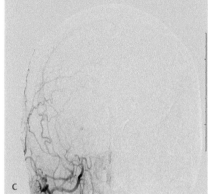
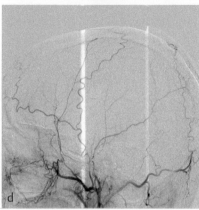

Fig. 22.2 Frontal **(a)** and lateral **(b)** views of a digital subtraction angiogram of the right external carotid artery prior to treatment with intra-arterial chemotherapy of a right lacrimal gland adenocystic carcinoma. Lacrimal branches of the right internal maxillary artery were superselected for intra-arterial chemotherapy administration. There is no significant tumor blush of the right lacrimal region. Control frontal **(c)** and lateral **(d)** angiography of the right ECA demonstrates a similar appearance of the parent vessel. (Photo credit: Priyank Khandelwal, MD.)

Patient was admitted for neoadjuvant IAC with cisplatin and Adriamycin on day 1 followed by IACC with Adriamycin for another 2 days. She was premedicated with decadron, Zofran, and Ativan, and started on Neulasta on treatment day 2.

22.2.3 Follow-up

Patient initially complained of right-sided tinnitus and tingling of the right head and extremities which dissipated by day 3. She had no hematologic alterations, cardiovascular changes, or nephrotoxicity. On her last clinic visit 5 years posttreatment, she is doing well. She complains of occasional dry eyes but denies blurry vision, headache, or local symptomatology.

22.3 Case Summary

What are the circumstances when IAC might be a reasonable treatment option?

22.3.1 Adenoid Cystic Carcinoma of the Lacrimal Gland

Adenoid cystic carcinoma (ACC) is a rare tumor of the oral and maxillofacial regions predominately found in the minor salivary glands,[1] but can occur in any secretory gland including the breast, cervix, esophagus, lungs, prostate, and lacrimal gland.[2] Lacrimal gland ACC carries a poor prognosis despite disfiguring wide local excision because of its propensity for perineural spread and distant temporal recurrence.[3] The current standard of care is radical orbitectomy, but eye-sparing procedures have been gaining support in the literature because of similar survival rates to radical surgical excision.[4]

Recurrence most commonly occurs locally.[5] For this reason, adjuvant radiation therapy and chemotherapy on top of surgical excision is considered the most promising treatment option.[6] A case report[7] and larger case series[8] have reported improved overall survival and decreased recurrence with IAC for lacrimal gland ACC followed by orbital exenteration, chemoradiation, and IV chemotherapy. Patients who completed treatment had a significantly higher 10-year disease-free survival when compared to the group undergoing conventional treatment (100 vs. 14.3%); however, this group excluded those who were not given IAC due to sacrifice of the lacrimal artery from excisional biopsy, precluding straightforward catheterization. IAC resulted in downstaging primary tumors with intracranial extension or temporal fossa involvement to disease limited to the intraorbital compartment. One major adverse event occurred in a patient who was treated through the ICA and sustained central retinal artery occlusion and complete vision loss prior to exenteration.

A smaller case series of four patients who underwent IAC followed by resection reported significant adverse effects including eye lid and globe necrosis, facial palsy, difficulty chewing, facial swelling, and neutropenia.[9] Three patients had total exenteration, and at follow-up (range 48–69 mo), there was no evidence of recurrence of metastases. The fourth patient had lacrimal gland resection alone and at 54 months was found to have local recurrence for which total exenteration was recommended.

Table 22.1 Untreated malignant gliomas: single IA agent series and trials

Study	Year	IA agent	N	CR	PR	MS (mo)
Yamashita	1983	ACNU	17 (GBM)	NR	NR	12.5 IA, 9 IV
Greenberg	1984	BCNU	36 (12 Grade III–IV, 24 grade I–II)	NR	NR	Prior surgery 13.5 Prior RT 6.5
Hochberg	1985	BCNU	79 (39 New)	NR	NR	12.5–13.5
Bashir	1988	BCNU	28 (Grade III–IV)	22.0	22.0	9.2
Greenberg	1988	BUdR	18 (GBM and AA)	17.0	28.0	22
Wolpert	1988	BCNU	10	NR	NR	No outcomes discussed
Clayman	1989	BCNU	15 (12 New)	33.3	6.7	19.2
Roosen	1989	ACNU	50 (42 New)	NR	57.1	14.2
Fauchon	1990	HeCNU	40 (33 GBM, 6 AA)	5.0	0.1	10.5 (GBM only)
Dropcho	1992	Cisplatin	22 (13 GBM, 9 AA)	NR	0.2	15.7
Mortimer	1992	Cisplatin	22	5.0	23.0	9.6–10.8
Vega	1992	ACNU	22 (4 GBM, 18 AA)	NR	NR	6
Shapiro	1992	BCNU IA vs. IV	315 (94 GBM IV, 111 GBM IA)	NR	NR	11.2 (IA), 14 (IV)
Chauveinc	1996	ACNU	27 (10 GBM, 17 AA)	NR	NR	10
Kochii	2000	ACNU IA vs. IV	82	NR	NR	14.8 (IA), 14 (IV)
Imbesi	2006	ACNU IA vs. IV	43	NR	NR	17 (IA), 20 (IV)

Abbreviations: AA, anaplastic astrocytoma; ACNU, nimustine; BCNU, carmustine; BUdR, bromodeoxyuridine; CR, complete response; GBM, glioblastoma multiforme; HeCNU, 1-(2-hydroxyethyl)-3-(2 chloroethyl)-3-nitrosourea; IA, intra-arterial; IV, intravenous; MS, median survival; NR, not recorded; PR, partial response—generally > 50% decrease in tumor volume; RT, radiotherapy.

Stage I and II disease or tumors less than 4 cm without extraparenchymal extension do well with globe preservation surgery and radiation, with local recurrence observed in those with greater residual tumor burden.[10] Given the high morbidity of orbital exenteration, globe-sparing surgery is gaining popularity with adjuvant proton radiation therapy or concurrent chemoradiation.[11] IAC may play a growing role in reducing microscopic tumor burden.

22.3.2 Intracranial Gliomas

For newly diagnosed malignant gliomas, the standard of treatment entails surgical resection with adjuvant chemoradiation,[12,13,14] yielding an overall survival of 15 months.[15,16] Methylated O[6]-methylguanine-DNA methyltransferase (MGMT)-positive histology confers a better prognosis with overall survival of 23.4 months.[17] IAC is currently utilized either in clinical trials or as off-label salvage therapy.[18]

There are four phase III randomized controlled trials (RCTs) comparing IA with systemic chemotherapy[19,20,21,22] in patients with newly diagnosed glioblastoma multiforme. All patients underwent surgical resection followed by radiation therapy with IA carmustine (BCNU),[19,21] nimustine (ACNU),[20] and carboplatin and ACNU.[22] These initial chemotherapeutic agents were chosen for their lipophilic properties.[23] IA therapy was administered through the internal carotid and vertebral arteries, and in some cases the dose was divided between arteries, if the tumor crossed arterial territories.[21] Three of the four studies were terminated at interim analysis. The trials' cumulative 469 patients successfully randomized showed no survival benefit for IAC.

Thousands of patients have been enrolled in phase I and II clinical trials testing the safety and efficacy of IAC for newly diagnosed as well as recurrent grade III to IV gliomas. Early small case series for newly diagnosed malignant gliomas focused on nitrosoureas (ACNU, BCNU, and hydroxyethyl-chloroethyl nitrosourea [HeCNU]) on the basis that lipophilic agents would facilitate passage across the blood–brain barrier. Leukoencephalopathy and ocular toxicity were common side effects, prompting combination therapy. Median survival ranges from 5 to 22 months (▶ Table 22.1, ▶ Table 22.2).

With recurrent tumors, overall survival is 25 weeks.[24] One multi-institutional RCT found a statistically significant survival benefit of IV PCNU over IA cisplatin (13 vs. 10 mo).[25] Although IV PCNU was associated with greater hematotoxicity, IA cisplatin led to greater renal toxicity, ototoxicity, and encephalopathy.

Similar to the literature on newly diagnosed malignant gliomas, early trials in the treatment of recurrent tumors (▶ Table 22.3) initially focused on nitrosoureas before moving toward platinum-based agents (cisplatin, carboplatin). Reports of ocular, hematologic, and neurologic toxicities likely spurred interest in immunologic agents and combination IA, IV, and PO therapy. In the recurrent tumor IA literature, there are more reports of these new agents as well as the use of hydrophilic compounds with adjuvant blood–brain barrier disruption (BBBD).[26] Despite greater patient volume and outcomes data, conclusions are difficult to make on the whole because of treatment and patient heterogeneity. Many studies include not only patients with various prior surgical, medical, and radiation histories but also add adjuvant or concurrent radiation in the treatment arm along with multiagent therapy (▶ Table 22.4).

Poor support to IA therapy may be related to the heterogeneity of the underlying pathology, toxicity of earlier chemotherapeutic agents, and poor patient selection. MGMT gene expression confers a particular benefit from temozolomide and may be used for patient selection for super selective intra-arterial chemotherapy (SSIAC) trials.[27,28] Other prognostic factors for survival include young age, good clinical performance status, extensive surgical resection, seizures, and histologic features.[29] In the highly selected populations undergoing IAC, it is difficult to surmise which patient characteristics predict a

Table 22.2 Untreated malignant gliomas: multi-IA agent series and trials

Study	Year	IA agent	N	CR	PR	MS (mo)
West	1983	BCNU IV vincristine, procarbazine	16	0.0	80.0	17.1
Madajewicz	1991	Cisplatin, etoposide	48 (13 new)	5.0	37.0	14 (GBM)
Watne	1991	BCNU IV vincristine, PO procarbazine	79 (19 AA, 60 GBM)	NR	NR	30 overall 10 GBM
Bobo	1992	BCNU and cisplatin	39 (21 AA, 18 GBM)	16.7	27.8	12.5
Watne	1993	BCNU IV vincristine, PO proarbazine	173 (35 AA, 138 GBM)	NR	NR	GBM 10, AA 57
Nakagawa	1994	Cisplatin, etoposide	7 (4 GBM, 3 AA)	25 (GBM) 33 (AA)	25 (GBM), 33 (AA)	5
Madajewicz	2000	Cisplatin, etoposide	83 (63 GBM, 20 AA)	5.6 (all), 8.9 (GBM)	42 (all), 41 (GBM)	20 before RT 7 concurrent RT
Silvani	2002	IA carboplatin and ACNU or IV cisplatin and BCNU	30	0.0	21 (IA), 33 (IV)	18.3 (IA), 18.6 (IV)

Abbreviations: AA, anaplastic astrocytoma; ACNU, nimustine; BCNU, carmustine; CR, complete response; GBM, glioblastoma multiforme; IA, intra-arterial; IV, intravenous; MS, median survival; NR, not recorded; PR, partial response—generally >50% decrease in tumor volume; RT, radiotherapy.

good response. In one series of 41 patients receiving IAC, 80% of which were glioblastomas (GBMs), half of the tumors were avascular and the other half very hypervascular on angiography. Hypervascularity was a statistically significant predictor of decreased survival.[30] Imaging related predictors of increased survival included small enhancing tumor volume, avascularity, and longer time to recurrence which was defined as clinical deterioration or more than 25% increase in tumor area on magnetic resonance imaging (MRI) (fluid-attenuated inversion recovery [FLAIR] hyperintensity or enhancement). Small tumor volume and avascularity are thought to be related as more aggressive tumors tend to more vascular because of increased microvessel density[31] and tumoral angiogenesis.[32]

Major hurdles in selective drug delivery include the angioarchitecture of GBMs which derive vascular supply from adjacent vascular territories or even the contralateral hemisphere.[23] Postcontrast enhancement on MRI typically underestimates the vascular territory involved, a finding overcompensated by T2 signal abnormalities.[33] Using FLAIR hyperintensity, 66% of tumors were supplied by both anterior and posterior territories and 10% were supplied by three arterial territories. This suggests that catheterization of a single intracranial artery is insufficient, and effective treatment likely involves superselection of branches in different vascular territories.

Most recent SSIAC case series have been performed in those with recurrent high-grade gliomas.[34,35,36] One group has published phase I and II clinical trials employing SSIAC with bevacizumab for recurrent glioblastoma.[34,35] IAC was administered with concomitant balloon occlusion of downstream parent vessels. Follow-up MRI at 1 month also demonstrated decrease in tumor volume as measured by FLAIR hyperintensity, perfusion volume, and enhancement. IAC conferred a median progression-free (PFS) and overall (MOS) survival of 10 and 8.8 months, respectively, which was comparable to prior studies using IV bevacizumab where medial PFS and MOS ranged 3.7–4.2 and 7.2–9.2 months, respectively.[37,38]

Qureshi et al reported a case series of 12 GBM patients treated with SSIAC carboplatin and nonapeptide H-Arg-Pro-Hyp-Gly-Thi-Ser-Pro-Tyr(Me)-ψ(CH2NH)-Arg-OH (RMP-7) for BBBD (discussed later). All were cases of recurrent GBM after gross total resection and chemoradiation. In the six patients with GBM for whom follow-up data was available, one-half demonstrated decreased tumor volume on MRI, defined as enhancement on T1-weighted images, at a median follow-up of 4.9 months. One-year survival for GBM patients was 45% (5 out of 11).[36]

SSIAC decreases nontarget drug delivery while increasing the tumor tissue dose, particularly those supplied by small distal branches. Superselective catheterization of the middle cerebral artery (MCA) was associated with fewer ocular toxicities.[39] In later studies employing SSIAC, there is a notable decrease in the incidence of seizures, leukoencephalopathy, and hematologic toxicities.[34,35,36] Interestingly, those receiving intraprocedural RMP-7 for BBBD had fewer neurological complications, though not statistically significant.[36]

The advantage of SSIAC is direct administration to the tumor bed to achieve high local concentrations. To decrease streaming, pulsatile dosing and spatial dose fractionation was used to deliver a more tailored dose for the territory supplied by a given artery. This accounts for individual variations in the circle of Willis so that dosing is based on arterial territory volume and not body weight or body surface area as a way to decrease neurologic complications from administering chemotherapy to normal tissues.[18]

Advances in the understanding of drug delivery have informed clinical trials. Initially postcontrast enhancement on MRI of the brain was used to indicate blood–brain barrier breakdown and support the use of IAC.[40] While degree of enhancement does reflect tissue uptake of chemotherapeutic drugs,[26] animal studies comparing MRI enhancement with drug uptake in tumor versus normal tissues have demonstrated unacceptably high doses in normal brain tissue as well as sys-

Table 22.3 Recurrent malignant gliomas: single IA agent series and trials

Study	Year	IA agent	N	CR	PR	MS (mo)
Lehane	1982	Cisplatin	10 (Grade III–IV)	0.0	80.0	4
Feun	1984	Cisplatin	35 (18 GBM, 3 AA)	0.0	28.6 (Grade II–IV)	NR
Greenberg	1984	BCNU	36 (31 Grade III–IV)	8.0	62–67	13–13.5
Hochberg	1985	BCNU	79 (25 Recurrent)	NR	NR	13.5
Feun	1987	Etoposide	28 (13 GBM, 1 AA)	0.0	0.0	NR
Johnson	1987	BCNU	20 (18 GBM)	0.0	10.0	8.7
Stewart	1987	PCNU	17 (8 GBM, 3 AA)	0.0	50 (GBM)	NR
Mahaley	1989	Cisplatin	40 (20 GBM, 14 AA)	0.0	18 (Overall)	4.1
Newton	1989	Cisplatin	12 (9 GBM or AA)	0.0	8.0	NR
Calvo	1989	Cisplatin	12 (8 GBM)	41.7	50.0	10
Roosen	1989	ACNU	50 (7 Recurrent)	NR	NR	6.1
Poisson	1990	HECNU	53 (30 GBM, 10 AA)	17 (GBM) 40 (AA)	13 (GBM) 10 (AA)	4.5 (GBM) 18 (AA)
Saris	1991	Cisplatin	10 (7 GBM, 3 AA)	10.0	0.0	NR
Bradac	1992	BCNU	17 (12 GBM, 5 AA)	0.0	29 (All AA)	6.7 (AA) 6 (GBM)
Stewart	1992	Carboplatin	15 (6 GBM, 1 grade II–III, 2 grade II)	0.0	0 (GBM) 33 (Grade II–III)	1.5
Vega	1992	ACNU	18 (6 GBM, 12 AA)	0 GBM 25 (AA)	33 (GBM) 17 (AA)	8
Hiesiger	1995	IA cisplatin vs. IV PCNU	311 (174 GBM)	NR	NR	10 (IA) 13 (IV)
Chow	2000	Carboplatin with cereport	46 (32 GBM, 9 AA)	NR	NR	NR (7.3–11.6)
Qureshi	2001	Carboplatin with RMP-7	24 (12 GBM, 6 AA)	8 (GBM)	8 (GBM) 17 (AA)	7 (GBM) 25.5 (AA)
Boockvar	2011	Bevacizumab and mannitol vs. IV bevacizumab	30 (26 GBM, 2 AA)	NR	NR	NR
Burkhardt	2012	IA bevacizumab and mannitol IV bevacizumab	14 GBM	0.0	57.0	10

Abbreviations: AA, anaplastic astrocytoma; ACNU, nimustine; BCNU, carmustine; CR, complete response; GBM, glioblastoma multiforme; IA, intra-arterial; IV, intravenous; MS, median survival; NR, not recorded; PR, partial response—generally > 50% decrease in tumor volume; RT, radiotherapy.

temically.[41] This has fueled research in local disruption of the blood–brain barrier to facilitate drug delivery.

Clinical trials employing IAC with BBBD are accruing patients and results are promising. The most commonly employed agent is hyperosmolar mannitol infused right before chemotherapy administration to induce osmotic shrinkage of the endothelial cells lining the capillaries to promote separation of tight junctions.[42] An alternative agent is lobradimil (also known as RMP-7 or Cereport), a bradykinin derivative that increases vascular permeability, and regadenoson an adenosine agonist causing transient BBBD.[43]

In addition to superselective catheterization, other strategies for efficient drug delivery include flow arrest to maximize drug extraction and minimize drug streaming. High cerebral blood flow and low drug concentrations hinder tissue uptake. Streaming can be overcome with injections of drug volumes greater than 20% of the background blood flow rate, injecting during diastole, or using catheters with side ports.[44,45,46] These delivery pharmacokinetics are studied using the Dedrick model of blood flow.[47]

Convection-enhanced drug delivery is another catheter-based strategy where catheters are directly implanted into the tumor bed. Drugs are pressure infused at a set concentration, rate, and duration across the leaky cytoarchitecture of growing tumor cells[48] and across pre-existing tracts of white matter edema.[49] Small phase I and II trials have experimented with monoclonal antibodies, liposomal vectors packaged for gene therapy, antisense oligonucleotides, and exotoxins.[50] However, early phase III trials were not able to demonstrate a survival benefit,[51] although PFS was significantly increased in the treatment arm, 17.7 versus 11.4 weeks.

Riina et al have reported the use of SSIAC with bevacizumab and mannitol for a malignant glioma in 2009 and for a malignant brainstem glioma in 2010 with decreased enhancement seen on follow-up MRI in both cases.[52,53] Numerous clinical trials have also described IAC in the treatment of diffuse intrinsic pontine gliomas (DIPGs),[54] esthesioneuroblastoma,[55] anaplastic oligodendrogliomas,[56] germ cell tumors,[57] cerebral metastatic disease. However, these treatments are entirely experimental.

Table 22.4 Recurrent malignant gliomas: multi-IA agent series and trials

Study	Year	IA agent	N	CR	PR	MS (mo)
West	1983	BCNU IV vincristine and procarbazine	25 (9 Recurrent)	0.0	22 (Recurrent)	5.1
Stewart	1984	Carmustine, cisplatin, teniposide	37 (17 GBM)	0.0	63.0	NR
Kapp	1985	BCNU and cisplatin	13 (6 GBM, 5 AA)	17 (GBM) 0 (AA)	17 (GBM) 80 (AA)	11
Stewart	1987	BCNU, teniposide, cisplatin IV teniposide, MTX, vincristine, bleomycin, procarbazine	26 (21 Grade III–IV)	0.0	48 (Grade III–IV)	4.1
Rogers	1991	Carmutine and cisplatin	43 (25 GBM, 17 AA)	0.0	20.0	9
Watne	1992	IA carmustine IV vincristine, oral procarbazine	79 (30 AA and GBM)	NR	62.0	6.5 GBM 20 AA
Stewart	1993	IA carmustine, cisplatin, teniposide IV cisplatin, teniposide, cytarabine vs. all IV	16 (10 GBM, 4 AA)	0.0	0.0	3.5 IA 3.1 IV
Nakagawa	1994	Cisplatin, etoposide	13 (11 GBM, 2 AA)	18 (GBM) 0 (AA)	9 (GBM) 0 (AA)	6
Doolittle	2000	IA carboplatin IV mannitol, cyclophosphamide, etoposide	73 (all GBM)	2.7	13.7	NR
Ashby	2001	IA cisplatin and oral etoposide	25 (11 GBM, 6 AA)	0	33 (AA) 0 (GBM)	5.5
Osztie	2001	IV carboplatin, etoposide IV cytoxan	Six optic pathway hypothalamic gliomas	0.0	67.0	12.5
Newton	2002	IA carboplatin, IV etoposide	25 (9 AA)	4.0	12.0	13.7
Fortin	2005	IA carboplatin IV etoposide and cyclophosphamide	31 (20 GBM, 6 AA)	6	51	9.1
Fortin	2014	IA carboplatin and melphalan	51 (all GBM)	3.9	43.1	11

Abbreviations: AA, anaplastic astrocytoma; ACNU, nimustine; BCNU, carmustine; CR, complete response; GBM, glioblastoma multiforme; IA, intra-arterial; IV, intravenous; MS, median survival; MTX, methotrexate; NR, not recorded; PR, partial response—generally > 50% decrease in tumor volume; RT, radiotherapy.

This limited availability has led to international controversy in the media for rare malignancies for which there is no accepted treatment.[58]

22.3.3 Primary CNS Lymphoma

Primary CNS lymphoma (PCNSL) accounts for less than 3% of all primary brain tumors.[59] Current treatment with combined chemoradiation has produced response rates ranging from 80 to 90%.[60] PCNSL is an ideal target for IAC due to its chemosensitivity. Early reports described improved response rates (85 vs. 50%) and better survival with chemotherapy prior to radiation compared to those receiving radiation first.[61] The authors noted a plateau in survival curves and postulated that some patients may be cured with chemotherapy and BBBD without radiation.

More recent studies employ BBBD techniques with 25% mannitol (▶ Table 22.5). Many discussions on BBBD are available,[62] and promising novel targets have been described.[63,64] The largest series reported treated 149 newly diagnosed patients with IA methotrexate with BBBD in a multi-institutional study.[65] Complete and partial response rates were 58% and 24%, respectively. Median survival was 3.1 years overall and 14 years in low-risk patients (age less than 60 y and high premorbid performance scores). One patient died from pulmonary embolism within 48 hours of treatment. Periprocedural complications included seizures in one-third of the patient population (9% of procedures), asymptomatic dissection in 11%, and permanent neurologic deficit from stroke in 3%, yielding a 0.2% risk of complication per procedure.

Smaller studies have demonstrated overall responses of 85 to 100% with complete response in over 50% of patients in all but one study.[66] Myelosuppression was the most common toxicity, seen in 69% of patients.[67] However, in the most experienced center, the most frequent side effect was focal seizure, which occurred in 9% of procedures, without long-term sequela. This is likely a result of well-tailored medical management, which includes pretreatment with anticonvulsants, atropine, sodium bicarbonate, and leucovorin to prevent seizures, bradycardia, tumor lysis syndrome, and myelosuppression, respectively.[68]

22.3.4 Intracranial Metastases

Intracranial metastases are the most common intracranial malignancy, occurring six to seven times more frequently than primary intracranial malignancies.[69] The allure of IAC applies for metastatic disease with the added benefit that the lesions

22

Table 22.5 Primary CNS lymphoma: IA agent series and case report

Study	Year	IA agent	N	CR	PR	MS (mo)
Neuwelt	1991	IA MTX, IV mannitol post-RT vs. pre-RT	30	70.0	30.0	17.8 post-RT vs. 44.5 pre-RT
Doolittle	2000	IA carboplatin IV mannitol, cyclophosphamide, etoposide	221 (53 PCNSL)	75.5	15.1	NR
Fortin	2005	IA carboplatin IV etoposide and cyclophosphamide	31 (8 PCNSL)	37.5	62.5	Not reached
Sonoda	2007	IA ACNU and RT	63	75.0	25.0	39
MacNealy	2008	IA MTX IV etoposide, cyclophosphamide, mannitol	Primary meningeal lymphoma case report	–	–	–
Angelov	2009	IA MTX, IV mannitol	149	57.8	24.2	37

Abbreviations: AA, anaplastic astrocytoma; ACNU, nimustine; BCNU, carmustine; CR, complete response; GBM, glioblastoma multiforme; IA, intra-arterial; IV, intravenous; MS, median survival; MTX, methotrexate; NR, not recorded; PCNSL, primary CNS lymphoma; PR, partial response—generally > 50% decrease in tumor volume; RT, radiotherapy.

tend to be well marginated rather than infiltrative. The earliest reported series were published from 1979 to 1987 using BCNU or PCNU for previously radiated intracranial metastases for a variety of primary malignancies including lung, breast, and melanoma.[70,71,72,73] While single-agent studies with small subsets of the population getting metastatic lesion treatment with cisplatin[74,75] and etoposide[76] were equivocal, when given in combination there was a 55 to 70% response.[66,77,78,79,80] Later studies[36,68] using IA platinum-based agents and IV etoposide also incorporated BBBD without significant improvement on the approximately 25% complete response rate reported in prior studies.

Fortin et al have reported the greatest overall median survival of 29.6 months in the second largest series: 11.2, 16.3, 42.3, and 8.1 months in patients with intracranial metastases from lung, lymphoma, ovarian, and breast cancer, respectively. Patients with systemic lymphoma received IA methotrexate with leucovorin and neupogen while all others received IA carboplatin. All patients received adjuvant etoposide and cyclophosphamide.[80] These findings are a significant improvement in the reported range of 2 to 7.1 months from the radiation therapy oncology group.[81]

22.3.5 Squamous Cell of the Head and Neck

There has been a resurgence in squamous cell carcinoma (SCC) with the increased prevalence of human papillomavirus (HPV), or HPV-positive SCC,[82] which responds well to chemotherapy and radiation compared to HPV-negative SCC.[83] For the purpose of this review, HPV-positive and HPV-negative status is not distinguished for the treatment of oropharyngeal SCC, and it should be noted that chemosensitivity of this subgroup may be an independent driver of the results in smaller trials.

While stage I and II SCC is treated with surgical resection,[84] stage III and IV disease entails adjuvant treatment with chemoradiation.[85] Induction chemoradiation prior to definite radiation or surgical excision has demonstrated lower rates of local recurrence,[86] as well as increased overall survival and lower prevalence of distant metastases at 5 years.[87] A recent meta-analysis found an 8 to 20% increase in overall survival with induction chemotherapy with locoregional (surgery, radiation, or both) treatment compared to locoregional treatment alone across 29 trials comprising over 5,000 patients.[88]

The first RCTs for IAC reported greater tumor response with IA methotrexate and radiation compared to radiation alone.[89,90] However, when evaluated by tumor subgroup, statistical significance persisted only in oral cavity tumors, 54% versus 27%.

Early case studies from the 1980s to mid-1990s on untreated advanced staged SCC of the head and neck relied heavily on IA and IV combinations comprising of bleomycin,[91,92,93,94,95] mitomycin,[96] methotrexate,[92,93,95,97] cisplatin,[91,93,94,97,98] vincristine,[92,93] and 5-fluorouracil.[91,93] Complete and partial responses are as high as 39%[93] and 65%,[94] respectively, and MOS ranged from 19 to 39 months.[95,96,97]

A multicenter RCT conducted by the European Organization for Research and Treatment of Cancer examined the effect of preoperative IAC with vincristine and bleomycin on survival for patients undergoing surgery. Most patients received postoperative radiation therapy. IAC conferred significantly increased survival when adjusting for T and N status overall and especially for those in the oropharyngeal cancer group: median survival, 7 versus 3 years, respectively. However, about one-quarter of the patients in the IA arm were not evaluated due to technical difficulties arising from catheter placement and/or maintenance.[99]

SSIAC was first described in 1985 in Japan[100] and the United States[91] in 1989. Case series with SSIAC report response rates over 90% with complete response rates of 25 to 50%.[101,102] Case series with long-term follow-up has been published in recurrent[91,101,111] and newly diagnosed[91,92,93,94,95,96,97,98] disease. Complete and partial responses ranged from 25 to 92% and 6 to 54%, respectively. These studies, largely published in the 1990s and early 2000s, used cisplatin[102,103,105,106,108,109,111,112,113] with doxetaxel,[107,110,114] paclitaxel,[104] and nedaplatin[107] arriving in later reports. Particularly in the later years, MOS has increased up to 5 years.[105,107] Clinical trials are actively recruiting for treatment with IA cetuximab.[115]

In the RADPLAT study, 213 patients received high-dose superselected IA cisplatin with thiosulfate for systemic neutralization, with a reported 80% complete and an 8% partial response rate.[105] Kaplan-Meier plot showed that 5-year estimated overall survival was 39%. Similarly, high response rates were seen with this protocol expanded across 11 institutions.[106] Unfortunately, these results did not bear out in an RCT comparing RADPLAT with IV cisplatin in a multicenter trial in the Netherlands with 236 patients. Overall complete response was 79% and 92% and 3-year survival was 51% and 47% for IA and IV, respectively. Taking into account high rates of feeding tube placements and transient ischemic attack (TIA), the authors concluded that IA chemoradiation is not superior to IV chemoradiation.[116]

Follow-up results published in 2010 reported greater overall survival favoring IA, 32% versus 20%, but the difference was not statistically significant.[117] For these reasons, momentum for high-dose IA cisplatin with sodium thiosulfate followed by radiotherapy has waned. Taking note of subgroup analyses from prior RCTs,[89,90] it may be time to fine-tune study design by differentiating advanced SCC by location for optimal treatment evaluation. The higher prevalence of SCC in Japan has not only spurned novel and highly tailored therapies[118] but also has facilitated this type of study. A second national undertaking of RADPLAT in Japan began in 2014 to evaluate effect on stage IV maxillary sinus cancer.[84]

1. *What are the attendant risks?*

Risks specific to IAC for intracranial malignancies are secondary to catheterization: dissection, hemorrhage, and stroke in addition to drug toxicity. In the most recent and largest case series comprising 3,583 procedures, one institution reported a 1.8% prevalence of MRI or angiographic findings of dissection, stenosis, occlusion, hemorrhage, lacunar stroke, and ischemic stroke. Less than half of these complications were symptomatic, yielding a prevalence of 0.8%.[119] This is consistent with the range of 0.9 to 5% and 0 to 4.9% for asymptomatic and symptomatic complications, respectively.[18,21,36,68,120] Drug toxicity in this patient population is most commonly manifest as seizures, 2 to 23% prevalence,[119,120,121] which has decreased with preprocedural Keppra.[68,119] Hematologic toxicity including neutropenia, thrombocytopenia, and anemia was seen in 75%. Using the National Cancer Institution Toxicity Criteria (Grade 0–4: 0 = no hematologic toxicity, 1 = mild, 2 = moderate, 3 = severe, and 4 = life-threatening), the incidence of grade 3 and 4 toxicity was 18.6% in the most recent cohort.[119]

Chemoprotection with sodium thiosulfate is used to prevent hearing loss in earlier trials.[122,123] N-acetyl cysteine has been studied in a phase I trial for IV versus IAC for its protective effects on both hearing and renal function.[123] Vision loss has also been reported (16% prevalence in one series Shapiro[21]) and can be minimized with selective IAC in the supraophthalmic segment to minimize inadvertent administration to the retina. A concomitant decrease in the reported prevalence treatment-related retinopathy has been shown.[124] Ocular and ototoxicities have decreased with the use of carboplatin, methotrexate, and biological agents like bevucizumab.[23]

For SSIAC in SCC, toxicities included nausea, hemifacial alopecia, mucositis, skin necrosis, mild hematologic toxicities,

and neurologic deficits. The authors of RADPLAT in 2005 noted a strikingly increased prevalence of grade 4 and 5 toxicities at inexperienced centers, particularly at the start of the trial, highlighting a substantial learning curve in the proper execution of the RADPLAT protocol, although no technical or protocol errors were identified upon review.[106] Compared to the reports for malignant gliomas, the incidence and long-term sequela are lower and better tolerated. Although less likely, catheter-related complications include cerebrovascular accidents, seizures leading to cardiopulmonary collapse and death, and external carotid artery (ECA) spasm precluding completion of treatment.[91] Others[105] argue that a 2.8% treatment-related mortality is not outside the range of that reported for chemoradiation in advanced head and neck cancer (5–18%).[125,126,127]

2. *What are the limitations?*

For lacrimal gland adenocystic carcinoma, intracranial metastases, and primary CNS lymphoma, the literature is largely anecdotal or limited to case series, and techniques are highly dependent on premorbid anatomy.

For malignant gliomas, the major limitation is absence of phase III trials demonstrating treatment benefit for malignant gliomas. While small phase I and II trials with newer chemotherapeutic agents are promising, the degree of variability owing to their uptake properties, adverse effect profiles, dosing regimens, as well as the various blood–brain barrier adjuncts being employed in these studies has likely hindered large-scale phase III trials. Heterogeneity of the treatment population in their age, histology, and prior treatment history also limits the generalizability of early trials. Finally, because of the idiosyncratic techniques for catheterization, tumor vascularity, and flow dynamics, large-scale trial design may not lend itself to true randomization and conformity of treatment.

While phase III trials have shown benefit of IAC in the treatment of SCC of the head and neck, these results are limited to the oropharyngeal and oral cavity subset. Like malignant gliomas, evidence suffers from similar issues of treatment and patient population heterogeneity.

22.4 Level of Evidence

IAC versus current standard of care for gliomas: Phase III does not support nitrosourea or early platinum-based chemotherapeutic agents in newly diagnosed malignant gliomas. Phase III trial does not support IA cisplatin for recurrent malignant gliomas (Class III; Level of Evidence A).

IAC versus current standard of care for high-grade head and neck SCCs: Early phase III trials demonstrated survival benefit when comparing IAC and radiation with radiation alone for oral cavity and oropharyngeal cancers, but not in other regions of the head and neck (Class IIA; Level of Evidence A).

Later phase III trial comparing high-dose super-selective IAC and radiation therapy with chemoradiation did not demonstrate IAC survival benefit for high-grade head and neck SCCs (Class III; Level of Evidence B).

IAC versus current standard of care for lacrimal gland ACC, intracranial metastases, and primary CNS lymphoma are limited to case reports (Class IIB; Level of Evidence C).

22.5 Landmark Papers

Kochii M, Kitamura I, Goto T, et al. Randomized comparison of intra-arterial versus intravenous infusion of ACNU for newly diagnosed patients with glioblastoma. J Neurooncol. 2000;49(1): 63–70.

Imbesi F, Marchioni E, Benericetti E, et al. A randomized phase III study: Comparison between intravenous and intraarterial AC-NU administration in newly diagnosed primary glioblastomas. Anticancer Res. 2006;26(1B):553–558.

Shapiro WR, Green SB, Burger PC, et al. A randomized comparison of intra-arterial versus intravenous BCNU, with or without intravenous 5-fluorouracil, for newly diagnosed patients with malignant glioma. J Neurosurg. 1992;76(5):772–781.

Silvani A, Eoli M, Salmaggi A, Erbetta A, Fariselli L, Boiardi A. Intra-arterial ACNU and carboplatin versus intravenous chemotherapy with cisplatin and BCNU in newly diagnosed patients with glioblastoma. Neurol Sci. 2002;23(5):219–224.

The four RCTs in the literature for IAC are related to the treatment of newly diagnosed glioblastoma multiforme.[19,20,21,22] But these were performed with nitrosourea agents that are no longer considered the standard of care, which currently are temozolomide and adjuvant radiation for newly diagnosed tumors and IV bevacizumab for recurrent GBM.[17,54] For recurrent tumors, Hiesiger reported no survival benefit for IA versus IV chemotherapy.[25] The current status of IAC literature for malignant gliomas with newer chemotherapy agents is limited to case series and phase I and II clinical trials.[12]

For the treatment of lacrimal gland ACC, primary CNS lymphoma, DIPG, aggressive oligodendrogliomas, recurrent and primary SCCs of the head and neck, current evidence is limited to case series and case–control studies. No RCTs and no landmark papers have been published to date.

22.6 Recommendations

Given the tumor stage with infiltrative growth, adjuvant IAC may be pursued to decrease local tumor burden. Depending on the response, the stage of the tumor may be downgraded sufficiently to warrant complete resection or eye-sparing surgery with radiotherapy.

22.7 Summary

1. IAC is an attractive treatment strategy but has not yet attained footing as an element in the standard of care of intracranial or head and neck malignancies outside of retinoblastoma.
2. Experimental applications include: ACC of the head and neck, high-grade SCCs of the head and neck, high-grade astrocytomas and oligodendrogliomas, intracranial lymphoma, and progressive DIPG but results of these treatments are limited to enrollment in clinical trials and are not available as first-line treatment in the absence of level I evidence.
3. Advances in catheter navigability and manipulation of the blood–brain barrier are promising in the development of novel IAC applications.

References

[1] Kokemueller H, Eckardt A, Brachvogel P, Hausamen JE. Adenoid cystic carcinoma of the head and neck: a 20 years experience. Int J Oral Maxillofac Surg. 2004; 33(1):25–31

[2] Dodd RL, Slevin NJ. Salivary gland adenoid cystic carcinoma: a review of chemotherapy and molecular therapies. Oral Oncol. 2006; 42(8):759–769

[3] Henderson JW. Past, present, and future surgical management of malignant epithelial neoplasms of the lacrimal gland. Br J Ophthalmol. 1986; 70(10): 727–731

[4] Polito E, Leccisotti A. Epithelial malignancies of the lacrimal gland: survival rates after extensive and conservative therapy. Ann Ophthalmol. 1993; 25 (11):422–426

[5] Wright JE, Rose GE, Garner A. Primary malignant neoplasms of the lacrimal gland. Br J Ophthalmol. 1992; 76(7):401–407

[6] Scheel JV, Schilling V, Kastenbauer E, Knöbber D, Böhringer W. Intra-arterial cisplatin and sequential radiotherapy. Long-term follow-up. Laryngorhinootologie. 1996; 75(1):38–42

[7] Meldrum ML, Tse DT, Benedetto P. Neoadjuvant intracarotid chemotherapy for treatment of advanced adenocystic carcinoma of the lacrimal gland. Arch Ophthalmol. 1998; 116(3):315–321

[8] Tse DT, Kossler AL, Feuer WJ, Benedetto PW. Long-term outcomes of neoadjuvant intra-arterial cytoreductive chemotherapy for lacrimal gland adenoid cystic carcinoma. Ophthalmology. 2013; 120(7):1313–1323

[9] Jang SY, Kim DJ, Kim CY, Wu CZ, Yoon JS, Lee SY. Neoadjuvant intra-arterial chemotherapy in patients with primary lacrimal adenoid cystic carcinoma. Cancer Imaging. 2014; 14:19

[10] Noh JM, Lee E, Ahn YC, et al. Clinical significance of post-surgical residual tumor burden and radiation therapy in treating patients with lacrimal adenoid cystic carcinoma. Oncotarget. 2016; 7(37):60639–60646

[11] Woo KI, Kim YD, Sa HS, Esmaeli B. Current treatment of lacrimal gland carcinoma. Curr Opin Ophthalmol. 2016; 27(5):449–456

[12] Newton HB. Intra-arterial chemotherapy of primary brain tumors. Curr Treat Options Oncol. 2005; 6(6):519–530

[13] Stupp R, Mason WP, van den Bent MJ, et al. European Organisation for Research and Treatment of Cancer Brain Tumor and Radiotherapy Groups, National Cancer Institute of Canada Clinical Trials Group. Radiotherapy plus concomitant and adjuvant temozolomide for glioblastoma. N Engl J Med. 2005; 352(10):987–996

[14] Hegi ME, Diserens AC, Gorlia T, et al. MGMT gene silencing and benefit from temozolomide in glioblastoma. N Engl J Med. 2005; 352(10):997–1003

[15] Andratschke N, Grosu AL, Molls M, Nieder C. Perspectives in the treatment of malignant gliomas in adults. Anticancer Res. 2001; 21(5):3541–3550

[16] Lefranc F, Rynkowski M, DeWitte O, Kiss R. Present and potential future adjuvant issues in high-grade astrocytic glioma treatment. Adv Tech Stand Neurosurg. 2009; 34:3–35

[17] Stupp R, Hegi ME, Mason WP, et al. European Organisation for Research and Treatment of Cancer Brain Tumour and Radiation Oncology Groups, National Cancer Institute of Canada Clinical Trials Group. Effects of radiotherapy with concomitant and adjuvant temozolomide versus radiotherapy alone on survival in glioblastoma in a randomised phase III study: 5-year analysis of the EORTC-NCIC trial. Lancet Oncol. 2009; 10(5):459–466

[18] Gobin YP, Cloughesy TF, Chow KL, et al. Intraarterial chemotherapy for brain tumors by using a spatial dose fractionation algorithm and pulsatile delivery. Radiology. 2001; 218(3):724–732

[19] Kochii M, Kitamura I, Goto T, et al. Randomized comparison of intra-arterial versus intravenous infusion of ACNU for newly diagnosed patients with glioblastoma. J Neurooncol. 2000; 49(1):63–70

[20] Imbesi F, Marchioni E, Benericetti E, et al. A randomized phase III study: comparison between intravenous and intraarterial ACNU administration in newly diagnosed primary glioblastomas. Anticancer Res. 2006; 26 1B:553–558

[21] Shapiro WR, Green SB, Burger PC, et al. A randomized comparison of intra-arterial versus intravenous BCNU, with or without intravenous 5-fluorouracil, for newly diagnosed patients with malignant glioma. J Neurosurg. 1992; 76(5):772–781

[22] Silvani A, Eoli M, Salmaggi A, Erbetta A, Fariselli L, Boiardi A. Intra-arterial ACNU and carboplatin versus intravenous chemotherapy with cisplatin and BCNU in newly diagnosed patients with glioblastoma. Neurol Sci. 2002; 23(5): 219–224

[23] Ellis JA, Banu M, Hossain SS, et al. Reassessing the role of intra-arterial drug delivery for glioblastoma multiforme treatment. J Drug Deliv. 2015; 2015:405735

[24] Nieder C, Adam M, Molls M, Grosu AL. Therapeutic options for recurrent high-grade glioma in adult patients: recent advances. Crit Rev Oncol Hematol. 2006; 60(3):181–193

[25] Hiesiger EM, Green SB, Shapiro WR, et al. Results of a randomized trial comparing intra-arterial cisplatin and intravenous PCNU for the treatment of primary brain tumors in adults: Brain Tumor Cooperative Group trial 8420A. J Neurooncol. 1995; 25(2):143–154

[26] Doolittle ND, Muldoon LL, Culp AY, Neuwelt EA. Delivery of chemotherapeutics across the blood-brain barrier: challenges and advances. Adv Pharmacol. 2014; 71:203–243

[27] Iaccarino C, Orlandi E, Ruggeri F, et al. Prognostic value of MGMT promoter status in non-resectable glioblastoma after adjuvant therapy. Clin Neurol Neurosurg. 2015; 132:1–8

[28] Wang Y, Chen X, Zhang Z, et al. Comparison of the clinical efficacy of temozolomide (TMZ) versus nimustine (ACNU)-based chemotherapy in newly diagnosed glioblastoma. Neurosurg Rev. 2014; 37(1):73–78

[29] Salminen E, Nuutinen JM, Huhtala S. Multivariate analysis of prognostic factors in 106 patients with malignant glioma. Eur J Cancer. 1996; 32A(11):1918–1923

[30] Chow KL, Gobin YP, Cloughesy T, Sayre JW, Villablanca JP, Viñuela F. Prognostic factors in recurrent glioblastoma multiforme and anaplastic astrocytoma treated with selective intra-arterial chemotherapy. AJNR Am J Neuroradiol. 2000; 21(3):471–478

[31] Leon SP, Folkerth RD, Black PM. Microvessel density is a prognostic indicator for patients with astroglial brain tumors. Cancer. 1996; 77(2):362–372

[32] Brem S. The role of vascular proliferation in the growth of brain tumors. Clin Neurosurg. 1976; 23:440–453

[33] Yohay K, Wolf DS, Aronson LJ, Duus M, Melhem ER, Cohen KJ. Vascular distribution of glioblastoma multiforme at diagnosis. Interv Neuroradiol. 2013; 19(1):127–131

[34] Boockvar JA, Tsiouris AJ, Hofstetter CP, et al. Safety and maximum tolerated dose of superselective intraarterial cerebral infusion of bevacizumab after osmotic blood-brain barrier disruption for recurrent malignant glioma. Clinical article. J Neurosurg. 2011; 114(3):624–632

[35] Burkhardt JK, Riina H, Shin BJ, et al. Intra-arterial delivery of bevacizumab after blood-brain barrier disruption for the treatment of recurrent glioblastoma: progression-free survival and overall survival. World Neurosurg. 2012; 77(1):130–134

[36] Qureshi AI, Suri MF, Khan J, et al. Superselective intra-arterial carboplatin for treatment of intracranial neoplasms: experience in 100 procedures. J Neurooncol. 2001; 51(2):151–158

[37] Friedman HS, Prados MD, Wen PY, et al. Bevacizumab alone and in combination with irinotecan in recurrent glioblastoma. J Clin Oncol. 2009; 27(28):4733–4740

[38] Kreisl TN, Kim L, Moore K, et al. Phase II trial of single-agent bevacizumab followed by bevacizumab plus irinotecan at tumor progression in recurrent glioblastoma. J Clin Oncol. 2009; 27(5):740–745

[39] Wolpert SM, Kwan ES, Heros D, Kasdon DL, Hedges TR, III. Selective delivery of chemotherapeutic agents with a new catheter system. Radiology. 1988; 166(2):547–549

[40] Liebner S, Fischmann A, Rascher G, et al. Claudin-1 and claudin-5 expression and tight junction morphology are altered in blood vessels of human glioblastoma multiforme. Acta Neuropathol. 2000; 100(3):323–331

[41] Jahnke K, Muldoon LL, Varallyay CG, et al. Efficacy and MRI of rituximab and methotrexate treatment in a nude rat model of CNS lymphoma. Neuro-oncol. 2009; 11(5):503–513

[42] Rapoport SI, Robinson PJ. Tight-junctional modification as the basis of osmotic opening of the blood-brain barrier. Ann N Y Acad Sci. 1986; 481:250–267

[43] Jackson S, Weingart J, Nduom EK, et al. The effect of an adenosine A2A agonist on intra-tumoral concentrations of temozolomide in patients with recurrent glioblastoma. Fluids Barriers CNS. 2018; 15(1):2–17

[44] Saris SC, Shook DR, Blasberg RG, et al. Carotid artery mixing with diastole-phased pulsed drug infusion. J Neurosurg. 1987; 67(5):721–725

[45] Saris SC, Blasberg RG, Carson RE, et al. Intravascular streaming during carotid artery infusions: demonstration in humans and reduction using diastole-phased pulsatile administration. J Neurosurg. 1991; 74(5):763–772

[46] Lutz RJ, Dedrick RL, Boretos JW, Oldfield EH, Blacklock JB, Doppman JL. Mixing studies during intracarotid artery infusions in an in vitro model. J Neurosurg. 1986; 64(2):277–283

[47] Dedrick RL. Arterial drug infusion: pharmacokinetic problems and pitfalls. J Natl Cancer Inst. 1988; 80(2):84–89

[48] Jain RK, di Tomaso E, Duda DG, Loeffler JS, Sorensen AG, Batchelor TT. Angiogenesis in brain tumours. Nat Rev Neurosci. 2007; 8(8):610–622

[49] Geer CP, Grossman SA. Interstitial fluid flow along white matter tracts: a potentially important mechanism for the dissemination of primary brain tumors. J Neurooncol. 1997; 32(3):193–201

[50] Vogelbaum MA, Iannotti CA. Convection-enhanced delivery of therapeutic agents into the brain. Handb Clin Neurol. 2012; 104:355–362

[51] Kunwar S, Chang S, Westphal M, et al. PRECISE Study Group. Phase III randomized trial of CED of IL13-PE38QQR vs Gliadel wafers for recurrent glioblastoma. Neuro-oncol. 2010; 12(8):871–881

[52] Riina HA, Knopman J, Greenfield JP, et al. Balloon-assisted superselective intra-arterial cerebral infusion of bevacizumab for malignant brainstem glioma: a technical note. Interv Neuroradiol. 2010; 16(1):71–76

[53] Riina HA, Fraser JF, Fralin S, Knopman J, Scheff RJ, Boockvar JA. Superselective intraarterial cerebral infusion of bevacizumab: a revival of interventional neuro-oncology for malignant glioma. J Exp Ther Oncol. 2009; 8(2):145–150

[54] Cohen K, Jones A, Raabe E, Pearl M. Highly selective intra-arterial chemotherapy for the treatment of progressive diffuse intrinsic pontine gliomas (DIPG). Neuro-oncol. 2014; 16 Suppl 3:iii29

[55] Watne K, Hager B. Treatment of recurrent esthesioneuroblastoma with combined intra-arterial chemotherapy: a case report. J Neurooncol. 1987; 5(1):47–50

[56] Guillaume DJ, Doolittle ND, Gahramanov S, Hedrick NA, Delashaw JB, Neuwelt EA. Intra-arterial chemotherapy with osmotic blood-brain barrier disruption for aggressive oligodendroglial tumors: results of a phase I study. Neurosurgery. 2010; 66(1):48–58, discussion 58

[57] Jahnke K, Kraemer DF, Knight KR, et al. Intraarterial chemotherapy and osmotic blood-brain barrier disruption for patients with embryonal and germ cell tumors of the central nervous system. Cancer. 2008; 112(3):581–588

[58] Hansen J. Why Aussies are heading to Mexico for brain cancer treatment. Daily Telegraph. https://www.dailytelegraph.com.au/news/nsw/why-aussies-are-heading-to-mexico-for-brain-cancer-treatment/news-story/eb0980e81d0edbab2bcafdb4d1d9bc01. Updated 2018. Accessed May 28, 2018

[59] Ostrom QT, Gittleman H, Liao P, et al. CBTRUS Statistical Report: Primary brain and other central nervous system tumors diagnosed in the United States in 2010–2014. Neuro-oncol. 2017; 19 suppl_5:v1–v88

[60] Shah GD, Yahalom J, Correa DD, et al. Combined immunochemotherapy with reduced whole-brain radiotherapy for newly diagnosed primary CNS lymphoma. J Clin Oncol. 2007; 25(30):4730–4735

[61] Dahlborg SA, Henner WD, Crossen JR, et al. Non-AIDS primary CNS lymphoma: first example of a durable response in a primary brain tumor using enhanced chemotherapy delivery without cognitive loss and without radiotherapy. Cancer J Sci Am. 1996; 2(3):166–174

[62] Siegal T, Zylber-Katz E. Strategies for increasing drug delivery to the brain: focus on brain lymphoma. Clin Pharmacokinet. 2002; 41(3):171–186

[63] Ponzoni M, Issa S, Batchelor TT, Rubenstein JL. Beyond high-dose methotrexate and brain radiotherapy: novel targets and agents for primary CNS lymphoma. Ann Oncol. 2014; 25(2):316–322

[64] Karathanasis E, Ghaghada KB. Crossing the barrier: treatment of brain tumors using nanochain particles. Wiley Interdiscip Rev Nanomed Nanobiotechnol. 2016; 8(5):678–695

[65] Angelov L, Doolittle ND, Kraemer DF, et al. Blood-brain barrier disruption and intra-arterial methotrexate-based therapy for newly diagnosed primary CNS lymphoma: a multi-institutional experience. J Clin Oncol. 2009; 27(21):3503–3509

[66] Fortin D, Desjardins A, Benko A, Niyonsega T, Boudrias M. Enhanced chemotherapy delivery by intraarterial infusion and blood-brain barrier disruption in malignant brain tumors: the Sherbrooke experience. Cancer. 2005; 103(12):2606–2615

[67] Sonoda Y, Matsumoto K, Kakuto Y, et al. Primary CNS lymphoma treated with combined intra-arterial ACNU and radiotherapy. Acta Neurochir (Wien). 2007; 149(11):1183–1189, discussion 1189

[68] Doolittle ND, Miner ME, Hall WA, et al. Safety and efficacy of a multicenter study using intraarterial chemotherapy in conjunction with osmotic opening of the blood-brain barrier for the treatment of patients with malignant brain tumors. Cancer. 2000; 88(3):637–647

[69] Newton HB. Primary brain tumors: review of etiology, diagnosis and treatment. Am Fam Physician. 1994; 49(4):787–797

[70] Cascino TL, Byrne TN, Deck MD, Posner JB. Intra-arterial BCNU in the treatment of metastatic brain tumors. J Neurooncol. 1983; 1(3):211–218

[71] Madajewicz S, West CR, Park HC, et al. Phase II study: intra-arterial BCNU therapy for metastatic brain tumors. Cancer. 1981; 47(4):653–657

[72] Yamada K, Bremer AM, West CR, Ghoorah J, Park HC, Takita H. Intra-arterial BCNU therapy in the treatment of metastatic brain tumor from lung carcinoma: a preliminary report. Cancer. 1979; 44(6):2000–2007

[73] Stewart DJ, Grahovac Z, Russel NA, et al. Phase I study of intracarotid PCNU. J Neurooncol. 1987; 5(3):245–250

[74] Feun LG, Wallace S, Stewart DJ, et al. Intracarotid infusion of cis-diamminedichloroplatinum in the treatment of recurrent malignant brain tumors. Cancer. 1984; 54(5):794–799

[75] Lehane DE, Bryan RN, Horowitz B, et al. Intraarterial cis-platinum chemotherapy for patients with primary and metastatic brain tumors. Cancer Drug Deliv. 1983; 1(1):69–77

[76] Feun LG, Lee YY, Yung WK, Savaraj N, Wallace S. Intracarotid VP-16 in malignant brain tumors. J Neurooncol. 1987; 4(4):397–401

[77] Madajewicz S, Chowhan N, Iliya A, et al. Intracarotid chemotherapy with etoposide and cisplatin for malignant brain tumors. Cancer. 1991; 67(11): 2844–2849

[78] Stewart DJ, Grahovac Z, Benoit B, et al. Intracarotid chemotherapy with a combination of 1,3-bis(2-chloroethyl)-1-nitrosourea (BCNU), cis-diaminedichloroplatinum (cisplatin), and 4'-O-demethyl-1-O-(4,6-O-2-thenylidenebeta-D-glucopyranosyl) epipodophyllotoxin (VM-26) in the treatment of primary and metastatic brain tumors. Neurosurgery. 1984; 15(6):828–833

[79] Newton HB, Slivka MA, Volpi C, et al. Intra-arterial carboplatin and intravenous etoposide for the treatment of metastatic brain tumors. J Neurooncol. 2003; 61(1):35–44

[80] Fortin D, Gendron C, Boudrias M, Garant MP. Enhanced chemotherapy delivery by intraarterial infusion and blood-brain barrier disruption in the treatment of cerebral metastasis. Cancer. 2007; 109(4):751–760

[81] Gaspar L, Scott C, Rotman M, et al. Recursive partitioning analysis (RPA) of prognostic factors in three Radiation Therapy Oncology Group (RTOG) brain metastases trials. Int J Radiat Oncol Biol Phys. 1997; 37(4):745–751

[82] Mehanna H, Beech T, Nicholson T, et al. Prevalence of human papillomavirus in oropharyngeal and nonoropharyngeal head and neck cancer: systematic review and meta-analysis of trends by time and region. Head Neck. 2013; 35(5):747–755

[83] Wang MB, Liu IY, Gornbein JA, Nguyen CT. HPV-positive oropharyngeal carcinoma: a systematic review of treatment and prognosis. Otolaryngol Head Neck Surg. 2015; 153(5):758–769

[84] Homma A, Onimaru R, Matsuura K, Robbins KT, Fujii M. Intra-arterial chemoradiotherapy for head and neck cancer. Jpn J Clin Oncol. 2016; 46(1): 4–12

[85] Shah JP, Gil Z. Current concepts in management of oral cancer: surgery. Oral Oncol. 2009; 45(4–5):394–401

[86] Domenge C, Hill C, Lefebvre JL, et al. French Groupe d'Etude des Tumeurs de la Tête et du Cou (GETTEC). Randomized trial of neoadjuvant chemotherapy in oropharyngeal carcinoma. French Groupe d'Etude des Tumeurs de la Tête et du Cou (GETTEC). Br J Cancer. 2000; 83(12):1594–1598

[87] Lefebvre JL, Chevalier D, Luboinski B, Kirkpatrick A, Collette L, Sahmoud T, EORTC Head and Neck Cancer Cooperative Group. Larynx preservation in pyriform sinus cancer: preliminary results of a European Organization for Research and Treatment of Cancer phase III trial. J Natl Cancer Inst. 1996; 88(13):890–899

[88] Furness S, Glenny AM, Worthington HV, et al. Interventions for the treatment of oral cavity and oropharyngeal cancer: chemotherapy. Cochrane Database Syst Rev. 2011(4):CD006386

[89] Arcangeli G, Nervi C, Righini R, Creton G, Mirri MA, Guerra A. Combined radiation and drugs: the effect of intra-arterial chemotherapy followed by radiotherapy in head and neck cancer. Radiother Oncol. 1983; 1(2):101–107

[90] Richard JM, Sancho H, Lepintre Y, Rodary J, Pierquin B. Intra-arterial methotrexate chemotherapy and telecobalt therapy in cancer of the oral cavity and oropharynx. Cancer. 1974; 34(3):491–496

[91] Lee YY, Dimery IW, Van Tassel P, De Pena C, Blacklock JB, Goepfert H. Superselective intra-arterial chemotherapy of advanced paranasal sinus tumors. Arch Otolaryngol Head Neck Surg. 1989; 115(4):503–511

[92] Claudio F, Cacace F, Comella G, et al. Intraarterial chemotherapy through carotid transposition in advanced head and neck cancer. Cancer. 1990; 65(7): 1465–1471

[93] Simunek A, Krajina A, Hlava A. Selective intraarterial chemotherapy of tumors in the lingual artery territory by a new approach. Cardiovasc Intervent Radiol. 1993; 16(6):392–395

[94] Sulfaro S, Frustaci S, Volpe R, et al. A pathologic assessment of tumor residue and stromal changes after intraarterial chemotherapy for head and neck carcinomas: a study on serial sections of the whole surgical specimen. Cancer. 1989; 64(5):994–1001

[95] Hollmann K, Mailath G, Rasse M, Kühlböck J, Stadler B. Regional chemotherapy of inoperable maxillofacial tumours combined with radiotherapy: long-term results. J Craniomaxillofac Surg. 1990; 18(2):88–90

[96] Andreasson L, Biörklund A, Mercke C, et al. Intra-arterial mitomycin C and intravenous bleomycin as induction chemotherapy in advanced head and neck cancer: a phase II study. Radiother Oncol. 1986; 7(1):37–45

[97] Cheung DK, Regan J, Savin M, Gibberman V, Woessner W. A pilot study of intraarterial chemotherapy with cisplatin in locally advanced head and neck cancers. Cancer. 1988; 61(5):903–908

[98] Frustaci S, Barzan L, Tumolo S, et al. Intra-arterial continuous infusion of cis-diamminedichloroplatinum in untreated head and neck cancer patients. Cancer. 1986; 57(6):1118–1123

[99] Richard JM, Kramar A, Molinari R, et al. Randomised EORTC head and neck cooperative group trial of preoperative intra-arterial chemotherapy in oral cavity and oropharynx carcinoma. Eur J Cancer. 1991; 27(7):821–827

[100] Hattori T, Hirano T, Toyoda S, Nakagawa T, Yamaguchi N, Sakakura Y. Superselective continuous intra-arterial infusion therapy via superficial temporal artery for head and neck tumors. Nippon Igaku Hoshasen Gakkai Zasshi. 1985; 45(7):1056–1058

[101] Imai S, Kajihara Y, Munemori O, et al. Superselective cisplatin (CDDP)-carboplatin (CBDCA) combined infusion for head and neck cancers. Eur J Radiol. 1995; 21(2):94–99

[102] Korogi Y, Hirai T, Nishimura R, et al. Superselective intraarterial infusion of cisplatin for squamous cell carcinoma of the mouth: preliminary clinical experience. AJR Am J Roentgenol. 1995; 165(5):1269–1272

[103] Rohde S, Kovács AF, Turowski B, Yan B, Zanella F, Berkefeld J. Intra-arterial high-dose chemotherapy with cisplatin as part of a palliative treatment concept in oral cancer. AJNR Am J Neuroradiol. 2005; 26(7):1804–1809

[104] Damascelli B, Cantù G, Mattavelli F, et al. Intraarterial chemotherapy with polyoxyethylated castor oil free paclitaxel, incorporated in albumin nanoparticles (ABI-007): Phase I study of patients with squamous cell carcinoma of the head and neck and anal canal: preliminary evidence of clinical activity. Cancer. 2001; 92(10):2592–2602

[105] Robbins KT, Kumar P, Wong FS, et al. Targeted chemoradiation for advanced head and neck cancer: analysis of 213 patients. Head Neck. 2000; 22(7): 687–693

[106] Robbins KT, Kumar P, Harris J, et al. Supradose intra-arterial cisplatin and concurrent radiation therapy for the treatment of stage IV head and neck squamous cell carcinoma is feasible and efficacious in a multi-institutional setting: results of Radiation Therapy Oncology Group Trial 9615. J Clin Oncol. 2005; 23(7):1447–1454

[107] Kobayashi W, Teh BG, Sakaki H, et al. Superselective intra-arterial chemoradiotherapy with docetaxel-nedaplatin for advanced oral cancer. Oral Oncol. 2010; 46(12):860–863

[108] Kerber CW, Wong WH, Howell SB, Hanchett K, Robbins KT. An organ-preserving selective arterial chemotherapy strategy for head and neck cancer. AJNR Am J Neuroradiol. 1998; 19(5):935–941

[109] Samant S, Robbins KT, Kumar P, Ma JZ, Vieira F, Hanchett C. Bone or cartilage invasion by advanced head and neck cancer: intra-arterial supradose cisplatin chemotherapy and concomitant radiotherapy for organ preservation. Arch Otolaryngol Head Neck Surg. 2001; 127(12):1451–1456

[110] Hayashi Y, Mitsudo K, Sakuma K, et al. Clinical outcomes of retrograde intra-arterial chemotherapy concurrent with radiotherapy for elderly oral squamous cell carcinoma patients aged over 80 years old. Radiat Oncol. 2017; 12(1):112

[111] Furusawa J, Homma A, Onimaru R, et al. Indications for superselective intra-arterial cisplatin infusion and concomitant radiotherapy in cases of hypopharyngeal cancer. Auris Nasus Larynx. 2015; 42(6):443–448

[112] Robbins KT, Storniolo AM, Kerber C, Seagren S, Berson A, Howell SB. Rapid superselective high-dose cisplatin infusion for advanced head and neck malignancies. Head Neck. 1992; 14(5):364–371

[113] Yokoyama J, Ohba S, Fujimaki M, Kojima M, Suzuki M, Ikeda K. Significant improvement in superselective intra-arterial chemotherapy for advanced paranasal sinus cancer by using indocyanine green fluorescence. Eur Arch Otorhinolaryngol. 2014; 271(10):2795–2801

[114] Yabuuchi H, Kuroiwa T, Tajima T, Tomita K, Ochiai N, Kawamoto K. Efficacy of intra-arterial infusion therapy using a combination of cisplatin and docetaxel for recurrent head and neck cancers compared with cisplatin alone. Clin Oncol (R Coll Radiol). 2003; 15(8):467–472

[115] Boockvar JA. Super-selective intraarterial infusion of cetuximab (erbitux) with or without radiation therapy for the treatment of unresectable

22

recurrent squamous cell carcinoma of the head and neck. https://clinical-trials.gov/ct2/show/NCT02438995?term=boockvar&rank=3

[116] Rasch CR, Hauptmann M, Schornagel J, et al. Intra-arterial versus intravenous chemoradiation for advanced head and neck cancer: results of a randomized phase 3 trial. Cancer. 2010; 116(9):2159–2165

[117] Heukelom J, Lopez-Yurda M, Balm AJ, et al. Late follow-up of the randomized radiation and concomitant high-dose intra-arterial or intravenous cisplatin (RADPLAT) trial for advanced head and neck cancer. Head Neck. 2016; 38 Suppl 1:E488–E493

[118] Nishino H, Takanosawa M, Kawada K, et al. Multidisciplinary therapy consisting of minimally invasive resection, irradiation, and intra-arterial infusion of 5-fluorouracil for maxillary sinus carcinomas. Head Neck. 2013; 35(6): 772–778

[119] Fortin D. Intra-arterial chemotherapy in the treatment of primary brain tumors. 2017

[120] Nakagawa H, Fujita T, Kubo S, et al. Selective intra-arterial chemotherapy with a combination of etoposide and cisplatin for malignant gliomas: preliminary report. Surg Neurol. 1994; 41(1):19–27

[121] Rogers LR, Purvis JB, Lederman RJ, et al. Alternating sequential intracarotid BCNU and cisplatin in recurrent malignant glioma. Cancer. 1991; 68(1):15–21

[122] Doolittle ND, Muldoon LL, Brummett RE, et al. Delayed sodium thiosulfate as an otoprotectant against carboplatin-induced hearing loss in patients with malignant brain tumors. Clin Cancer Res. 2001; 7(3):493–500

[123] Dósa E, Heltai K, Radovits T, et al. Dose escalation study of intravenous and intra-arterial N-acetylcysteine for the prevention of oto- and nephrotoxicity of cisplatin with a contrast-induced nephropathy model in patients with renal insufficiency. Fluids Barriers CNS. 2017; 14(1):26

[124] Clocchlatti L, Cartei G, Lavaroni A, et al. Intra-arterial chemotherapy with carboplatin (CBDCA) and vepesid (VP16) in primary malignant brain tumours: preliminary findings. Interv Neuroradiol. 1996; 2(4):277–281

[125] Kies MS, Haraf DJ, Athanasiadis I, et al. Induction chemotherapy followed by concurrent chemoradiation for advanced head and neck cancer: improved disease control and survival. J Clin Oncol. 1998; 16(8):2715–2721

[126] Rosen F, Vokes EE, Lad T, et al. Phase II study of amonafide in the treatment of patients with advanced squamous cell carcinoma of the head and the neck. An Illinois Cancer Center study. Invest New Drugs. 1995; 13(3):249–252

[127] Vokes EE, Kies M, Haraf DJ, et al. Induction chemotherapy followed by concomitant chemoradiotherapy for advanced head and neck cancer: impact on the natural history of the disease. J Clin Oncol. 1995; 13(4):876–883

22

23 Spinal Metastases Embolization

Andrew S. Griffin and L. Fernando Gonzalez

Abstract

Preoperative transarterial embolization of metastatic spinal tumors is routinely performed for hypervascular tumors to reduce intraoperative blood loss. The data on efficacy of preoperative embolization is somewhat limited due to mostly small, retrospective series. In this chapter we review the available literature and highlight some of the key studies to try and better understand the utility of preoperative embolization for spinal metastases.

Keywords: spinal metastases, spinal neoplasms, transarterial embolization, spinal angiography, intraoperative bleeding

23.1 Goals

1. Review the indications, technique, and complications of transarterial embolization of spinal tumors in the setting of a case example.
2. Analyze the literature evaluating the efficacy of preoperative embolization of spinal metastases in reducing intraoperative blood loss during tumor resection surgery.
3. Review other factors that may influence success of transarterial embolization such as degree of embolization,

timing of surgery following embolization, and tumoral histology.

23.2 Case Example

23.2.1 History of Present Illness

A 51-year-old male with a history of renal cell carcinoma presented with 6 months of progressive back pain. He denied any neurologic symptoms including loss of bowel or bladder function, weakness, numbness, or paresthesias. He underwent a CT and MRI which demonstrated a pathologic fracture of the L1 vertebral body.

Past medical history: Renal cell carcinoma diagnosed 9 months earlier, currently on chemotherapy. Prior deep venous thrombosis, not currently on anticoagulation.

Past surgical history: Prior left hydrocele repair.

Family history: Sister with colon cancer.

Social history: None.

Review of systems: As per the above.

Neurological examination: Unremarkable.

Imaging studies: See ▸ Fig. 23.1 and ▸ Fig. 23.2.

In ▸ Fig. 23.1a–d, computed tomography (CT) demonstrates a lytic lesion in the posterior vertebral body and left pedicle of

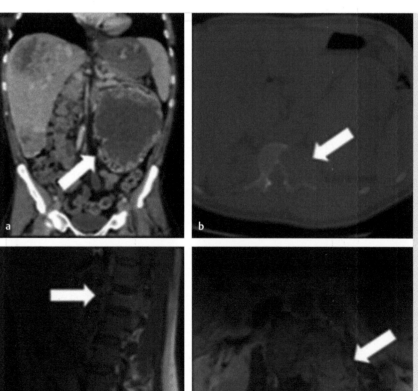

Fig. 23.1 Contrast-enhanced coronal CT image of the abdomen and pelvis demonstrates a large necrotic mass arising from the left kidney (*white arrow*, a). Axial image reformatted in bone windows from the same CT shows a lytic lesion in L1 involving the posterior vertebral body and pedicle (*white arrow*, b). Sagittal T1-weighted post-contrast MRI of the lumbar spine shows a pathologic fracture of the L1 vertebral body (*white arrow*, c). Axial T1-weighted post-contrast MRI demonstrates an enhancing mass involving the posterior left L1 vertebral body and pedicle with ventral epidural tumor extension and invasion into adjacent paraspinal soft tissues (*white arrow*, d).

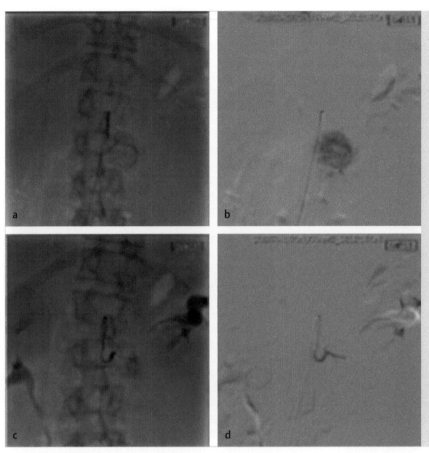

Fig. 23.2 Anteroposterior (AP) views of the spinal angiogram at the level of L1 demonstrates hypervascularity and tumoral blush in the region of the known left L1 vertebral body and pedicle metastasis (**a** and **b**). AP views of the spinal angiogram at the level of L1 postparticle and coil embolization of the L1 tumor demonstrates no residual tumoral vascularity (**c** and **d**).

the L1 vertebral body. Magnetic resonance imaging (MRI) shows the lesion is enhancing and T2 hyperintense. There is epidural tumor extension resulting in left lateral recess stenosis and severe left neural foraminal narrowing. In ▶ Fig. 23.2a–d, spinal angiogram at the level of L1 demonstrates tumoral blush of hypervascular L1 vertebral body metastasis. Follow-up spinal angiography status postparticle and coil embolization of the L1 tumor demonstrates no residual tumoral vascularity.

23.2.2 Treatment Plan

Findings are consistent with metastatic renal cell carcinoma to the lumbar spine. The patient was offered radiation therapy, radiosurgery, or surgery preceded by transarterial embolization. The patient decided to proceed with preoperative embolization and surgery.

23.2.3 Follow-up

The patient underwent complete transarterial embolization of the metastatic lesion at L1. The next day he underwent a transpedicular L1 corpectomy with cage reconstruction and T11 to L3 pedicle screw fixation and fusion. The patient tolerated the embolization and surgery well and experienced a marked improvement in his pain. His neurological status remained intact. He was restarted on chemotherapy shortly after surgery.

Unfortunately the patient already had widespread metastatic disease and succumbed to his illness 8 months later.

23.3 Case Summary

1. *What are the treatment options for this patient's spinal tumor?*
The spine is the most common site of osseous metastatic disease and affects up to 40% of cancer patients, thought to be a result of its close proximity to regional venous and lymphatic drainage pathways.[1,2] Spinal metastases can cause significant morbidity with up to 10% of patients suffering from cord compression.[3] Currently, the standard of care for treatment of spinal metastases is radiotherapy.[4] However for patients with mechanical instability or radioresistant tumors, surgery is indicated. Surgical treatment is aimed at pain control and preservation of mechanical and neurologic function.[5]

2. *What are the purposes of transarterial embolization of tumors?*
Surgery in patients with hypervascular tumors may be hazardous due to excessive blood loss. One technique for reducing intraoperative blood loss is preoperative transarterial embolization. Preoperative embolization not only reduces blood loss but may allow for more complete tumor resection and shorter intraoperative time.[6,7,8,9,10] Embolization may also be indicated in patients with unresectable tumors as it can help to reduce pain and slow growth.[11] A less common

application is in cases where a large vessel is encased within the tumor confines (i.e., vertebral artery). In order to have an en-bloc resection of the tumor, it may be necessary to deconstruct this vessel after showing patency of the contralateral vessel.

3. *What spinal tumors can be treated with transarterial embolization?*

Preoperative embolization is described for a wide variety of tumors including those known to be at high risk for intraoperative hemorrhage such as thyroid carcinoma, renal cell carcinoma, and melanoma but also for more common malignancies such as breast, prostate, and lung carcinoma.[12,13] Embolization has also been successfully used in patients with hypervascular primary bone tumors such as aneurysmal bone cysts, hemangiomas, giant cell tumors, and chordomas.[14,15,16,17]

4. *What is the technique for embolization of spinal tumors?*

Spinal arterial embolizations should be performed under general anesthesia with somatosensory-evoked potential (SSEP) monitoring. A preshaped guide catheter is used to access the corresponding bilateral segmental arteries, including two levels above and below the lesion. Angiography through the guide catheter is performed to identify tumor feeders, arterial supply to the spinal cord, and normal en passage vessels. Based on the configuration and origin of the feeder artery as well as the embolysate that will be used for the particular case, the microcatheter is selected. Once the microcatheter is in position, embolic material is delivered into the feeding pedicle.

5. *What embolic agents are available for use and what are the pros and cons of each?*

a) PVA (Polyvinyl Alcohol)

1. PVA was first introduced as an intravascular embolization agent in 1975 and is now routinely used for preoperative spinal tumor embolization.[7,10,18,19] PVA particles are formed from PVA foam sheets and are available in sizes ranging from 100 to 1,100 mm. PVA particles adhere to the vessel wall and result in slow flow, causing thrombus formation and eventual angionecrosis.[20] When using PVA, the preferred method of delivery is direction infusion into the pedicle supplying the tumor. If that vessel is unable to be catheterized and PVA must be injected from a more proximal vessel, flow control techniques can be used to direct particles into the tumor pedicle while avoiding normal branches. Post-embolization angiography is obtained immediately after embolization to evaluate for any residual angiographic blush or nontarget embolization.

b) NBCA (n-butyl cyanoacrylate)

1. NBCA is a low-viscosity cyanoacrylate glue that forms a polymer upon contact with ionic mediums such as water or blood. It is FDA approved for embolization of cerebral AVMs but is used off-label for tumor embolization.[7,21,22,23] NBCA is injected together with lipiodol under fluoroscopic guidance. NBCA is very adherent, which requires a rapid infusion time and can make the delivery difficult to control. The two main complications are nontarget embolization and catheter retention. These complications can be minimized by injecting rapidly and flushing the catheter with a nonheparinized 5% dextrose solution, which is nonionic and delays polymerization of NBCA within the catheter tip upon contact with blood or saline.[24]

c) Onyx

1. Onyx is a liquid embolic agent that has been successfully used for preoperative spinal tumor embolization.[13,25,26] It is composed of a polymer (ethylene-vinyl alcohol) dissolved in dimethyl sulfoxide (DMSO) that forms a cast within vessels upon contact with blood. It is a useful alternative to PVA when the tumor pedicle is close to the anterior spinal artery, and there is a risk of nontarget particle embolization. Onyx is available in two formulations (Onyx 18 and Onyx 34). Onyx 34 is higher viscosity and used primarily for high flow lesions such as AV malformations. The Onyx 18 formulation is used for tumor embolization because the lower viscosity results in better distal vascular penetration. Onyx is prepared per the manufacturer instructions, which involves agitation of the Onyx vials for 20 minutes and priming of the dead space of the microcatheter (typically an Echelon or Marathon microcatheter) with DMSO. Onyx is subsequently injected into the microcatheter under the blank roadmap technique. A small plug often forms along the distal tip of the microcatheter, which is desirable because it prevents retrograde reflux. Unlike NBCA, Onyx is nonadhesive. This decreases the chances of gluing the microcatheter in place and allows for a slow administration that can be evaluated angiographically in real-time. Onyx is administered until the vascular pedicle is occluded.

6. *What are the potential complications of transarterial embolization?*

The most clinically significant complication of transarterial embolization in the spine is nontarget embolization, which can result in ischemia and infarction of the spinal cord.[27,28] The true incidence of this complication is not known, likely because it occurs infrequently and is underreported. To prevent this complication, superselective catheterization and vigilant inspection of the pre-embolization angiograms must be performed to avoid spinal and radiculomedullary arteries and identify any intersegmental anastomoses. The neurological status of the patient should be monitored throughout the procedure and frequent angiograms should be obtained to evaluate for nontarget flow. For cervical tumors that are supplied by branches of the vertebral arteries, vertebrobasilar strokes from nontarget embolization are a risk.[8] If the tumor pedicle cannot be selectively catheterized, flow diversion via temporary balloon occlusion of the vertebral artery can be performed to protect against nontarget embolization. Although less common since the development of hydrophilic and detachable-tip microcatheters, catheter retention remains a potential complication of transarterial embolization with liquid embolics.[29,30] For adhesives such as NBCA, there is a risk gluing the microcatheter to the vessel wall due to reflux along the microcatheter tip.[31] With the use of Onyx, the chance of catheter retention is lower since Onyx is nonadhesive. However, the microcatheter is still at risk for retention due to encasement within the Onyx cast.[32] There is no literature currently available regarding the management of retained catheters within the spine possibly related to the short distance from the guide catheter to the target site. For retained catheters within cerebral lesions, the catheters are usually retrieved endovascularly or surgically,[33,34,35] although in some cases they have been left in place without ill-effect.[31,32]

Other complications are common to all catheter angiographic procedures and include access site sequelae (groin hematoma, pseudoaneurysm, or AV fistula), radiation exposure, iodinated contrast (acute kidney injury, anaphylaxis), and vascular injury (spasm, dissection, rupture).

7. *What is the postprocedure care for embolization patients and when should surgery be performed?*

A neurological examination should be performed after the procedure to assess for any neurologic changes. Patients are admitted to the neurological intensive care unit overnight for observation and pain management. Patients undergo frequent neurological checks to monitor for any change in their neurologic status as postembolization edema may occur, resulting in myelopathy.[36,37] They are also monitored for postembolization syndrome. Although postembolization syndrome most commonly occurs after solid organ embolization, it has been reported to occur in patients treated with spinal tumor embolization.[38] It is a self-limited syndrome consisting of fever, nausea, vomiting, pain, and leukocytosis. It usually manifests within 72 hours after the procedure and resolves after a week following supportive treatment. The optimal timing of when to perform surgery after embolization is somewhat debated, but most authors advocate for surgical resection within 72 hours of the embolization procedure to prevent angiogenesis.[9,39] In cases where the spinal canal is compromised by the tumor, the embolization may worsen the local edema and compress the cord even further, ultimately requiring an earlier surgical resection.

23.4 Level of Evidence

Treatment options for metastatic spinal neoplasm: Surgery with preoperative transarterial embolization (Class IIa, Level of Evidence B).

Types of spinal metastases that are amenable to treatment with transarterial embolization: Renal cell carcinoma (Class Ia, Level of Evidence B).

Timing of surgery after embolization: The patient underwent surgery within 24 hours after the embolization procedure (Class IIb, Level of Evidence C).

Degree of embolization: Complete embolization is noninferior to partial embolization (Class IIa, Level of Evidence B).

23.5 Landmark Papers

Embolization of spinal tumors was first described in 1974 and is now common practice for patients with hypervascular tumors.[40] A number of studies have described lower rates of intraoperative hemorrhage following transarterial embolization, with some authors reporting blood loss reductions of up to 50%.[6,8,28,41] However, the literature supporting the utility of preoperative embolization remains controversial, with multiple studies showing transarterial embolization does not affect intraoperative blood loss.[42,43,44] There are a number of potential reasons for these conflicting results. Currently available studies on spinal tumor embolization are mostly retrospective reviews and case series limited by small patient cohorts and a lack of control groups. Furthermore, there is marked heterogeneity in tumor histology, tumor size, and tumor location, as well as surgical technique. The primary end point for most of the studies is intraoperative blood loss, which is challenging to measure. The volume of fluid in the suction canisters can be easily determined but is often a mix of blood and other fluids used for flushing and cleaning the operative field during the surgery. Furthermore, quantifying blood left behind in the surgical field as well as contained within surgical sponges and towels is subjective. Given all these different variables and a somewhat subjective primary end point, it is not surprising that the literature is not definitive regarding the efficacy of transarterial embolization. Two recent meta-analyses attempted to reconcile all these different findings and determined that preoperative embolization does result in decreased intraoperative blood loss for both renal cell carcinoma and mixed primary tumor groups.[45,46] However, the first prospective randomized controlled trial on the subject was recently published in 2015, and it did not show any benefit to preoperative embolization.[47] In this section, we critically analyze some of the most robust studies to date that have evaluated the efficacy of spinal tumor embolization.

Olerud C, Jónsson H Jr, Löfberg AM, Lörelius LE, Sjöström L. Embolization of spinal metastases reduces peroperative blood loss. 21 patients operated on for renal cell carcinoma. Acta Orthop Scand 1993;64(1):9–12.

Olerud et al conducted a retrospective review of 21 patients that underwent 29 surgeries for renal cell carcinoma metastases to the spine.[48] Preoperative embolization with PVA and/or gelatin sponge was performed in slightly less than half (11) of the cases. All surgeries were performed within 24 hours of the embolization procedure and surgical technique involved both anterior and posterior approaches. The primary outcome was intraoperative blood loss, which was calculated based on blood volume in suction canisters, surgical sponges, and an estimate of blood in the operating field. They reported an average blood loss of 4,300 mL among embolized patients compared to 6,200 mL in nonembolized patients.

This work was one of the earliest, well-designed studies in the preoperative spinal tumor embolization literature. They evaluated only patients with renal cell carcinoma, which eliminates potential confounding variables when evaluating heterogenous groups of patients with multiple tumor types. Renal cell carcinoma is known to be one of the most hypervascular tumors and is the most commonly included tumor type in analyses of preoperative embolization. This study also had a control group of patients that did not undergo preoperative embolization. Many prior works have not had control groups and simply compared average blood loss of a group of embolized patients to the average blood loss in the literature, but this is inaccurate as surgical and blood loss measurement techniques are variable.[7,8]

Kato, Sato Shi, et al. Preoperative embolization significantly decreases intraoperative blood loss during palliative surgery for spinal metastasis. Orthopedics 2012; 35(9): e1389–e1395.

Kato et al[49] conducted a retrospective review of 46 patients that underwent palliative surgical decompression over a decade. Preoperative embolization was performed in 23 of the

46 patients using a combination of coils, PVA, and gelatin sponge. Tumor vascularity was graded as mild, moderate, or extensive, and the degree of embolization was characterized as partial or complete. Tumor histology was variable, with lung, breast, and prostate accounting for the majority of malignancies. Surgical decompression and stabilization was performed via a posterior approach and was performed within 72 hours of the embolization procedure. There was no difference in intraoperative blood loss among patients undergoing surgery within the first 24 hours compared to those undergoing surgery within 24 to 72 hours. The average intraoperative blood loss was 520 mL in the embolization group compared to 1,128 mL in the nonembolization group ($p < 0.05$). There was a trend toward high intraoperative blood loss among the tumors with increased vascularity and among those that were incompletely embolized but the differences were not statistically significant.

This study is important because it was one of the first to evaluate efficacy of preoperative embolization among a population with heterogenous tumor histology that included a control group. The surgical approach was the same among the two groups as was the distribution of tumor histology. There was no significant difference in blood loss among the tumors that were incompletely embolized, which is line with multiple previous studies.[44,50] Often times, complete embolization is not possible because the tumor pedicle also supplies a radiculomedullary artery. This work suggests incomplete embolization is still superior to nonembolization.

Clausen C, Dahl B, Frevert SC, Hansen LV, Nielsen MB, Lönn L. Preoperative embolization in surgical treatment of spinal metastases: single-blind, randomized controlled clinical trial of efficacy in decreasing intraoperative blood loss. J Vasc Interv Radiol 2015;26(3):402–412.

Clausen et al conducted the first randomized controlled trial evaluating the efficacy of transarterial embolization in reducing intraoperative blood loss. They randomized patients with symptomatic cord compression to undergo spinal angiography with embolization ($n = 23$) or spinal angiography alone ($n = 22$) within 48 hours prior to wide laminectomy with posterior stabilization. A combination of coils, PVA, and/or gelatin sponge was used for embolization. More than 10 different tumor histologies were included, with the majority (56%) composed of patients with lung or breast cancer. The vascularity of the metastases on angiography was graded as none, moderate, or pronounced. In the embolization group, tumors with moderate or pronounced hypervascularity were embolized. The end point of the embolization was complete obliteration of all feeder arteries supplying the tumor. Patients subsequently underwent posterior decompression and fusion. The primary outcome was intraoperative blood loss, which was calculated as the volume of blood in suction containers and weight of surgical sponges. Secondary outcomes were perioperative blood loss, need for red blood cell transfusion, and surgery time. They did not find a significant difference among intraoperative blood loss or need for transfusion, although preoperative embolization did result in a 27% reduction in operative time.

While this is the first and only randomized controlled trial of preoperative transarterial embolization for spinal metastases, there are a number of limitations to this study. First, this was a small cohort of patients and the study was terminated prior to reaching its planned sample size. A subgroup analysis found that for patients with hypervascular tumors, there was a statistically significant decrease in intraoperative blood loss of 260 mL. While the authors state that this amount is not clinically significant, this represents almost 40% of the mean blood loss. The average blood loss in this study was only 676 mL, approximately one-third the average blood loss of 1,828 mL cited in a meta-analysis of surgical patients with spinal metastases.[51] The low mean blood loss in this study is likely multifactorial; patients were included in this cohort regardless of tumor vascularity, and tranexamic acid was administered preoperatively. Furthermore, the surgical technique was relatively simple with only laminectomy and posterior decompression performed. Many prior studies demonstrating lower intraoperative hemorrhage following preoperative embolization have been in the context of complex surgical techniques involving corpectomies and combined approaches.[12,28,50] Finally, only 7% of patients in this cohort had renal cell carcinoma, which is known to be one of the most hypervascular tumors.

23.6 Recommendations

As the treatment of primary cancers continues to improve, the number of patients living with spinal metastases is increasing. Surgery is part of a multimodality treatment strategy involving chemotherapy and radiation that can decrease neurological morbidity and mortality.[52] Surgery is associated with multiple potential complications including massive blood loss, particularly those involving hypervascular tumors. Preoperative tumor embolization may decrease intraoperative blood loss, facilitate surgical resection, and shorten procedure times; however, the data is controversial. This is in large part because most of the studies to date are retrospective, single-center studies composed of various embolization strategies. The timing of preoperative embolization and use of different embolics is variable across the studies, which makes it difficult to draw any definitive conclusions. A meta-analysis of preoperative embolization was conducted by Griessenauer et al in 2016.[46] They reviewed results of 1,305 patients across 37 studies, all of which were retrospective (level III evidence). Renal cell carcinoma comprised almost 50% of all cases, and complete or near complete devascularization was achieved in nearly 70% of cases (defined as at least an 80% reduction in tumor vascularity). There was no difference in efficacy among different embolic agents, and there was a trend toward decreased blood loss in the more recent studies. This is likely a combination of improved neurointerventional, radiation and minimally invasive surgical techniques. There was a low overall complication rate of 3.1%. Although the data is limited, current literature suggests preoperative embolization of spinal tumors is safe, feasible, and may aid in surgical resection. It should be considered as an adjunctive therapy, particularly for hypervascular tumors.

23.7 Summary

1. There is controversy in the literature regarding the efficacy of preoperative transarterial embolization for spinal metastases.
2. Data suggests that preoperative tumor embolization reduces blood loss in patients with hypervascular tumors such as renal cell carcinoma and shortens intraoperative time.

3. Partial embolization is superior to no embolization at all.
4. There is no high-level evidence to support transarterial embolization in patients with avascular tumors.

References

[1] Maccauro G, Spinelli MS, Mauro S, Perisano C, Graci C, Rosa MA. Physiopathology of spine metastasis. Int J Surg Oncol. 2011; 2011:107969

[2] Wong DA, Fornasier VL, MacNab I. Spinal metastases: the obvious, the occult, and the impostors. Spine. 1990; 15(1):1–4

[3] Klimo P, Jr, Schmidt MH. Surgical management of spinal metastases. Oncologist. 2004; 9(2):188–196

[4] Lutz S, Berk L, Chang E, et al. American Society for Radiation Oncology (ASTRO). Palliative radiotherapy for bone metastases: an ASTRO evidence-based guideline. Int J Radiat Oncol Biol Phys. 2011; 79(4):965–976

[5] Barzilai O, Fisher CG, Bilsky MH. State of the art treatment of spinal metastatic disease. Neurosurgery. 2018; 82(6):757–769

[6] Manke C, Bretschneider T, Lenhart M, et al. Spinal metastases from renal cell carcinoma: effect of preoperative particle embolization on intraoperative blood loss. AJNR Am J Neuroradiol. 2001; 22(5):997–1003

[7] Shi HB, Suh DC, Lee HK, et al. Preoperative transarterial embolization of spinal tumor: embolization techniques and results. AJNR Am J Neuroradiol. 1999; 20(10):2009–2015

[8] Wilson MA, Cooke DL, Ghodke B, Mirza SK. Retrospective analysis of preoperative embolization of spinal tumors. AJNR Am J Neuroradiol. 2010; 31(4): 656–660

[9] Gellad FE, Sadato N, Numaguchi Y, Levine AM. Vascular metastatic lesions of the spine: preoperative embolization. Radiology. 1990; 176(3):683–686

[10] Patsalides A, Leng LZ, Kimball D, et al. Preoperative catheter spinal angiography and embolization of cervical spinal tumors: outcomes from a single center. Interv Neuroradiol. 2016; 22(4):457–465

[11] Ozkan E, Gupta S. Embolization of spinal tumors: vascular anatomy, indications, and technique. Tech Vasc Interv Radiol. 2011; 14(3):129–140

[12] Robial N, Charles YP, Bogorin I, et al. Is preoperative embolization a prerequisite for spinal metastases surgical management? Orthop Traumatol Surg Res. 2012; 98(5):536–542

[13] Ghobrial GM, Chalouhi N, Harrop J, et al. Preoperative spinal tumor embolization: an institutional experience with Onyx. Clin Neurol Neurosurg. 2013; 115(12):2457–2463

[14] Mindea SA, Eddleman CS, Hage ZA, Batjer HH, Ondra SL, Bendok BR. Endovascular embolization of a recurrent cervical giant cell neoplasm using N-butyl 2-cyanoacrylate. J Clin Neurosci. 2009; 16(3):452–454

[15] Mavrogenis AF, Rossi G, Calabrò T, Altimari G, Rimondi E, Ruggieri P. The role of embolization for hemangiomas. Musculoskelet Surg. 2012; 96(2): 125–135

[16] Terzi S, Gasbarrini A, Fuiano M, et al. Efficacy and safety of selective arterial embolization in the treatment of aneurysmal bone cyst of the mobile spine: a retrospective observational study. Spine. 2017; 42(15):1130–1138

[17] Yang H, Zhu L, Ebraheim NA, et al. Surgical treatment of sacral chordomas combined with transcatheter arterial embolization. J Spinal Disord Tech. 2010; 23(1):47–52

[18] Breslau J, Eskridge JM. Preoperative embolization of spinal tumors. J Vasc Interv Radiol. 1995; 6(6):871–875

[19] Tadavarthy SM, Moller JH, Amplatz K. Polyvinyl alcohol (Ivalon): a new embolic material. Am J Roentgenol Radium Ther Nucl Med. 1975; 125(3): 609–616

[20] Davidson GS, Terbrugge KG. Histologic long-term follow-up after embolization with polyvinyl alcohol particles. AJNR Am J Neuroradiol. 1995; 16(4) Suppl:843–846

[21] Mattamal GJUS. US FDA perspective on the regulations of medical-grade polymers: cyanoacrylate polymer medical device tissue adhesives. Expert Rev Med Devices. 2008; 5(1):41–49

[22] Awad AW, Almefty KK, Ducruet AF, et al. The efficacy and risks of preoperative embolization of spinal tumors. J Neurointerv Surg. 2016; 8(8):859–864

[23] Rossi G, Mavrogenis AF, Rimondi E, Braccaioli L, Calabrò T, Ruggieri P. Selective embolization with N-butyl cyanoacrylate for metastatic bone disease. J Vasc Interv Radiol. 2011; 22(4):462–470

[24] Hill H, Chick JFB, Hage A, Srinivasa RN. N-butyl cyanoacrylate embolotherapy: techniques, complications, and management. Diagn Interv Radiol. 2018; 24(2): 98–103

[25] Clarençon F, Di Maria F, Cormier E, et al. Onyx injection by direct puncture for the treatment of hypervascular spinal metastases close to the anterior spinal artery: initial experience. J Neurosurg Spine. 2013; 18(6):606–610

[26] Ladner TR, He L, Lakomkin N, et al. Minimizing bleeding complications in spinal tumor surgery with preoperative Onyx embolization via dual-lumen balloon catheter. J Neurointerv Surg. 2016; 8(2):210–215

[27] Cloft HJ, Jensen ME, Do HM, Kallmes DF. Spinal cord infarction complicating embolisation of vertebral metastasis: a result of masking of a spinal artery by a high-flow lesion. Interv Neuroradiol. 1999; 5(1):61–65

[28] Berkefeld J, Scale D, Kirchner J, Heinrich T, Kollath J. Hypervascular spinal tumors: influence of the embolization technique on perioperative hemorrhage. AJNR Am J Neuroradiol. 1999; 20(5):757–763

[29] Paramasivam S, Altschul D, Ortega-Gutiarrez S, Fifi J, Berenstein A. N-butyl cyanoacrylate embolization using a detachable tip microcatheter: initial experience. J Neurointerv Surg. 2015; 7(6):458–461

[30] Oztürk MH, Unal H, Dinç H. Embolization of an AVM with acrylic glue through a new microcatheter with detachable tip: an amazing experience. Neuroradiology. 2008; 50(10):903–904

[31] Niimi Y, Berenstein A, Setton A. Complications and their management during NBCA embolization of craniospinal lesions. Interv Neuroradiol. 2003; 9 Suppl 1:157–164

[32] Qureshi AI, Mian N, Siddiqi H, et al. Occurrence and management strategies for catheter entrapment with Onyx liquid embolization. J Vasc Interv Neurol. 2015; 8(3):37–41

[33] Kelly ME, Turner RT, Gonugunta V, Rasmussen PA, Woo HH, Fiorella D. Monorail snare technique for the retrieval of an adherent microcatheter from an onyx cast: technical case report. Neurosurgery. 2008; 63:89

[34] Alamri A, Hyodo A, Suzuki K, et al. Retrieving microcatheters from Onyx casts in a series of brain arteriovenous malformations: a technical report. Neuroradiology. 2012; 54(11):1237–1240

[35] Walcott BP, Gerrard JL, Nogueira RG, Nahed BV, Terry AR, Ogilvy CS. Microsurgical retrieval of an endovascular microcatheter trapped during Onyx embolization of a cerebral arteriovenous malformation. J Neurointerv Surg. 2011; 3(1):77–79

[36] Cloft HJ, Dion JE. Preoperative and palliative embolization of vertebral tumors. Neuroimaging Clin N Am. 2000; 10(3):569–578

[37] Smith TP, Gray L, Weinstein JN, Richardson WJ, Payne CS. Preoperative transarterial embolization of spinal column neoplasms. J Vasc Interv Radiol. 1995; 6(6):863–869

[38] Facchini G, Di Tullio P, Battaglia M, et al. Palliative embolization for metastases of the spine. Eur J Orthop Surg Traumatol. 2016; 26(3):247–252

[39] Kumar N, Tan B, Zaw AS, et al. The role of preoperative vascular embolization in surgery for metastatic spinal tumours. Eur Spine J. 2016; 25(12):3962–3970

[40] Benati A, Dalle Ore G, Da Pian R, Bricolo A, Maschio A, Perini S. Transfemoral selective embolisation in the treatment of some cranial and vertebro-spinal vascular malformations and tumours: preliminary results. J Neurosurg Sci. 1974; 18(4):233–238

[41] Wirbel RJ, Roth R, Schulte M, Kramann B, Mutschler W. Preoperative embolization in spinal and pelvic metastases. J Orthop Sci. 2005; 10(3):253–257

[42] Qiao Z, Jia N, He Q. Does preoperative transarterial embolization decrease blood loss during spine tumor surgery? Interv Neuroradiol. 2015; 21(1):129–135

[43] Thiex R, Wu I, Mulliken JB, Greene AK, Rahbar R, Orbach DB. Safety and clinical efficacy of Onyx for embolization of extracranial head and neck vascular anomalies. AJNR Am J Neuroradiol. 2011; 32(6):1082–1086

[44] Jackson RJ, Loh SC, Gokaslan ZL. Metastatic renal cell carcinoma of the spine: surgical treatment and results. J Neurosurg. 2001; 94(1) Suppl:18–24

[45] Luksanapruksa P, Buchowski JM, Tongsai S, Singhatanadgige W, Jennings JW. Systematic review and meta-analysis of effectiveness of preoperative embolization in surgery for metastatic spine disease. J Neurointerv Surg. 2018; 10 (6):596–601

[46] Griessenauer CJ, Salem M, Hendrix P, Foreman PM, Ogilvy CS, Thomas AJ. Preoperative embolization of spinal tumors: a systematic review and meta-analysis. World Neurosurg. 2016; 87:362–371

[47] Clausen C, Dahl B, Frevert SC, Hansen LV, Nielsen MB, Lönn L. Preoperative embolization in surgical treatment of spinal metastases: single-blind, randomized controlled clinical trial of efficacy in decreasing intraoperative blood loss. J Vasc Interv Radiol. 2015; 26(3):402–12

[48] Olerud C, Jónsson H, Jr, Löfberg AM, Lörelius LE, Sjöström L. Embolization of spinal metastases reduces peroperative blood loss: 21 patients operated on for renal cell carcinoma. Acta Orthop Scand. 1993; 64(1):9–12

23

[49] Kato S, Murakami H, Minami T, et al. Preoperative embolization significantly decreases intraoperative blood loss during palliative surgery for spinal metastasis. Orthopedics. 2012; 35(9):e1389-e1395

[50] Prabhu VC, Bilsky MH, Jambhekar K, et al. Results of preoperative embolization for metastatic spinal neoplasms. J Neurosurg. 2003; 98(2) Suppl:156–164

[51] Chen Y, Tai BC, Nayak D, et al. Blood loss in spinal tumour surgery and surgery for metastatic spinal disease: a meta-analysis. Bone Joint J. 2013; 95-B(5): 683–688

[52] Patchell RA, Tibbs PA, Regine WF, et al. Direct decompressive surgical resection in the treatment of spinal cord compression caused by metastatic cancer: a randomised trial. The Lancet. 2005; 366(9486):643-648

23

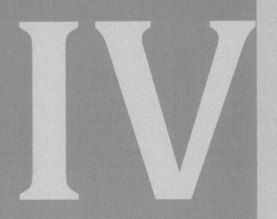

Section IV

Miscellaneous

IV

24 Balloon Test Occlusions

Arun P. Amar, Parampreet Singh, and Phillip Bonney

Abstract

Carotid artery sacrifice is a necessary adjunct in the treatment of a variety of vascular lesions as well as head and neck malignancies. Balloon test occlusion (BTO) is an important test to assess risk of ischemic complication following carotid sacrifice. In this chapter, we will discuss the indications, techniques, and complications associated with BTO.

Keywords: balloon test occlusion, angiogram, endovascular, SPECT, carotid

24.1 Goals

1. Understand the indications for balloon test occlusion (BTO).
2. Analyze standard techniques for BTO.
3. Evaluate the nuances and complications associated with this procedure.
4. Review adjunct modalities aimed at improving prediction of ischemic complications with BTO.

24.2 Case Example 1

24.2.1 History of Present Illness

A 62-year-old, right-handed woman presented with a 1-year history of persistent right-sided ear discharge. Imaging revealed a mass involving the right external auditory canal extending to the petrous bone with involvement of the petrous segment of the right internal carotid artery (ICA). A biopsy confirmed squamous cell carcinoma. The patient was scheduled to undergo a resection of the tumor with possible right ICA sacrifice.

Past medical history: Hypothyroidism, hyperlipidemia, colon cancer.

Past surgical history: Partial colectomy for colorectal carcinoma.

Family history: Noncontributory.

Social history: Noncontributory.

Review of systems: As per the above.

Neurological examination: Unremarkable.

Imaging studies: Right external auditory canal mass with provided history of squamous cell carcinoma. There is extension into the middle ear cavity, right condylar fossa and destruction of the anterior petrous portion of the temporal bone (▶ Fig. 24.1a).

24.2.2 Treatment Plan

Given the possibility of potential sacrifice of the right ICA during surgery, the patient underwent a preoperative BTO with hypotensive challenge followed by HMPAO SPECT (hexamethylpropyleneamine oxime single-photon emission computed tomography). The study was negative clinically, angiographically, and on SPECT scan (▶ Fig. 24.1).

24.2.3 Follow-up

Following BTO, the patient underwent a successful resection of her tumor without requiring carotid sacrifice.

24.3 Case Example 2

24.3.1 History of Present Illness

A 63-year-old, right-handed woman was referred by her primary physician after imaging for headache work-up revealed a 2-cm left ICA cavernous aneurysm with intradural extension. The patient was referred for a BTO prior to therapeutic ICA occlusion for treatment of this partially thrombosed giant aneurysm.

Past medical history: Hypertension, hyperlipidemia, obesity.

Past surgical history: None.

Family history: Negative for aneurysms or subarachnoid hemorrhage.

Social history: Noncontributory.

Review of systems: As per the above.

Neurological examination: Unremarkable.

Imaging studies: Computed tomography angiography (CTA) showed a large, partially thrombosed, left ICA cavernous segment aneurysm (▶ Fig. 24.2a).

24.3.2 Treatment Plan

Given the size, morphology, and partial thrombosis of the aneurysm, both endovascular embolization and open clip ligation were deemed high risk. Permanent occlusion of the carotid was therefore planned. A BTO with HMPAO SPECT study was performed to evaluate the safety of left carotid occlusion. The study was negative clinically and angiographically; however, on HMPAO SPECT imaging subtle asymmetry was noted, suggestive of hypoperfusion rendering an overall intermediate risk status.

24.3.3 Follow-up

Following the BTO, the patient underwent a successful surgical ligation of the left cervical ICA, and an intracranial superficial temporal artery to middle cerebral artery (STA-MCA) bypass was performed due to the findings of the HMPAO SPECT scan (▶ Fig. 24.2). There were no ischemic complications.

24.4 Case Example 3

24.4.1 History of Present Illness

A 68-year-old, right-handed man presented with progressive left-sided hearing loss and facial weakness. Imaging revealed a mass involving the left temporal bone and ear canals. Biopsy confirmed a squamous cell carcinoma, and the patient was planned to undergo a temporal bone resection with parotidectomy and possible left ICA sacrifice.

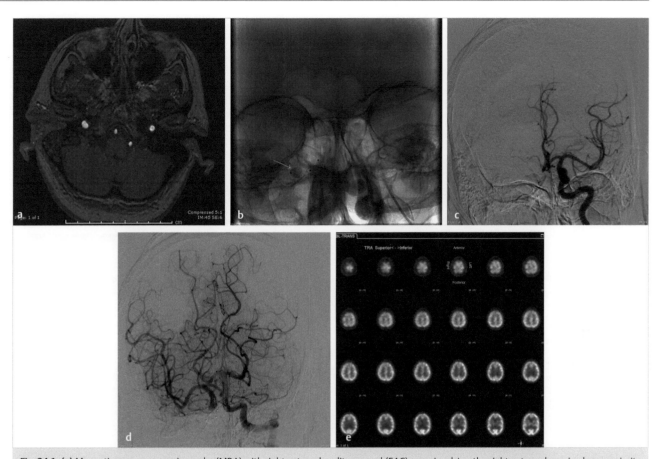

Fig. 24.1 (a) Magnetic resonance angiography (MRA) with right external auditory canal (EAC) mass involving the right petrous bone in close proximity to the right internal carotid artery (ICA). (b) Balloon microcatheter inflated in the right petrous ICA. (c) Contralateral ICA run with balloon microcatheter inflated in the right petrous ICA with minimal filling across the anterior communicating artery. (d) Posterior circulation run with balloon microcatheter inflated in the right petrous ICA, with robust filling of the left internal carotid via a posterior communicating artery. (e) Follow-up HMPAO SPECT (hexamethylpropyleneamine oxime single-photon emission computed tomography) shows symmetric filling of the bilateral hemispheres. (Representative imaging for both cases 1 and 3.)

Past medical history: Hypertension, hyperlipidemia, hypothyroidism.
Past surgical history: None.
Family history: Noncontributory.
Social history: Noncontributory.
Review of systems: As per the above.
Neurological examination: Left-sided sensorineural hearing loss and subtle left nasolabial flattening (House-Brackmann scale 2). The remainder of the neurological examination was unremarkable.
Imaging studies: Mass associated with the left external auditory canal, middle ear cavity, and mastoid temporal bone with superior extension into the middle cranial fossa, as well as anterior-inferior extension into the temporomandibular joint (▶ Fig. 24.3a).

24.4.2 Treatment Plan

Given the possible need for intraoperative left ICA sacrifice, the patient underwent BTO of the left ICA with hypotensive challenge and HMPAO SPECT study. The study was negative clinically, angiographically, and on SPECT scan (▶ Fig. 24.3).

24.4.3 Follow-up

Following the BTO, the patient underwent a successful resection of his tumor without requiring carotid sacrifice.

24.5 Level of Evidence

BTO is an important test for prediction of ischemic complications following a permanent carotid occlusion.

The sensitivity of BTO is increased with addition of adjunctive modalities such as hypotensive challenge, HMPAO SPECT, positron emission tomography (PET), magnetic resonance imaging (MRI), and transcranial Doppler (TCD), among others. Majority of evidence for these procedures are based on observational case series and expert opinion only (Level of Evidence C).

24.6 Case Summaries

1. *What is the purpose of BTO?*
   Elective carotid sacrifice is necessary in certain clinical settings involving resection of head and neck tumors and in complex vascular lesions, such as fistulas or large aneurysms.

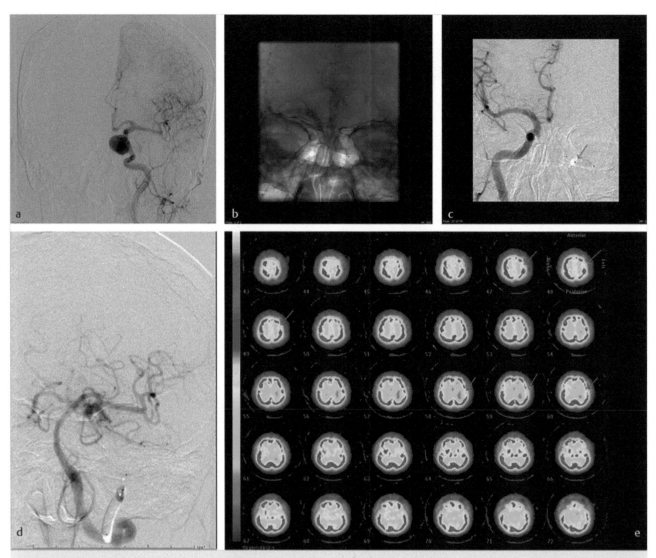

Fig. 24.2 **(a)** Left internal carotid artery (ICA) cavernous segment aneurysm (> 2 cm) with intradural extension. **(b)** A balloon microcatheter inflated in the petrous left ICA. **(c)** Right ICA angiogram with occluded left ICA (petrous segment, *white arrow*). No significant cross-filling noted. **(d)** Posterior circulation angiogram with balloon inflated in the petrous left ICA, demonstrating robust filling of the left ICA via a posterior communicating artery. **(e)** Subtle asymmetry noted in the HMPAO SPECT (hexamethylpropyleneamine oxime single-photon emission computed tomography) scan predominantly in the left frontoparietal regions (*white arrows*) following completion of the balloon test occlusion (BTO).

ICA ligations are associated with ischemic complications in 49% of patients. Similarly, in common carotid artery occlusions, ischemic complications were noted in 28% of patients[1,2,3] with a mortality of about 12%.[4] These complications may arise due to poor collateral circulation across the circle of Willis, inadequate reserve despite good collateral flow, and thromboembolism. However, with favorable anatomy, vessel sacrifice can be asymptomatic. BTO is an endovascular angiographic procedure which simulates an arterial occlusion in a controlled environment to predict ischemic complications.

2. *What are the procedural complications and associated prevention strategies associated with BTO?*

The major complications associated with BTOs may be asymptomatic or symptomatic vessel injury and/or transient or persistent ischemic events. The largest BTO case series to date by the Ouciversity of Pittsburgh reported asymptomatic

events in 1.6% of patients and symptomatic events in 1.6% (1.2% transient and 0.4% permanent).[5] Similar results have been reported by others which are within the range for diagnostic angiography alone.[6,7] The major preventative strategies include correct sizing of the balloon and preinflation heparinization.

3. *What adjunctive modalities are used with BTO to increase sensitivity and specificity?*

The common adjunctive modalities to improve predictions of ischemic complications include clinical testing with a simulated hypotensive challenge, TCD ultrasonography, Xenon-enhanced computed tomography, O-15 labeled PET, or 99mTc-HMPAO SPECT. The literature on these techniques is discussed below.

4. *What are the common causes of ischemic complications and preventative strategies following permanent occlusions in patients with a negative BTO?*

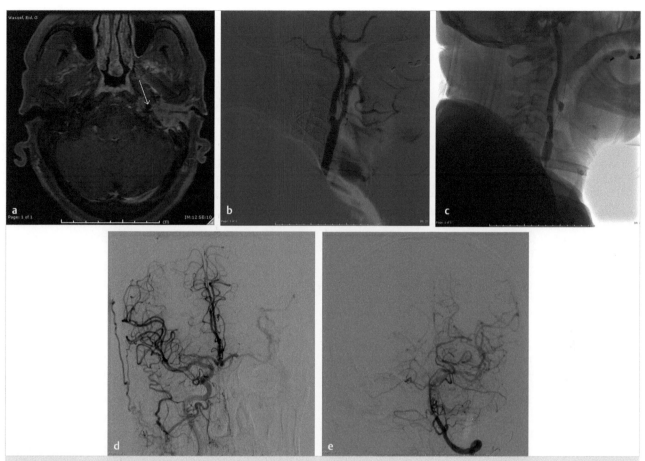

Fig. 24.3 **(a)** Magnetic resonance imaging (MRI) T1 with contrast showing left temporal bone mass in close proximity to the left petrous internal carotid artery (ICA) (*arrow*). **(b)** A high-grade stenosis in the left ICA origin which poses technical difficulties and risk of embolizing the plaque intracranially during passage of a balloon microcatheter. A dual balloon setup is employed as seen in the next image. **(c)** Dual balloon setup with a balloon guide catheter (8F Stryker Flowgate) inflated in the left common carotid artery, and a balloon microcatheter (4-mm Scepter XC) inflated in the right external carotid artery with stagnant flow in the left ICA. **(d)** Contralateral ICA angiogram demonstrating delayed arterial cross-filling on the left through the anterior communicating artery. **(e)** A posterior circulation angiogram demonstrating good filling in the arterial phase via a robust posterior communicating artery.

Following a negative BTO, there is still a 4.7 to 25% risk of ischemic complications, depending upon the adjunct modality.[4,5,8,9,10] The major causes of these ischemic complications include both hemodynamic insufficiency and thromboembolism. A rescue bypass has been utilized to correct hemodynamic complications with success.[11,12] Short-term anticoagulation or antiplatelet therapy can be considered following permanent occlusions to reduce risk of stump embolism.[13] There are, however, no evidence-based guidelines for these strategies.

24.7 Landmark Papers

Serbinenko FA. Balloon catheterization and occlusion of major cerebral vessels. J Neurosurg 1974;41(2):125–145.

Prior to the introduction of formal BTO,[14] methods to determine the functional adequacy of the circle of Willis involved indirect cerebral blood flow (CBF) measurements such as angiography with manual compression, ICA stump pressure measurements, and oculoplethysmography (OPG).[15] However, these techniques had several limitations, including inconsistencies in applied manual pressure and variations in the pressure of the injected dye during an angiogram. Stump pressure measurements were proven unreliable in carotid endarterectomy case series models.[16] Similarly, OPG measured flow indirectly by measuring the flow in the ophthalmic artery.

In his groundbreaking paper, Serbinenko used self-designed, silicone balloon catheters for temporary occlusion of more than 300 vessels. One hundred and eighty-seven of these cases involved occlusion of the ICA. His procedure involved direct puncture of the carotid artery for introduction of the balloon catheter which was then flow navigated to various portions of the ICA. He reported only two complications out of his over 300 temporary balloon occlusions due to unexplained thrombosis of the middle cerebral artery. Unfortunately, both of these cases resulted in the patients' death.

While this is the original study demonstrating the feasibility of BTOs, it served as an introduction to the technique rather than a rigorous, controlled validation of it. While Serbinenko successfully provided a very detailed manual on the use of BTO in various pathologies and locations within the extra- and intracranial cerebrovasculature and successfully introduced the practice of BTO to the neurosurgical community, he did not provide any information concerning the predictive value of the study following permanent occlusion.

De Vries EJ, Sekhar LN, Horton JA, et al. A new method to predict safe resection of the internal carotid artery. Laryngoscope 1990;100(1):85–88.

With the incorporation of clinical BTO in the 1980s, prediction of ischemic complications from vessel occlusions were markedly improved, with nearly 100% prediction of ischemic complication for patients failing the test.[5,15,17] However, a significant percentage of patients, up to 10%, had strokes despite passing the clinical BTO.[4,8,9,18,19,20]

In light of an insufficient negative predictive value of a clinical BTO, authors reported benefits of adding CBF analysis to improve risk prediction.[4,21,22] The initial case series on BTO with Xenon-enhanced CT (Xe-CT) for CBF analysis was published by Vries et al in 1990.[15] The authors defined compromised flow as less than 20 mL/100 mg/min based on prior data.[23] Their case series demonstrated less than 3% incidence of ischemic complications following permanent carotid occlusion in patients that passed BTO with Xe-CT. Similarly, Linskey et al demonstrated an approximately 3% risk of ischemia when BTO was paired with Xe-CT scan.[4] In Sen et al's series of ICA bypass patients, ischemic complications were seen in 7% of patients that passed both clinical and Xe-CT components of BTO, 56% of patients who passed the clinical component of BTO but failed Xe-CT (with a CBF less than 30 mL/100 mg/min), and 100% of patients who failed both.[17]

One of the technical limitations associated with using Xe-CT is the need to deflate the balloon, move the patient to a Xenon CT scanner, and re-inflate the balloon for Xe-CT. This adds significantly to the overall procedural complexity and risk. Administration of 133 radioactive Xenon followed by gamma activity measurements using cranial probes has also been described to assess CBF.[24,25] While this method can be completed in the angiography suite, 133 radioactive Xenon does not provide regional blood flow information and may be less sensitive than newer methods.

Matsuda H, Higashi S, Asli IN, et al. Evaluation of cerebral collateral circulation by technetium-99 m HM-PAO brain SPECT during Matas test: report of three cases. J Nucl Med 1988;29 (10):1724–1729.

99 m Technetium HMPAO is a lipophilic radiotracer with a half-life of about 6 hours. It readily crosses the blood–brain barrier and is converted into a hydrophilic form, leading to contrast retention between normal and abnormal brain for up to 2 hours. The earliest report using HMPAO SPECT to assess CBF was published by Matsuda et al during manual compression. The findings in this initial study of three cases correlated well with the collateral status of the downstream occluded vessel, as observed on direct cerebral angiography.[26] Used as an adjunct with BTO, HMPAO SPECT has been shown to add useful information to stratify risk after permanent carotid occlusion.[27,28] Monsein et al compared HMPAO SPECT scans at baseline followed by scans performed with BTO. The authors noted that patients with no change between baseline and test occlusion SPECT imaging had adequate collaterals to sustain flow after a permanent occlusion of the artery.[29] These initial studies validated the negative predictive value of this adjunct test. Efforts to quantify CBF more objectively have since been pursued to

correlate with clinical intolerance to vessel sacrifice. One study reported that a reduction in CBF to less than 85% of baseline in the MCA territory is associated with ischemic complications.[30] Other authors have utilized similar approaches to calculate asymmetry indices for specific regions of interest on SPECT imaging. Similar cutoffs of 10 to 15% correlated well with ischemic complications after permanent occlusion.[31,32,33]

Brunberg JA, Frey KA, Horton JA, Deveikis JP, Ross DA, Koeppe RA. [15O]H2O positron emission tomography determination of cerebral blood flow during balloon test occlusion of the internal carotid artery. AJNR Am J Neuroradiol 1994;15(4):725–732.

Despite the advantages of using Xe-CT or SPECT for CBF analysis in conjunction with BTO, these studies lacked specificity, as the semiquantitative asymmetry analysis was associated with high rates of false-positive results.[21] PET, which allows quantitative CBF analysis, improved both the sensitivity and specificity of a clinical BTO.[4,21,22,34,35]

PET technology in neuroimaging makes use of O-15 labeled compounds to determine a variety of physiologic variables including CBF, cerebral blood volume (CBV), oxygen extraction fraction (OEF), and cerebral metabolic rate of oxygen ($CMRO_2$). These variables can then be utilized for assessing ischemia in both acute and chronic cerebrovascular disease states.

The first report employing PET during BTO for prediction of ischemia after permanent occlusion was published by Brunberg et al using [15O]H2O. This study showed that patients with CBF reduction to 25 to 35 mL/100 g/min during balloon occlusion are at risk for developing cerebral infarction after permanent ICA occlusion.[36] Similar findings were reported by Murphy et al.[37] Overall PET scans were more reliable than other available modalities; however, the prolonged inflation of the balloon during the entirety of the PET scan may pose significant procedural risks.

A more recent study utilized a novel dual tracer autoradiographic (DRAG) method in PET scans as an adjunct to BTO for shortening the PET examination period. The authors employed use of sequential administration of dual tracers of $^{15}O_2$ and $C^{15}O_2$ during a single PET scan, followed by computation of CBF and $CMRO_2$ autoradiographically.[34] This protocol reduced the time of scan from 1 hour to 15 minutes. The study further consolidated the previously established CBF critical values and introduced the use of $OEF/CMRO_2$ ratio to further predict ischemic complications. Despite the promise of PET scans with BTO, these novel protocols are not available at most institutions. Furthermore, requirement of reinflation of the balloon outside of the angiography lab and prolonged balloon inflation times have limited the utilization of PET studies with BTO.

Schneweis S, Urbach H, Solymosi L, Ries F. Preoperative risk assessment for carotid occlusion by transcranial Doppler ultrasound. J Neurol Neurosurg Psychiatry 1997 May;62(5):485–489.

Another adjunctive test employed TCD ultrasonography to assess CBF. Early studies demonstrated that TCD velocities can be correlated with CBF as assessed simultaneously on Xe-CT following carotid occlusion.[38] Schneweiss et al validated the use of TCD with BTO. They concluded that a drop in the mean velocities of more than 30% was associated with clinical manifestations during temporary occlusion.[39] The addition of acetazolamide potentially not only made the test more reliable by exhausting cerebral autoregulation but also increased the risk of ischemic injury during the trial.

Another case series of 32 patients demonstrated that a reduction in both mean velocity and pulsatility index (PI) greater than 50% was associated with neurological deficits. A reduction of up to 30%, however, had no significant ischemic complications. For patients with an intermediate reduction between 30 and 50% in mean velocity and PI, motor vasoreactivity (representative of cerebrovascular autoregulation following voluntary motor activity) was used to further stratify risk.[40] Similar results were noted in another study reviewing changes in MCA velocities in 22 patients undergoing percutaneous transluminal angioplasty of the ICA. A greater than 50% drop in velocities was associated with transient or persistent neurological deficits.[41] In a study of carotid balloon occlusion monitored with electroencephalogram (EEG), SPECT, and TCDs, a drop of up to 40% in mean TCD velocity was not associated with changes in EEG, SPECT, or clinical examination. However, a drop greater than 40% was correlated with changes in each of these.[42] Based upon the available data, TCD velocity reductions > 30% may predict higher risks of ischemic complications.

van Rooij WJ, Sluzewski M, Slob MJ, Rinkel GJ. Predictive value of angiographic testing for tolerance to therapeutic occlusion of the carotid artery. AJNR Am J Neuroradiol 2005;26(1):175–178.

Abud DG, Spelle L, Piotin M, Mounayer C, Vanzin JR, Moret J. Venous phase timing during balloon test occlusion as a criterion for permanent internal carotid artery sacrifice. AJNR Am J Neuroradiol 2005;26(10):2602–2609.

A simple adjunct which can be performed during test occlusion is assessment of collateral status. Evaluation of cortical venous delay on the occluded side compared to the contralateral control was used to assess collateral circulation.[43,44,45] van Rooij et al followed 74 patients who underwent BTO prior to therapeutic carotid occlusion. Synchronous venous filling with < 0.5 seconds delay was the cutoff criteria for a negative angiographic BTO. Only 1 patient in 51 therapeutic occlusions of the carotid artery following a negative study developed a transient, hemiparesis with hypoperfusion infarcts on follow-up imaging. However, two patients with ruptured aneurysms died from diffuse vasospasm following permanent occlusion.[44]

Similarly, Abud et al showed that a venous delay of < 3 seconds on a BTO angiogram was associated with low risk of ischemic hemodynamic complications following permanent vessel occlusion. One of the three patients in this study with venous delay > 3 seconds had a border zone ischemic stroke following permanent occlusion.[43] More recently, venous delay on angiogram was compared with HMPAO SPECT imaging in 56 patients. Twenty-six patients had no hypoperfusion on SPECT with an average 0.5 seconds of venous delay. Of these, eight went on to have carotid occlusions with no ischemic complications. Patients with mild hypoperfusion on SPECT had an average 0.65 seconds of venous delay and patients with moderate-to-severe hypoperfusion on SPECT had an average of 1.08 seconds of delay.[45] These results suggested a cutoff closer to 0.5 seconds in contrast to reports of negative results with up to 3 seconds of venous delay. There is risk of significant inter-rater variability due to the lack of objective assessment of venous delay time on angiograms.

Tanaka F, Nishizawa S, Yonekura Y, et al. Changes in cerebral blood flow induced by balloon test occlusion of the internal carotid artery under hypotension. Eur J Nucl Med 1995;22(11):1268–1273.

While the adjuncts above are useful in stratifying risk profiles, the role of blood pressure was not taken into account. Paterman et al noted an incidence of ischemic strokes in patients following BTO with a symmetric SPECT, related to intraoperative hypotension.[27] Similarly, Eckard et al reported that patients with both symmetric and asymmetric SPECT perfusion patterns presented with delayed strokes.[46]

Tanaka et al reviewed changes in CBF using SPECT following induced hypotension during a BTO. The study was remarkable for 20 to 40% reduction in ipsilateral CBF during the hypotensive challenge. While the patients remained asymptomatic during the study, the authors identified significant alterations of CBF during hypotension in many patients who would otherwise have normal HMPAO SPECT BTOs.[47] Linskey et al similarly noted three risk profiles, including low risk in patients passing both clinical and imaging studies and high risk in patients failing both studies. Moderate-risk patients passed the clinical study but demonstrated asymmetry with Xe perfusion and were noted to have ischemic complications following carotid occlusion.[4]

Unfortunately, these adjunctive tests lacked specificity in predicting ischemic outcomes.[21] Furthermore, these quantitative tests reviewed hemodynamic profile in a controlled environment and may not accurately predict stroke risk during periods of physiologic stress states.

24.8 Recommendations

BTO is an important diagnostic tool to determine the feasibility of therapeutic occlusion of vessels supplying the brain. While multiple quantitative and qualitative methods have described this procedure, there is no clear consensus regarding the best adjunctive test to determine the safety of permanent occlusion. Many of the adjunctive methods that quantitatively measure CBF following temporary occlusion are difficult to perform and require sophisticated instruments which are not readily available within the angiography suite. This introduces potential risks during patient transport and inflation and deflation of balloons outside of the angiography suite. In addition, the thresholds used to determine success in quantitative studies directly corresponds with the predictive value of the test. These reports all rely on retrospective data as the basis for their assessments. As of yet, no randomized, controlled studies have been performed on BTOs to determine which of these modalities provides the best sensitivity and/or specificity for immediate and delayed ischemic events following artery sacrifice. In addition, given the advances in neurointerventional tools, the role of deconstructive treatments will likely continue to diminish as more reconstructive tools are developed.

24.9 Summary

1. BTO can help predict ischemic complication from carotid artery sacrifice.
2. Standard BTO involves clinical, angiographic, and an adjunctive measurement of cerebral perfusion (Xe CT, PET, SPECT, etc.).
3. The complication rate is similar to that of a diagnostic cerebral angiogram with the most common complications including stroke and dissection.

4. The risk of ischemic complications after a negative BTO is between 4 and 30% and may be caused by hypoperfusion or thromboembolism.

References

[1] Nishioka H. Results of the treatment of intracranial aneurysms by occlusion of the carotid artery in the neck. J Neurosurg. 1966; 25(6):660–704

[2] Swearingen B, Heros RC. Common carotid occlusion for unclippable carotid aneurysms: an old but still effective operation. Neurosurgery. 1987; 21(3): 288–295

[3] Winn HR, Richardson AE, Jane JA. Late morbidity and mortality of common carotid ligation for posterior communicating aneurysms: a comparison to conservative treatment. J Neurosurg. 1977; 47(5):727–736

[4] Linskey ME, Jungreis CA, Yonas H, et al. Stroke risk after abrupt internal carotid artery sacrifice: accuracy of preoperative assessment with balloon test occlusion and stable xenon-enhanced CT. AJNR Am J Neuroradiol. 1994; 15(5):829–843

[5] Mathis JM, Barr JD, Jungreis CA, et al. Temporary balloon test occlusion of the internal carotid artery: experience in 500 cases. AJNR Am J Neuroradiol. 1995; 16(4):749–754

[6] Meyers PM, Thakur GA, Tomsick TA. Temporary endovascular balloon occlusion of the internal carotid artery with a nondetachable silicone balloon catheter: analysis of technique and cost. AJNR Am J Neuroradiol. 1999; 20(4): 559–564

[7] Dion JE, Gates PC, Fox AJ, Barnett HJ, Blom RJ. Clinical events following neuroangiography: a prospective study. Stroke. 1987; 18(6):997–1004

[8] Vazquez Añon V, Aymard A, Gobin YP, et al. Balloon occlusion of the internal carotid artery in 40 cases of giant intracavernous aneurysm: technical aspects, cerebral monitoring, and results. Neuroradiology. 1992; 34(3):245–251

[9] Higashida RT, Halbach VV, Dowd C, et al. Endovascular detachable balloon embolization therapy of cavernous carotid artery aneurysms: results in 87 cases. J Neurosurg. 1990; 72(6):857–863

[10] Dare AO, Chaloupka JC, Putman CM, Fayad PB, Awad IA. Failure of the hypotensive provocative test during temporary balloon test occlusion of the internal carotid artery to predict delayed hemodynamic ischemia after therapeutic carotid occlusion. Surg Neurol. 1998; 50(2):147–155, discussion 155–156

[11] Ibrahim TF, Jahromi BR, Miettinen J, et al. Long-term causes of death and excess mortality after carotid artery ligation. World Neurosurg. 2016; 90:116–122

[12] Pancucci G, Potts MB, Rodríguez-Hernández A, Andrade H, Guo L, Lawton MT. Rescue bypass for revascularization after ischemic complications in the treatment of giant or complex intracranial aneurysms. World Neurosurg. 2015; 83(6):912–920

[13] Whisenant JT, Kadkhodayan Y, Cross DT, III, Moran CJ, Derdeyn CP. Incidence and mechanisms of stroke after permanent carotid artery occlusion following temporary occlusion testing. J Neurointerv Surg. 2015; 7(6):395–401

[14] Serbinenko FA. Balloon catheterization and occlusion of major cerebral vessels. J Neurosurg. 1974; 41(2):125–145

[15] de Vries EJ, Sekhar LN, Horton JA, et al. A new method to predict safe resection of the internal carotid artery. Laryngoscope. 1990; 100(1):85–88

[16] Kelly JJ, Callow AD, O'Donnell TF, et al. Failure of carotid stump pressures: its incidence as a predictor for a temporary shunt during carotid endarterectomy. Arch Surg. 1979; 114(12):1361–1366

[17] Sen C, Sekhar LN. Direct vein graft reconstruction of the cavernous, petrous, and upper cervical internal carotid artery: lessons learned from 30 cases. Neurosurgery. 1992; 30(5):732–742, discussion 742–743

[18] Fox AJ, Viñuela F, Pelz DM, et al. Use of detachable balloons for proximal artery occlusion in the treatment of unclippable cerebral aneurysms. J Neurosurg. 1987; 66(1):40–46

[19] Weil SM, van Loveren HR, Tomsick TA, Quallen BL, Tew JM, Jr. Management of inoperable cerebral aneurysms by the navigational balloon technique. Neurosurgery. 1987; 21(3):296–302

[20] Andrews JC, Valavanis A, Fisch U. Management of the internal carotid artery in surgery of the skull base. Laryngoscope. 1989; 99(12):1224–1229

[21] Yonas H, Linskey M, Johnson DW, et al. Internal carotid balloon test occlusion does require quantitative CBF. AJNR Am J Neuroradiol. 1992; 13(4):1147–1152

[22] Witt JP, Yonas H, Jungreis C. Cerebral blood flow response pattern during balloon test occlusion of the internal carotid artery. AJNR Am J Neuroradiol. 1994; 15(5):847–856

[23] Yonas H, Gur D, Good BC, et al. Stable xenon CT blood flow mapping for evaluation of patients with extracranial-intracranial bypass surgery. J Neurosurg. 1985; 62(3):324–333

[24] Leech PJ, Miller JD, Fitch W, Barker J. Cerebral blood flow, internal carotid artery pressure, and the EEG as a guide to the safety of carotid ligation. J Neurol Neurosurg Psychiatry. 1974; 37(7):854–862

[25] Holmes AE, James IM, Wise CC. Observations on distal intravascular pressure changes and cerebral blood flow after common carotid artery ligation in man. J Neurol Neurosurg Psychiatry. 1971; 34(1):78–81

[26] Matsuda H, Higashi S, Asli IN, et al. Evaluation of cerebral collateral circulation by technetium-99m HM-PAO brain SPECT during Matas test: report of three cases. J Nucl Med. 1988; 29(10):1724–1729

[27] Peterman SB, Taylor A, Jr, Hoffman JC, Jr. Improved detection of cerebral hypoperfusion with internal carotid balloon test occlusion and 99mTc-HMPAO cerebral perfusion SPECT imaging. AJNR Am J Neuroradiol. 1991; 12(6): 1035–1041

[28] Moody EB, Dawson RC, III, Sandler MP. 99mTc-HMPAO SPECT imaging in interventional neuroradiology: validation of balloon test occlusion. AJNR Am J Neuroradiol. 1991; 12(6):1043–1044

[29] Monsein LH, Jeffery PJ, van Heerden BB, et al. Assessing adequacy of collateral circulation during balloon test occlusion of the internal carotid artery with 99mTc-HMPAO SPECT. AJNR Am J Neuroradiol. 1991; 12(6):1045–1051

[30] Ryu YH, Chung TS, Lee JD, et al. HMPAO SPECT to assess neurologic deficits during balloon test occlusion. J Nucl Med. 1996; 37(4):551–554

[31] Kaminogo M, Ochi M, Onizuka M, Takahata H, Shibata S. An additional monitoring of regional cerebral oxygen saturation to HMPAO SPECT study during balloon test occlusion. Stroke. 1999; 30(2):407–413

[32] Tansavatdi K, Dublin AB, Donald PJ, Dahlin B. Combined balloon test occlusion and SPECT analysis for carotid sacrifice: angiographic predictors for success or failure? J Neurol Surg B Skull Base. 2015; 76(4):249–251

[33] Palestro CJ, Sen C, Muzinic M, Afriyie M, Goldsmith SJ. Assessing collateral cerebral perfusion with technetium-99m-HMPAO SPECT during temporary internal carotid artery occlusion. J Nucl Med. 1993; 34(8):1235–1238

[34] Kawai N, Kawanishi M, Shindou A, et al. Cerebral blood flow and metabolism measurement using positron emission tomography before and during internal carotid artery test occlusions: feasibility of rapid quantitative measurement of CBF and OEF/CMRO(2). Interv Neuroradiol. 2012; 18(3):264–274

[35] Field M, Jungreis CA, Chengelis N, Kromer H, Kirby L, Yonas H. Symptomatic cavernous sinus aneurysms: management and outcome after carotid occlusion and selective cerebral revascularization. AJNR Am J Neuroradiol. 2003; 24(6):1200–1207

[36] Brunberg JA, Frey KA, Horton JA, Deveikis JP, Ross DA, Koeppe RA. [15O]H2O positron emission tomography determination of cerebral blood flow during balloon test occlusion of the internal carotid artery. AJNR Am J Neuroradiol. 1994; 15(4):725–732

[37] Murphy KJ, Payne T, Jamadar DA, Beydoun A, Frey KA, Brunberg JA. Correlation of continuous EEG monitoring with [O-15]H2O positron emission tomography determination of cerebral blood flow during balloon test occlusion of the internal carotid artery: experience in 34 cases. Interv Neuroradiol. 1998; 4(1):51–55

[38] Kofke WA, Brauer P, Policare R, Penthany S, Barker D, Horton J. Middle cerebral artery blood flow velocity and stable xenon-enhanced computed tomographic blood flow during balloon test occlusion of the internal carotid artery. Stroke. 1995; 26(9):1603–1606

[39] Schneweis S, Urbach H, Solymosi L, Ries F. Preoperative risk assessment for carotid occlusion by transcranial Doppler ultrasound. J Neurol Neurosurg Psychiatry. 1997; 62(5):485–489

[40] Eckert B, Thie A, Carvajal M, Groden C, Zeumer H. Predicting hemodynamic ischemia by transcranial Doppler monitoring during therapeutic balloon occlusion of the internal carotid artery. AJNR Am J Neuroradiol. 1998; 19(3): 577–582

[41] Eckert B, Thie A, Valdueza J, Zanella F, Zeumer H. Transcranial Doppler sonographic monitoring during percutaneous transluminal angioplasty of the internal carotid artery. Neuroradiology. 1997; 39(3):229–234

[42] Keller E, Ries F, Grünwald F, et al. Multimodal carotid occlusion test for determining risk of infarct before therapeutic internal carotid artery occlusion. Laryngorhinootologie. 1995; 74(5):307–311

[43] Abud DG, Spelle L, Piotin M, Mounayer C, Vanzin JR, Moret J. Venous phase timing during balloon test occlusion as a criterion for permanent internal carotid artery sacrifice. AJNR Am J Neuroradiol. 2005; 26(10):2602–2609

[44] van Rooij WJ, Sluzewski M, Slob MJ, Rinkel GJ. Predictive value of angiographic testing for tolerance to therapeutic occlusion of the carotid artery. AJNR Am J Neuroradiol. 2005; 26(1):175–178

[45] Snelling BM, Sur S, Shah SS, et al. Venous phase timing does not predict SPECT results during balloon test occlusion of the internal carotid artery. World Neurosurg. 2017; 102:229–234

[46] Eckard DA, Purdy PD, Bonte FJ. Temporary balloon occlusion of the carotid artery combined with brain blood flow imaging as a test to predict tolerance prior to permanent carotid sacrifice. AJNR Am J Neuroradiol. 1992; 13(6): 1565–1569

[47] Tanaka F, Nishizawa S, Yonekura Y, et al. Changes in cerebral blood flow induced by balloon test occlusion of the internal carotid artery under hypotension. Eur J Nucl Med. 1995; 22(11):1268–1273

24

25 Wada and Selective Wada Tests

Rachel Jacobs, Nitin Agarwal, Brian T. Jankowitz, and Bradley A. Gross

Abstract

The Wada test has been considered the gold standard for lateralizing language and memory function in the presurgical workup of patients with epilepsy. It has further evolved in its applications in its superselective form with applicability to a plethora of cerebrovascular pathology. This chapter reviews historical manuscripts and provides a review of the approach with a critical analysis of its utility in the era of advanced noninvasive imaging modalities.

Keywords: Wada test, epilepsy, sodium amobarbital

25.1 Goals

1. Present the frequency, clinical indications, and methods of Wada testing and its associated complications.
2. Compare the literature on use of Wada and noninvasive approaches.
3. Analyze the validity of Wada testing for language determination and memory function.
4. Review the literature on posterior cerebral artery (PCA) and superselective Wada.

25.2 Case Example

25.2.1 History of Present Illness

A 53-year-old, left-handed man on aspirin with a history of traumatic brain injury presents for surgical consideration of his medically refractory complex partial epilepsy with secondary generalization since the age of 15 after a motor vehicle accident. The patient reports his seizures start with right eye deviation, head deviation to the right, ringing noises in his ears, "feeling funny," and unusual odor perception. He continues to have bilateral upper extremity tremors as a side effect from his Depakote. He complains of residual weakness in his right leg and numbness that affects his right foot and palm after a stroke in 2000. A Wada test was recommended prior to a potential left temporal lobectomy.

> *Past medical history*: Mitral valve prolapse, aortic stenosis, cerebrovascular accident, right-sided eye trauma (status postprosthesis).
> *Past surgical history*: Appendectomy, right eye removed, C3–C5 fusion.
> *Family history*: Noncontributory, no family history of seizures.
> *Social history*: 30-pack-year smoking history, social alcohol usage, no drugs of abuse.
> *Review of systems*: As per the history of present illness.
> *Neurological examination*: Remarkable for a mild right facial droop, decreased hearing bilaterally, and mild right hemiparesis (4+/5). He has a noticeable tremor of the left greater than right on outstretched upper extremities.
> *Imaging studies*: See ▶ Fig. 25.1.

25.2.2 Treatment Plan

The patient underwent selective catheterization and angiography of the bilateral internal carotid arteries (ICAs) followed by administration of 125 mg of sodium Amytal in the left ICA and 200 mg of sodium Amytal in the right ICA followed by language and memory testing and subsequent Mynx closure of right common femoral artery. Wada testing affirmed that the patient harbored a left hemisphere language representation and left memory dominance. After performance of the Wada test, a frontotemporal grid was implanted with depth electrodes into the hippocampus. Surgical resection was subsequently performed after mapping the location of the seizure focus more definitively.

25.2.3 Follow-up

The patient tolerated the Wada test without complication. He initially underwent placement of a frontotemporal grid with depth electrodes into the hippocampus and subsequent resection of the seizure focus. At 1-year follow-up evaluation, the patient has been seizure-free since his surgery.

25.3 Case Summary

1. *What would you report as the most common complications associated with the Wada test?*
   The complication rate associated with angiography and has been reported to range from 0.3% to nearly 11% of patients.[1,2,3,4,5] Most complications are associated with the

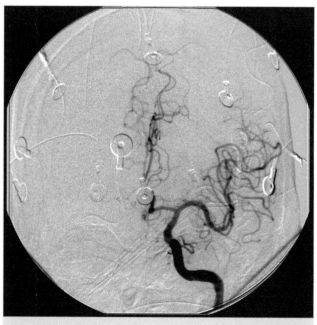

Fig. 25.1 Anteroposterior (AP) angiographic run performed of the patient's left internal carotid artery prior to injection of amobarbital for Wada testing.

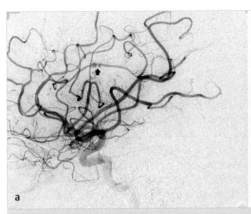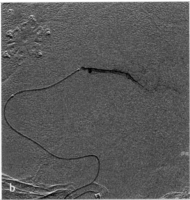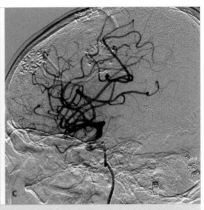

Fig. 25.2 (a) Carotid angiography delineates a pseudoaneurysm of the pericallosal anterior cerebral artery (ACA) (lateral view, *arrow*). Superselective angiography prior to injection of Amytal demonstrates the aneurysm. **(b)** Control angiography after Onyx embolization demonstrates obliteration of the aneurysm with Onyx casting the lesion (lateral view, **c**, *arrow*).

angiogram and not with the injection of amobarbital itself; thus, the main source of complications is thromboemboli. Other sources of morbidity include dissections and groin complications. As modern reports cite lower and lower rates of complications, one would expect a commensurate rate for the Wada test as well.

2. *What patient factors would you consider when deciding on your recommendations for Wada testing?*
   Both patient's age and medical comorbidities are important patient factors when deciding on Wada testing. Neurologic complications are significantly more common in patients 55 years of age or older and in patients with cardiovascular disease.[3] In the study by Loddenkemper et al, older age was a risk factor for stroke (47 years as compared with 32 years) and dissection (52 years as compared with 32 years), whereas younger age (21 years as compared with 32 years) was a risk factor for seizures.[4]

3. *In which cases may the Wada test be omitted prior to surgical resection?*
   Although decisions should be made on a case-by-case basis, the Wada test may possibly be omitted in the preoperative evaluation in a patient with right temporal lobe epilepsy if there is an evidence of typical left hemispheric language dominance from functional imaging.[1] Also, combined structural and functional imaging in conjunction with neuropsychological testing could be used as opposed to the Wada testing for patients at high risk of memory decline.[6] Some centers consider functional magnetic resonance imaging (fMRI) to be a reasonable "triage test," and Wada testing is indicated when fMRI does not provide straightforward left lateralization.[7] As functional imaging improves and resultant ambiguity decreases, the use of the Wada test may become reserved for a narrower patient population.

4. *Can the Wada test be more broadly applied?*
   Wada tests may also be performed superselectively to identify clinically relevant neurologic deficits. This procedure can be employed to detect eloquent cortex perfused by feeding arteries, and therefore prior to embolization, one can anticipate potential neurologic deficits. The following case demonstrates utilization of the superselective Wada.
   A 43-year-old male who previously underwent craniotomy for resection of a left frontal glioma and subsequent radiation

was found to have an anterior cerebral artery (ACA) pseudoaneurysm on follow-up imaging, confirmed angiographically (► Fig. 25.2a). The patient underwent superselective Wada testing with 30 mg of intra-arterial sodium amobarbital infused into the right pericallosal artery resulting in no discernible neurologic changes (► Fig. 25.2b). He thus underwent embolization of the pseudoaneurysm and parent vessel with Onyx 34 without complication (► Fig. 25.2c).
Imaging studies: See ► Fig. 25.2.

25.4 Level of Evidence

Given the patient's refractory epilepsy, left-handedness and potential need for temporal lobectomy, a Wada test is a safe and effective test to facilitate determination of language and memory dominance (Class 4).

25.5 Landmark Papers

25.5.1 Original Wada Papers

Wada J. A new method for the determination of the side of cerebral speech dominance: a preliminary report of the intra-carotid injection of sodium Amytal in man. Med Biol 1949;14:221–222.

Any discussion of landmark papers on the Wada test must include the original work of Juhn A. Wada in his development of the intracarotid amobarbital procedure (IAP).[8,9,10,11] While studying seizure mechanisms and searching for a method to allow unilateral electroconvulsive shock therapy for psychosis during the course of several studies in 1948, Juhn Wada used intracarotid injection of sodium amobarbital and metrazol to investigate how epileptic discharge spreads between the hemispheres of the brain.[11] It was determined that this technique could be utilized to assess the lateralization of cerebral speech dominance as sodium amobarbital induced a temporary aphasia when the dominant cerebral hemisphere was injected. This technique was tested on 80 patients in Japan from 1948 to 1954 without any reported complications. The procedure described by Wada would become the standard test in the presurgical assessment for resection of an epileptic focus for the treatment of medically intractable epilepsy.

Perria L, Rosadini G, Rossi GF. Determination of side of cerebral dominance with amobarbital. Arch Neurol 1961;4:173–181.

In 1961, Perria et al set out to establish the validity of the IAP and to standardize results.12 Perria et al established conditions that must be satisfied before interpreting results from the method utilized by Wada. These conditions included: (1) the dose of amobarbital that produces an effect when injected into the carotid must not produce any effect when administered intravenously; (2) the action of the drug be confined to the hemisphere ipsilateral to the side of the intracarotid injection; and (3) the EEG and all the clinical phenomena are correlated. On the basis of these conditions, Perria et al looked for changes in EEG activity, speech production, plantar reflex, knee jerk, and emotional state. They reached the conclusion that speech disturbances combined with depressive-type emotional reactivity shows the drug is acting on the dominant hemisphere, whereas lack of speech deficits with euphoric-type emotional reactivity shows the drug is acting on the nondominant hemisphere. These clinical effects can only be analyzed when the EEG activity, reflexes, and motor power are also lateralized.

Jack CR, Jr., Nichols DA, Sharbrough FW, Marsh WR, Petersen RC. Selective posterior cerebral artery Amytal test for evaluating memory function before surgery for temporal lobe seizure. Radiology 1988;168:787–793.

When the Wada test is intended for use prior to selective amygdalohippocampectomy, the reliability of the IAP has been questioned. In most patients, the ICA perfuses the uncus, amygdala, and anterior hippocampus, but not the posterior two-thirds of the hippocampus.[13] Due to this inadequate perfusion of mediobasal temporal lobe structures with the ICA method, in 1988, Jack et al injected sodium amobarbital selectively into the PCA to distribute the sodium amobarbital solely within the hippocampus for selective testing of memory function, depicting favorable procedures in 38 of 45 patients.[14] The significant correlation between performance during memory testing during the PCA-amobarbital procedure and pre- and postoperative results was significant only for left-sided operations and injections, which the authors suggest signifies that the left PCA-amobarbital procedure simulates the outcomes of resection on memory performance and verbal learning.

Urbach H, Klemm E, Linke DB, et al. Posterior cerebral artery Wada test: sodium Amytal distribution and functional deficits. Neuroradiology 2001;43:290–294.

In the study by Urbach et al, the authors sought to assess sodium amobarbital distribution in the PCA Wada test and to relate it to the neurological deficits that occurred during the test.[13] The PCA Wada test was performed in 14 patients with medically intractable temporal lobe epilepsy. Eighty mg of sodium amobarbital and 14.8 MBq ^{99m}Tc-hexamethylpropylene-amine oxime (HMPAO) (due to the lipophilic nature of HMPAO, the distribution of the radiotracer reflects that of sodium amobarbital) were simultaneously injected into the P2-segment of the PCA, and distribution of sodium amobarbital was determined with high-resolution single-photon emission computed tomography (SPECT). In all patients, SPECT demonstrated the HMPAO/sodium amobarbital combination was distributed throughout the parahippocampal gyrus, hippocampus, and occipital lobe (including the calcarine area), and in 11 cases was also seen in the thalamus. Selective amygdalohippocampectomy

was subsequently carried out in nine of the 14 patients, none of whom showed a major postoperative decline in memory.

Rauch RA, Vinuela F, Dion J, et al. Preembolization functional evaluation in brain arteriovenous malformations: the superselective Amytal test. AJNR American journal of neuroradiology 1992;13:303–308.

During the analysis of vascular anomalies such as aneurysms and arteriovenous malformations (AVMs), superselective angiography is useful in providing accurate architecture on angiography.[15] The combination of pretreatment Wada testing with arterial occlusion proves a helpful instrument, providing dynamic, functional, and anatomic data about the vascular territory of the vessel to be catheterized. In the endovascular treatment of an aneurysm located in eloquent cortex with possible speech and language involvement, a superselective Wada test can be used to determine the safety of vascular sacrifice.[16] Injection of sodium amobarbital or lidocaine to detect feeding vessels to the spinal cord in primates[17] and in humans[18] has similarly been described.

Rauch et al reported on 109 superselective Wada tests that were performed with 30-mg injections of sodium amobarbital prior to embolization of an AVM to reproduce the subsequent injection of contrast and embolic material.[19] The vascular territory of the vessels studied included middle cerebral artery in 32 patients, anterior cerebral artery in 13 patients, and PCA in 18 patients. There were 23 positive tests (associated with changes in the neurologic examination or EEG) following sodium amobarbital injection. There were no reported adverse long-term effects of the 109 injections as the focal effects of the sodium amobarbital completely dissipated after 10 minutes. The authors conclude that determining positive tests can facilitate decision making as to which vessels can be embolized without inducing permanent neurologic deficits.

25.6 Recommendations

Debate continues regarding the reliability, predictive value, and safety of the Wada test. Though the Wada test is considered the gold standard in lateralizing language and memory function in the presurgical work-up of patients with epilepsy, the test's reliability and predictive value has been called into question with respect to postoperative memory decline.[20,21,22] Evaluation of the Wada test is additionally limited, as clinical indications differ among epilepsy centers, and no universally accepted standardized protocol exists.[23]

Haag et al evaluated Wada test practice from 2000 to 2005 as well as clinicians' attitudes toward the test.[1] Twenty-six German, Swiss, Austrian, and Dutch epilepsy centers were asked to report on the use of the Wada test, providing information on 1,421 Wada tests. Wada test frequency significantly decreased throughout the study period from 282 tests in 2000 to 210 in 2005 despite an increase in surgical resection during this time. Seventy-three percent of the test centers utilized the classic procedure with ICA injection and bilateral consecutive investigation of both hemispheres, and test protocols were similar, even though no universal standard protocol exists.

A total of 15 complications were reported by Haag et al with an overall complication rate of 1.09% (range of 0–20% across centers). Loddenkemper et al reviewed 677 consecutive patient charts for complications during the IAP, reporting a complication rate of 10.9% (74 patients).[4] These observed complications included encephalopathy (7.2%), seizures (1.2%), strokes (0.6%), transient ischemic attacks (0.6%), localized hemorrhage at the catheter insertion site (0.6%), and carotid artery dissections (0.4%). The authors found that older patients were more susceptible to the complication of stroke or dissection, whereas younger patients more frequently had seizures.

In the study by Haag et al, clinicians rated the Wada test as having good reliability and validity for language determination, whereas respondents estimated the reliability and validity of the Wada test for memory lateralization as moderate to low.[1] In a study to estimate the retest reliability of the IAP for language and memory lateralization, 1,249 consecutive tests on 1,190 Cleveland Clinic patients were retrospectively reviewed.[24] Retesting yielded reproducible results in language lateralization in all but one patient; however, repeated memory test results were less consistent across tests, and memory lateralization was unreliable in 63% of the patients.

Less invasive alternatives such as fMRI have emerged. fMRI measures neuronal activity indirectly through changes in blood oxygenation-level dependent contrast.[25] Many imaging studies have estimated the validity of fMRI as an alternative to Wada test, finding an overall discordance rate of approximately 15%.[26,27,28] Part of this discrepancy between fMRI and Wada test results involves fMRI's role as a marker of brain activation compared to the IAP as a measure of brain inactivation. Inactivation techniques rather than activation techniques better mimic surgical intervention as a region activated in fMRI might be compensated for after its removal during the operation.[25] Further, unlike the Wada test, fMRI cannot determine whether a structure has an essential role in language processing, only if it is involved. Other possible proposed alternatives to the Wada test include methods like synthetic aperture magnetometry,[29] functional transcranial Doppler sonography,[30] and infrared spectroscopy.[31] As reported by Haag et al, clinicians do not feel confident relying exclusively on the results of these noninvasive, mostly activation-based imaging techniques in all patients.[1]

Superselective Wada has ongoing utility in identifying potential deficits that may result from embolization.[32] Pretreatment with superselective Wada may facilitate prediction of neurological deficits, providing patient-specific information to determine treatment outcomes as functional anatomy related to chronic brain lesions may vary from traditional anatomy.

25.7 Summary

"A surgeon is never justified in carrying out any formidable procedure involving the areas of the brain responsible for speech if any doubt remains as to the side of the speech control."

— Walter Dandy

1. The intracarotid sodium amobarbital procedure still holds an important role in the presurgical evaluation of patients with medically intractable seizures, given its validity and reliability.
2. The Wada test can correctly determine atypical individual language dominance but has more ambiguous prognostic value for postoperative memory deficits.

3. Superselective Wada testing has ongoing applications for a plethora of cerebrovascular pathology.

References

[1] Haag A, Knake S, Hamer HM, et al. Arbeitsgemeinschaft für Prächirurgische Epilepsiediagnostik und Operative Epilepsietherapie e.V. The Wada test in Austrian, Dutch, German, and Swiss epilepsy centers from 2000 to 2005: a review of 1421 procedures. Epilepsy Behav. 2008; 13(1):83–89

[2] Fifi JT, Meyers PM, Lavine SD, et al. Complications of modern diagnostic cerebral angiography in an academic medical center. J Vasc Interv Radiol. 2009; 20(4):442–447

[3] Willinsky RA, Taylor SM, TerBrugge K, Farb RI, Tomlinson G, Montanera W. Neurologic complications of cerebral angiography: prospective analysis of 2,899 procedures and review of the literature. Radiology. 2003; 227(2):522–528

[4] Loddenkemper T, Morris HH, Möddel G. Complications during the Wada test. Epilepsy Behav. 2008; 13(3):551–553

[5] Beimer NJ, Buchtel HA, Glynn SM. One center's experience with complications during the Wada test. Epilepsia. 2015; 56(8):e110–e113

[6] Kemp S, Prendergast G, Karapanagiotidis T, et al. Concordance between the Wada test and neuroimaging lateralization: Influence of imaging modality (fMRI and MEG) and patient experience. Epilepsy Behav. 2018; 78:155–160

[7] Bauer PR, Reitsma JB, Houweling BM, Ferrier CH, Ramsey NF. Can fMRI safely replace the Wada test for preoperative assessment of language lateralisation? A meta-analysis and systematic review. J Neurol Neurosurg Psychiatry. 2014; 85(5):581–588

[8] Wada J. A new method for the determination of the side of cerebral speech dominance: a preliminary report of the intra-carotid injection of sodium Amytal in man. Igaku To Seibutsugaku. 1949; 14:221–222

[9] Wada J. An experimental study on the neural mechanism of the spread of epileptic impulse. Folia Psychiatr Neurol Jpn. 1951; 4(4):289–301

[10] Wada J, Kirikae T. Neurological contribution to induced unilateral paralysis of human cerebral hemisphere: special emphasis on experimentally induced aphasia. Hokkaido Igaku Zasshi. 1949; 24:1–10

[11] Wada J, Rasmussen T. Intracarotid injection of sodium Amytal for the lateralization of cerebral speech dominance: 1960. J Neurosurg. 2007; 106(6):1117–1133

[12] Perria L, Rosadini G, Rossi GF. Determination of side of cerebral dominance with amobarbital. Arch Neurol. 1961; 4:173–181

[13] Urbach H, Klemm E, Linke DB, et al. Posterior cerebral artery Wada test: sodium Amytal distribution and functional deficits. Neuroradiology. 2001; 43(4):290–294

[14] Jack CR, Jr, Nichols DA, Sharbrough FW, Marsh WR, Petersen RC. Selective posterior cerebral artery Amytal test for evaluating memory function before surgery for temporal lobe seizure. Radiology. 1988; 168(3):787–793

[15] Rajpal S, Moftakhar R, Bauer AM, Turk AS, Niemann DB. Superselective Wada test for ruptured spontaneous fusiform middle cerebral artery aneurysm: a technical case report. J Neurointerv Surg. 2011; 3(3):237–241

[16] Deveikis JP. Sequential injections of amobarbital sodium and lidocaine for provocative neurologic testing in the external carotid circulation. AJNR Am J Neuroradiol. 1996; 17(6):1143–1147

[17] Doppman JL, Girton M, Oldfield EH. Spinal Wada test. Radiology. 1986; 161(2):319–321

[18] Horton JA, Latchaw RE, Gold LH, Pang D. Embolization of intramedullary arteriovenous malformations of the spinal cord. AJNR Am J Neuroradiol. 1986; 7(1):113–118

[19] Rauch RA, Vinuela F, Dion J, et al. Preembolization functional evaluation in brain arteriovenous malformations: the superselective Amytal test. AJNR Am J Neuroradiol. 1992; 13(1):303–308

[20] Simkins-Bullock J. Beyond speech lateralization: a review of the variability, reliability, and validity of the intracarotid amobarbital procedure and its nonlanguage uses in epilepsy surgery candidates. Neuropsychol Rev. 2000; 10(1):41–74

[21] Lineweaver TT, Morris HH, Naugle RI, Najm IM, Diehl B, Bingaman W. Evaluating the contributions of state-of-the-art assessment techniques to predicting memory outcome after unilateral anterior temporal lobectomy. Epilepsia. 2006; 47(11):1895–1903

[22] Helmstaedter C, Kurthen M. Validity of the WADA test. Epilepsy Behav. 2002; 3(6):562–563

[23] Jones-Gotman M, Rouleau I, Snyder PJ. Clinical and research contributions of the intracarotid amobarbital procedure to neuropsychology. Brain Cogn. 1997; 33(1):1–6

25

[24] Loddenkemper T, Morris HH, Lineweaver TT, Kellinghaus C. Repeated intracarotid amobarbital tests. Epilepsia. 2007; 48(3):553–558

[25] Klöppel S, Büchel C. Alternatives to the Wada test: a critical view of functional magnetic resonance imaging in preoperative use. Curr Opin Neurol. 2005; 18 (4):418–423

[26] Szaflarski JP, Gloss D, Binder JR, et al. Practice guideline summary: use of fMRI in the presurgical evaluation of patients with epilepsy: Report of the Guideline Development, Dissemination, and Implementation Subcommittee of the American Academy of Neurology. Neurology. 2017; 88(4):395–402

[27] Dym RJ, Burns J, Freeman K, Lipton ML. Is functional MR imaging assessment of hemispheric language dominance as good as the Wada test? A meta-analysis. Radiology. 2011; 261(2):446–455

[28] Janecek JK, Swanson SJ, Sabsevitz DS, et al. Language lateralization by fMRI and Wada testing in 229 patients with epilepsy: rates and predictors of discordance. Epilepsia. 2013; 54(2):314–322

[29] Hirata M, Kato A, Taniguchi M, et al. Determination of language dominance with synthetic aperture magnetometry: comparison with the Wada test. Neuroimage. 2004; 23(1):46–53

[30] Knecht S, Deppe M, Ebner A, et al. Noninvasive determination of language lateralization by functional transcranial Doppler sonography: a comparison with the Wada test. Stroke. 1998; 29(1):82–86

[31] Watson NF, Dodrill C, Farrell D, Holmes MD, Miller JW. Determination of language dominance with near-infrared spectroscopy: comparison with the intracarotid amobarbital procedure. Seizure. 2004; 13(6):399–402

[32] Tawk RG, Tummala RP, Memon MZ, Siddiqui AH, Hopkins LN, Levy EI. Utility of pharmacologic provocative neurological testing before embolization of occipital lobe arteriovenous malformations. World Neurosurg. 2011; 76(3–4):276–281

25

26 Venous Sinus Stenting for Intracranial Hypertension

Matthew R. Sanborn and Matthew Johnson

Abstract

Intracranial hypertension has long been considered an idiopathic disease. Advances in endovascular evaluation and management, however, increasingly suggest that venous hypertension plays a role in its pathogenesis, with many patients exhibiting signs of venous stenosis located within the cerebral venous sinuses. Venous sinus stenting for the treatment of intracranial hypertension has become an accepted treatment for patients that have failed more conservative management. Although long-term follow-up is lacking, recent studies suggest that, in carefully selected patients, this treatment option compares favorably to traditional invasive treatments such as ventriculoperitoneal shunting.

Keywords: intracranial hypertension, venous sinus stenosis, venous sinus stenting, pseudotumor cerebri, pulsatile tinnitus, transverse sinus, sigmoid sinus

26.1 Goals

1. Review the literature that informs current understanding of the pathogenesis of intracranial hypertension.
2. Critically analyze the literature on the treatment options for intracranial hypertension.
3. Review the literature that evaluates outcomes of treatment of intracranial hypertension with venous sinus stenting.

26.2 Case Example

26.2.1 History of Present Illness

A 27-year-old female presented with 8 months of progressive daily headaches, rated a 7/10 on the visual analog pain scale. She developed blurry vision and subsequent ophthalmological examination revealed bilateral papilledema, Frisen grade II. She denied pulsatile tinnitus.

A lumbar puncture was performed in the lateral decubitus position with a measured opening pressure of 27 cm H_2O. She developed a postlumbar puncture headache requiring epidural blood patch and subsequently noted transient improvement in her headaches and vision for several days.

The patient had attempted diet and weight loss without success. She had transient improvement in her headaches with acetazolamide but was unable to tolerate the side effects. She underwent a trial of topiramate without improvement.

Past medical history: Polycystic ovarian syndrome, anxiety, irritable bowel syndrome, ocular migraine.

Past surgical history: Cholecystectomy, dilatation, and curettage of uterus.

Family history: Noncontributory.

Social history: Denies alcohol or tobacco use.

Neurological examination: Unremarkable.

Imaging studies: Magnetic resonance venography (MRV) demonstrated a dominant right transverse sinus with signal dropout at the transverse sigmoid junction along with a nondominant left transverse sinus with signal dropout at the left transverse sigmoid junction (▶ Fig. 26.1a, b).

26.2.2 Treatment Plan

Treatment options were discussed in depth with the patient, including optic nerve sheath fenestration (ONSF), cerebrospinal fluid (CSF) diversion, and venography with potential venous sinus stenting. She elected to pursue venography and possible venous sinus stenting. Venography was performed under light conscious sedation. This confirmed a hypoplastic left transverse sinus with focal narrowing at the transverse-sigmoid junction (▶ Fig. 26.2a) as well as a dominant right transverse sinus with focal narrowing at the transverse-sigmoid junction (▶ Fig. 26.2b). Venous pressure manometry was performed showing a pressure of 21 mm Hg in the superior sagittal sinus, 21 mm Hg in the right transverse sinus, 14 mm Hg in the left transverse sinus, 7 mm Hg in the left sigmoid sinus, and 9 mm Hg in the right sigmoid sinus.

Given the pressure gradient of 12 mm Hg in the dominant transverse sinus, the patient was offered transverse sinus stenting, and she elected to proceed. She was placed on 325 mg of aspirin and 75 mg of clopidogrel for 7 days and subsequently underwent uneventful placement of a stent within the right transverse sigmoid junction (▶ Fig. 26.3).

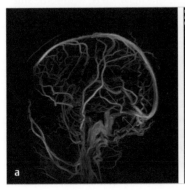
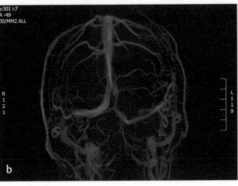

Fig. 26.1 Magnetic resonance venography (MRV) of the brain lateral **(a)** and anteroposterior (AP) **(b)** views showing a dominant right transverse sinus with a nondominant left transverse sinus. There is signal dropout at the bilateral transverse-sigmoid junctions suggesting venous stenosis.

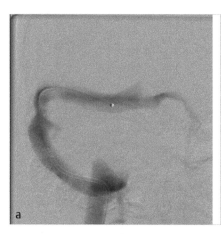
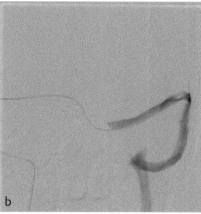

Fig. 26.2 Venography of the right (**a**) and left (**b**) transverse sinuses, anteroposterior (AP) views confirming narrowing bilaterally at the transverse-sigmoid junction.

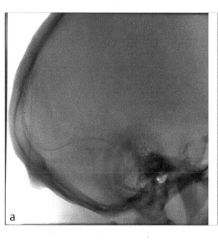
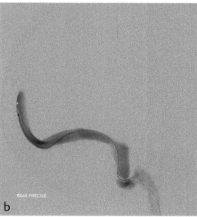

Fig. 26.3 Lateral unsubtracted (**a**) and subtracted (**b**) angiography following placement of a stent within the right transverse-sigmoid junction. There is a significantly improved caliber and flow following stent placement.

26.2.3 Follow-up

The patient developed the expected postoperative headache that resolved after 10 to 14 days. She was maintained on aspirin and clopidogrel for 6 months at which point a CTA demonstrated wide patency of the stent and the clopidogrel was discontinued. At her 1-year follow-up, her papilledema had resolved, and she was no longer suffering from headaches.

26.3 Case Summary

1. *What are the criteria for diagnosis of idiopathic intracranial hypertension?*
   While multiple classification and diagnostic schemes have been proposed for intracranial hypertension,[1,2,3] the most widely cited and adopted criteria for the diagnosis of idiopathic intracranial hypertension are the modified Dandy criteria, proposed by Smith in 1985 (► Table 26.1).[4] These criteria include signs and symptoms of increased intracranial pressure (such as papilledema and headache) in the setting of CSF pressure of greater than 200 mm of water relative to the level of the left atrium in a patient that is alert and oriented with no localizing neurological findings (except possible cranial nerve VI palsy). In addition, there can be no evidence of abnormalities within the ventricular system and no other obvious source of increased intracranial pressure. For CSF pressures of 200 to 250 mm H_2O, at least one of the following is also required: pulse synchronous tinnitus, cranial nerve VI palsy, Frisen grade II papilledema, MRV with

transverse sinus stenosis/collapse, partially empty sella or optic nerve sheath with filled out CSF spaces on magnetic resonance imaging (MRI), echography for drusen negative. This patient meets the modified Dandy criteria for the diagnosis of idiopathic intracranial hypertension.

2. *What are the treatment options for idiopathic intracranial hypertension?*
   a) Diet and exercise/weight loss:
      In the absence of fulminant papilledema or progressive visual changes, treatment options begin with diet and lifestyle modification. In 1974, Newborg demonstrated a complete reversal of papilledema in all of nine patients with a very low-calorie (400–1000 calories per day) and low-sodium (less than 100 mg/d) diet with accompanying fluid restriction.[5] More recent studies have shown improvements with less draconian diets, with some studies showing reversal of symptoms in patients who are able to lose 5 to 10% of total body weight.[6]
   b) Carbonic anhydrase inhibitors:
      The Idiopathic Intracranial Hypertension Treatment Trial (IIHTT) was the first randomized, controlled trial examining the use of acetazolamide and weight loss for treatment of vision loss related to idiopathic intracranial hypertension. Patients were randomized to weight loss and placebo or weight loss and acetazolamide with a primary outcome measure of perimetric mean deviation (PMD). Secondary outcomes included safety, quality of life, change in Frisen scale papilledema grade, weight loss, and headache disability.

Table 26.1 Modified Dandy criteria for intracranial hypertension

Modified Dandy criteria for intracranial hypertension

1. Signs and symptoms of increased intracranial pressure

2. Absence of localizing findings on neurological examination

3. Absence of deformity, displacement, or obstruction of the ventricular system and otherwise normal neurodiagnostic studies, except for evidence of increased CSF pressure; abnormal neuroimaging except for empty sella, optic nerve sheath with filled out CSF spaces, and smooth-walled non-flow-related venous sinus stenosis or collapse should lead to another diagnosis

4. Awake and alert

5. No other cause of increased intracranial pressure present

For CSF opening pressure of 200–250 mm water at least one of the following is required:

– Pulse synchronous tinnitus

– Cranial nerve VI palsy

– Frisen grade II papilledema

– Echography for drusen-negative and no other disc anomalies mimicking disc edema present

– MRV with lateral sinus collapse/stenosis

– Partially empty sella on coronal or sagittal views and optic nerve sheaths with filled-out CSF spaces next to globe on T2-weighted axial scans

Abbreviations: CSF, cerebrospinal fluid; MRV, magnetic resonance venography.

The study was able to demonstrate significant improvements in visual field, CSF opening pressure, papilledema, and quality of life in the acetazolamide and weight-loss groups when compared to the placebo and weight-loss groups. The study did not find a significant improvement in headache severity.

c) Bariatric surgery:

Given the success of weight loss in ameliorating symptoms of intracranial hypertension it is unsurprising that bariatric surgery has been suggested as an invasive treatment option for refractory intracranial hypertension. In a study of 24 morbidly obese females (mean BMI 47) with headaches and elevated opening pressure on lumbar puncture who underwent gastric surgery, 18 of the 19 patients not lost to follow-up at 1 year demonstrated resolution of headache. Only 12 of the patients had papilledema preoperatively and this improved following surgery. Two patients later regained weight with return of symptoms.[7] A meta-analysis comparing bariatric surgery and nonsurgical weight loss for treatment of symptoms of intracranial hypertension including a total of 65 patients undergoing surgery and 277 without surgery showed that 100% of the patients with papilledema in the surgical group improved and 90.2% had a reduction in headaches, whereas nonsurgical weight loss led to a reduction in papilledema in 66.7% and an improvement in headache symptoms in 23.2%.[8]

d) Optic nerve sheath fenestration (ONSF):

Multiple retrospective case series speak to the utility of ONSF in arresting visual deterioration in intracranial hypertension.[9,10,11,12] In one representative study, 54% of eyes had stabilization of visual acuity following ONSF, with 22% showing improvement and visual deterioration in 24% of operated eyes.[11] These results are in alignment with other studies.[10] Although there is a broad agreement on the utility of ONSF for stabilization of visual loss, it seems to be less effective for ameliorating headaches than other surgical interventions. One systematic review found that only 36% of patients had improvement in headaches with ONSF compared to 62.5% with ventriculoperitoneal

shunting, 75.2% with lumboperitoneal shunting, and 82.9% with venous stenting.[13] Complications can be seen in up to 40% and, although mostly minor disorders of ocular motility, approximately 5% were central retinal artery occlusion with subsequent loss of vision.[14]

e) CSF diversion:

CSF diversion has been the most widely adopted invasive intervention for intracranial hypertension. Shunting for intracranial hypertension increased 350% between 1988 and 2002.[15] Despite its widespread use there are no randomized, controlled trials to guide treatment; and evidence, similar to the other interventions discussed, remains largely limited to retrospective case series. While CSF diversion is generally effective at arresting vision loss or improving vision, its effect on headaches is more variable. Sinclair et al showed that, while visual acuity improved at 6 and 12 months following CSF diversion, 68% of patients had persistent headaches at 6 months and 79% at 2 years.[16]

CSF diversion generally is performed using either ventriculoperitoneal (VP) or lumboperitoneal (LP) shunts. There are multiple other possible configurations, such as ventriculoatrial and ventriculopleural, but these remain less commonly utilized or reserved for second-line procedures. Some studies have shown that LP shunts have a 2.5-fold risk of requiring revision.[17]

f) Subtemporal decompression:

Although initially used by Dandy as the treatment of choice for idiopathic intracranial hypertension, subtemporal decompression has largely fallen out of favor as a first-line surgical treatment for intracranial hypertension. In a retrospective study of eight patients undergoing subtemporal decompression for intracranial hypertension, Kessler et al demonstrated arrest of deterioration in visual fields in all eight patients, although five subsequently required CSF diversion for intractable headaches.[18]

g) Venous sinus stenting:

Recognition that dural sinus thrombosis can cause symptoms of intracranial hypertension dates back to at least 1951.[19] It was not until 2001, however, that Higgins reported the first use of a venous stent for treatment of intracranial hypertension.[20] Multiple case series have since demonstrated the efficacy of venous sinus stenting in treating select cases of intracranial hypertension.[21,22,23,24,25,26]

Meta-analysis comparing CSF diversion and venous sinus stenting in medically refractory intracranial hypertension demonstrated that, among patients undergoing venous sinus stenting, 78% experienced improvement in vision, 83% showed improvement in headache, and 97% showed improvement in papilledema. These numbers compare favorably to ONSF (59% improvement in vision, 44% improvement in headache, and 80% improvement in papilledema) and CSF diversion (54% improvement in vision, 80% improvement in vision, and 70% improvement in papilledema).[27]

3. *What factors would you consider in making treatment recommendations?*

a) Presence and characteristics of venous stenosis on MRV:
Farb et al found that 90% of patients with intracranial hypertension have stenosis of the venous sinuses. They furthermore differentiated between two distinct types of stenosis: intrinsic and extrinsic. Intrinsic stenosis manifests as "marginated," well-demarcated filling defects within the sinus—likely reflecting arachnoid granulation. Extrinsic stenosis are smooth, tapered areas of narrowing thought to reflect external compression (e.g., from swollen brain parenchyma).[28]

While both extrinsic and intrinsic stenoses have responded to stenting, some authors have found that clinical recurrence has a predilection for extrinsic stenosis with many of these occurring in the setting of stenosis proximal to the stent.[29] Other authors have noted a greater mean improvement in opening pressure following venous stenting in patients with intrinsic stenosis compared to extrinsic stenosis.

Anatomical variation is the rule rather than the exception in the venous sinuses, with hypoplasia or focal stenosis of one side being a common and likely incidental finding. This has led most groups to perform venography to better characterize any potential stenosis seen on noninvasive imaging as well as manometry evaluate the physiologic significance of any abnormalities prior to proceeding with stent placement.

b) Venography and manometry:
Venography, typically using a 0.027-inch microcatheter, allows not only for better anatomical characterization of problem areas but also for dynamic evaluation of flow characteristics. By connecting the microcatheter to a manometer with "0 mm Hg" pressure standardized to the midaxillary line, venous pressure can be assessed throughout the venous sinus system. General anesthesia has a significant and highly variable effect on venous manometry and should be avoided during manometry.[30] While the practice of performing manometry to define a pressure gradient across an area of stenosis is ubiquitous, there is no evidence-based data to suggest that a particular threshold can accurately predict a positive clinical response. Values represented in the literature vary from 4 mm Hg[31] to 15 mm Hg[32] with many larger series using a cutoff of 8 mm Hg.[20]

c) Severity of papilledema and vision loss:
There is little data to support any particular treatment algorithm. In general, most patients benefit from a trial of weight loss and diet—advancing to treatment with carbonic anhydrase inhibitors before consideration is given to more invasive treatment options. The exception are patients with moderate-to-severe visual loss and high-grade papilledema (often defined as mean deviation on automated perimetry greater than −5 dB).[33]

Acute vision loss in the setting of intracranial hypertension is unusual and is a surgical emergency. CSF diversion should be performed emergently, either with lumbar puncture as a temporizing measure or proceeding directly to shunt placement. CSF diversion should be performed emergently, with consideration given to high-volume lumbar puncture if shunting emergently is not feasible.[34]

d) Headaches:
Headaches are often the chief complaint of patients with intracranial hypertension. The efficacy of different treatment modalities in ameliorating this disabling symptom varies widely. Small studies have shown improvement in headache severity and frequency with an aggressive (< 425 kcal/d) weight-loss regimen.[35] ONSF has widely variable results in headache management. In a series of 86 patients, only 13% reported improvement in headache at follow-up.[36] With ventriculoperitoneal shunting up to 95% of patients have significant improvement in headache symptoms at 1 month; however, severe headaches recur in 19% by 12 months and 48% at 36 months.[16] Venous stent placement compares favorably to other treatment modalities in alleviating headaches. Rates of symptomatic improvement in larger studies range from 69.2%[37] to 93%[20] with a meta-analysis highlighting improvement in 83%.[26]

4. *What would you recommend for this patient?*
This patient has failed conservative management with intractable headaches, vision changes, and papilledema despite attempts at weight loss and therapy with a carbonic anhydrase inhibitor. Her MRV suggested a possible venous stenosis on her dominant side with hypoplasia of the transverse sinus on the contralateral side.

Bariatric surgery is reserved for appropriate, morbidly obese candidates. Although this patient is overweight, she is not morbidly obese. ONSF is unreliable in treating headaches and, with headaches being a dominating symptom in this patient, there are better interventional options. CSF diversion and venography with an eye toward venous stenting are both reasonable options. We tend to offer VP shunting over LP shunting simply because of the higher failure rate of LP shunts. After extensive discussion with the patient regarding the relative merits of CSF diversion and stenting, the patient elected to proceed with venous sinus stenting. She underwent venography with manometry under conscious sedation, which confirmed a venous stenosis on the right with an associated venous pressure gradient. She was then started on aspirin and clopidogrel and underwent venous stent placement 7 days later.

5. *What follow-up is needed for patients with intracranial hypertension?*

There is no particular accepted follow-up protocol. We perform a computed tomography (CT) venogram at 6 months and, if there is no evidence of new or recurrent stenosis, allow the patient to discontinue clopidogrel and maintain them on aspirin indefinitely.

26.4 Level of Evidence

Medical management: Acetazolamide is safe and well tolerated up to 4 g/d and, combined with weight loss, is more effective than weight loss alone for the treatment of vision loss, papilledema, increased intracranial pressure, and quality of life (Class I, Level of Evidence B).

Weight loss: Weight loss can help improve symptoms associated with intracranial hypertension, including headache and papilledema (Class IIa, Level of Evidence C).

ONSF: It is effective at treating papilledema with more variable effects on headaches (Class IIa, Level of Evidence B).

CSF diversion: CSF diversion is an effective treatment for intracranial hypertension refractory to medical management (Class IIa, Level of Evidence B).

Venous sinus stenting: Stenting of stenotic areas of the intracranial venous sinuses associated with pressure gradients is effective at treating headache, vision changes, and pulsatile tinnitus (Class IIa, Level of Evidence B).

26.5 Landmark Papers

Satti SR, Leishangthem L, Chaudry MI. Meta-Analysis of CSF diversion procedures and dural venous sinus stenting in the setting of medically refractory idiopathic intracranial hypertension. AJNR Am J Neuroradiol. 2015; 36:1899–1904.

In this meta-analysis, Satti et al compared results in patients with intracranial hypertension undergoing ONSF, CSF diversion, and venous sinus stenting. Data extraction encompassed peer-reviewed publications between 1988 and 2014 and resulted in 18 studies with 712 patients for ONSF, 17 studies with 435 patients for CSF diversion, and 8 studies with 136 patients for venous stenting.

Venous sinus stenting compared favorably to CSF diversion and ONSF in this analysis, with better rates of improvement in vision (78% for venous stenting, 54% in CSF diversion, and 59% in ONSF), headache (83% improved in venous stenting, 80% in CSF diversion, and 44% in ONSF), and papilledema (97% improved in venous stenting, 70% in CSF diversion, and 80% in ONSF). Additional procedures were performed in 14.8% of patients undergoing ONSF, 43% in CSF diversion, and 10.3% in venous stenting.

Major complications were reported in 1.5% of ONSF cases, 7.6% of CSF diversion, and 2.9% of venous stent cases, while minor complications were reported in 16.4%, 32.9%, and 4.4%, respectively.

As in all meta-analyses, this paper suffers from a lack of homogeneity of the data. ONSF data, for example, was largely, and unsurprisingly, focused on vision—with results on both visual acuity and visual fields available for a majority of included patients. CSF diversion and venous stenting studies, by

contrast subsumed both visual fields and visual acuity under the heading of "visual acuity changes" and, even then, data was only available from 193 of 435 patients. Similarly, although 60% of the 712 patients included for analysis in the ONSF study reported headache, data on improvement in headache were available for only 127 patients.

The Nordic Idiopathic Intracranial Hypertension Group Writing Committee. Effect of acetazolamide on visual function in patients with idiopathic intracranial hypertension and mild visual loss. JAMA 2014;311(16):1641–1651.

The list of randomized, controlled, double-blind trials addressing treatment of intracranial hypertension is short. The Nordic group[38] has attempted to address this with the IIHTT. In this multicenter, randomized, controlled trial, patients with intracranial hypertension and mild visual loss (mean perimetric deviation between −2 dB and −7 dB) were randomized to either a low-sodium weight-reduction diet and placebo or the same diet with acetazolamide (up to a maximum of 4 g/d) for 6 months.

One hundred sixty-five patients were enrolled (161 women and 4 men). Eighty-six were randomized to acetazolamide, while 79 received placebo. The planned primary outcome measure was the change in PMD at 6 months in the most affected eye. Secondary outcomes included papilledema grade change (using the Frisen scale), quality of life, headache disability, and weight loss.

While both the treatment groups saw improvement in PMD over the 6 months, the acetazolamide group experienced a modestly greater improvement (95% CI, 0 to −1.43 dB; $p = 0.050$). Similarly, there was a significant improvement in Frisen grade in the acetazolamide group compared to placebo and in quality-of-life measures (a difference of 8.33 on the Visual Function Questionnaire 25 [VFQ-25] in the acetazolamide group versus a difference of 1.98 in the placebo group). Interestingly, there was no significant treatment effect between the two groups in headache disability (measured by the HIT-6 score) or in visual acuity.

While well designed, this study was necessarily limited in scope. Although the study shows a convincing, if modest, benefit to acetazolamide in addition to diet compared to diet alone in improving PMD, papilledema, and quality of life, no discernable benefit was seen for visual acuity and headache. For many, severe headache is the presenting, and most disabling, complaint. The fact that 69% of patients in the acetazolamide group and 68% of patients in the placebo group had persistent headaches at 6 months highlights a need for additional therapy in a substantial subset of this patient population. The pressing question of the best intervention for addressing refractory cases of intracranial hypertension remains unresolved.

Ahmed RM, Wilkinson M, Parker GD, et al. Transverse sinus stenting for idiopathic hypertension: a review of 52 patients and of model predictions. AJNR Am J Neuroradiol 2011;32(8):1408–1414.

In the first, large retrospective series of intracranial hypertension patients treated with venous stenting, Ahmed and colleagues[39] reported on their experiences with 52 patients. They utilized modified Dandy criteria for diagnosis of intracranial hypertension, although six patients had headache without papilledema but high CSF pressures. Treated patients ranged in age from 10 to 64 years, with mean 34. In keeping with the demographics of intracranial hypertension 47 of the 52 patients were females and 47 had BMI over 30.

Their study went on for 9 years during which 80 patients were evaluated with manometry and venography. Of those 80 patients, 52 met criteria, which was arbitrarily defined as a transverse sinus stenosis with a trans-stenosis gradient of > /= 8 mm Hg. Cerebral venography and manometry was performed under light sedation—either via femoral vein or right internal jugular access. Venous stenting was subsequently performed under general endotracheal anesthesia.

Ahmed et al reported that, following stent placement, papilledema resolved in all 46 patients in whom it was present preoperatively. Out of 43 patients who reported headache preoperatively, 8 still had "some headaches" following stent placement; 6 of these went on to have additional stent placement with ultimate resolution of headaches in 5 of these 8. Preoperatively 19 patients reported transient visual obscuration, 17 reported pulsatile tinnitus, and 6 reported diplopia. All these resolved following stent placement. Prior to stent placement, 30 of the 46 patients with papilledema had significant visual field loss on quantitative perimetry. Seven of these defects persisted following stent placement. Complications included allergic reactions to antiplatelet medications in two patients and two patients with stent-related hemorrhages necessitating craniotomy—both of whom made a full recovery. Transient hearing loss was reported in an additional two patients. Six patients required multiple stent placement.

Importantly, they also differentiated intrinsic from extrinsic stenosis in their patients. The former, which they suggest is a primary lesion, appears radiographically as a focal, discrete obstruction while the latter has a smooth, tapered appearance and was postulated to be a result of compression of the distensible portions of the transverse sinus by increased intracranial pressure. While both intrinsic and extrinsic morphologies were successfully treated with stenting, five of the six patients requiring restenting exhibited extrinsic stenosis. The authors opined that patients with extrinsic stenosis may benefit from a longer stent construct.

While this study was the first large published series demonstrating benefit from venous sinus stenting in the treatment of intracranial hypertension, its retrospective nature and use of predominantly subjective outcome criteria limit its applicability to generating evidence-based guidelines.

26.6 Recommendations

There are no standard guidelines for the treatment of intracranial hypertension. In fact, there is a paucity of any high-quality data guiding management of intracranial hypertension. In the absence of fulminant papilledema or vision loss, weight loss and diet remain the cornerstone of treatment and should be attempted, if possible, before other, more aggressive, interventional treatments are attempted. The IIHTT provided the first randomized, controlled evidence that acetazolamide together with weight loss is more effective than weight loss alone in ameliorating many of the symptoms of intracranial hypertension.[3]

While there is a widespread agreement that progressive vision loss or high-grade papilledema is an indication for surgical intervention, there is a persistent controversy about how more aggressive, interventional treatments should be approached. There are currently no randomized, controlled, prospective studies to recommend one treatment as standard of care. A single, retrospective case series directly compared ONSF to CSF diversion and was unable to show a difference in postoperative visual acuity; headache improvement was not documented.[40] While meta-analysis supports a role for venous sinus stenting in the treatment of intracranial hypertension, further randomized, controlled trials are necessary to guide treatment protocols.

26.7 Summary

1. Idiopathic intracranial hypertension is defined by the modified Dandy criteria.
2. In the absence of fulminant papilledema, treatment options begin with weight loss and carbonic anhydrase inhibitors, such as acetazolamide.
3. More invasive options for treatment are reserved for failure of medical management and include ONSF, CSF diversion, gastric bypass, and venous sinus stenting.
4. There is no-high level evidence to support use of one invasive treatment over another. While some meta-analysis suggest venous sinus stenting, in appropriately chosen patients, compares favorably to other invasive options, further well-designed clinical trials are warranted.

References

[1] Friedman DI, Liu GT, Digre KB. Revised diagnostic criteria for the pseudotumor cerebri syndrome in adults and children. Neurology. 2013; 81(13):1159–1165

[2] Friedman DI, McDermott MP, Kieburtz K, et al. NORDIC IIHTT Study Group. The idiopathic intracranial hypertension treatment trial: design considerations and methods. J Neuroophthalmol. 2014; 34(2):107–117

[3] Wall M, Corbett JJ. Revised diagnostic criteria for the pseudotumor cerebri syndrome in adults and children. Neurology. 2014; 83(2):198–199

[4] Smith JL. Whence pseudotumor cerebri? J Clin Neuroophthalmol. 1985; 5(1):55–56

[5] Newborg B. Pseudotumor cerebri treated by rice reduction diet. Arch Intern Med. 1974; 133(5):802–807

[6] Johnson LN, Krohel GB, Madsen RW, March GA, Jr. The role of weight loss and acetazolamide in the treatment of idiopathic intracranial hypertension (pseudotumor cerebri). Ophthalmology. 1998; 105(12):2313–2317

[7] Sugerman HJ, Felton WL, III, Sismanis A, Kellum JM, DeMaria EJ, Sugerman EL. Gastric surgery for pseudotumor cerebri associated with severe obesity. Ann Surg. 1999; 229(5):634–640, discussion 640–642

[8] Manfield JH, Yu KK-H, Efthimiou E, Darzi A, Athanasiou T, Ashrafian H. Bariatric surgery or non-surgical weight loss for idiopathic intracranial hypertension? A systematic review and comparison of meta-analyses. Obes Surg. 2017; 27(2):513–521

[9] Goh KY, Schatz NJ, Glaser JS. Optic nerve sheath fenestration for pseudotumor cerebri. J Neuroophthalmol. 1997; 17(2):86–91

[10] Obi EE, Lakhani BK, Burns J, Sampath R. Optic nerve sheath fenestration for idiopathic intracranial hypertension: a seven year review of visual outcomes in a tertiary centre. Clin Neurol Neurosurg. 2015; 137(137):94–101

[11] Pineles SL, Volpe NJ. Long-term results of optic nerve sheath fenestration for idiopathic intracranial hypertension: earlier intervention favours improved outcomes. Neuroophthalmology. 2013; 37(1):12–19

[12] Acheson JF, Green WT, Sanders MD. Optic nerve sheath decompression for the treatment of visual failure in chronic raised intracranial pressure. J Neurol Neurosurg Psychiatry. 1994; 57(11):1426–1429

[13] Lai LT, Danesh-Meyer HV, Kaye AH. Visual outcomes and headache following interventions for idiopathic intracranial hypertension. J Clin Neurosci. 2014; 21(10):1670–1678

[14] Plotnik JL, Kosmorsky GS. Operative complications of optic nerve sheath decompression. Ophthalmology. 1993; 100(5):683–690

[15] Curry WT, Jr, Butler WE, Barker FG, II. Rapidly rising incidence of cerebrospinal fluid shunting procedures for idiopathic intracranial hypertension in the United States, 1988–2002. Neurosurgery. 2005; 57(1):97–108, discussion 97–108

[16] Sinclair AJ, Kuruvath S, Sen, D, Nightingale PG, Burdon M, Flint G. Is cerebrospinal fluid shunting in idiopathic intracranial hypertension worthwhile? A 10-year review. Cephalgia. 2011 Dec; 31(16):1627-1633

[17] McGirt MJ, Woodworth G, Thomas G, Miller N, Williams M, Rigamonti D. Cerebrospinal fluid shunt placement for pseudotumor cerebri-associated intractable headache: predictors of treatment response and an analysis of long-term outcomes. J Neurosurg. 2004; 101(4):627–632

[18] Kessler LA, Novelli PM, Reigel DH. Surgical treatment of benign intracranial hypertension: subtemporal decompression revisited. Surg Neurol. 1998; 50(1):73–76

[19] Ray BS, Dunbar HS. Thrombosis of the dural venous sinuses as a cause of pseudotumor cerebri. Ann Surg. 1951; 134(3):376–386

[20] Higgins JN, Owler BK, Cousins C, Pickard JD. Venous sinus stenting for refractory benign intracranial hypertension. Lancet. 2002; 359(9302):228–230

[21] Ahmed RM, Wilkinson M, Parker GD, et al. Transverse sinus stenting for idiopathic intracranial hypertension: a review of 52 patients and of model predictions. AJNR Am J Neuroradiol. 2011; 32(8):1408–1414

[22] Asif H, Craven C, Siddiqui A, Shah S. Idiopathic intracranial hypertension: 120-day clinical, radiological, and manometric outcomes after stent insertion into the dural venous sinus. J Neurosurg. 2017; •••:1–9

[23] Kumpe DA, Bennett JL, Seinfeld J, Pelak VS, Chawla A, Tierney M. Dural sinus stent placement for idiopathic intracranial hypertension. J Neurosurg. 2012; 116(3):538–548

[24] Ducruet AF, Crowley RW, McDougall CG, Albuquerque FC. Long-term patency of venous sinus stents for idiopathic intracranial hypertension. J Neurointerv Surg. 2014; 6(3):238–242

[25] Donnet A, Metellus P, Levrier O, et al. Endovascular treatment of idiopathic intracranial hypertension: clinical and radiologic outcome of 10 consecutive patients. 2008; 70(8):641–647

[26] Dinkin M, Patsalides A. Venous sinus stenting in idiopathic intracranial hypertension: results of a prospective trial. J Neuroophthalmol. 2016; 0:1–9

[27] Satti SR, Leishangthem L, Chaudry MI. Meta-analysis of CSF diversion procedures and dural venous sinus stenting in the setting of medically refractory idiopathic intracranial hypertension. AJNR Am J Neuroradiol. 2015; 36(10):1899–1904

[28] Farb RI, Vanek I, Scott JN, et al. Idiopathic intracranial hypertension: the prevalence and morphology of sinovenous stenosis. Neurology. 2003; 60(9):1418–1424

[29] Ahmed RM, Parker GD, Halmagyi GM. Letters to the editor: stenting and idiopathic intracranial hypertension. J Neurosurg. 2012; 117(6):1205–, author reply 1205–1206

[30] Raper DMS, Buell TJ, Chen C-J, Ding D, Starke RM, Liu KC. Intracranial venous pressures under conscious sedation and general anesthesia. J Neurointerv Surg. 2017; 9(10):986–989

[31] Radvany MG, Solomon D, Nijjar S, et al. Visual and neurological outcomes following endovascular stenting for pseudotumor cerebri associated with transverse sinus stenosis. J Neuroophthalmol. 2013; 33(2):117–122

[32] Smith KA, Peterson JC, Arnold PM, Camarata PJ, Whittaker TJ, Abraham MG. A case series of dural venous sinus stenting in idiopathic intracranial hypertension: association of outcomes with optical coherence tomography. Int J Neurosci. 2017; 127(2):145–153

[33] Wall M. Idiopathic intracranial hypertension. Neurol Clin. 2010; 28(3):593–617

[34] Elder BD, Goodwin CR, Kosztowski TA, et al. Venous sinus stenting is a valuable treatment for fulminant idiopathic intracranial hypertension. J Clin Neurosci. 2015; 22(4):685–689

[35] Sinclair AJ, Burdon MA, Nightingale PG, et al. Low energy diet and intracranial pressure in women with idiopathic intracranial hypertension: prospective cohort study. BMJ. 2010; 341:c2701

[36] Banta JT, Farris BK. Pseudotumor cerebri and optic nerve sheath decompression. Ophthalmology. 2000; 107(10):1907–1912

[37] Satti SR, Leishangthem L, Spiotta A, Chaudry MI. Dural venous sinus stenting for medically and surgically refractory idiopathic intracranial hypertension. Interv Neuroradiol. 2017; 23(2):186–193

[38] The Nordic Idiopathic Intracranial Hypertension Group Writing Committee. Effect of acetazolamide on visual function in patients with idiopathic intracranial hypertension and mild visual loss. JAMA 2014;311(16):1641–1651

[39] Ahmed RM, Wilkinson M, Parker GD, et al. Transverse sinus stenting for idiopathic hypertension: a review of 52 patients and of model predictions. AJNR Am J Neuroradiol 2011;32(8):1408–1414

[40] Fonseca PL, Rigamonti D, Miller NR, Subramanian PS. Visual outcomes of surgical intervention for pseudotumour cerebri: optic nerve sheath fenestration versus cerebrospinal fluid diversion. Br J Ophthalmol. 2014; 98(10):1360-1363

26

27 Epistaxis

Stepan Capek, Jeyan S. Kumar, Michael F. Stiefel, M. Yashar S. Kalani, and Min S. Park

Abstract

Endovascular embolization (EE) is a widely accepted treatment option for refractory cases of posterior epistaxis. EE is considered a safe and effective treatment modality, with stroke risk approximately 1% and efficacy of 90% or more; however, available literature lacks quality, prospective studies. Only a few comparable studies exist, with surgical ligation of the sphenopalatine artery being the main comparator. The published literature should be interpreted with caution to understand the appropriate indications for the procedure.

Keywords: epistaxis, embolization, ligation, PVA, endovascular, interventional, radiology

27.1 Goal

1. Review and critically analyze the literature that supports endovascular embolization (EE) for intractable epistaxis in adults.

27.2 Case Example

27.2.1 History of Present Illness

A 36-year-old male presented to an outside hospital with acute left-sided epistaxis. The patient underwent unilateral nasal packing and was discharged home. He re-presented later the same day with recurrent epistaxis despite nasal packing and was transferred to our facility. On presentation he was hypertensive with SBP > 170. The patient was evaluated by ENT and a clear source of hemorrhage could not be identified upon nasal inspection due to uncontrolled bleeding.

   Past medical history: No significant PMH.
   Past surgical history: No significant PSH.
   Family history: No significant FH.
   Social history: Spanish speaking.
   Review of systems: Noncontributory.
   Neurological examination: Unremarkable.
   Imaging studies: Endoscopy, angiography (see ▶ Fig. 27.1).

27.2.2 Treatment

The patient underwent embolization of the left distal internal maxillary artery utilizing PVA particles (355–500 μm) (▶ Fig. 27.1). The procedure was uncomplicated and no underlying vascular pathology was identified.

27.2.3 Follow-up

The patient was seen in follow-up in 1 month and reported a self-limited episode of epistaxis on the contralateral side, which lasted only a few minutes, but he did not have a recurrent epistaxis on the ipsilateral side. He denied any stroke-like or other neurological symptoms.

27.3 Case Summary

1. *When should a patient with intractable epistaxis be treated?*
   The primary source of epistaxis should be identified; patients with anterior epistaxis are not typically candidates for endovascular management; however, patients with intractable posterior epistaxis should be considered for arterial embolization. Anterior epistaxis is typically controlled with topical agents and/or anterior nasal packing. If these fail, next step is direct cauterization or ligation of the anterior or posterior ethmoidal artery.[1] The ethmoidal arteries arise from the ophthalmic artery and embolization would carry a high risk of major complications. If a posterior source is suspected and the patient failed initial conservative management including nasal packing and attempted cauterization/ligation, a more invasive procedure as EE is a reasonable consideration.[1,2,3]

2. *What determines the treatment modality?*
   Two definite treatment options are available for intractable posterior epistaxis: EE and surgical ligation of the sphenopalatine artery (typically "endoscopic sphenopalatine artery ligation"—ESPAL). Our patient was not a candidate for ESPAL due to difficult visualization and, respectively, patients with connections between the internal maxillary artery (IMAX)

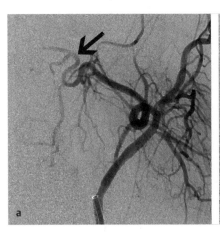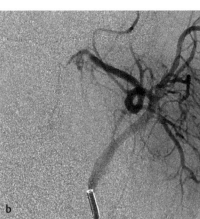

Fig. 27.1 Digital subtraction angiography of a left distal external carotid artery in the anteroposterior (AP) view, before **(a)** and after **(b)** embolization of the distal internal maxillary artery. The pre-embolization injection demonstrates the sphenopalatine artery **(a**, *arrow*), which is absent on the postembolization run **(b)**.

27

and intracranial circulation are not candidates for embolization due to the significantly increased risk of a major neurologic complication.[3] Patient's comorbidities should be taken into consideration as EE is typically done under conscious sedation/local anesthesia, while ESPAL requires general anesthesia. On the contrary, decreased renal function could preclude EE. However, if a patient is a candidate for surgical, as well as endovascular treatment, there are no prospective controlled trials to support one over the other.[4] Caution is needed in interpreting available evidence. Published literature consists mostly of single-center retrospective studies with heterogenous methodology and inconsistent outcome reporting,[4] only a few of which compared both treatment options. The two largest studies[5,6] utilized the National Inpatient Sample database and did not report bleeding control rate or recurrences. Other studies have reported similar success rates for both techniques with an average success rate of 88% and range of 71 to 100% for EE.[4] ESPAL may be associated with a higher rate of minor complications,[7] but EE is associated with significantly higher stroke risk of 0.9% compared to 0.1% with surgical ligation.[5]

Cost of the procedure may also be a consideration when deciding on treatment. The largest study to date[5] comparing 4,440 embolization patients versus 64,289 surgical ligation patients demonstrated EE to be significantly more expensive, with mean hospital charges of $50,372 versus $17,367 in the surgical group, a trend seen in other studies as well.[8,9]

3. *What vessels should be embolized and what agent should be used?*

   If laterality can be determined, then embolization of the ipsilateral IMAX is often sufficient.[10,11] Majority of the patients, however, receive bilateral IMAX embolization,[12,13,14] which should be indicated carefully, as there is a linear association between the number of treated vessels and the rate of minor complications.[15]

   PVA particles of various sizes are the most frequently used agent, but there is no evidence to support one agent over another.

27.4 Class of Recommendation and Level of Evidence

27.4.1 Indications for Embolization

For patients, who fail initial conservative management and/or packing, EE is a reasonable treatment option (Class I, Level of Evidence C).

27.4.2 Embolization versus Surgical Ligation

No conclusive evidence to support one treatment modality over the other.

27.4.3 Embolization Technique

No conclusive evidence to support one technique over the other.

27.4.4 Embolization Target

Embolization of a distal ipsilateral maxillary artery is often times sufficient, and an increased number of treated vessels are associated with increased number of minor complications (Class IIb, Level of Evidence C).

27.4.5 Treatment Risks

Embolization is associated with approximately 1% risk of stroke, which is significantly higher than surgical ligation. Embolization is not associated with increased mortality compared with other treatment options (Class IIb, Level of Evidence B).

27.4.6 Cost-Effectiveness

Embolization is associated with higher hospital charges than other treatment options (Class IIb, Level of Evidence B).

27.5 Landmark Papers

Sokoloff J, Wickbom I, McDonald D, Brahme F, Goergen TG, Goldberger LE. Therapeutic percutaneous embolization in intractable epistaxis. Radiology 1974 May;111:285–287.[2]

Sokoloff et al reported the first two cases of successful embolization for intractable epistaxis, although their technique differed significantly from current standard practice of superselective microcatheterization of a distal internal maxillary artery. In both cases, they embolized the external carotid artery "near the internal maxillary artery origin" with Gelfoam particles.

Swords C, Patel A, Smith ME, Williams RJ, Kuhn I, Hopkins C. Surgical and interventional radiological management of adult epistaxis: systematic review. J Laryngol Otol 2017 Dec;131:1108–1130.[12]

The largest systematic review comparing embolization versus surgical ligation reviewed 34 reports relating to EE and found significant limitations in the published literature. No randomized controlled trials were available. The vast majority of the reviewed literature consisted of single-center retrospective studies with significant heterogeneity preventing meta-analysis. Overall success rate of EE in the pooled data was 88% (range 71–100%), which was comparable or better than those for surgical management. Across all series there was an approximately 10% risk of ischemic temporofacial pain, 1.1% risk of stroke, and 0.3% risk of blindness.

Brinjikji W, Kallmes DF, Cloft HJ. Trends in epistaxis embolization in the United States: a study of the Nationwide Inpatient Sample 2003–2010. J Vasc Intervent Radiol 2013 Jul 1;24:969–973.[7]

The largest retrospective study to date utilized the National Inpatient Sample (NIS) database resulting in inherent limitations due to the lack of detailed clinical data. The database does not contain data on success rate, the principal outcome measure. Another major caveat is that the "surgical" group included "cauterization" codes; hence, many of the "different patients" are likely one and the same patient initially treated by cauterization and then transferred to a higher institution for additional treatment (i.e., embolization). Acknowledging the limitations, the study reviewed epistaxis cases performed between 2003 and 2010, during which 64,289 patients underwent surgical ligation and 4440 patients underwent embolization. The embolization

27

group had a significantly higher risk of stroke, albeit still low (0.9% vs. 0.1%). The mortality was not statistically different between the groups, but the embolization procedure was associated with higher hospital charges ($50,372 vs. $17,367 in the surgical group).

Tseng EY, Narducci CA, Willing SJ, Sillers MJ. Angiographic embolization for epistaxis: a review of 114 cases. Laryngoscope 1998 Apr;108:615–619.[4]

The largest retrospective study with reported outcomes detailed 114 embolization cases in 107 patients. Although the authors reviewed cases performed in 1990 to 1995, they described standard superselective embolization of the distal internal maxillary artery utilizing PVA particles. A unilateral internal maxillary artery embolization was performed in 70 cases with a 93% success rate. However, success rate is poorly defined in the study. This is in contrast with more recent studies, which report that the vast majority of patients underwent bilateral IMAX embolization. The series reports two stroke events with a final major long-term complication rate of 0.9%.

27.6 Recommendations

Major difficulty with forming recommendations stems from the lack of quality, prospective trials. EE is an effective and widely accepted treatment option for patients with idiopathic posterior epistaxis, who fail initial treatment. Based on the current evidence, no formal recommendations to use EE over another treatment options exist; however, EE has been utilized more and more frequently. This likely reflects several factors: (1) increased availability of EE related to increasing number of stroke centers, (2) ability to avoid general anesthesia, (3) use of EE as a bail-out procedure after failed cauterization/ligation, and (4) provider preference.

The most frequently utilized embolic agent is PVA particles. Based on the provider's preference, Onyx or coils may be an acceptable alternative. However, permanent embolisates or coils may preclude redo embolization in case of recurrent epistaxis. There is no robust evidence to support one agent over another. Cyanoacrylate glues are not widely reported.

The current literature reflects significant differences in standard practice. Some providers start with embolization of a single vessel, if a source of bleeding can be localized. Others embolize bilateral internal maxillary arteries routinely. The reported success rates between unilateral and bilateral embolization appear to be similar. A single study reported an association between the number of treated vessels and minor complications.[7]

27.7 Summary

1. EE is a reasonable treatment option for intractable posterior epistaxis, but there is no conclusive evidence to support EE over surgery.
2. Overall risk of stroke is low for EE, but still higher than for surgical treatment options. Respectively, surgery seems to be associated with higher rate of minor complications. There is no difference in mortality between EE and other treatments.

References

[1] Krulewitz NA, Fix ML. Epistaxis. Emerg Med Clin North Am. 2019; 37(1): 29–39

[2] Siniluoto TM, Leinonen AS, Karttunen AI, Karjalainen HK, Jokinen KE. Embolization for the treatment of posterior epistaxis: an analysis of 31 cases. Arch Otolaryngol Head Neck Surg. 1993; 119(8):837–841

[3] Reyre A, Michel J, Santini L, et al. Epistaxis: the role of arterial embolization. Diagn Interv Imaging. 2015; 96(7–8):757–773

[4] Swords C, Patel A, Smith ME, Williams RJ, Kuhn I, Hopkins C. Surgical and interventional radiological management of adult epistaxis: systematic review. J Laryngol Otol. 2017; 131(12):1108–1130

[5] Brinjikji W, Kallmes DF, Cloft HJ. Trends in epistaxis embolization in the United States: a study of the Nationwide Inpatient Sample 2003–2010. J Vasc Interv Radiol. 2013; 24(7):969–973

[6] Villwock JA, Jones K. Recent trends in epistaxis management in the United States: 2008–2010. JAMA Otolaryngol Head Neck Surg. 2013; 139(12):1279–1284

[7] Cullen MM, Tami TA. Comparison of internal maxillary artery ligation versus embolization for refractory posterior epistaxis. Otolaryngol Head Neck Surg. 1998; 118(5):636–642

[8] Strong EB, Bell DA, Johnson LP, Jacobs JM. Intractable epistaxis: transantral ligation vs. embolization: efficacy review and cost analysis. Otolaryngol Head Neck Surg. 1995; 113(6):674–678

[9] Klotz DA, Winkle MR, Richmon J, Hengerer AS. Surgical management of posterior epistaxis: a changing paradigm. Laryngoscope. 2002; 112(9):1577–1582

[10] Tseng EY, Narducci CA, Willing SJ, Sillers MJ. Angiographic embolization for epistaxis: a review of 114 cases. Laryngoscope. 1998; 108(4 Pt 1):615–619

[11] Baloch MA, Awan MS, Resident HN. Angioembolization in itractable epistaxis: a tertiary care experience. J Pak Med Assoc. 2012; 62(3):254–256

[12] Christensen NP, Smith DS, Barnwell SL, Wax MK. Arterial embolization in the management of posterior epistaxis. Otolaryngol Head Neck Surg. 2005; 133(5):748–753

[13] Robinson AE, McAuliffe W, Phillips TJ, Phatouros CC, Singh TP. Embolization for the treatment of intractable epistaxis: 12 month outcomes in a two centre case series. Br J Radiol. 2017; 90(1080):20170472

[14] Huyett P, Jankowitz BT, Wang EW, Snyderman CH. Endovascular embolization in the treatment of epistaxis. Otolaryngol Head Neck Surg. 2019; 160(5): 822–828

[15] Gottumukkala R, Kadkhodayan Y, Moran CJ, Cross WT, III, Derdeyn CP. Impact of vessel choice on outcomes of polyvinyl alcohol embolization for intractable idiopathic epistaxis. J Vasc Interv Radiol. 2013; 24(2):234–239

27

28 Venolymphatic Malformations of the Head and Neck

Rulon Hardman and Claire Kaufman

Abstract

Treatment of venolymphatic malformations is primarily based on expert opinion and retrospective small cohort studies. While there are some safety trials and cohort studies published, few randomized, controlled trials comparing various treatment options are available. However, despite the lack of scientific evidence, awareness of these conditions is needed to appropriately diagnose and triage patients. Appropriate diagnosis, characterization, and referral to specialty centers will allow for organized trials to be performed in this disease. Vascular malformations are prevalent in 1 to 4% of the population, but it is still treated as an orphan disease. Practitioners should know the presentation of these lesions, their differential diagnosis, imaging findings, appropriate work-up, and treatment options to develop a multidisciplinary treatment plan.

Keywords: venous malformation, lymphatic malformation, sclerotherapy, sotradecol, ethanol

28.1 Goals

1. To understand the types of vascular malformations and their clinical presentations.
2. Review available sclerotherapy agents and any data to support their use in venolymphatic malformations.
3. Understand emerging medical therapies of medical management for venolymphatic malformations.
4. Review available literature regarding the treatment and follow-up of venolymphatic malformations.

28.2 Case Examples

28.2.1 Case Example 1

History of Present Illness

A 29-year-old Pacific Islander male with increasing facial swelling over the past few years presents for evaluation. The swelling is in the left face from the temple to the submandibular region. His swelling is associated with dull pain. He reports his pain can range from 2/10 at baseline up to 8/10 when he has upper respiratory infections.

Past medical history: No other medical conditions.
Family history: Noncontributory.
Social history: Married with two children. Works in construction. Denies smoking and alcohol or illicit drug use.
Physical examination: Left facial swelling over the mandible and extending up the lateral left face. No discoloration to the skin, no palpable pulse.
Imaging studies: See ▶ Fig. 28.1.

Treatment Plan

The imaging and presentation of this patient is that of a venolymphatic malformation. Treatment plan is focused on the resolution of pain in this patient, with a hope of additional cosmetic improvement. Treatment often requires three to four treatment sessions, which needs to be explained to the patient and an expected treatment plan written out for the treatment course. Treatment involved percutaneous sclerotherapy over three treatments (▶ Fig. 28.2). Mixed agent sclerotherapy using bleomycin (Blenoxane) and sodium tetradecyl sulfate foam (STS, Sotradecol, Angiodynamics) was employed.

Follow-up

The patient's pain resolved after the second treatment. Cosmetic swelling improved over the treatments, and the patient felt comfortable with his appearance after three treatments. He did develop a minor complication of chemical cellulitis after the second treatment, which was treated with oral cephalexin with a good result. Patients are followed up in the clinic as there is a high level of recurrence with these lesions after 8 to 10 years.

28.2.2 Case Example 2

History of Present Illness

A 26-year-old Ph.D. student from Iran presented with a forehead/scalp lesion. Patient has had this soft lesion as long as he can remember. The lesion is not painful. He had a magnetic resonance imaging (MRI) 8 years ago of the lesion, but the physicians he encountered did not believe there was any possible treatment of the lesion.

Past medical history: No other medical conditions.
Family history: Noncontributory.
Social history: Currently in graduate school. Nonsmoker. Occasional alcohol use.
Physical examnation: 4-cm round, soft mass at the left forehead/scalp extending into the hairline. Mass is not mobile on the calvarium and is nonpulsatile but has a bluish discoloration.
Imaging studies: See ▶ Fig. 28.3.

Treatment Plan

The imaging appearance of internal flow voids and contrast enhancement on gadolinium MRI confirm this to be a venous malformation. Typically, therapy is reserved for painful masses. Other indications for treatment include disfigurement, consumption coagulopathy, respiratory compromise, and bleeding. Treatment plan includes percutaneous sclerotherapy and possible surgical resection. Considering the surrounding structures is important for any malformation treatment, but especially of scalp and oropharynx lesions. Venous drainage pathways may be difficult to control, and treatment may cause thrombosis of cerebral venous structures. Oropharynx lesions may cause enough swelling to obstruct the airway. Percutaneous sclerotherapy with bleomycin was used in this lesion (▶ Fig. 28.4). There is a plan for surgical resection after venous sclerotherapy. Possible other treatments for venous malformations include radiofrequency or cryoablation.[1,2]

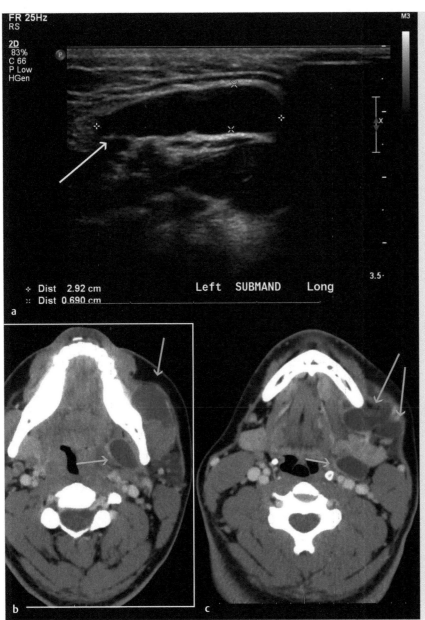

Fig. 28.1 Case 1: A 29-year-old male with left facial swelling and pain. The lesion is submandibular and extends along the mandibular angle. **(a)** B-mode ultrasound. An anechoic lesion is seen below the mandible (*yellow arrow*). There was no flow seen within the mass. **(b,c)** Axial computed tomography (CT) contrast-enhanced images showing the patient's submandibular mass (*green arrows*). CT is usually not the imaging modality of choice but was performed by the referring provider. There is no internal enhancement of the lesion that crosses compartments of the neck. Peripheral enhancement of the lesion is present.

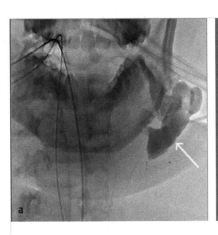
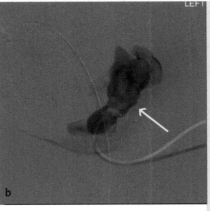

Fig. 28.2 Case 1: Treatment of the left facial lymphatic malformation. **(a,b)** The lesion is a lobulated macrocystic lymphatic malformation (*yellow arrow*). The patient underwent sclerotherapy of the lesion over three separate sessions. The first treatment session involved injecting 180 mg of STS (Sotradecol) percutaneously through a 21-gauge needle. A second needle was placed to vent the lesion. The second treatment involved similar protocol of accessing the malformation using a 21-gauge needle under ultrasound guidance. A mixture of 8 Units of bleomycin and contrast was injected and left to dwell for 30 minutes, then drained from the malformation. During the third treatment, a small drain was placed and sclerotherapy was performed using Sotradecol followed by bleomycin.

28

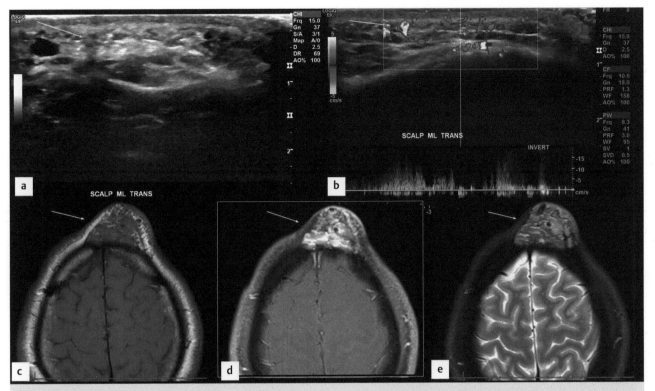

Fig. 28.3 Case 2: A 26-year-old male with a soft mass on the forehead. The mass is not painful but is cosmetically deforming. **(a)** B-mode ultrasound images of the malformation demonstrate a few large spaces within the mass (*green arrow*). **(b)** Ultrasound image demonstrates internal low velocity flow voids. Diagnosis of venous malformation is made based on the ultrasound. Magnetic resonance imaging (MRI) is performed to determine the depth of the lesion, bone involvement, and plan locations for needle placement during treatment. MRI images of this venous malformation are typical for venous malformations (*yellow arrows*). **(c)** T1-weighted (T1W) images show the mass is isointense to muscle. Internal enhancement is present on post-gadolinium T1 W images in venous malformations **(d)**. Both venous malformations and lymphatic malformations are hyperintense on T2 W images **(e)**.

28

Follow-up

Even after surgical resection, patients should be followed annually due to the high probability of recurrence. Additional treatment should be based on the same considerations as the first treatment, namely, controlling pain and improving deformity.

28.3 Case Summary

1. *What imaging is indicated to evaluate vascular malformations?*

   Plain films play a little role in diagnosing and evaluating vascular malformations.[3] In some cases, plain film can demonstrate bone loss associated with malformations, such as in Gorham disease (lymphatic malformation that is associated with bone resorption). Ultrasound is the first-line imaging modality to evaluate venolymphatic malformations.[3] Ultrasound can exclude high-flow malformations such as arterial venous malformations. Ultrasound can often distinguish between venous and lymphatic malformations. Initial evaluation should be with b-mode (2D gray-scale imaging). Phleboliths can often be seen, which are pathognomonic for a vascular malformation. Phleboliths are most often seen in venous malformations, although they can be seen in lymphatic malformations with prior internal hemorrhage. Duplex ultrasound may show flow within vascular malfor-

mations. However, at least 15% of venous malformations will have no internal flow by ultrasound.[3,4]

Computed tomography (CT) has a little role in evaluating venolymphatic malformations. The malformations tend to be of the same soft tissue density as surrounding tissues, making full evaluation of the extent of the malformation difficult. MRI has become the mainstay for evaluating the extent, depth, and character of venolymphatic malformations.[5,6] MRI protocols include T1, T2, and contrast-enhanced images in at least two orthogonal planes. Contrast-enhanced MRI has a 100% sensitivity and 95% specificity of distinguishing vascular malformations from other lesions.[7] Venous malformations tend to have internal enhancement on contrast-enhanced images, but no flow voids on T2 images. Lymphatic malformations tend to have no internal enhancement but have an enhancing rim. MRI is also helpful to plan needle placement for therapy[8] and follow-up treatment response.

2. *Which vascular lesions require or respond to treatment?*

   Treatment of arteriovenous malformations (AVMs) differs from that of venolymphatic malformations. When approaching an AVM of the head and neck, the goal of therapy can be to aid with pain and deformity. Patients can present with heart failure with high-flow lesions, and airway compromise when they involve the airway. Often, therapy involves a team of otolaryngologists, plastic surgeons, vascular surgeons, and interventional radiologists in addition to the

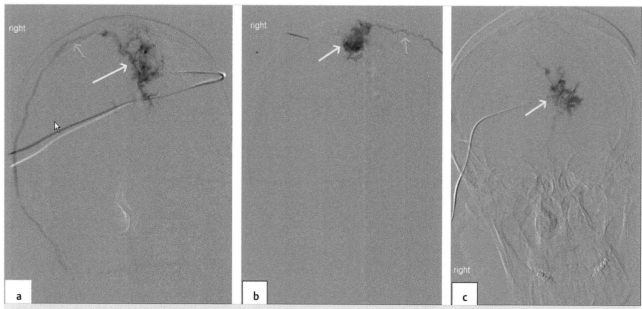

Fig. 28.4 Case 2: Digital subtraction images during treatment. A 25-gauge needle was placed under ultrasound-guidance into the venous malformation (*yellow arrow*). Images **(a)** and **(b)** show draining veins from the mass. Sclerotherapy without compressing these draining veins could lead to scalp necrosis, pulmonary emboli, or intracranial venous thrombosis. The draining veins were compressed **(c)** and the venous malformation was treated with 2 Units of bleomycin.

neurosurgeon.[3,8] Percutaneous sclerotherapy prior to resection may be needed to minimize bleeding during surgery. Treatment strategy for AVM is beyond the scope of this chapter but involves treating the nidus of the malformation with sclerosants such as ethanol or liquid embolics, such as n-butyl-cyanoacrylate glue (Histoacryl Blau, B Braun Medical, Sempach, Schweiz).

Venous and lymphatic malformations do not resolve spontaneously, and if symptomatic, will require treatment. Common indications for treatment include pain, deformity, bone loss, airway compromise, consumptive coagulopathy, or for lymphatic malformations, recurrent infections. Venous malformations can activate the coagulation cascade, perhaps by slow flow through the lesion. The activated coagulation leads to an elevated D-dimer and consumption of platelets. This condition is seen in 42% of patients with venous malformations.[9] Lymphatic and venous malformations do tend to respond to percutaneous sclerotherapy, with reported rates ranging from 50 to 100% overall response.[10] Macrocystic lymphatic malformations tend to have the best response. Microcystic lymphatic malformations tend not to respond as well to percutaneous sclerotherapy.

3. *What medical therapies are available to treat venolymphatic malformations?*

Several medical therapies have been pursued for venolymphatic malformations, but the mammalian target of rapamycin (mTOR) inhibitor, Sirolimus, has the most promise at this time. Several randomized trials are in process to confirm the outcomes of Sirolimus treatment.

Symptomatic control has been attempted with heparin in venous malformations.[11] Thrombus that occurs in venous malformations is unlikely to result in symptomatic pulmonary emboli in patients due to the superficial nature of these lesions, but recurrent thromboses are bothersome to some

patients. Prophylactic heparin or low-molecular-weight heparin can be used to reduce these thrombosis events. Lymphatic malformations are prone to infection, and sometimes require antibiotic treatment for cellulitis, usually cephalexin. Propranolol is helpful in hemangiomas but has little benefit for venolymphatic malformations. Sildenafil has had mixed results in cohort studies but may have some symptom relief by its effect on smooth muscle.[12]

Sirolimus is a tyrosine kinase inhibitor of the mTOR pathway, which is involved in the angiogenesis and the PI3K-AKT pathway.[13] Sirolimus was first reported to have effect in a case series of six patients, five with microcystic lymphatic malformations.[13] All patients had response to the treatment. Adams et al have subsequently performed a prospective analysis of 57 patients treated with Sirolimus for various vascular malformations.[14] Partial response was noted in 83% after 6 treatments and 85% after 12 treatments. Currently, there are phase II (NCT00975819, NCT02509468) and phase III (NCT02638389) trials testing Sirolimus in venolymphatic malformations. See ▸ Fig. 28.5.

4. *What sclerotherapy agent should be used in venous and lymphatic malformations?*

The type of sclerosant and method of application of the sclerotherapy varies throughout the literature. Unfortunately, most reports are small population retrospective studies and have mixed location of sclerosant administration, few in the head and neck. Common agents that are used for sclerotherapy include ethanol, bleomycin, STS (or Sotradecol), doxycycline, OK-432, polidocanol, and ethanolamine.

Ethanol is the first and the most commonly reported sclerosant in all malformations. Ethanol denatures proteins, which destroys the vascular wall endothelium. Ethanol also causes thrombosis. In their systematic review of studies on head and neck malformations, Horbach et al found 6 studies that

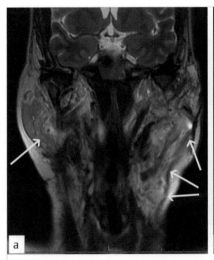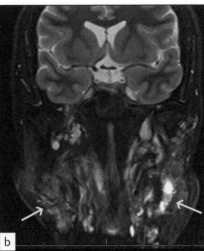

Fig. 28.5 A 33-year-old male with an extensive mixed microcystic/macrocystic lymphatic malformation spanning through the compartments of the neck and face. He received several treatments as a teenager, including sclerotherapy and surgery. Given the extensive microcystic areas of the malformation, decision was made to trial Sirolimus. He was started on Sirolimus, with a target trough level between 10 and 15 ng/mL. He experienced hypertension and a rash along his legs; so the trough target was reduced to 5 to 10 ng/mL. **(a)** T2-weighted (T2W) magnetic resonance imaging (MRI) before Sirolimus treatment demonstrates an extensive malformation along the entire left face and extending down the left neck (*yellow arrows*). There is also malformation at the right buccal tissues. **(b)** T2 W MRI image after Sirolimus treatment shows significant reduction in the malformation at all spaces. He also had a significant cosmetic improvement.

met criteria in 327 patients.[10] The overall response was between 84 and 100%. However, it is important to note that ethanol has the highest reported complication rate, with studies showing up to 61% of patients having complications.[15]

Sotradecol is the next most used agent in vascular malformations in all sites. Sotradecol is a strong detergent, which breaks down the cellular lipid bilayer. Sotradecol is often applied as a foam, as described by Tessari.[16] Horbach et al could only find two studies that met criteria for STS in head and neck. The reports showed overall response rates of 100% and no complications, but few patients are included (*n* = 12).[10]

Bleomycin is a chemotherapy agent that was found to have sclerosing properties on the endothelium. Several groups prefer to use bleomycin, believing it to be less caustic in sensitive areas such as the head and neck. Horbach et al found five studies on bleomycin, with 70 to 100% overall response rate.[10] Bleomycin had higher recurrence rates in a study when compared to ethanol.[15] A subtype of bleomycin, pingyangmycin, has mostly been studied in China. Pingyangmycin reports are the largest in the literature in head and neck sclerotherapy, with 8 studies in 693 patients. The overall response rate is > 95% with complete response rates of 48 to 100% described. Quality of the reports has been questioned as the groups only report a 2% adverse event rate.

OK-432 (Picibanil) is a lyophilized group A streptococcus pyogenes with low virulence which is incubated with benzyl-penicillin. High-volume groups report good response to therapy in lymphatic malformations,[11,17] but the agent was not approved by the FDA and therefore is not available in the United States. Overall response rate in nine studies was 50 to 95%.[10] Complications were reported in 0 to 30% of patients.[10]

Polidocanol is also a detergent agent. Two studies are evaluated by Horbach et al in 39 patients.[18] The overall response rate was 100%, but in small studies.

Doxycycline also has been reported in 2 studies involving 22 patients.[18] The overall response rate was 67 to 100%.

Doxycycline was reported to cause zero complications in the reports but was used predominantly in lymphatic malformations.[19]

5. *When is surgery indicated for venolymphatic malformations?*
A systemic review by Van der Vleuten reported only a single study with at least 10 patients.[20] Zhong et al reported retrospective outcomes of 10 patients with head and neck malformations,[21] with a 90% clinical success in their series. Surgical management in isolation is difficult in these lesions.[8,22,23,24,25] Malformations are prone to bleeding, which can limit evaluation of the surgical field, leave residual malformation, and lead to injury of critical structures. A combined approach usually involving percutaneous sclerotherapy of the venous malformation or macrocystic components of lymphatic malformations prior to resection is now advocated. Surgical resection goals then involve debulking, with the knowledge that additional therapy by sclerotherapy can be pursued in the future if needed. Lee et al have described their surgical approach using a multidisciplinary team, which involves 15 different specialties. Of their patient cohort, about 10% of the patients had surgical management of their vascular malformations, with 72% receiving concurrent sclerotherapy.[26] This study reported nine minor complications in the surgical group.[26]

28.4 Level of Evidence

Imaging: Ultrasound should be used as a first-line modality to establish the diagnosis of high-flow versus low-flow vascular malformation. Contrast-enhanced MRI is then used for treatment planning and to determine the depth of the malformation (Class I, Level of Evidence: C).

Which lesions require treatment: Common indications for treatment of venolymphatic malformations of the head and neck include pain, deformity, or recurrent infection. Other reasons for treatment include airway compromise, bleeding, ulceration, consumptive coagulopathy, and bone loss (Class I, Level of Evidence: C).

Medical therapy of venolymphatic malformations: Complex malformations that will not respond well to percutaneous or

28

surgical management may be treated with Sirolimus. Microcystic lymphatic malformations have the most data for this therapy (Class IIB, Level of Evidence: B).

Choosing a sclerotherapy agent: A variety of sclerotherapy agents are available for lymphatic and venous malformations, including ethanol, STS, ethanolamine, OK-432, polidocanol, bleomycin, and doxycycline. Retrospective and prospective studies show efficacy with all of these agents, but no randomized, controlled trials are available to suggest superiority of any agent (Class IIB, Level of Evidence: C).

Surgery for venolymphatic malformations: Surgical debulking plays a role in head and neck venolymphatic malformations, especially involving the oropharynx and tongue (Class IIB, Level of Evidence: C).

28.5 Landmark Papers

Mulliken JB, Glowacki J. Hemangiomas and vascular malformations in infants and children: a classification based on endothelial characteristics. Plast Reconstr Surg 1982;69(2):412–422.

Mulliken and Glowacki provided one of the first real attempts to characterize and group the common vascular malformations that can be encountered.[27] Before the report by Mulliken, the literature was peppered with different terms for vascular lesions, leading to confusion and no consensus in reporting treatment strategies. The nomenclature of vascular malformations varied from interosseous AVM, cirsoid aneurysm, serpentine aneurysm, angioma, hemangioma, verrucous hemangioma, capillary hemangioma, nevus flammeus, nevus angiectoides, capillary telangiectasia angioma arteriole racemosum, and several others. Mulliken describes that these malformations were often blamed on the mother during the 19th century with names of the lesions such as "naevus maternus" and "stigma metrocelis." The vascular lesions were thought to be "produced by the longing of the mother for particular things, or her aversion to them; hence these marks resemble mulberries, strawberries, grapes, pines, bacon, etc."[28,29]

Mulliken divided vascular malformations into hemangiomas and malformations based on pathology results from 49 operative specimens. The malformations were further classified as capillary, venous, arterial, lymphatic, and fistulae.[29]

The International Society for the Study of Vascular Anomalies (ISSVA) used Mulliken's work to develop the ISSVA classification in 1996.[30] The classification system was updated in 2014.[31] Physicians should use these terms to describe vascular malformations.

Yakes WF, Luethke JM, Parker SH, et al. Ethanol embolization of vascular malformations. Radiographics 1990;10(5):787–796.

Yakes' first series of percutaneous sclerotherapy was published in 1989 in *Radiology*.[32] The report is a landmark paper in that it describes the first series of patients treated with percutaneous sclerotherapy using 98% ethanol. We choose to detail his second report, however, as the 1989 paper was using ethanol only in AVMs. The follow-up report in 1990 in *Radiographics* involved 20 patients, 9 of whom had venous malformations.[33] Up to this point, surgery had been the mainstay for treatment of vascular malformations. Surgery was subject to poor results, with high failure rates and complications from bleeding. Ethanol was injected transcatheter or percutaneous into the central area of the malformation (nidus). The venous outflow was blocked using coils, tourniquets, and occlusion balloons. The 20 patients in the study underwent 83 procedures. All nine of the venous malformations showed thrombosis of the malformation by venography or ultrasound. Yakes et al reported a 13% complication rate.[33]

All subsequent series have been variations of the treatments described by Yakes et al. Various sclerosants have been studied including: ethanol, STS, bleomycin, picibanil (OK-432), polidocanol, ethanolamine, and doxycycline.

Adams DM, Trenor CC 3rd, Hammill AM, et al. Efficacy and safety of sirolimus in the treatment of complicated vascular anomalies. Pediatrics 2016;137(2):e2015.

Options for medical therapy in venolymphatic malformations were basically nonexistent until 2011. Patients were prescribed heparin or low-molecular-weight heparin to prevent thrombus within the malformation, but this had no effect on the underlying lesion.[8] Hammill et al was the first to describe a series of six patients in whom they tried the drug Sirolimus.[13] The patient group included five patients with microcystic lymphatic malformations and one patient with kaposiform hemangioendothelioma with Kasbach-Merritt phenomenon. All six of these patients had response to treatment with Sirolimus. The results of this series led to other phase II and phase III trials of Sirolimus in venolymphatic malformations.

Genetic investigation into vascular malformations has shown that common mutations in vascular malformations involve the PIK3-AKT pathway.[34] Klippel-Trenaunay syndrome involves mutation of the PIK3CA gene. Lymphedema syndromes and familial lymphedema syndrome involve the VEFG3 pathway. Other heritable vascular malformation syndromes involve PTEN and AKT pathway alterations. Sirolimus is an inhibitor of mTOR, which regulates the PIK3-AKT pathway.[35] The drug prevents downstream protein synthesis, thereby decreasing cell proliferation and angiogenesis.

Adams et al treated 57 patients with various vascular anomalies with Sirolimus. The majority of the patients had variations of lymphatic malformations. Patients received 0.8 mg/m^2 dosing twice daily with titration to maintain trough level between 10 and 15 ng/mL. Planned therapy was 12 courses. Fifteen patients did not complete the therapy; this was due to progressive disease in eight patients, drug toxicity in two patients, refusal in two patients, and physician's decision to stop the medication in two patients. Forty-seven patients (83%) had partial response after 6 courses, which increased to 45 patients (85%) after 12 courses. There were no complete responses, but only one had progression of disease in the cohort of patients that completed the study. Toxicity from the Sirolimus was blood/marrow suppression in 27%. Other toxicities all were less than 3%, including infection, pulmonary/respiratory compromise, and gastrointestinal disturbance.

These studies by Hammill and Adams show the first real promising medical therapy, especially for difficult to treat microcystic lymphatic malformations.

28.6 Recommendations

Venolymphatic malformations are uncommon enough that most physicians are not familiar or comfortable with these lesions, but common enough that a busy neurosurgical practice will see at least one to two of these lesions yearly. The treatment planning for venolymphatic malformations should involve a multidisciplinary team, including surgeons, anesthesiologists, and radiologists. Imaging work-up starts with duplex ultrasound and subsequent MRI evaluation with contrast.

For most lesions, percutaneous sclerotherapy is the first-line treatment modality. Ethanol has the best efficacy in the treatment of venous and lymphatic malformations, but nontarget embolization is associated with pulmonary hypertension, pulmonary embolism, and skin necrosis. Sclerotherapy with ethanol should only be performed by practitioners trained in using the agent, under general anesthesia (GA), and with pulmonary artery monitoring via a Swan-Ganz catheter. Given the risks of ethanol sclerotherapy, most practitioners will choose to only use ethanol for lesions refractory to other sclerosants. STS, bleomycin, and polidocanol are treatment choices for venous malformations. Doxycycline and bleomycin may give good results in lymphatic malformations with potentially a safer side-effect profile.

Sclerotherapy should be performed under GA. Sclerotherapy is often very painful, and GA is desired to avoid patient discomfort and movement during the procedure. GA is also very important for lesions near the airway. Some lesions in the posterior oropharynx may even require prolonged intubation until the procedural associated edema resolves.

Surgery is often used for debulking and in conjunction with sclerotherapy. Sclerotherapy reduces the overall mass of the lesions and reduces blood loss, making surgical procedures more feasible and safe. The mTOR inhibitor Sirolimus can be used in complex malformations, especially microcystic lymphatic malformations. Randomized trials should be available over the next few years to confirm preliminary results of Sirolimus treatment.

Overall, additional trials are needed to delineate the optimal treatment protocol for venolymphatic malformations.

28.7 Summary

1. Venolymphatic malformations remain underdiagnosed and/or misdiagnosed. Successful treatment is based on consensus opinion and best outcomes are likely from multidisciplinary approach at high-volume centers.
2. There is no high-level evidence to support one treatment over other options. Current practice is for percutaneous sclerotherapy as first-line therapy when it is possible. Given the lack of evidence showing superiority of one agent over another, the agent used for sclerotherapy is best determined by the performing physician.
3. Medical therapies focused on specific mutation pathways may play a greater role in the treatment of vascular malformations in the future.

References

[1] Garg S, Kumar S, Singh YB. Intralesional radiofrequency in venous malformations. Br J Oral Maxillofac Surg. 2015; 53(3):213–216
[2] Cornelis FH, Marin F, Labrèze C, et al. Percutaneous cryoablation of symptomatic venous malformations as a second-line therapeutic option: a five-year single institution experience. Eur Radiol. 2017; 27(12):5015–5023
[3] Lee BB, Bergan J, Gloviczki P, et al. International Union of Phlebology (IUP). Diagnosis and treatment of venous malformations. Consensus document of the International Union of Phlebology (IUP)-2009. Int Angiol. 2009; 28 (6):434–451
[4] Legiehn GM, Heran MK. Venous malformations: classification, development, diagnosis, and interventional radiologic management. Radiol Clin North Am. 2008; 46(3):545–597, vi
[5] Moukaddam H, Pollak J, Haims AH. MRI characteristics and classification of peripheral vascular malformations and tumors. Skeletal Radiol. 2009; 38 (6):535–547
[6] Konez O, Burrows PE. Magnetic resonance of vascular anomalies. Magn Reson Imaging Clin N Am. 2002; 10(2):363–388, vii
[7] van Rijswijk CS, van der Linden E, van der Woude H-J, van Baalen JM, Bloem JL. Value of dynamic contrast-enhanced MR imaging in diagnosing and classifying peripheral vascular malformations. AJR Am J Roentgenol. 2002; 178(5):1181–1187
[8] Lee BB, Baumgartner I, Berlien P, et al. International Union of Phlebology. Diagnosis and treatment of venous malformations. Consensus document of the International Union of Phlebology (IUP): updated 2013. Int Angiol. 2015; 34(2):97–149
[9] Dompmartin A, Acher A, Thibon P, et al. Association of localized intravascular coagulopathy with venous malformations. Arch Dermatol. 2008; 144(7):873–877
[10] Horbach SE, Lokhorst MM, Saeed P, de Goüyon Matignon de Pontouraude CM, Rothová A, van der Horst CM. Sclerotherapy for low-flow vascular malformations of the head and neck: a systematic review of sclerosing agents. J Plast Reconstr Aesthet Surg. 2016; 69(3):295–304
[11] Burrows PE. Endovascular treatment of slow-flow vascular malformations. Tech Vasc Interv Radiol. 2013; 16(1):12–21
[12] Horbach SE, Jolink F, van der Horst CM. Oral sildenafil as a treatment option for lymphatic malformations in PIK3CA-related tissue overgrowth syndromes. Dermatol Ther (Heidelb). 2016; 29(6):466–469
[13] Hammill AM, Wentzel M, Gupta A, et al. Sirolimus for the treatment of complicated vascular anomalies in children. Pediatr Blood Cancer. 2011; 57(6):1018–1024
[14] Adams DM, Trenor CC, III, Hammill AM, et al. Efficacy and safety of sirolimus in the treatment of complicated vascular anomalies. Pediatrics. 2016; 137(2):e20153257
[15] Spence J, Krings T, TerBrugge KG, Agid R. Percutaneous treatment of facial venous malformations: a matched comparison of alcohol and bleomycin sclerotherapy. Head Neck. 2011; 33(1):125–130
[16] Tessari L, Cavezzi A, Frullini A. Preliminary experience with a new sclerosing foam in the treatment of varicose veins. Dermatol Surg. 2001; 27(1):58–60
[17] Burrows PE, Lasjaunias PL, Ter Brugge KG, Flodmark O. Urgent and emergent embolization of lesions of the head and neck in children: indications and results. Pediatrics. 1987; 80(3):386–394
[18] Horbach SE, Rigter IM, Smitt JHS, Reekers JA, Spuls PI, van der Horst CM. Intralesional bleomycin injections for vascular malformations: a systematic review and meta-analysis. Plast Reconstr Surg. 2016; 137(1):244–256
[19] Burrows PE, Mitri RK, Alomari A, et al. Percutaneous sclerotherapy of lymphatic malformations with doxycycline. Lymphat Res Biol. 2008; 6(3–4):209–216
[20] van der Vleuten CJ, Kater A, Wijnen MH, Schultze Kool LJ, Rovers MM. Effectiveness of sclerotherapy, surgery, and laser therapy in patients with venous malformations: a systematic review. Cardiovasc Intervent Radiol. 2014; 37 (4):977–989
[21] Zhong LP, Ow A, Yang WJ, Hu YJ, Wang LZ, Zhang CP. Surgical management of solitary venous malformation in the midcheek region. Oral Surg Oral Med Oral Pathol Oral Radiol. 2012; 114(2):160–166
[22] Lee B-B, Do YS, Yakes W, Kim DI, Mattassi R, Hyon WS. Management of arteriovenous malformations: a multidisciplinary approach. J Vasc Surg. 2004; 39(3):590–600
[23] Kim JY, Kim DI, Do YS, et al. Surgical treatment for congenital arteriovenous malformation: 10 years' experience. Eur J Vasc Endovasc Surg. 2006; 32(1):101–106
[24] Malan E. Surgical problems in the treatment of congenital arterio-venous fistulae. J Cardiovasc Surg (Torino). 1965; 5(6):251–255
[25] Belov S, Loose DA. Surgical treatment of congenital vascular defects. Int Angiol. 1990; 9(3):175–182
[26] Lee BB. Critical issues in management of congenital vascular malformation. Ann Vasc Surg. 2004; 18(3):380–392
[27] Mulliken JB, Glowacki J. Classification of pediatric vascular lesions. Plast Reconstr Surg. 1982; 70(1):120–121
[28] Hooper R. Lexicon Medicum (Medical Dictionary). Vol. 1. New York; 1841
[29] Mulliken JB, Glowacki J. Hemangiomas and vascular malformations in infants and children: a classification based on endothelial characteristics. Plast Reconstr Surg. 1982; 69(3):412–422
[30] Enjolras O. Classification and management of the various superficial vascular anomalies: hemangiomas and vascular malformations. J Dermatol. 1997; 24(11):701–710

28

[31] Dasgupta R, Fishman SJ. ISSVA classification. Paper presented at: seminars in pediatric surgery2014

[32] Yakes WF, Haas DK, Parker SH, et al. Symptomatic vascular malformations: ethanol embolotherapy. Radiology. 1989; 170(3 Pt 2):1059–1066

[33] Yakes WF, Luethke JM, Parker SH, et al. Ethanol embolization of vascular malformations. Radiographics. 1990; 10(5):787–796

[34] Keppler-Noreuil KM, Rios JJ, Parker VE, et al. PIK3CA-related overgrowth spectrum (PROS): diagnostic and testing eligibility criteria, differential diagnosis, and evaluation. Am J Med Genet A. 2015; 167A(2):287–295

[35] Boon LM, Hammer J, Seront E, et al. Rapamycin as novel treatment for refractory-to-standard-care slow-flow vascular malformations. Plast Reconstr Surg. 2015; 136 4S:38

29 Chronic Subdural Hematoma Embolization

Joseph Carnevale, Justin Schwarz, Alexander Ramos, Jacob Goldberg, Thomas Link, and Jared Knopman

Abstract

Chronic subdural hematomas (cSDH) are a common pathology encountered routinely in clinical practice, particularly in the elderly population. This pathology is historically difficult to treat due to the comorbidities inherent in this patient population and the high rate of recurrence following surgical evacuation. The decision to manage conservatively with serial imaging versus surgical evacuation (twist drill craniotomy, burr-holes, or craniotomy) remains controversial and depends on patient symptomatology, radiographic findings, and patient comorbidities. A novel, multidisciplinary approach involving neurosurgeons and neurointerventionalists has recently shown promise in the treatment of cSDH. Embolization of the middle meningeal artery (MMA) is a safe procedure that has shown potential efficacy in decreasing the size of cSDH when performed as a stand-alone procedure and limiting cSDH recurrence following surgical evacuation.

Keywords: chronic subdural hematoma, embolization, middle meningeal artery

29.1 Goals

1. Review and understand the symptomatology and natural history of chronic subdural hematomas (cSDH).
2. Review the current management strategies of cSDH and how it applies to the treatment decision for this pathology.
3. Critically analyze the limited literature that evaluates the utility of middle meningeal artery (MMA) embolization for cSDH.

29.2 Case Example

29.2.1 History of Present Illness

A 74-year-old female presents with a progressive headache and gait imbalance over 3 to 4 weeks. She endorses a fall from standing with head strike approximately 6 weeks ago while gardening with no loss of consciousness. The headache is predominantly right-sided, dull, constant, and not positional. The headache has been worsening over the last week, prompting her to seek medical care in the emergency department. She denies any weakness, numbness, tingling, seizures, or other significant neurologic complaints.

Past medical history: Hypertension, hyperlipidemia, hypothyroidism, coronary artery disease on aspirin 81 mg daily, ovarian cancer (no evidence of disease).
Past surgical history: Cesarean section (1971), hysterectomy and bilateral oophorectomy (1992).
Family history: Denies any relevant familial history.
Social history: One to two glasses of wine per week, former smoker, no illicit substance use.
Review of systems: As per the above.

Examination: Awake, alert, oriented to name, location, and date. Cranial nerves II–XII intact and symmetric, motor examination is grossly symmetric and strong, no drift.
Imaging studies: See ▶ Fig. 29.1a.

29.2.2 Treatment Plan

Given the size of the patient's cSDH, treatment was recommended. The patient and her family adamantly wanted to avoid an open surgical procedure, including twist drill craniotomy, burr-hole drainage, and craniotomy. The patient was neurologically intact and had only moderate headaches. MMA embolization was offered with the understanding that any worsening of symptoms or radiologic characteristics would warrant surgical evacuation. The patient underwent a right MMA embolization using polyvinyl alcohol particles under local anesthesia (▶ Fig. 29.2). She was discharged home the next day following a stable noncontrast head computed tomography (CT).

29.2.3 Follow-up

The patient did very well after MMA embolization for her right cSDH. Following discharge on postprocedural day 1, the patient had gradual improvement of her headaches and gait. Her 2- and 4-week postprocedural follow-up head CTs demonstrated a reduction of her right cSDH, with complete resolution by 6 weeks postprocedure (▶ Fig. 29.1). At her 6-week follow-up appointment, she had no headaches and was able to resume aspirin 81 mg daily for her coronary artery disease.

29.3 Case Summary

1. *What are the general characteristics, symptomatology, and pathophysiology cSDH?*
   cSDH is an intracranial, extra-axial collection of chronic blood products that accumulates in the subdural space. It causes mass effect on the adjacent cerebral cortex, resulting in a variety of neurologic symptoms and signs. cSDH occur in 13.4 per 100,000 individuals annually, with a dramatic increase in patients older than 65 years. In the elderly population, the incidence is 58.1 per 1,00,000, a nearly 20-fold increase over the general population.[1,2,3,4,5,6,7,8,9,10]
   On presentation, patients and patient caretakers commonly complain of headache, confusion, language difficulty, gait instability, unilateral weakness, and/or seizures. cSDH can also be asymptomatic depending on the time course over which they develop and the degree of the patient's brain atrophy. It is not uncommon for large cSDH to be fairly asymptomatic relative to their size. On noncontrast CT imaging, cSDH appear hypodense and are most often located along the cerebral convexity. Trace hyperdensities within cSDH are indicative of small acute blood products and commonly septations or membranes can be visualized on CT. Classic teaching states that SDH are due to tearing of bridging veins, which can be under tension in the elderly, atrophic

29

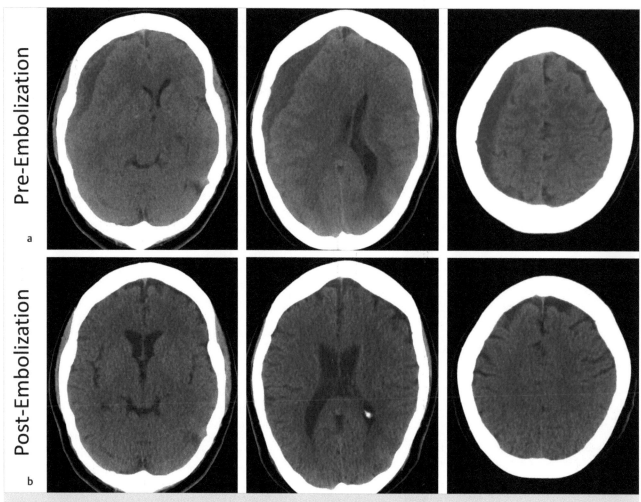

Fig. 29.1 **(a)** Computed tomography (CT) head noncontrast reveals an approximately 1.3-cm right chronic subdural hematoma (cSDH) with minimal acute blood products and 9 mm of right to left midline shift. **(b)** CT head noncontrast demonstrates complete resolution of the right cSDH and midline shift 6 weeks following right middle meningeal artery (MMA) embolization.

brain. Current studies suggest that the pathophysiology of cSDH is more complex. Most cSDH begin as acute subdural hematomas, which evoke an inflammatory response. Within days, there is perihematoma inflammation and neovascularization with permeable endothelial gap junctions, which can lead to rehemorrhage or accumulation of new blood products causing cSDH enlargement. Simply removing the cSDH may only provide temporary clinical and radiographic improvement but not address the causative neovascularization that leads to reaccumulation. With our aging patient population, managing cSDH surgically requires durable and innovative measures to treat the underlying pathophysiology to curtail cSDH recurrence.[11,12,13,14,15,16,17,18] Recurrence of cSDH occurs frequently regardless of the surgical procedure, with rates ranging from 5 to 37% after evacuation.[1]

2. *What role does MMA embolization play in management of cSDH?*
   MMA embolization has emerged as a safe, minimally invasive intervention for newly diagnosed or recurrent cSDH. By eliminating the neovascularization that contributes to cSDH by embolization, the progression and recurrence of cSDH is halted.[12,13,14,15,16,17,18,19,20] Early case reports and recent case

series have demonstrated encouraging results, specifically in regard to early brain re-expansion and decreased hematoma recurrence.[20,21,22,23] These studies examine MMA embolization as either a primary, stand-alone treatment or an intervention following recurrence. In 2018, our group published the largest case series to date of MMA embolization for stand-alone treatment of newly diagnosed cSDH, prophylaxis following surgical evacuation, and for recurrence following surgical evacuation.[1] Overall, current literature examining MMA embolization reports a notable decline in the rate of cSDH recurrence down to 3.6% with an exceptionally low rate of procedural complications.[10]

3. *What patient and radiographic factors would you consider when deciding on observation or treatment for cSDH?*
   Traditionally, cSDH management has been determined by cSDH size and patient symptomatology. If the cSDH is small and the patient is relatively asymptomatic, conservative management with observation and sequential imaging is favored. If the cSDH is very large or if there are neurologic deficits referable to the cSDH, surgical evacuation is usually more appropriate. There are multiple surgical options that vary in their level of invasiveness. The least invasive is twist

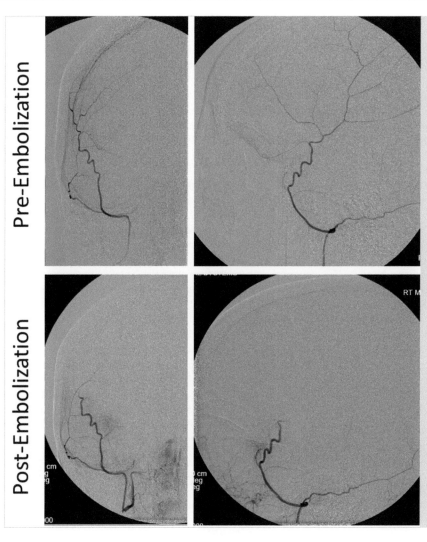

Pre-Embolization

Post-Embolization

Fig. 29.2 Cerebral angiography and embolization of the right middle meningeal artery (MMA). Frontal and lateral projections of the right MMA injections pre- and postembolization demonstrate successful embolization. There is a robust chronic subdural hematoma (cSDH) blush demonstrated on the preembolization images that is not evident on postembolization angiography. There is no significant ophthalmic anastomosis demonstrated.

29

drill craniotomy under moderate sedation, whereas the most invasive is a craniotomy under general anesthesia. The type of surgical procedure chosen is determined by the operator's preference and by the patient's history and symptomatology. In 1981, Markwalder et al presented a clinical criteria to classify cSDH based on patient symptoms. Grade 0 patients are asymptomatic, while Grade 1 patients are alert, oriented, with only mild symptoms, such as headache. Grade 2 patients are drowsy or disoriented, with neurologic deficits, including hemiparesis. Grade 3 patients are stuporous with severe focal signs such as hemiplegia, and Grade 4 patients are comatose.[24] Typically, asymptomatic patients can be observed with serial imaging, as long as their cSDH are not of a radiographic size to warrant surgical evacuation.

It is important to understand the radiologic factors that could indicate a higher likelihood of cSDH worsening or recurrence following treatment. In 2001, Nakaguchi et al suggested a radiological classification of cSDH used in predicting rate of postoperative recurrence based on imaging characteristics of the hematoma. Recurrence was shown to be highest in the cSDH with acute bleeding along a vascular membrane, corresponding to the proposed pathophysiology of cSDH reaccumulation.[25,26,27] In these cases, a potentially more invasive

surgical evacuation could be pursued to attempt to eliminate these vascular membranes, or adjunct MMA embolization could be considered.

As with all candidates for surgery, the age and medical comorbidities of the patient need to be carefully considered in the context of the patient's symptoms. Any patient with a neurologic deficit from a cSDH should undergo surgical evacuation. A patient with only mild-to-moderate symptoms, such as a headache, can be treated more conservatively with observation alone or potentially stand-alone MMA embolization. An elderly patient with multiple medical comorbidities on antiplatelet/anticoagulant medications and an asymptomatic or mildly symptomatic cSDH may be better served by close observation, MMA embolization alone, or twist drill craniotomy followed by MMA embolization, as opposed to undergoing a higher risk craniotomy.

4. *When is MMA embolization appropriate?*

Although surgical evacuation is the historical treatment of cSDH, MMA embolization could provide a significant benefit to patients by decreasing hematoma recurrence following evacuation or decreasing the need for surgical evacuation. Despite the early published success of MMA embolization in cSDH, this procedure remains controversial. The majority of the studies are small-volume, retrospective case series and, thus, are unable to show superiority of MMA embolization compared to surgical evacuation. A randomized, controlled clinical trial is needed to further define the promising role of MMA embolization in cSDH management.

In our institution we rigorously counsel patients and their families about the experimental nature of the procedure and perform stand-alone MMA embolization only on patients with Markwalder Grade 0 or 1 cSDH. Patients with higher Markwalder cSDH grade or with neurologic deficit from cSDH first undergo surgical evacuation followed by MMA embolization in an attempt to prevent recurrence.

5. *What treatment would you recommend for this patient's chronic subdural hematoma?*

The patient in the above case was recommended for stand-alone MMA embolization due to the patient's intact neurologic status and relatively mild symptoms. Surgical evacuation alone or surgical evacuation with adjunctive MMA embolization is also reasonable, given the relatively large size of the cSDH. If stand-alone MMA embolization is performed, the patient and patient's family must be thoroughly counseled on potential need for urgent surgical evacuation in the event of radiographic worsening or clinical deterioration.

29.4 Level of Evidence

MMA embolization for chronic subdural hematoma: MMA embolization alone potentially decreases cSDH as a stand-alone treatment and potentially reduces postevacuation cSDH recurrence (Class 3A, Level of Evidence C).

Currently, multiple randomized clinical trials evaluating MMA embolization are underway to further advance the evidence and wide ranging acceptance of this promising minimally invasive neuroendovascular procedure for cSDH.[28,29,30]

29.5 Landmark Papers

Link TW, Boddu S, Paine SM, Kamel H, Knopman J. Middle meningeal artery embolization for chronic subdural hematoma: a series of 60 cases. Neurosurgery 2018 Nov 9.

This represents the first, most widely cited, and largest case series examining the role of MMA embolization for cSDH. Link et al. retrospectively analyzed their experience with MMA embolization for cSDH at New York Presbyterian Hospital from 2015 to 2018. This identified 60 cases of cSDH in 48 patients who underwent MMA embolization. The authors separated these patients into three groups: (1) upfront embolization for previously untreated cSDH; (2) embolization for cSDH recurrence after surgical evacuation; and (3) prophylactic embolization following surgical evacuation. Overall 91.1% (41/45) of patients were able to avoid surgery with clinical improvement and decrease in subdural width on repeat imaging without complication. Numerous other groups have started to examine the potential benefit of MMA embolization in a challenging pathology and patient population. This is the landmark paper that has started a nationwide push toward a much anticipated multicenter, randomized, controlled, clinical trial evaluating the utility of MMA embolization for cSDH.

29.6 Recommendations

cSDH represent a difficult clinical entity to manage due to its predominance in the elderly and medically complex patient population and the high recurrence rates following surgical evacuation. The role of MMA embolization for cSDH remains controversial due to the lack of high quality evidence, but case series have shown an exciting potential benefit of MMA embolization as a stand-alone treatment for newly diagnosed cSDH or as a surgical adjunct to prevent recurrence following surgical evacuation.

Given the lack of high-quality evidence, patients and their families must be appropriately educated and consented as to appropriately manage their expectations. If stand-alone MMA embolization is performed, patients must be closely followed in the outpatient setting and informed that radiographic worsening or clinical deterioration could require urgent or emergent surgical evacuation. Care must also be taken to minimize potential procedural risk, including the dangers of inadvertent embolization of the petrosal branch of the MMA or the ophthalmic artery via an MMA-ophthalmic anastomosis.

Ideal stand-alone MMA candidates are neurologically intact patients with otherwise mild-to-moderate symptomatology, who are reliable and compliant with appropriate clinical follow-up. Adjunctive MMA embolization can be performed in all patients undergoing surgical evacuation as long as care is taken to minimize any potential procedural complication. Prospective randomized control trials are forthcoming and will further elucidate the role of MMA embolization in cSDH management.

29.7 Summary

1. cSDH represent a difficult pathology to treat, given their high rate of recurrence in a medically complex patient population.
2. MMA embolization is a safe procedure that has shown potential efficacy in decreasing the size of cSDH when performed as a stand-alone procedure.
3. MMA embolization is potentially useful in lowering the recurrence rate of cSDH in patients requiring cSDH surgical evacuation.
4. MMA embolization remains controversial and further investigation with prospective randomized trials is needed.

References

[1] Link TW, Boddu S, Paine SM, Kamel H, Knopman J. Middle meningeal artery embolization for chronic subdural hematoma: a series of 60 cases. Neurosurgery. 2018

[2] Liu W, Bakker NA, Groen RJ. Chronic subdural hematoma: a systematic review and meta-analysis of surgical procedures. J Neurosurg. 2014; 121 (3):665–673

[3] Xu CS, Lu M, Liu LY, et al. Chronic subdural hematoma management: clarifying the definitions of outcome measures to better understand treatment efficacy. A systematic review and meta-analysis. Eur Rev Med Pharmacol Sci. 2017; 21(4):809–818

[4] Almenawer SA, Farrokhyar F, Hong C, et al. Chronic subdural hematoma management: a systematic review and meta-analysis of 34,829 patients. Ann Surg. 2014; 259(3):449–457

[5] Ivamoto HS, Lemos HP, Jr, Atallah AN. Surgical treatments for chronic subdural hematomas: a comprehensive systematic review. World Neurosurg. 2016; 86:399–418

[6] Gernsback J, Kolcun JP, Jagid J. To drain or two drains: recurrences in chronic subdural hematomas. World Neurosurg. 2016; 95:447–450

[7] Xu C, Chen S, Yuan L, Jing Y. Burr-hole irrigation with closed-system drainage for the treatment of chronic subdural hematoma: a meta-analysis. Neurol Med Chir (Tokyo). 2016; 56(2):62–68

[8] Abboud T, Dührsen L, Gibbert C, Westphal M, Martens T. Influence of antithrombotic agents on recurrence rate and clinical outcome in patients operated for chronic subdural hematoma. Neurocirugia (Astur). 2018; 29(2):86–92

[9] Weigel R, Hohenstein A, Schilling L. Vascular endothelial growth factor concentration in chronic subdural hematoma fluid is related to computed tomography appearance and exudation rate. J Neurotrauma. 2014; 31(7):670–673

[10] Waqas M, Vakhari K, Weimer PV, Hashmi E, Davies JM, Siddiqui AH. Safety and effectiveness of embolization for chronic subdural hematoma: systematic review and case series. World Neurosurg. 2019; 126:228–236

[11] Weir B, Gordon P. Factors affecting coagulation: fibrinolysis in chronic subdural fluid collections. J Neurosurg. 1983; 58(2):242–245

[12] Killeffer JA, Killeffer FA, Schochet SS. The outer neomembrane of chronic subdural hematoma. Neurosurg Clin N Am. 2000; 11(3):407–412

[13] Jafari N, Gesner L, Koziol JM, Rotoli G, Hubschmann OR. The pathogenesis of chronic subdural hematomas: a study on the formation of chronic subdural hematomas and analysis of computed tomography findings. World Neurosurg. 2017; 107:376–381

[14] Tanaka T, Kaimori M. Histological study of vascular structure between the dura mater and the outer membrane in chronic subdural hematoma in an adult. No Shinkei Geka. 1999; 27(5):431–436

[15] Hong HJ, Kim YJ, Yi HJ, Ko Y, Oh SJ, Kim JM. Role of angiogenic growth factors and inflammatory cytokine on recurrence of chronic subdural hematoma. Surg Neurol. 2009; 71(2):161–165, discussion 165–166

[16] Kitazono M, Yokota H, Satoh H, et al. Measurement of inflammatory cytokines and thrombomodulin in chronic subdural hematoma. Neurol Med Chir (Tokyo). 2012; 52(11):810–815

[17] Link Thomas W., et al. Middle meningeal artery embolization for recurrent chronic subdural hematoma: a case series. World Neurosurgery. 2018; 118:e570-e574.

[18] Shono T, Inamura T, Morioka T, et al. Vascular endothelial growth factor in chronic subdural haematomas. J Clin Neurosci. 2001; 8(5):411–415

[19] Link TW, Rapoport BI, Paine SM, Kamel H, Knopman J. Middle meningeal artery embolization for chronic subdural hematoma: endovascular technique and radiographic findings. Interv Neuroradiol. 2018; 24(4):455–462

[20] Link TW, Boddu S, Marcus J, et al. Middle meningeal artery embolization as treatment for chronic subdural hematoma: a case series. Oper Neurosurg (Hager-stown). 2018; 14(5):556–562

[21] Hashimoto T, Ohashi T, Watanabe D, et al. Usefulness of embolization of the middle meningeal artery for refractory chronic subdural hematomas. Surg Neurol Int. 2013; 4(1):104

[22] Tempaku A, Yamauchi S, Ikeda H, et al. Usefulness of interventional embolization of the middle meningeal artery for recurrent chronic subdural hematoma: five cases and a review of the literature. Interv Neuroradiol. 2015; 21(3):366–371

[23] Kim E. Embolization therapy for refractory hemorrhage in patients with chronic subdural hematomas. World Neurosurg. 2017; 101:520–527

[24] Markwalder TM, Steinsiepe KF, Rohner M, Reichenbach W, Markwalder H. The course of chronic subdural hematomas after burr-hole craniostomy and closed-system drainage. J Neurosurg. 1981; 55(3):390–396

[25] Nakaguchi H, Tanishima T, Yoshimasu N. Factors in the natural history of chronic subdural hematomas that influence their postoperative recurrence. J Neurosurg. 2001; 95(2):256–262

[26] Chon KH, Lee JM, Koh EJ, Choi HY. Independent predictors for recurrence of chronic subdural hematoma. Acta Neurochir (Wien). 2012; 154(9):1541–1548

[27] Srivatsan A, Mohanty A, Nascimento FA, et al. Middle meningeal artery embolization for chronic subdural hematoma: meta-analysis and systematic review. World Neurosurg. 2018

[28] Middle Meningeal Artery (MMA) Embolization Compared to Traditional Surgical Strategies to Treat Chronic Subdural Hematomas (cSDH) - Full Text View - ClinicalTrials.gov. https://clinicaltrials.gov/ct2/show/NCT04095819. Accessed December 31, 2020

[29] Middle Meningeal Artery Embolization for Treatment of Chronic Subdural Hematoma - Full Text View - ClinicalTrials.gov. https://clinicaltrials.gov/ct2/show/NCT03307395. Accessed December 31, 2020

[30] Middle Meningeal Artery Embolization for Chronic Subdural Hematoma - Full Text View - ClinicalTrials.gov. https://clinicaltrials.gov/ct2/show/NCT04065113. Accessed December 31, 2020

29

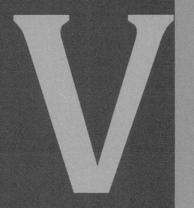

Section V

Spine Interventions

30 Spinal Dural Arteriovenous Fistulas and Malformations

Abdullah H. Feroze, Guilherme Barros, Rajeev Sen, I. Joshua Abecassis, Melanie Walker, Danial K. Hallam, Basavaraj V. Ghodke, Louis J. Kim, and Michael R. Levitt

Abstract

Spinal vascular malformations are a rare but treatable cause of spinal cord hemorrhage, myelopathy, and associated morbidity. Both clinical presentation and ideal treatments for such lesions vary widely, primarily due to variations in anatomy and associated angioarchitecture. A variety of mechanisms including venous hypertension/congestion, hemorrhage, vascular steal, and mass effect underlie the mechanism of arteriovenous shunting in spinal vascular malformations and their associations with neurologic insult and decline. Given their complexity, many attempts have been made to classify such malformations, with two major systems (the American/French/English connection and the Spetzler system). With the advent and evolution of both microsurgical and endovascular techniques, the ability to diagnose and manage such lesions through conservative management, radiotherapy, microsurgical extirpation, and endovascular obliteration continues to evolve.

Keywords: spinal vascular malformations, dural arteriovenous malformations, Foix-Alajouanine syndrome, spinal arteriovenous fistulas, dural arteriovenous fistulas

30.1 Goals

1. To review the literature that forms the basis of our understanding of the natural history of spinal dural arteriovenous fistulas (dAVFs).
2. To provide clinically relevant details regarding the anatomy, clinical presentation, and radiographic features unique to spinal arteriovenous fistulas (AVFs), their diagnosis, and subsequent management via endovascular and open techniques.
3. To review the major publications that classify presentations of spinal AVFs based upon location, angiographic features, and other variables.

30.2 Case Example

30.2.1 History of Present Illness

A 30-year-old Caucasian woman presents to the emergency department with progressive, episodic lower back pain with radiation to her neck and bilateral hips. She notes a history of low-grade lower back pain over the past several years but notes particularly discomfort over the past 24 hours with concomitant photophobia and headache. She denies any recent illness, exposure to ill contacts, or exotic travel. She also denies any other neurologic symptoms.

Past medical/surgical history: Negative for history of prior intracranial hemorrhage, hypertension, polycystic kidney disease, collagen vascular disease, or blood dyscrasias.

Family history: Negative for any history of cerebral aneurysms or other intracranial pathology.

Social history: Employed as local schoolteacher. Denies use of tobacco or illicit substances.

Review of systems: Negative with exceptions as aforementioned.

Physical examination: Notable for photophobia and reported 7/10 headache. Fully alert and oriented. Cranial nerves II–XII intact. Strength 5/5 in all testable upper and lower extremities with exception of 4/5 strength in bilateral hip flexors. 2 + deep tendon reflexes in biceps and Achilles distribution. Evidence of negative Brudzinski sign but positive Kernig sign. Sensation grossly intact to light touch but evidence of difficulty with proprioception in bilateral lower extremities.

Laboratory studies: Lumbar puncture performed within the emergency department is notable for positive subarachnoid panel but without evidence of leukocytosis or albuminocytologic dissociation. Complete blood cell count, electrolyte panel, and coagulation studies otherwise within normal limits.

Imaging: Noncontrast head computed tomography (CT) negative for evidence of acute intracranial pathology. Magnetic resonance imaging (MRI) of the thoracolumbar spine demonstrates prominent flow voids dorsal to the conus medullaris at T12 (► Fig. 30.1a).

30.2.2 Treatment Plan and Follow-up

Based upon irregularities noted above concerning for possible spinal vascular malformation, the patient underwent formal diagnostic spinal angiography that demonstrated a conus medullaris arteriovenous malformation (AVM) fed by the left T11 intercostal, right L1, and right L2 intercostal arteries (► Fig. 30.1b–d). The patient subsequently underwent T12-L1 laminectomies for resection of the AVM (► Fig. 30.1e). She was discharged on postoperative day 3 to inpatient rehabilitation and was evaluated in clinic 6 weeks postoperatively without deficit. She remains asymptomatic 2 years from initial presentation.

30.3 Case Summary

30.3.1 Introduction

Spinal arteriovenous malformations (sAVMs) represent a rare and challenging neurosurgical entity characterized by abnormal connections between spinal arteries and veins, estimated to comprise approximately 4% of all intradural spinal cord lesions.[1] Despite their rarity, accurate and timely diagnosis is of tantamount importance as they are associated with a wide variety of morbidity, including radiculopathy, weakness, paresthesias, sensory deficits, loss of bowel and bladder function, and paraplegia.[2] More recent advances in radiographic technology have allowed for more accurate diagnoses via noninvasive modalities such as MRI and magnetic resonance angiography (MRA), but spinal angiography remains the gold standard for analysis of anatomical, architectural, and morphological features of the lesions.

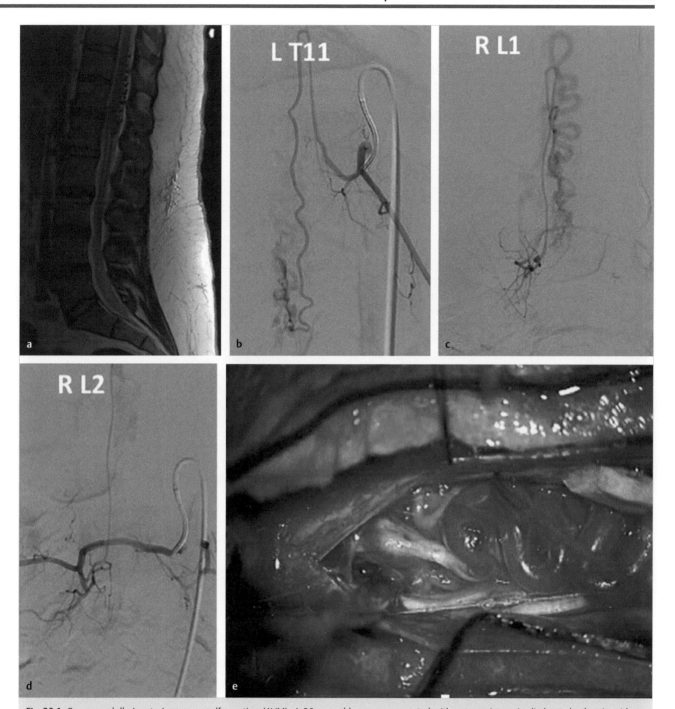

Fig. 30.1 Conus medullaris arteriovenous malformation (AVM). A 30-year-old woman presented with progressive, episodic lower back pain with radiation to her neck and bilateral hips with concomitant photophobia and headache. Magnetic resonance imaging (MRI) of the thoracolumbar spine demonstrated prominent flow voids dorsal to the conus medullaris at T12 **(a)**. Lumbar puncture yielded evidence of subarachnoid hemorrhage. Formal angiography demonstrated a conus medullaris AVM fed by the left T11 intercostal, right L1, and right L2 intercostal arteries **(b–d)**. The patient underwent T12-L1 laminectomies for resection of the AVM **(e)**.

30.3.2 History

In 1888, Gaupp first published his findings of what seems to be most consistent with a dural arteriovenous fistula (dAVF), characterizing the lesion as "hemorrhoids" of the pia mater. Shortly thereafter, in 1890, Berenbruch made similar observations of a lesion most consistent with a spinal vascular malformation. In 1911, Fedor Krause was first to describe visualization intraoperatively of a spinal vascular malformation during a laminectomy, and Charles Elsberg became the first surgeon to document attempted resection of such a lesion, in 1916. Foix and Alajouanine in 1926 described their observations of rapid neurologic decline secondary to sAVM thrombosis, now recognized as subacute necrotic myelopathy or Foix-Alajouanine syndrome.[3]

30

30.3.3 Incidence

While not as common as brain AVFs and AVMs, spinal AVFs account for 70% of all spinal arteriovenous shunts. Several classification systems have been devised based upon anatomical location, vascular features, genetics, and types of shunts involved (nidus vs. fistula) in an attempt to distinguish the subtypes of such lesions, the major systems of which are described in further detail below.[4,5,6,7,8,9,10] While such pathologies typically manifest independent of any syndromic correlate, spinal dAVFs and dAVMs have been linked with hereditary hemorrhagic telangiectasia or Osler-Weber-Rendu disease and associated genes *HHT1* and *HHT2*.

30.3.4 Anatomy

In order to understand and appreciate both the pathophysiology of various manifestations of sAVMs, an understanding of spinal anatomy and its evolution is required. The work of Adamkiewicz in 1881 was the first comprehensive treatise on the subject of spinal cord vascularization. Significant further advances in spinal vascular anatomy came with the advent of spinal angiography and work by Doppman, Djindjian, and Lazorthes.[11] Building on such work, the work of Lasjaunias et al further improved our understanding of anatomy of both normal spinal angioarchitecture and development as well as that central to pathologies such as spinal vascular malformations, allowing for modern day treatments in the form of microsurgical resection and endovascular obliteration.[12]

From a basic level, the aorta derives from the heart and branches into segmental arteries, which further subdivide into spinal radicular and medullary arteries. The medullary artery subsequently bifurcates into anterior and posterior divisions, which then merge to form the anterior spinal artery coursing through the pia of the anterior median fissure and posterior spinal arteries coursing through the pia of the posterolateral sulci. The cervicothoracic spinal cord is supplied by a number of segmental vessels from the aorta as well as subclavian and both internal and external carotid arteries. The midthoracic spinal cord is supplied from segmental vessels deriving from the aorta, but due to lack of the lack of anastomotic redundancy that the cervicothoracic cord enjoys, stands at a higher risk of possible infarction. Separately, the thoracolumbar cord is supplied by segmental vessels from the abdominal aorta and iliac arteries.

While previous classification systems described spinal anatomical nomenclature based upon spinal artery location (i.e., posterior, anterior, and posterolateral distributions), the Lasjaunias classification sought to differentiate radicular arteries by regions of supply, including radiculopial, radiculomedullary, and radicular. Via posterior radicular arteries, the radiculopial arteries supply the dorsolateral superficial pial system and nerve root. Via anterior radicular arteries, the radiculomedullary arteries supply the anterior superficial pial system, nerve root, and the gray matter of the spinal cord. Spinal radicular arteries at every segmental level supply the neighboring nerve root and adjacent dura but not the spinal cord itself.

The anterior spinal artery, originating from bilateral vertebral arteries, travels along the anterior medial fissure with additional contributions from 2 to 14 (on average, 6) segmental radiculomedullary arteries to supply the anterior two-thirds of the spinal cord. Of note, during embryological development, each radicular artery gives rise to its own respective radiculomedullary artery to supply the spinal cord, although the number of radicular arteries subsequently diminishes by postnatal life. This anterior circulatory supply gives rise to multiple sulcocommissural arteries within the ventral sulcus to supply the central gray matter and portions of peripheral white matter.[13] The largest of the anterior radiculomedullary arteries is the artery of Adamkiewicz (arteria radiculomedullaris magna), which arises close to the thoracolumbar enlargement, typically between T9 and L1. The posterior one-third of the spinal cord (i.e., the dorsolateral pial supply or centripetal system) relies upon circulation from the posterior spinal arteries, which derive origination from the posterior inferior cerebellar artery and intradural portion of the vertebral artery in addition to contributions from over a dozen radiculopial branches.[14] This network supplies radial arteries that circumferentially course along the spinal cord to anastomose with the ventral system, allowing for axially oriented perforating branches into white matter. Ultimately, both anterior and posterior spinal circulation anastomoses at the conus medullaris via two anastomotic semicircles known as the "arcade" of the cone.[15]

The spinal venous system begins with radially oriented intrinsic veins and small superficial pial veins leading into superficial longitudinal medial spinal cord veins. Ultimately, these drain with significant transmedullary anastomoses into larger vein tributaries mimicking the arterial system (anterior and posterior medial spinal veins) which reach the extraspinal veins and epidural plexus (also known as Batson plexus). Anteriorly draining sulcal veins and posterior draining radial veins drain into the coronal venous plexus through the pia and through medullary veins into epidural veins, which drain into the dural sleeve of the dorsal nerve root. The spinal venous system is unique, in that it is a valveless system and, as such, does not prevent retrograde flow—a key consideration in fistula formation and pathophysiology as congestion throughout the entire circuit can manifest in myelopathy.

30.3.5 Diagnosis

Clinical Presentation

While the potential for presenting complaints underlying spinal vascular malformations may be broad and often nonspecific, most common presentations remain related to venous congestion and hypertension. Symptoms may include paraparesis and sensory disturbances manifesting in ill-defined lower back pain, sensory loss, ataxia, loss of bowel and/or bladder control, as well as sexual dysfunction. Rarely, spinal vascular malformations may present with spinal cord hemorrhage or subarachnoid hemorrhage, even potentially within the intracranial space in the setting of cervical spine malformations.[16] A variety of imaging modalities, both invasive and noninvasive, remain available to clinicians to allow for distinction of such symptoms secondary to spinal vascular malformations rather than to other entities that may present with similar constellations of symptoms, such as spinal stenosis and neurogenic claudication.

Imaging Modalities

Magnetic resonance imaging and magnetic resonance angiography

Conventional magnetic resonance imaging

As the most common initial imaging modality obtained for the evaluation of sAVMs, most MRI protocols comprise of T1- and T2-weighted imaging in axial and sagittal planes along with short tau inversion recovery (STIR) sequences in the sagittal plan. While variation exists in appearance secondary to underlying particular anatomical considerations of different subclassifications of spinal malformations, the conventional MRI appearance of lesions such as dAVFs involves T1-hypointense, T2-hyperintense enlargement of the distal spinal cord secondary to pial vascular engorgement and associated T2-hypointense vascular flow voids. Diffuse parenchymal enhancement may also be seen on contrast-enhanced T1-weighted images. Of note, the presence of T2-hyperintense cord expansion and enhancement may also be seen in other pathologies, including neoplasms, infection, demyelination, and inflammation.

Spinal magnetic resonance angiography

While the gold standard test to allow for localization of spinal vascular malformations is diagnostic spinal angiography, noninvasive methods for localization such as spinal MRA have become more informative. With advances in technique and resolution, the ability to perform noninvasive, dynamic, and time-resolved MRA examinations to allow for further insight in the extent of AVMs to guide management and potential treatment has become far more available over the past decade. Reliant of multiphasic image acquisition after an initial intravenous bolus of gadolinium-based contrast, nonenhanced images serve as a roadmap for superimposed contrast-enhanced images over a function of time to allow for malformation location and potential for focusing catheter angiography to the appropriate level of interest. Recent analyses of MRA fidelity suggest the modality to be capable of identifying underlying spinal vascular malformations in 75 to 80% of patients who ultimately undergo formal diagnostic catheter angiography.[3] For this indication, the hallmark finding on dynamic contrast-enhanced MRA is simultaneous opacification of spinal radicular artery branches and large perimedullary veins.

Computed tomography (CT)

Conventional CT and CT angiography

In the diagnosis of spinal vascular malformations, CT tends to be less useful than MR due to decreased contrast resolution in the evaluation of soft tissue. Conventional CT may demonstrate diffuse enlargement of the spinal cord with possible diffuse pial vascular enhancement in the region of underlying spinal vascular malformations. While CT angiography allows for improved identification of lesions with fistulous connections such as dAVFs, it appears to be somewhat less reliable for localization than contrast-enhanced MRA.[17] However, in instances where there exists a contraindication to MRI, such as the presence of medication pumps, spinal cord stimulators, or retained foreign bodies, CT myelography may be of significant diagnostic relevance.

Diagnostic catheter angiography

Catheter angiography serves as the gold standard technique for the evaluation of spinal vascular malformations, given its ability to provide for identification of arterial inflow, venous outflow, and means for both localization of and access to lesions that might be deemed amenable to endovascular treatment. Angiography also allows for localization of normal structures such as the anterior spinal artery (artery of Adamkiewicz), which serves as the dominant source of arterial inflow of thoracic and upper lumbar cord and may precipitate anterior cord ischemia and subsequent paraparesis in the setting of inadvertent embolization.

A full diagnostic spinal angiogram requires selective catheterization of each intercostal artery bilaterally as well as potentially subclavian arteries and associated branches including internal and external carotid arteries, thyrocervical and costocervical trunks, vertebral arteries, and internal iliac arteries in the setting of suspected cervical or lumbar involvement. Such a systematic approach may lead to long procedure times, administration of high volumes of contrast load, and high radiation doses, so in appropriate settings, preprocedure localization with noninvasive imaging such as dynamic MRA for spinal vascular malformations may be deemed appropriate.

30.3.6 Treatment

With the advent of new and more sophisticated imaging modalities, more incidental spinal dAVFs may be encountered in clinical practice. While in certain circumstances observation alone may be reasonable in the absence of neurologic symptoms, consideration of microsurgical or endovascular obliteration of incidental lesions is common and often best practice as it is widely recognized that even asymptomatic lesions may very promptly lead to significant symptom development.[18] Once a lesion becomes symptomatic, early treatment is of paramount importance, as permanent disability may result in patients with long-standing symptoms lacking intervention. No prospective, randomized trials exist comparing microsurgical extirpation to endovascular embolization of such lesions given significant variability in malformation angioarchitecture, but both modalities prove to be viable and safe options in particular conditions under the care of experienced surgeons. Radiosurgery may also be employed in limited cases.

30.3.7 Classification Systems

Features of spinal vascular malformations and their distinct anatomic locations allow for classification and differentiation to inform and guide clinical management. While three major systems for differentiation of such lesions are used by clinicians today, including the American/French/English connection, the Hôpital Bicêtre classification, and the Spetzler system, a number of various additional systems have been used spanning as early as the mid-19th century.[19] The most common system, the Spetzler classification system, is discussed below.

Spetzler Classification System

In 2002, Spetzler et al expanded upon the prior American/English/French system by further delineating the specific anatomic locations of spinal AVFs and AVMs, with the addition of

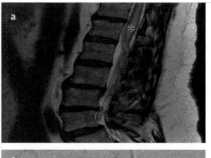
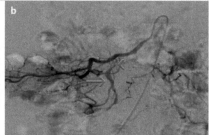
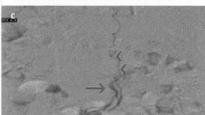
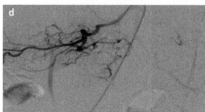

Fig. 30.2 Conus medullaris extradural arteriovenous fistula (AVF). A 57-year-old man presented with complaints of progressive lower back pain, lower extremity weakness, and urinary incontinence. T2-weighted sagittal magnetic resonance imaging (MRI) of the lumbar spine demonstrated congestive edema of the conus medullaris (*asterisk*) with abnormal perimedullary flow voids **(a)**. Spinal angiography demonstrated evidence of a fistulous connection (*arrowhead*) between right L3 segmental artery and epidural venous pouch (*arrow*) **(b)**. Further selective spinal angiogram runs revealed an epidural fistulous pouch (*arrow*) with ascending perimedullary drainage (*arrowheads*) **(c)**. The epidural fistulous pouch was successfully embolized without evidence of residual fistula **(d)**.

categories for spinal aneurysms, neoplastic vascular lesions (e.g., cavernous malformations and hemangioblastomas), and the previously unrecognized separate entity of AVMs of the conus medullaris (► Fig. 30.2). Specifically, spinal cord malformations were subclassified into types I through IV representing dural AVFs, glomus AVMs, juvenile AVMs, and pial AVFs, respectively. This system was subsequently refined by Kim and Spetzler in 2006, whereby AVFs and AVMs were recognized as separate entities.[7]

Type I: Dural arteriovenous fistulas (dAVFs)

Thought to be the most common of spinal dural vascular malformations (70–80%) that can manifest in either the extradural or intradural space, the pathophysiology underlying dAVFs was first proposed by Aminoff and colleagues in 1974.[2,20] Secondary to high-pressure arterial blood flow entering into a valveless venous system in the absence of intervening capillary beds to allow for capacitance, high pressure is transmitted to underlying spinal cord parenchyma, often resulting in progressive myelopathy and other symptoms including spinal hypoperfusion, hypoxia, and edema. Such type I malformations are created when a radiculomeningeal artery feeds directly into a radicular vein, most often found in men between the fifth and eighth decades of life and typically in a dural root sleeve of the thoracolumbar spine.[21,22,23] No clear consensus exists regarding the pathogenesis of dAVFs, but a number of hypotheses have been proposed. Most common of these hypothesis is that of the thrombosis and subsequent venous hypertension pathway, where (1) dural sinus thrombosis leads to impaired sinus drainage, (2) subsequent development of fistulous channels between thromboses sinus and dural arteries, and (3) recanalization of the dural sinus allowing for direct arterial shunting into the sinus from dural arteries.

The main objective involves obliteration of the fistulous connection with restoration of normal anterograde arterial flow and venous drainage, whether by open surgical or endovascular means. Surgical obliteration of such fistulous connections often involve hemilaminectomy or laminectomy for isolation and ligation of the draining vein, with success rates reported to be as high as 98% and minimal rates of associated morbidity.[24] However, at many institutions, endovascular management and

obliteration also remains a mainstay of treatment, particular when a single feeding artery is identified and the arteriovenous connection is direct rather than diffuse.[15]

More recent work by Spetzler et al has aimed to further subdivide these lesions into extradural and intradural types and those located dorsally versus ventrally. Briefly, intradural dorsal AVFs are thought to represent the most common type of spinal AVF, usually occurring in the thoracic region (► Fig. 30.3). Separately, intradural ventral AVFs, as fistulous connections between the anterior spinal artery and enlarged venous network, have been subclassified into types A, B, and C. Type A lesions are small lesions fed by one feeder, whereas type B lesions are larger lesions with a major feeder from the anterior spinal artery and minor feeders at the fistula level. In contrast, type C lesions are giant, multipedicled lesions with high flow and the associated proclivity for vascular steal from intrinsic spinal cord arterial supply. Small lesions (type A and B) are typically managed microsurgically, while giant multipedicled spinal dAVFs are typically targeted via embolization given their complex angioarchitecture.

Type II: Glomus arteriovenous malformations (AVMs)

Accounting for approximately 15 to 20% of spinal vascular malformations, glomus AVMs comprise a tight nidus of blood vessels within a short segment of the spinal cord. Found intradurally, such lesions may be intramedullary or extramedullary with intraparenchymal extension and found throughout the spinal axis, although their location is typically within the cervicomedullary junction. Associated nidal aneurysms are common. Patients with glomus AVMs are at risk for acute neurologic compensation secondary to risk of edema, mass effect, and hemorrhage, with rebleed rates approximated to be 10% within the first month and 40% within the first year after initial hemorrhage.[25]

Type III: Juvenile arteriovenous malformations (AVMs)

With a similar clinical presentation to that of glomus AVMs with the risk of acute neurologic decompensation secondary to

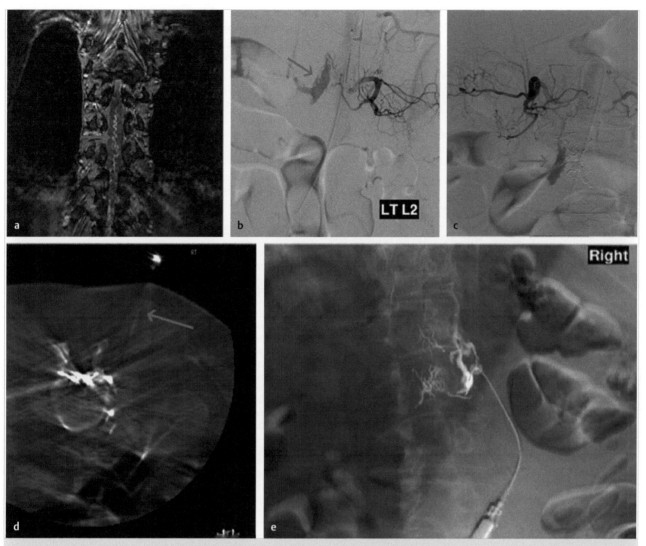

Fig. 30.3 Thoracolumbar extradural arteriovenous fistula (AVF). A 42-year-old man presented with progressive myelopathy with coronal contrast-enhanced magnetic resonance angiography (MRA) of the thoracic spine demonstrating a large perimedullary draining vein (**a**, *arrow*). Spinal angiography of left L2 segmental artery demonstrates feeding of epidural fistulous pouch (*arrow*) with faint arterial feeders from incomplete contrast reflux into the left L1 segmental artery (**b**, *arrowhead*). Repeat spinal angiography after previous embolization of left L1-L2 feeders and surgical disconnection of fistula demonstrates persistent fistulous pouch (*arrow*) fed by branches of the right L1 segmental artery (**c**, *arrowhead*). XperCT of lumbar spine during percutaneous embolization shows hyperdense previous embolization material and the fluoroscopically guided needle (**d**, *arrow*). Percutaneous embolization of the residual fistula was achieved with nBCA (n-butyl-2-cyanoacrylate) glue injection (**e**).

edema, mass effect, or hemorrhage, the juvenile variant of spinal AVMs consists of a loose nidus of vessels fed typically by multiple sources. Such lesions, also termed extradural-intradural or metameric AVMs, comprise of both intradural and extradural locations and may be either intramedullary or extramedullary in nature. Typically, in addition to spinal cord and canal involvement, they involve nerve roots, bone, muscle, and skin. As suggested by their moniker, juvenile AVMs present at higher rates in children and young adults but may also present in older subpopulations. Such lesions can be quite diffuse in anatomical presentation and involve adjacent vertebral bodies. Complete involvement of an entire somite level by such an AVM is termed as Cobb syndrome.

Type IV: Pial arteriovenous fistulas (AVFs)

Type IV intradural AVFs are direct fistulas between the anterior or posterior spinal arteries and draining veins, typically presenting within younger patients. Based upon the type and degree of arterial supply, such pial AVFs can be divided into three separate subtypes: Type IVa AVFs rely upon arterial supply from a single artery from the anterior spinal artery, type IVb AVFs rely upon arterial supply from both anterior and posterior spinal arteries to create multiple fistulas, and type IVc AVFs fistulas rely upon arterial supply from multiple arteries supplied from both anterior and posterior spinal arteries to allow for the creation of a giant fistula.

30.4 Level of Evidence

Imaging modality: While diagnostic cerebral angiography remains the gold standard for evaluation of spinal dAVFs, contrast-enhanced MRA may help to localize the lesion. CT angiography appears to have the lowest utility in the work-up for this disease (Class I, Level of Evidence C).

Treatment: Consideration for treatment of spinal dAVFs must be given strong weight, given the potential for even asymptomatic lesions to progress and result in neurological compromise (Class I, Level of Evidence C).

Surgical ligation: Open ligation of the intradural, arterialized vein is, oftentimes, a straightforward and elegant treatment for spinal dAVF (Class I, Level of Evidence C).

Endovascular embolization: Embolization of spinal dAVFs have become more popular with advances in catheter and embolysate technology (Class I, Level of Evidence C).

30.5 Landmark Papers

Aminoff MJ, Logue V. Clinical features of spinal vascular malformations. Brain 1974;97(1):197–210.

One of the original descriptions of spinal vascular lesions and their clinical features.

Borden JA, Wu JK, Shucart WA. A proposed classification for spinal and cranial dural arteriovenous fistulous malformations and implications for treatment. J Neurosurg 1995;82(2):166–179.

A classification scheme for both cranial and spinal dAVFs that is still commonly referred to by many neurointerventionalists.

Foix C, Alajouanine T. La myelite necrotique subaigue. Rev Neurol (Paris) 1926;2:1–42.

The original paper published nearly a century ago describing Foix-Alajouanine syndrome.

Kim LJ, Spetzler RF. Classification and surgical management of spinal arteriovenous lesions: arteriovenous fistulae and arteriovenous malformations. Neurosurgery 2006;59(5 Suppl 3):S195–201; discussion S193–113.

Based upon many years of personal experience and management strategies by the authors, this publication serves as the basis of the most referenced modern classification of spinal dAVFs and dAVMs.

Krings T. Vascular malformations of the spine and spinal cord: anatomy, classification, treatment. Clin Neuroradiol 2010;20(1): 5–24.

The author herein presents a rather detailed review of various sAVMs, relevant anatomy, and various means of attempted subclassification.

Oldfield EH, Doppman JL. Spinal arteriovenous malformations. Clin Neurosurg 1988;34:161–183.

An older paper on the topic of sAVMs that presents early classification and management of such lesions.

30.6 Summary

1. Spinal vascular malformations are rare lesions that pose often interesting clinical scenarios with potentially devastating morbidity if unrecognized or misdiagnosed. Early treatment is paramount due to correlation between duration of symptoms before treatment and neurologic outcome.

2. Clinical presentation can be vague, often leading to delays in evaluation, diagnosis, and treatment. Imaging characteristics are quite specific and can guide physicians in definitive treatment by radiosurgery, microsurgery, or endovascular management.

3. Surgical resection of spinal vascular malformations continues to remain the mainstay of treatment, particularly given the fact that such approaches are almost always definitive and curative. When performed by experienced surgeons, operative risks are low.

4. In the setting of more diffuse or surgically challenging lesions, endovascular intervention and radiotherapy are increasingly effective and available modalities of treatment.

References

[1] Veznedaroglu E, Nelson PK, Jabbour PM, Rosenwasser RH. Endovascular treatment of spinal cord arteriovenous malformations. Neurosurgery. 2006; 59(5) Suppl 3:S202–S209, discussion S3–S13

[2] Aminoff MJ, Logue V. Clinical features of spinal vascular malformations. Brain. 1974; 97(1):197–210

[3] Lindenholz A, TerBrugge KG, van Dijk JM, Farb RI. The accuracy and utility of contrast-enhanced MR angiography for localization of spinal dural arteriovenous fistulas: the Toronto experience. Eur Radiol. 2014; 24(11):2885–2894

[4] Bao YH, Ling F. Classification and therapeutic modalities of spinal vascular malformations in 80 patients. Neurosurgery. 1997; 40(1):75–81

[5] Borden JA, Wu JK, Shucart WA. A proposed classification for spinal and cranial dural arteriovenous fistulous malformations and implications for treatment. J Neurosurg. 1995; 82(2):166–179

[6] Geibprasert S, Pereira V, Krings T, et al. Dural arteriovenous shunts: a new classification of craniospinal epidural venous anatomical bases and clinical correlations. Stroke. 2008; 39(10):2783–2794

[7] Kim LJ, Spetzler RF. Classification and surgical management of spinal arteriovenous lesions: arteriovenous fistulae and arteriovenous malformations. Neurosurgery. 2006; 59(5) Suppl 3:S195–S201, discussion S3–S13

[8] Rodesch G, Lasjaunias P. Spinal cord arteriovenous shunts: from imaging to management. Eur J Radiol. 2003; 46(3):221–232

[9] Rosenblum B, Oldfield EH, Doppman JL, Di Chiro G. Spinal arteriovenous malformations: a comparison of dural arteriovenous fistulas and intradural AVMs in 81 patients. J Neurosurg. 1987; 67(6):795–802

[10] Spetzler RF, Detwiler PW, Riina HA, Porter RW. Modified classification of spinal cord vascular lesions. J Neurosurg. 2002; 96(2) Suppl:145–156

[11] Lazorthes G, Gouazé A, Djindjian R. Vascularisation et circulation de la moelle épinière: anatomie, physiologie, pathologie, angiographie. Paris: Masson; 1973

[12] Lasjaunias JC, Berenstein A. Functional vascular anatomy of brain, spinal cord, and spine. In: Surgical neuroangiography. New York, NY: Springer-Verlag; 1990

[13] Oldfield EH, Doppman JL. Spinal arteriovenous malformations. Clin Neurosurg. 1988; 34:161–183

[14] Krings T, Geibprasert S. Spinal dural arteriovenous fistulas. AJNR Am J Neuroradiol. 2009; 30(4):639–648

[15] Krings T, Thron AK, Geibprasert S, et al. Endovascular management of spinal vascular malformations. Neurosurg Rev. 2010; 33(1):1–9

[16] Kai Y, Hamada J, Morioka M, Yano S, Mizuno T, Kuratsu J. Arteriovenous fistulas at the cervicomedullary junction presenting with subarachnoid hemorrhage: six case reports with special reference to the angiographic pattern of venous drainage. AJNR Am J Neuroradiol. 2005; 26(8):1949–1954

[17] Oda S, Utsunomiya D, Hirai T, et al. Comparison of dynamic contrast-enhanced 3 T MR and 64-row multidetector CT angiography for the localization of spinal dural arteriovenous fistulas. AJNR Am J Neuroradiol. 2014; 35 (2):407–412

[18] Sato K, Terbrugge KG, Krings T. Asymptomatic spinal dural arteriovenous fistulas: pathomechanical considerations. J Neurosurg Spine. 2012; 16(5): 441–446

[19] Abecassis IJ, Osbun JW, Kim L. Classification and pathophysiology of spinal vascular malformations. Handb Clin Neurol. 2017; 143:135–143

[20] Kendall BE, Logue V. Spinal epidural angiomatous malformations draining into intrathecal veins. Neuroradiology. 1977; 13(4):181–189

30

[21] Krings T. Vascular malformations of the spine and spinal cord: anatomy, classification, treatment. Clin Neuroradiol. 2010; 20(1):5–24

[22] Jellema K, Canta LR, Tijssen CC, van Rooij WJ, Koudstaal PJ, van Gijn J. Spinal dural arteriovenous fistulas: clinical features in 80 patients. J Neurol Neurosurg Psychiatry. 2003; 74(10):1438–1440

[23] Fugate JE, Lanzino G, Rabinstein AA. Clinical presentation and prognostic factors of spinal dural arteriovenous fistulas: an overview. Neurosurg Focus. 2012; 32(5):E17

[24] Steinmetz MP, Chow MM, Krishnaney AA, et al. Outcome after the treatment of spinal dural arteriovenous fistulae: a contemporary single-institution series and meta-analysis. Neurosurgery. 2004; 55(1):77–87, discussion 87–88

[25] Gross BA, Du R. Spinal glomus (type II) arteriovenous malformations: a pooled analysis of hemorrhage risk and results of intervention. Neurosurgery. 2013; 72(1):25–32, discussion 32

30

31 Vertebro/Kyphoplasty for Osteoporotic Fractures

Justin E. Costello and Troy A. Hutchins

Abstract

In total, 700,000 known osteoporotic vertebral compression fractures (VCFs) occur annually in the United States. The actual incidence is likely higher as only an estimated third of all fractures are clinically diagnosed.[1] Osteoporotic VCFs can lead to significant disability and morbidity and are associated with increased risk of comorbidity-related mortality.[2] Percutaneous vertebral augmentation (PVA) techniques have been used for 30 years as adjuncts to medical management for pain palliation in VCFs. However, controversy exists in the literature regarding appropriate patient selection and clinical benefit compared to medical management.[3] A working knowledge of the current evidence is necessary for the neurointerventionalist to appropriately select patients who are most likely to benefit from PVA and to provide up-to-date information to referring clinicians and patients during consultation.

Keywords: kyphoplasty, vertebroplasty, percutaneous vertebral augmentation, vertebral compression fractures, osteoporosis

31.1 Goals

1. Review the literature regarding our basic understanding of percutaneous vertebral augmentation (PVA) for osteoporotic vertebral compression fractures (VCFs), emphasizing indications, contraindications, and potential complications.
2. Understand appropriate patient selection and effects of timing of intervention relative to fracture age when treating osteoporotic VCFs with PVA.
3. Critically analyze the literature regarding efficacy of pain palliation with PVA compared to medical management for osteoporotic VCFs.
4. Review advantages and disadvantages of vertebroplasty (VP) versus kyphoplasty (KP) for treating osteoporotic VCFs.
5. Review the current literature regarding mortality risk for patients with osteoporotic VCFs treated with PVA compared to those managed medically.

31.2 Case Example

31.2.1 History of Present Illness

A 77-year-old Caucasian female presents with 5 weeks unchanged lower back pain, which began suddenly after bending over in the garden. Initial magnetic resonance imaging (MRI) demonstrates a T11 VCF with associated marrow edema (▶ Fig. 31.1). Her pain is rated as an 8 out of 10 on visual analog scale (VAS), despite several weeks of conservative treatment, including bracing and oral pain medications. Her activities of daily living are severely limited by pain, and she spends most of her days in bed or in a chair. She denies neurologic deficit, bowel/bladder incontinence, or fevers.

> *Past medical history*: Osteoporosis (T score: –2.7), no history of cancer, steroid use, unexplained weight loss, active infection, bleeding disorder, or anticoagulant therapy.

Past surgical history: Hysterectomy for uterine leiomyomas.
Family history: Noncontributory.
Social history: No IV drug use, nonsmoker.
Review of systems: As per the above.
Physical examination: Antalgic gait, tender to palpation lower back T11 level, neurologically intact.
Imaging studies: See ▶ Fig. 31.1.

In ▶ Fig. 31.1(a–c) Sagittal T2, short tau inversion recovery (STIR), and T1-weighted MR images of the thoracic spine demonstrate a T11 compression fracture. There is 75% vertebral body height loss, with diffuse edema signal on STIR images (▶ Fig. 31.1b), consistent with acute fracture. Fracture line is also evident on T1-weighted imaging (▶ Fig. 31.1c). There is minimal retropulsed fragmentation, with intact posterior longitudinal ligament (▶ Fig. 31.1a).

31.2.2 Treatment Plan

After review of potential benefits, risks, and other treatment options, the patient elected to undergo treatment of the T11 compression with PVA. The T11 vertebral body was accessed via bilateral transpedicular approach (▶ Fig. 31.2). Following manual drilling (▶ Fig. 31.2), KP balloons containing saline and contrast are inflated to create small cavities within the vertebral body (▶ Fig. 31.3a). Cement is then injected slowly into the vertebral body and monitored in real time. A small amount of cement leakage is seen within the T10-T11 disc space (▶ Fig. 31.3b), an incidental finding that does not increase risk of adjacent-level vertebral fracture.

31.2.3 Follow-up

The patient did well with decreased use of pain medications and back brace at 2 weeks and VAS pain score reduced to 2/10. She also showed increased mobility and at 4 weeks was able to return to gardening, with no residual pain or dysfunction. Follow-up radiographs demonstrated maintained vertebral body height with no new fracture or deformity.

31.3 Case Summary

1. *What are the key indications and contraindications that should be assessed in this patient prior to performing PVA?*
   a) Preprocedural imaging assessment:
      In the setting of an osteoporotic VCF, MRI is the most important imaging modality for preprocedural assessment.[4] MRI should demonstrate an acute vertebral body compression deformity with marrow edema on STIR images (▶ Fig. 31.1b). MRI may also delineate unstable VCFs with significant retropulsed osseous fragmentation or posterior longitudinal ligament injury. Careful review of prior imaging immediately prior to PVA is important for planning of vertebral body access and for potential identification of new VCFs during the procedure.

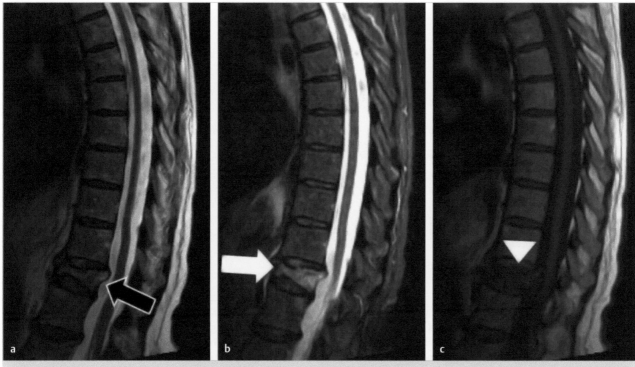

Fig. 31.1 Sagittal T2 (**a**), sagittal short tau inversion recovery (STIR) (**b**), and sagittal T1 (**c**) images of the thoracic spine. An acute T11 compression fracture is present with 75% height loss and diffuse marrow edema signal (*white arrow*). Fracture line is also evident on T1 imaging (*arrowhead*). There is minimal retropulsed fragmentation with intact posterior longitudinal ligament (*black arrow*). Further vertebral height loss or increased retropulsed fragmentation (than that depicted in this case) are relative contraindications to percutaneous vertebral augmentation (PVA).

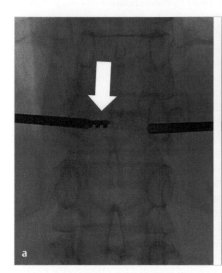
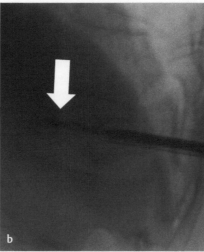

Fig. 31.2 Intraoperative fluoroscopic images from T11 kyphoplasty show T11 vertebral access via bilateral transpedicular approach (**a,b**). Care should be taken to not breach the medial pedicle cortex with transpedicular needle insertion. On the left, a drill has been advanced within the vertebral body (*arrows*) to accommodate the kyphoplasty balloon needle. Ideally, the drill should be advanced close to midline of the vertebral body on anteroposterior image (**a**) and near the anterior third of the vertebral body on lateral image (**b**). The right transpedicular access needle has already been placed and similarly drilled.

31

b) Pain must be attributed to the vertebral fracture:
Appropriate patient selection is essential as lower back pain is very common, with multiple potential etiologies.[5] Pain should be new, focal, and localized to the treatment vertebral level on physical examination.[4,6] Pain will typically worsen with weight-bearing without radicular symptoms.[4,6] Pain levels should be severe enough to impair activities of daily living and can be quantified with questionnaires or the VAS.[4] It is also recommended that patients have failed conservative management, including use of analgesics and back bracing. Pain severity score, impact on activities of daily living, clinical examination, and failed conservative management should be documented prior to treatment.

c) Absolute contraindications:
Absolute contraindications for PVA include irreversible coagulopathy, allergy to cement or contrast agent, and active infection, including local cellulitis, discitis-osteomyelitis, epidural abscess, or systemic infection.[7] PVA should be postponed in patients with a fever or suspected sepsis.

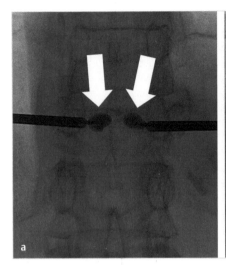
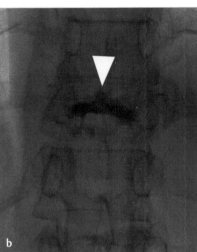

Fig. 31.3 Intraoperative fluoroscopic images from T11 kyphoplasty show interval insertion of bilateral kyphoplasty balloon needles. The balloons have been inflated with saline and contrast (*arrows*) to create small cavities for cement injection. Care should be taken not to breach the vertebral end-plate cortices during balloon inflation, to minimize cement leakage. After removal of the balloons, cement injection was performed slowly with real-time monitoring. There is symmetric cement dispersion within the vertebral body **(b)** with a small amount of cement leak within the T10-T11 disc interspace (*arrowhead*).

d) Relative contraindications:

Advanced vertebral collapse is a relative contraindication to PVA.[7] Usually at least 25% vertebral height is required to safely perform PVA. Unstable vertebral fractures with significant retropulsed fragmentation and fractures causing neurologic symptoms should generally not be treated with PVA.[7] Patients who are unable to lie prone are usually not candidates for PVA.

2. *What are the most common complications of vertebral augmentation in the setting of osteoporotic VCF?*

a) Cement leakage:

Cement leakage is the most common complication, reported in up to 88% of patients with PVA,[8] though the actual rate of cement leak is likely much lower. More importantly, the majority of cement leaks are asymptomatic and of no clinical significance, occurring within the paravertebral soft tissues or disc space (▶ Fig. 31.3b). There has been a controversy regarding disc cement leaks and higher risk of adjacent-level compression fractures[9,10,11,12]; however, recent randomized controlled studies, the VERTOS II[13] and VERTOS IV[14,15] trials, found no increased risk of adjacent-level vertebral fracture following PVA. The authors of the VERTOS IV study concluded that adjacent-level VCFs following PVA are the result of osteoporotic disease and not related to vertebral cementation.

Uncommonly, cement leaks can occur in the epidural space, neural foramina, paravertebral veins, or vertebral venous plexus, where there is potential for clinically relevant complications. The overall rate of symptomatic neurologic compromise following PVA for osteoporotic compression fracture is rare and reported at < 1%.[7] To minimize this risk, bone cement filling must be performed slowly and carefully monitored with real-time fluoroscopy.

Cement pulmonary embolism is common following PVA and reported to occur in 3.5 to 23% of osteoporotic compression fractures.[16] The majority of pulmonary emboli related to PVA involve subsegmental pulmonary arteries and are asymptomatic.[16]

b) Other complications:

Other potential complications are reported to occur at <1%, including infection, significant hemorrhage, allergic reaction, fracture, symptomatic hemothorax or pneumothorax, and death.[7] During PVA, intravenous antibiotic prophylaxis is recommended for immunocompromised patients; however, there is no consensus for antibiotic administration in immunocompetent patients.[17]

3. *Is PVA effective for treatment of osteoporotic VCF? Are there additional PVA treatment considerations?*

a) PVA effectiveness:

For treatment of osteoporotic VCFs, PVA has been shown to result in effective (and often immediate) pain relief through multiple prior studies.[13,18,19,20,21] The most recent randomized controlled studies conferring PVA effectiveness for osteoporotic VCFs include the fracture reduction evaluation (FREE),[19] VP versus conservative treatment in acute osteoporotic compression fractures (VERTOS II),[13] and safety and efficacy of VP for acute painful osteoporotic fractures (VAPOUR)[20] trials.

The FREE (published in 2009) and VERTOS II (published in 2010) trials prospectively compared PVA to medical management for treatment of acute osteoporotic VCFs. Both studies concluded superior pain relief at 1 month for patients treated with PVA versus medical management. Pain relief was also durable for 1 year or greater in both PVA treatment groups. The main criticism of both studies was lack of blinding and potential for placebo effect in the PVA treatment group.

The VAPOUR trial (published in 2016) prospectively compared PVA to a PVA sham procedure for treatment of acute osteoporotic VCFs. The study concluded superior pain relief for PVA versus the placebo procedure. Patients were followed to 6 months after the procedure and the primary end point of the study was pain below 4 out of 10 at 14 days postintervention.

b) PVA timing:

For treatment of osteoporotic VCF, PVA has been shown to be most effective for recent vertebral fractures.[13,18,19,20,21]

The VERTOS II[13] and VAPOUR[20] trials only included patients with vertebral fractures < 6 weeks old. The FREE[19] trial showed benefit for PVA treatment of subacute vertebral fractures < 3 months old. A recent single-arm prospective study, the EVOLVE[21] trial (published in 2019) also demonstrated pain benefit for PVA treatment of osteoporotic VCFs up to 4 months old.

Currently, there is no randomized controlled data to support effective pain palliation from PVA for chronic VCFs (> 4 months old), and medical management should be considered as the first-line therapy in these patients. An upcoming study, the VERTOS V trial,[22] which is not yet published, is currently investigating the efficacy of VP for patients with persistent pain and chronic unhealed osteoporotic VCFs.

c) Vertebroplasty (VP) versus kyphoplasty (KP):

Both VP and KP involve similar percutaneous vertebral access using trocar systems; however, in KP, balloon-assisted cavities are created prior to cement injection. Clinical outcomes are similar for patients treated with VP or KP. A recent meta-analysis and systematic review of the literature[23] found no difference in pain control for osteoporotic VCFs treated with VP or KP.

However, because of the balloon-assisted cavities, cement control can be easier during KP and studies have found that the rate of cement leak is significantly lower for KP compared to VP.[23] As stated previously, most cement leaks are of no clinical significance, with most occurring in the paravertebral or disc spaces. Thus, the benefit of decreased cement leaks with KP is likely marginal.

Studies have also found significantly decreased kyphotic wedge angles and increased vertebral body height restoration in patients treated with KP versus VP.[23] However, as with cement leaks, the clinical benefit of height restoration has not been well validated and it may also be clinically insignificant. More studies are needed to further investigate KP vertebral height restoration, particularly in the setting of advanced VCFs (> 50% vertebral height loss).

d) Cement injection volume:

There has been controversy regarding the effect of PVA injection volume and its relationship to treatment outcomes. Two studies published in 2012 (prospective follow-up study, 196 painful osteoporotic compression fractures)[24] and 2016 (retrospective review, 108 patients)[25] have suggested better pain relief with higher VP cement injection volumes, albeit at the detriment of higher rate of cement leaks. An additional retrospective study published in 2006 (158 patients)[26] concluded no clinical benefit for higher VP cement injection volumes and emphasized maximum safe filling of vertebral bodies.

4. *Is PVA more effective than conservative medical management for treatment of acute osteoporotic VCFs?*

a) 2009 NEJM sham procedure studies:

In 2009, two randomized controlled multicenter studies were published in the *New England Journal of Medicine*[27,28] comparing VP to a sham placebo procedure for treatment of osteoporotic VCFs. Although one study reported a trend for better pain relief in the VP versus placebo group (64% pain controlled in VP group at 1 month vs. 48% in placebo group),[27] both the studies concluded that there was no statistically significant difference in short-term pain relief between the two groups. At the time, these studies incited much debate in the medical community as to the efficacy and appropriateness of PVA for treatment of osteoporotic VCFs.

Both studies had limitations, primarily patient selection with inclusion of chronic osteoporotic VCFs. Both study designs randomized treatment for patients with VCFs < 1 year in age. In the study by Kallmes et al,[27] 36% of VCFs were > 6 months old and edema on MRI was not a requirement for study participants. In the study by Buchbinder et al,[28] 25% of VCFs were > 3 months old and physical examination was not required for study participants.

b) VAPOUR study:

The VAPOUR trial,[20] published in 2016 by Clark et al, also randomized patients to either VP or a placebo sham procedure. The major difference in study design versus the 2009 NEJM studies was patient selection. The VAPOUR trial only included patients (120) with fracture ages of < 6 weeks and nearly 80% of study participants had fracture ages of < 3 weeks. Baseline VAS and numeric-rated score for pretreatment pain assessment were also greater, 7 out of 10 or more in all study participants. The study found statistically significant pain relief for the VP treatment group versus the placebo group at both 2 weeks and 6 months follow-up. Also, many of the patients in the study were admitted inpatients (57%) and the study found a reduced mean hospital stay of 5.5 days for the VP treatment group.

c) VERTOS IV study:

VERTOS IV, published in 2018 by Firanescu et al,[14] was the latest randomized controlled study to compare VP to a placebo sham procedure. The study included 180 patients with VCF, pain up to 9 weeks, marrow edema on MRI, and VAS pain scores of 5 or greater. Pain scores were subsequently followed at day 1, week 1, and months 1, 3, 6, and 12 following VP or placebo procedure. The study concluded no significance in pain relief between the VP treatment and placebo groups at all follow-up time points.

d) *Where do we stand now?*

The study designs, with inclusion of chronic VCFs, calls into question the validity of the 2009 NEJM vertebroplasty sham studies. However, two subsequent randomized controlled studies with similar placebo sham procedures, VAPOUR and VERTOS IV, included only acute or subacute fractures, with conflicting results regarding VP pain control. Thus, it is important to understand the key differences in these two studies.

The placebo sham procedure in the VAPOUR study included conscious sedation, anesthetic injection into the subcutaneous soft tissues only, and did not use a polymethyl methacrylate (PMMA) kit to produce a cement smell. For the VERTOS IV sham procedure, there was infiltration of both the subcutaneous soft tissues and pedicle periosteum, without conscious sedation, and the PMMA kit emitted a smell during the procedure. Greater than 80% of placebo patients believed they had received cement during the VERTOS IV study, versus 46% in VAPOUR, leading authors of VERTOS IV to raise the possibility of increased placebo effect in the VERTOS IV sham control

31

group. VERTOS IV has also suggested a potential therapeutic benefit from pedicle periosteal infiltration of anesthetic.

Patient selection was also different between the two studies. The VAPOUR study included only fracture ages of < 6 weeks and most (80%) were < 3 weeks old. VERTOS IV included fracture ages of up to 9 weeks, with a median fracture age of 6.1 weeks for VP patients. Preprocedure pain score criteria were higher for VAPOUR (at least 7 out of 10 pain score) versus VERTOS IV (at least 5 out of 10 pain score). VAPOUR also had a large proportion of hospital inpatients (57%) as part of the study, whereas VERTOS IV included only outpatients.

These differences in study designs highlight the importance of patient selection when performing VP for osteoporotic VCFs. VCFs treated with VP should be < 6 weeks in age and preprocedure pain score should be severe (at least 7 out of 10 VAS), with a failed course of conservative therapy. An additional, similarly designed randomized trial, the VP with a sham procedure for painful acute osteoporotic vertebral fractures (VOPE) trial,[29] has yet to be published. Comparison of VOPE to VAPOUR and VERTOS IV will be useful, when available.

5. *Does PVA confer a mortality benefit in patients with acute osteoporotic VCF?*

Increased mortality risk, estimated at 2 to 42% for 12 months, for patients following an osteoporotic VCF can be substantial. Multiple large retrospective studies have concluded a significant long-term mortality benefit for patients with osteoporotic VCFs treated by PVA.

In 2010, a retrospective database study[30] of 5,766 non-neoplastic VCFs found a significantly lower in-hospital mortality rate for patients treated with KP compared to conservative management (0.3 vs. 1.6%). Improved measures of hospital discharge were also identified with a higher rate of discharge to home for KP patients compared to conservative management (38.4 vs. 21%). Similar mortality benefit was demonstrated by three subsequent large retrospective studies.[31,32,33] In a Taiwanese study,[33] the risk of respiratory failure was also significantly lower for the VP group, suggesting that pulmonary impairment may contribute to increased mortality in patients treated with conservative management.

31.4 Level of Evidence

PVA efficacy: Given the patient's clinical presentation (focal pain onset < 6 weeks, > 7/10 VAS pain score) and imaging findings (vertebral compression deformity and edema on MRI), treatment with PVA is a reasonable approach for pain control. Because there is controversy regarding PVA effectiveness versus medical management when comparing the VAPOUR and VERTOS IV randomized controlled studies, stringent patient selection is crucial prior to PVA treatment (Class I, Level of Evidence A).

PVA safety: With the patient's imaging findings, we can expect a very low risk for major complication following PVA (Class I, Level of Evidence A).

Chronic osteoporotic VCFs: Currently, there is no quality randomized controlled studies to support PVA for treatment of osteoporotic VCFs > 3 to 4 months in age. Medical management should remain standard-of-care treatment in these patients at this time. An upcoming study, the VERTOS V trial,[22] is currently investigating the efficacy of VP for patients with chronic unhealed osteoporotic VCFs (Class III, Level of Evidence C).

Progressive height loss and adjacent-level fractures following PVA: Recent randomized controlled studies have concluded less vertebral height loss following PVA. Also, there is no increased risk of adjacent-level vertebral fractures following PVA (Class I, Level of Evidence A).

Mortality benefit of PVA for osteoporotic VCFs: Several large retrospective cohort studies have concluded a mortality benefit for PVA treatment versus medical management. This mortality benefit could be related to improved respiratory function following PVA (Class III, Level of Evidence C).

31.5 Landmark Papers

Voormolen MH, Mali WP, Lohle PN, et al. Percutaneous vertebroplasty compared with optimal pain medication treatment: short-term clinical outcome of patients with subacute or chronic painful osteoporotic vertebral compression fractures. The VERTOS study. AJNR Am J Neuroradiol 2007;28:555–560

This was the first randomized controlled trial comparing VP to medical management for treatment of painful osteoporotic VCFs. Patients were 50 years old or greater with VCF-related back pain. Patients had to have persistent focal tenderness on examination despite 6 weeks, but no longer than 6 months, of medical therapy. They also had at least 15% vertebral height loss, bone density T-score less than −2.0, and evidence of bone marrow edema on spine MRI. Patients with poor cardiopulmonary status, ongoing systemic infection, osteomyelitis, spondylodiscitis, and radicular and/or cord compression symptoms were excluded.

Eighteen patients were randomized to the VP group and 16 to medical management. All patients were evaluated at 1 day and 2 weeks with VAS. In addition, before and 2 weeks after start of treatment, Quality of Life Questionnaire of the European Foundation for Osteoporosis (QUALEFFO) and Roland-Morris Disability (RMD) questionnaire scores were obtained. At 1 day posttreatment, patients in the VP group used less analgesics and had statistically significant, improved VAS scores (mean 2.3 decrease) compared to medical management group (mean 0.5 decrease). At 2 weeks, VP group patients had less mean VAS that was not statistically significant but showed better QUALEFFO and RMD scores and used less analgesics. Fourteen patients from the medical management group crossed over to VP group at 2 weeks.

Authors concluded from this early randomized controlled trial that improved pain, mobility, and function are immediate after percutaneous VP and significantly better in the short term compared to medical management. They realistically recognized the limitations of the small sample size and the high rate of patient crossover, making long-term follow-up impossible. This study served as a foundation for the development of future randomized controlled trials.

Wardlaw D, Cummings SR, Van Meirhaeghe J, et al. Efficacy and safety of balloon kyphoplasty compared with nonsurgical care for vertebral compression fracture (FREE): a randomised controlled trial. Lancet 2009;373:1016–1024.

A follow-up randomized controlled study published by Wardlaw et al in February 2009 (FREE study) compared KP ($n = 149$) to medical management ($n = 151$) for patients with VCF. Ninety-nine percent of patients in both treatment groups had VCFs secondary to osteoporosis, whereas 1% were related to multiple myeloma or metastatic disease. To be included in the study, the patients had to have at least 1 VCF with 15% or greater height loss, edema on MRI, and associated pain score of 4 out of 10 or greater. The primary outcome of the study was change in short-form (SF)-36 physical component summary (PCS) score (0–100) at 1 month follow-up. The PCS takes into account pain control and physical disability.

The study found statistically significant improved PCS scores for the KP group versus control group, with two adverse events for the KP group (hematoma and urinary tract infection). This led the authors to conclude that KP is an effective-and-safe procedure for treatment of patients with acute vertebral fractures. A subsequent publication on the same patients in 2011 demonstrated sustained (and statistically significant) pain relief for the KP group versus control group at 24 months, although the overall PCS score was not statistically different at 24 months. While the patient sample size was much greater ($n = 300$) compared to VERTOS ($n = 34$), the main limitation of the FREE study was lack of blinding and potential for placebo effect in the KP treatment group.

Buchbinder R, Osborne RH, Ebeling PR, et al. A randomized trial of vertebroplasty for painful osteoporotic vertebral fractures. N Engl J Med 2009;361:557–68

Kallmes DF, Comstock BA, Patrick MS, et al. A randomized trial of vertebroplasty for osteoporotic spinal fractures. N Engl J Med 2009;361:569–579.

These landmark studies were published together in the *New England Journal of Medicine* in August 2009 and are important for two main reasons. These were the first *placebo-controlled,* randomized trials to assess effectiveness of VP for improving pain and function in patients with painful osteoporotic VCFs. Second, both studies suggested that VP was no better than placebo for improvement in pain and pain-related disability in patients with osteoporotic VCFs.

The study by Buchbinder et al randomized 78 patients with osteoporotic VCFs to either VP or a VP sham procedure. To qualify for the study, patients had to have one or two VCFs, back pain for less than 12 months, and evidence of lack of healing by MRI (either fracture line, marrow edema, or both). The primary end point of the study was overall pain at 3 months, with pain scores also being assessed at 1 week, 1 month, and 6 months. Exclusion criteria were similar to the VERTOS study.

The study by Kallmes et al randomized 131 patients with osteoporotic VCFs to either VP or a VP sham procedure. To qualify for the study, patients had to be 50 years or older, one to three painful osteoporotic VCFs, failed medical management, and a pain intensity of at least 3 on scale of 0 to 10. Fractures had to be less than 1 year old as indicated by duration of pain, and only fractures of uncertain age by clinical assessment underwent MRI or bone scan. The average pain duration prior to treatment was 16 weeks for the VP group and 20 weeks for the sham treatment group. Exclusion criteria were similar to the VERTOS study. Patients were allowed to crossover to the other study group at 1 month.

The sham procedure by Buchbinder et al included periosteal infiltration of anesthetic within the pedicle and insertion of a blunt needle to the pedicle, followed by light tapping. The sham procedure by Kallmes et al included only verbal and physical cues, such as pressure on the patient's back. Both sham procedures opened the methacrylate monomer to simulate the odor associated with mixing PMMA.

Although there was a trend toward higher rate of clinically meaningful pain relief in the study by Kallmes et al (64 vs. 48%, $p = 0.06$), both studies concluded that there was no statistically significant difference in pain control or physical function between the two treatment groups. In the study by Buchbinder et al, reduction in pain score at 3 months (the primary end point of the study) was 2.6 +/– 2.9 for the VP group and 1.9 +/– 3.3 for the sham group.

The main limitation of both studies is the inclusion of chronic osteoporotic VCFs, which are not currently thought to respond as well to PVA compared to acute VCFs. Also, the study by Kallmes et al included patients with pain scores of 3 out of 10 or greater. Patients with lower pain scores are also not currently felt to respond as well to VP, as those with severe pain (> 7 out of 10). Interestingly, in the study by Kallmes et al, there was a significantly higher rate of crossover for the sham group (51 vs. 13%, $p = < 0.0001$), suggesting a decreased perceived treatment effect for the control group.

Klazen CA, Venmans A, de Vries J, et al. Percutaneous vertebroplasty is not a risk factor for new osteoporotic compression fractures: results from VERTOS II. AJNR Am J Neuroradiol 2010; 31:1447–1450.

VERTOS II was published by Klazen et al in 2010, following the NEJM sham studies. It had a similar study design as the FREE study, randomizing 431 patients with osteoporotic VCF to either VP or conservative medical management. The key difference between the two studies was patient selection, with VERTOS II only including patients with back pain for 6 weeks or less (and edema on MRI), whereas the FREE study only used edema on MRI as inclusion criterion, without specifying pain duration. Baseline pain score was also slightly higher for VERTOS II, at least 5 out of 10 or higher.

With a larger sample size and more stringent patient selection, VERTOS II found significantly greater pain relief for the VP group versus control group at both 1 month (−5.2 vs. −2.7 VAS scores) and 1 year (−5.7 vs. −3.7 VAS scores) follow-up, with no serious complications. The authors concluded that VP was effective and safe for treatment of acute osteoporotic VCFs, with sustained pain relief at 1 year. The main criticism of VERTOS II was similar to the FREE study: lack of blinding and potential for placebo effect in the VP treatment group.

Clark W, Bird P, Gonski P, et al. Safety and efficacy of vertebroplasty for acute painful osteoporotic fractures (VAPOUR): a multicentre, randomised, double-blind, placebo-controlled trial. Lancet 2016;388:1408–1416.

The VAPOUR study, published by Clark et al in 2016, randomized 120 patients with osteoporotic VCFs to either VP or a VP sham procedure. This trial was a modification of the 2009 NEJM study protocol by Kallmes et al (with two authors from that study included in the VAPOUR study). To be included in the study, patients had to be older than 60 years (mean age for VP and control groups was 80 and 81), back pain of less than 6 weeks duration, confirmation of recent fracture on MRI, and numeric rated scale (NRS) pain score of 7 or greater out of 10. Approximately 80% of patients in the study had a vertebral fracture age of 2 to 3 weeks and nearly 60% were hospital inpatients. The mean baseline NRS pain score was 8.6 for both study groups prior to treatment.

The sham procedure included conscious sedation, subcutaneous lidocaine injection *without* periosteal anesthetic infiltration, and manual tapping on the skin to mimic PVA. No PMMA was opened during the sham procedure to emit a cement smell.

Patients were followed at 3 days, 14 days, and 1, 3, and 6 months after the procedure. The primary outcome measure was NRS pain score at 14 days after the procedure. Duration of hospital stay was also recorded for inpatients. At 14 days, the number of patients with NRS pain score reduction less than 4 out of 10 was 24/55 patients in the VP group and 12/57 patients in the sham group ($p = 0.011$). Pain reduction was durable and statistically improved in favor of the VP group at all time points up to 6 months.

Mean hospital stay for the VP group was 5.5 days less than the sham procedure group. Follow-up radiographs revealed less vertebral height loss at the fracture site for the VP treatment group compared to the sham group (27% with subsequent vertebral height loss vs. 63%). Two serious events were reported in the VP group and two in the control group (serious events in the control group were related to progressive vertebral height loss). The authors concluded, "VP is superior to placebo intervention for pain reduction in patients with acute osteoporotic spinal fractures of less than 6 weeks in duration."

Firenescu CE, de Vries J, Lodder P, et al. Vertebroplasty versus sham procedure for painful acute osteoporotic vertebral compression fractures (VERTOS IV): randomised sham controlled clinical trial. BMJ 2018;360:k1551.

The VERTOS IV study was subsequently published in 2018 and was also a randomized controlled trial comparing VP to a sham procedure for treatment of osteoporotic VCFs. One hundred and eighty patients were randomized in the study, with inclusion criteria being 50 years or more in age (mean age for VP and control groups was 74.7 and 76.9), back pain for up to 6 weeks, pain score of 5 or greater on a VAS, and bone marrow edema on MRI. Due to lack of recruitment, inclusion criteria were later expanded to include patients with pain up to 9 weeks in duration. All study participants were outpatients.

The sham procedure included anesthetic infiltration of the subcutaneous soft tissues and pedicle periosteum. No conscious sedation was performed and PMMA cement was mixed, emitting a smell during the sham procedure.

The main outcome of the study was reduction in VAS scores at day 1, week 1, and months 1, 3, 6, and 12. Secondary outcomes included changes in quality of life and Roland-Morris disability scores during the 12 months of follow-up. The study found statistically significant pain relief for both treatment groups; however, they did not differ from each other at all time points. There was also no statistically significant difference in patient disability between the two groups following the procedures. The authors concluded "percutaneous vertebroplasty did not result in statistically significantly greater pain relief than a sham procedure during 12 months' follow-up among patients with acute osteoporotic vertebral compression fractures."

A secondary analysis of the VERTOS IV data, published in 2019,[15] reported no statistical difference in new vertebral fractures (adjacent-level or distant vertebral fractures) following VP or the sham procedure (31 new fractures in the VP group and 28 new fractures in the sham group). The study also found that further height loss was significantly less common and less severe in the VP group versus the sham group (8% of patients in the VP group vs. 45% in the sham group). Authors concluded that risk of further vertebral height loss is significantly less in the VP group and VP does not increase the risk of subsequent adjacent or distant VCFs.

Zampini JM, White AP, McGuire KJ. Comparison of 5766 vertebral compression fractures treated with or without kyphoplasty. Clin Orthop Relat Res 2010;468:1773–1780.

In this large retrospective review, 5,766 admissions for treatment of thoracolumbar VCFs were analyzed using the Nationwide Inpatient Sample database. There were several findings in the study in favor of KP, including a greater likelihood of routine discharge to home (38.4 vs. 21.0% for nonoperative treatment), a lower rate of discharge to skilled nursing (26.1 vs. 34.8% for nonoperative treatment), and a lower rate of in-hospital mortality (0.3 vs. 1.6% for nonoperative treatment). KP was associated with higher cost of hospitalization (mean $37,231 KP vs. $20,112 for nonoperative treatment), though the authors suggested that the initial higher cost of KP treatment may be offset by the reduced use of posthospital medical resources. The main conclusion of the study was that "KP may accelerate the return of independent patient function, as indicated by improved measures of hospital discharge." This study is mainly limited by its retrospective design.

Lin JH, Chien LN, Tsai WL, et al. Early vertebroplasty associated with a lower risk of mortality and respiratory failure in aged patients with painful vertebral compression fractures: a population based cohort study in Taiwan. Spine J 2017;17:1310–1318.

Several additional large retrospective database studies have been subsequently published, with similar conclusions of mortality benefit for patients treated with PVA.[31,32,33] Most recently, a study by Lin et al in 2017 reviewed 7,097 elderly patients with painful osteoporotic VCFs (1,773 VP patients and 5,324 non-VP patients) from the National Health Insurance Research Database in Taiwan from 2000 through 2013. The study found a significant difference in survival curves of mortality in favor of the VP group versus non-VP group. The incidence of death at 1 year was 0.46 per 100 person-months for the VP group and 0.63 per 100 person-months for non-VP group. Elevated risk of respiratory failure was also reported in the non-VP group (Hazard ratio: 2.48, 95% CI: 1.50–4.11, $p = <0.001$). Because of the potential mortality and respiratory benefits with the VP group, the authors concluded that VP should be considered a priority for the aged patients with painful VCFs requiring admission and analgesics. This study is also mainly limited by its retrospective design.

31.6 Recommendations

PVA has been performed for 30 years as adjunct therapy for painful compression fractures and has been shown to be a safe procedure with low complication rates. Although PVA effectiveness for pain palliation in osteoporotic VCFs remains controversial, particularly with recent publication of the VERTOS IV trial, the summation of current literature emphasizes the need for stringent patient selection prior to performing PVA. Patients that have been shown to benefit most from PVA are those with *acute* osteoporotic VCFs, at least < 6 weeks in age, and possibly < 3 weeks old. Also, from results of the VAPOUR study, patients with high baseline pain scores, 7 or above out of 10 VAS, and hospital inpatients may also benefit more from treatment with PVA.

Another advantage of PVA, as best demonstrated in VERTOS IV, is protection against progressive vertebral body height loss, which can be a significant cause of patient morbidity. While not validated by Level I randomized controlled studies, several large retrospective cohort studies have also concluded a mortality and respiratory function benefit for elderly patients with osteoporotic VCFs treated with PVA. These factors should also be considered, depending on patient age and comorbidities.

31.7 Summary

1. Effective and safe PVA treatment of osteoporotic VCFs has been demonstrated through multiple prior randomized controlled studies.
2. When comparing recent VAPOUR and VERTOS IV studies, there is a controversy as to effectiveness of PVA versus medical management for pain palliation in osteoporotic VCFs. However, these studies highlight the need for stringent patient selection prior to PVA treatment.
3. Other potential benefits of PVA for osteoporotic VCFs include protection against progressive vertebral height loss (Level 1 evidence) and decreased mortality (Level III evidence).
4. There is no increased risk of adjacent or distant VCFs following treatment with PVA (Level 1 evidence).

References

[1] Wong CC, McGirt MJ. Vertebral compression fractures: a review of current management and multimodal therapy. J Multidiscip Healthc. 2013; 6:205–214
[2] Hoshino M, Takahashi S, Yasuda H, et al. Balloon kyphoplasty versus conservative treatment for acute osteoporotic vertebral fractures with poor prognostic factors: propensity-score-matched analysis using data from two prospective multicenter studies. Spine. 2019; 44(2):110–117
[3] Chandra RV, Maingard J, Asadi H, et al. Vertebroplasty and kyphoplasty for osteoporotic vertebral fractures: what are the latest data? AJNR Am J Neuroradiol. 2018; 39(5):798–806
[4] Shaibani A, Ali S, Bhatt H. Vertebroplasty and kyphoplasty for the palliation of pain. Semin Intervent Radiol. 2007; 24(4):409–418
[5] Golob AL, Wipf JE. Low back pain. Med Clin North Am. 2014; 98(3):405–428
[6] Stallmeyer MJZG. Patient evaluation and selection. In: Mathis JM, Belkoff SM, eds. Percutaneous vertebroplasty. New York: Springer-Verlag; 2002:41–60
[7] Baerlocher MO, Saad WE, Dariushnia S, Barr JD, McGraw JK, Nikolic B, Society of Interventional Radiology Standards of Practice Committee. Quality improvement guidelines for percutaneous vertebroplasty. J Vasc Interv Radiol. 2014; 25(2):165–170
[8] Venmans A, Klazen CA, van Rooij WJ, de Vries J, Mali WP, Lohle PN. Postprocedural CT for perivertebral cement leakage in percutaneous vertebroplasty is not necessary: results from VERTOS II. Neuroradiology. 2011; 53(1):19–22
[9] Baroud G, Heini P, Nemes J, Bohner M, Ferguson S, Steffen T. Biomechanical explanation of adjacent fractures following vertebroplasty. Radiology. 2003; 229(2):606–607, author reply 607–608
[10] Lin EP, Ekholm S, Hiwatashi A, Westesson PL. Vertebroplasty: cement leakage into the disc increases the risk of new fracture of adjacent vertebral body. AJNR Am J Neuroradiol. 2004; 25(2):175–180
[11] Voormolen MH, Lohle PN, Juttmann JR, van der Graaf Y, Fransen H, Lampmann LE. The risk of new osteoporotic vertebral compression fractures in the

year after percutaneous vertebroplasty. J Vasc Interv Radiol. 2006; 17(1):71–76
[12] Hierholzer J, Fuchs H, Westphalen K, Baumann C, Slotosch C, Schulz R. Incidence of symptomatic vertebral fractures in patients after percutaneous vertebroplasty. Cardiovasc Intervent Radiol. 2008; 31(6):1178–1183
[13] Klazen CA, Venmans A, de Vries J, et al. Percutaneous vertebroplasty is not a risk factor for new osteoporotic compression fractures: results from VERTOS II. AJNR Am J Neuroradiol. 2010; 31(8):1447–1450
[14] Firanescu CE, de Vries J, Lodder P, et al. Vertebroplasty versus sham procedure for painful acute osteoporotic vertebral compression fractures (VERTOS IV): randomised sham controlled clinical trial. BMJ. 2018; 361:k1551
[15] Firenescu CE, de Vries J, Lodder P, et al. Percutaneous vertebroplasty is no risk factor for new vertebral fractures and protects against further height loss (VERTOS IV). Cardiovasv Intervent Radiol. 2019;doi:10.1007/s00270-019-02205-w
[16] Krueger A, Bliemel C, Zettl R, Ruchholtz S. Management of pulmonary cement embolism after percutaneous vertebroplasty and kyphoplasty: a systematic review of the literature. Eur Spine J. 2009; 18(9):1257–1265
[17] Gangi A, Buy X. Percutaneous bone tumor management. Semin Intervent Radiol. 2010; 27(2):124–136
[18] McGirt MJ, Parker SL, Wolinsky JP, Witham TF, Bydon A, Gokaslan ZL. Vertebroplasty and kyphoplasty for the treatment of vertebral compression fractures: an evidenced-based review of the literature. Spine J. 2009; 9(6):501–508
[19] Wardlaw D, Cummings SR, Van Meirhaeghe J, et al. Efficacy and safety of balloon kyphoplasty compared with non-surgical care for vertebral compression fracture (FREE): a randomised controlled trial. Lancet. 2009; 373(9668):1016–1024
[20] Clark W, Bird P, Gonski P, et al. Safety and efficacy of vertebroplasty for acute painful osteoporotic fractures (VAPOUR): a multicentre, randomised, double-blind, placebo-controlled trial. Lancet. 2016; 388(10052):1408–1416
[21] Beall DP, Chambers MR, Thomas S, et al. Prospective and multicenter evaluation of outcomes for quality of life and activities of daily living for balloon kyphoplasty in the treatment of vertebral compression fractures: The EVOLVE Trial. Neurosurgery. 2019; 84(1):169–178
[22] Carli D. A trial of vertebroplasty for painful chronic osteoporotic vertebral fractures (VERTOS V). https://clinicaltrials.gov/ct2/show/ NCT01963039. Accessed May 1, 2019
[23] Wang B, Zhao CP, Song LX, Zhu L. Balloon kyphoplasty versus percutaneous vertebroplasty for osteoporotic vertebral compression fracture: a meta-analysis and systematic review. J Orthop Surg Res. 2018; 13(1):264
[24] Nieuwenhuijse MJ, Bollen L, van Erkel AR, Dijkstra PD. Optimal intravertebral cement volume in percutaneous vertebroplasty for painful osteoporotic vertebral compression fractures. Spine. 2012; 37(20):1747–1755
[25] Fu Z, Hu X, Wu Y, Zhou Z. Is there a dose–response relationship of cement volume with cement leakage and pain relief after vertebroplasty? Dose Response. 2016; 14(4):1559325816682867
[26] Kaufmann TJ, Trout AT, Kallmes DF. The effects of cement volume on clinical outcomes of percutaneous vertebroplasty. AJNR Am J Neuroradiol. 2006; 27 (9):1933–1937
[27] Kallmes DF, Comstock BA, Heagerty PJ, et al. A randomized trial of vertebroplasty for osteoporotic spinal fractures. N Engl J Med. 2009; 361(6):569–579
[28] Buchbinder R, Osborne RH, Ebeling PR, et al. A randomized trial of vertebroplasty for painful osteoporotic vertebral fractures. N Engl J Med. 2009; 361 (6):557–568
[29] Hansen E, Simony A, Rousing R, et al. Vertebroplasty compared with a sham-procedure for painful acute osteoporotic vertebral fractures (VOPE). https:// clinicaltrials.gov/ct2/show/NCT01537770. Accessed May 1, 2019
[30] Zampini JM, White AP, McGuire KJ. Comparison of 5766 vertebral compression fractures treated with or without kyphoplasty. Clin Orthop Relat Res. 2010; 468(7):1773–1780
[31] Edidin AA, Ong KL, Lau E, Kurtz SM. Morbidity and mortality after vertebral fractures: comparison of vertebral augmentation and nonoperative management in the Medicare population. Spine. 2015; 40(15):1228–1241
[32] Lange A, Kasperk C, Alvares L, Sauermann S, Braun S. Survival and cost comparison of kyphoplasty and percutaneous vertebroplasty using German claims data. Spine. 2014; 39(4):318–326
[33] Lin JH, Chien LN, Tsai WL, Chen LY, Chiang YH, Hsieh YC. Early vertebroplasty associated with a lower risk of mortality and respiratory failure in aged patients with painful vertebral compression fractures: a population-based cohort study in Taiwan. Spine J. 2017; 17(9):1310–1318

31

32 Vertebro/Kyphoplasty for Metastatic Spine Fractures

Justin E. Costello and Troy A. Hutchins

Abstract

The management of spinal osseous metastatic disease requires a multidisciplinary approach. For painful uncomplicated osseous metastases to the spine, radiation therapy remains the treatment of choice for palliative treatment. However, there are limitations and potential complications of radiation therapy. Pain relief from external beam radiation is often a delayed response.[1] Also, patients who receive radiation therapy to a pre-existing pathologic fracture or vertebral segment that has had prior radiation are at higher risk for developing a new compression fracture at that level.[2] Newer ablative radiation therapy techniques (stereotactic body radiation therapy) are also associated with a higher risk of subsequent vertebral compression fracture.[3] In selected patients with osseous metastatic disease, percutaneous vertebral augmentation (PVA), with or without adjunctive tumor control interventions, may be an appropriate treatment choice and can offer advantages compared to radiation therapy alone. Therefore, it is important for the neurointerventionalist to understand the current literature regarding the use of PVA for treatment of pathologic compression fractures, as well as its limitations and potential complications.

Keywords: vertebroplasty, kyphoplasty, spine radiofrequency ablation, spinal metastases, multiple myeloma

32.1 Goals

1. Review the literature regarding the basic understanding of percutaneous vertebral augmentation (PVA) for metastatic lesions, emphasizing indications, contraindications, and potential complications.
2. Critically analyze the literature regarding the efficacy of PVA for spinal osseous metastases.
3. Understand when PVA is most appropriate in the setting of painful vertebral metastases.
4. Review current literature regarding use of PVA combined with radiation therapy or radiofrequency ablation (RFA).
5. Review the current literature pertaining to PVA for high-risk patients.

32.2 Case Example

32.2.1 History of Present Illness

A 62-year-old Caucasian male is referred for evaluation of a new painful L1 compression fracture. He has a history of multiple osseous metastases in the setting of advanced renal cell carcinoma, diagnosed a few years prior. He has received previous palliative external beam radiation to the lumber spine. The patient has been pain-free until 2 weeks prior, when he experienced sudden lower back pain while bending forward. Subsequent lumbar spine imaging revealed a new L1 compression fracture. His pain was rated as 8 out of 10 in severity and interfered with his activities of daily living. The patient attempted conservative therapy, including bracing and opioids, without relief of symptoms. He denies any lower extremity radicular symptoms, weakness, or saddle anesthesia.

Past medical history: COPD, knee osteoarthritis. No history of bleeding disorders.

Past surgical history: Bilateral total knee replacement.

Family history: Noncontributory.

Social history: Quit smoking 15 years prior; 10 pack/year smoking history.

Review of systems: As per the above.

Neurological examination: The patient is focally tender to palpation over the midline lower back, near the L1 level. Otherwise, unremarkable.

Imaging studies: See ▶ Fig. 32.1a–d. In this figure, sagittal computed tomography (CT) and sagittal T1, T2, and short tau inversion recovery (STIR) magnetic resonance (MR) images of the lumbar spine demonstrate an L1 compression fracture with 60% vertebral body height loss and an underlying osteolytic lesion on CT. High signal is seen on STIR images, consistent with acute marrow edema. There is no retropulsed fragmentation or vertebral cortical destruction. There are mild degenerative changes of the lumbar spine without evidence of high-grade spinal canal stenosis or nerve root impingement.

32.2.2 Treatment Plan

After review of potential risks and benefits, the patient elected to undergo treatment of the L1 compression with PVA and RFA. The L1 vertebral body was accessed via left unipediculate approach (▶ Fig. 32.2a, b). An RFA probe was then advanced into the L1 vertebral body and RFA was performed (▶ Fig. 32.2c). The RFA probe was removed and replaced with a vertebroplasty needle. Subsequent injection of polymethylmethacrylate (PMMA) shows adequate filling of the L1 vertebral body without evidence of cement leak (▶ Fig. 32.2d).

32.2.3 Follow-up

The patient did well after the L1 vertebroplasty and RFA procedure. He reported an immediate decrease in pain following treatment. Follow-up MR imaging 6 months after the procedure reveals no progression of the L1 fracture or tumor progression. The patient remained without lower back pain at time of the 6-month follow-up examination.

32.3 Case Summary

1. *What are the key indications and contraindications that should be assessed in this patient prior to performing PVA?*
   a) *Osteolytic* vertebral lesion:
      In the setting of osseous metastatic disease, CT is an important imaging modality for patient preassessment. CT should demonstrate an osteolytic vertebral lesion,[4] typically with associated vertebral height loss. The vertebral cortex should also be evaluated for evidence of cortical

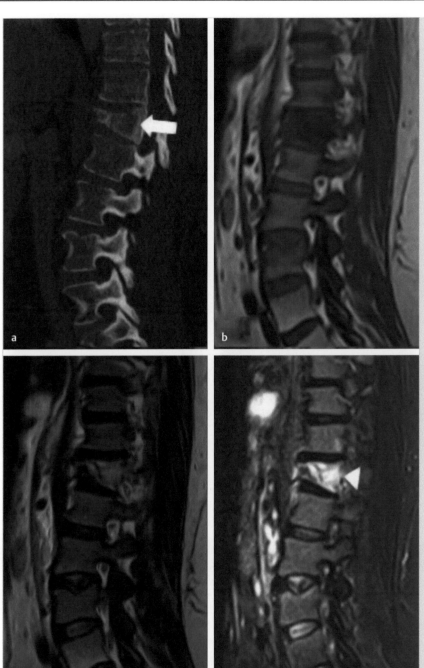

Fig. 32.1 Sagittal noncontrast computed tomography (CT) **(a)** sagittal T1 **(b)**, sagittal T2 **(c)**, and sagittal short tau inversion recovery (STIR) **(d)** images of the lumbar spine. An acute L1 compression fracture is present with 60% height loss, associated osteolytic lesion (*white arrow*), and diffuse marrow edema signal (*white arrowhead*). There is no posterior cortex destruction on CT or epidural disease on magnetic resonance imaging (MRI).

32

destruction or fracture instability. MRI is additionally recommended as part of the patient preassessment.[5] Vertebral marrow edema on STIR sequences (▶ Fig. 32.1c) indicates that the compression fracture is acute and MRI may better delineate epidural or foraminal tumor extension. Comparison with prior imaging is also important to help determine fracture acuity.

b) *Pain* must be attributed to the osteolytic vertebral fracture:

As described in the previous chapter, patient selection is essential.[5,6,7] Patients with metastatic disease may have back pain from multiple sources and physical examination should localize symptoms to the vertebral treatment level.

Pain levels should be severe enough to impair activities of daily living and new radicular symptoms should not be present. Pain severity score, impact on activities of daily living, clinical examination, and failed conservative management should be documented prior to treatment.

c) Absolute contraindications:

Absolute contraindications for PVA include irreversible coagulopathy, allergy to cement or contrast agent, and active infection, including local cellulitis, discitis-osteomyelitis, epidural abscess, or systemic infection.[4] PVA should be postponed in patients with a fever or suspected sepsis.

d) Relative contraindications:

Advanced vertebral collapse is a relative contraindication

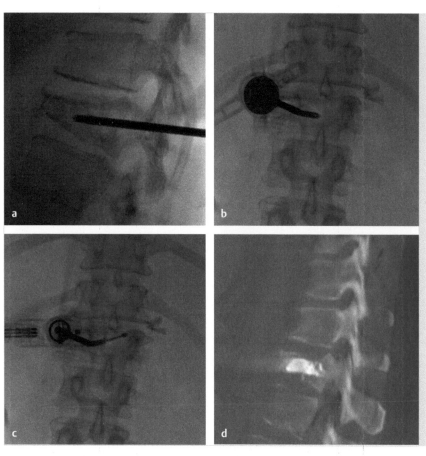

Fig. 32.2 Intraoperative fluoroscopic images from L1 vertebroplasty and radiofrequency ablation (RFA) show L1 vertebral access via left unilateral transpedicular approach **(a,b)**. After L1 vertebral access, RFA was performed **(c)**, followed by unipediculate vertebroplasty. Intraoperative 3D rotational images show adequate L1 vertebral filling with cement material, without evidence of cement leak **(d)**.

to PVA.[4] At least 25% vertebral height is usually required to safely perform PVA. Purely osteoblastic lesions are also a relative contraindication, due to limitations in vertebral access and cement distribution within the vertebral body. Vertebral lesions with posterior cortex breakthrough, unstable fractures, and fractures causing neurologic symptoms should generally not be treated with PVA.[4] However, with highly skilled neurointerventionalists, these are not considered absolute contraindications (see section below regarding high-risk patients). Finally, patients who are unable to lie prone are usually not candidates for PVA.

2. *What are the most common complications of vertebral augmentation in the setting of osseous metastases?*
   The overall complication rate is higher with PVA for metastatic compression fractures compared to osteoporotic compression fractures, estimated at approximately 10% (1–3% with osteoporotic compression fractures).[8] This increase in morbidity may be related to destruction of the vertebral body or medical condition of the cancer patient; however, most of these complications are minor or transient.[5]

   a) Cement leakage:
   As with osteoporotic vertebral compression fractures (VCFs), cement leakage is the most common complication following PVA for metastatic VCFs.[9] Similarly, the majority of cement leaks are of no clinical significance, including disc cement leaks, which, although controversial,[10,11,12,13] have been recently shown to *not* increase risk for adjacent-level vertebral fractures.[14]

Cement leaks can also occur in the epidural space, neural foramina, paravertebral veins, or vertebral venous plexus, where there is a higher incidence of clinically relevant complications. The overall rate of symptomatic neurologic compromise following PVA for metastatic compression fracture is < 2%,[4] and potentially higher in patients with vertebral cortical destruction. To minimize this risk, bone cement filling must be performed slowly and carefully monitored with real-time fluoroscopy. If foraminal cement material is encountered in the polymerization phase, targeted foraminal saline injection may be of benefit to prevent radiculopathy secondary to heating.[15]

Cement pulmonary embolism is common following PVA, occurring in 3.5 to 23% of osteoporotic VCFs,[16] with theoretical higher incidence with metastatic compression fractures due to tumor vascularity. The majority of cement pulmonary emboli are incidentally discovered on follow-up chest imaging and asymptomatic. No specific treatment is recommended for these patients, other than clinical follow-up.[16] Less than 1% of cement pulmonary emboli will be central or symptomatic (▶ Fig. 32.3c).[7,16] In these patients, therapy is recommended according to current thrombotic pulmonary embolism treatment guidelines.[16]

b) Other complications:
Other potential complications are reported to occur at <1%, including infection, significant hemorrhage, allergic reaction, fracture, symptomatic hemothorax or pneumothorax, and death.[4] During PVA, intravenous antibiotic

32

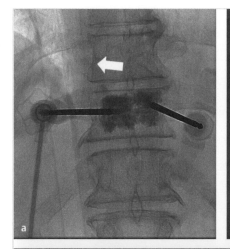
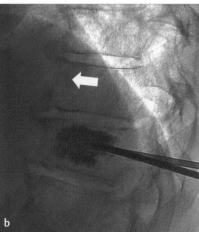
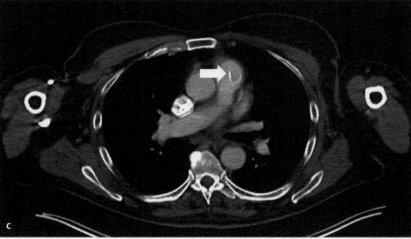

Fig. 32.3 Posterior-anterior and lateral intraoperative fluoroscopic images obtained during bilateral transpedicular kyphoplasty **(a,b)**. Cement leak within a paravertebral vein is present (*white arrows*). Follow-up surveillance PET-CT (positron emission tomography–computed tomography) images in the same patient demonstrate curvilinear high-attenuation filling defect within the main pulmonary artery **(c)**, consistent with cement pulmonary embolism (PE), a rare complication, occurring in < 1%. Because the cement PE is central (*arrow*), treatment should be considered according to current thrombotic PE treatment guidelines.

prophylaxis is recommended for immunocompromised patients; however, there is no consensus for antibiotic administration in immunocompetent patients.[1]

3. *Under fluoroscopic guidance, how should the vertebral body be accessed for injection of PMMA cement material in this patient?*

In this patient, the best method for vertebral access is by transpedicular approach (▶ Fig. 32.4a). Transpedicular access allows for the easiest recognition of anatomic landmarks and reduces the risk of nerve injury or cement leak.[5,8] Often this is performed by bilateral transpedicular access; however, Kim et al[17] have demonstrated similar efficacy and safety using a unipediculate approach. If the pedicle is infiltrated with tumor or is too small, parapedicular or posterolateral approaches (▶ Fig. 32.4b–c) can be used, though these may be associated with higher risk of paraspinous hematoma, pneumothorax, or foraminal cement leak.[5] Also, in the cervical spine, an anterolateral approach is used to avoid injury to the carotid or jugular vasculature.

4. *What is the difference between kyphoplasty and vertebroplasty techniques, and does one confer benefits over the other in this patient?*

Both vertebroplasty and kyphoplasty involve similar percutaneous vertebral access using trocar systems; however, in kyphoplasty, balloon-assisted cavities are created prior to cement injection. Clinical outcomes are similar for patients treated with vertebroplasty or kyphoplasty. A recent systematic review by Sadeghi-Naini et al[18] concluded that there were no clear benefits of vertebroplasty versus kyphoplasty in the setting of metastatic vertebral lesions; thus, treatment method is typically based upon operator experience and preference. Several studies have reported improved vertebral height restoration using kyphoplasty (versus vertebroplasty)[19,20,21]; however, this has not been shown to be clinically significant. Prior literature also mentions the need for general anesthesia when performing kyphoplasty, but these procedures are routinely performed with local anesthetic and conscious sedation.[8]

5. *Based on prior literature, is PVA effective for pain control in patients with a pathologic compression fracture?*

Vertebroplasty and kyphoplasty have been shown to rapidly alleviate pain secondary to VCFs with underlying osseous metastatic disease.[9] The body of evidence for PVA treatment of pathologic compression fractures is mostly based upon observational studies. Numerous single-arm prospective and retrospective studies have demonstrated decreased pain intensity from baseline following either vertebroplasty or kyphoplasty for compression fractures related to multiple myeloma or other metastatic cancers.[22,23,24,25,26,27,28,29,30,31,32,33,34] A statistically significant decrease in pain severity has been reported in 70 to 92% of patients,[4] with pain severity assessed at 12 hours up to 3 years following PVA.[22,23,24,25,26,27,28,29,30,31,32,33,34,35,36]

32

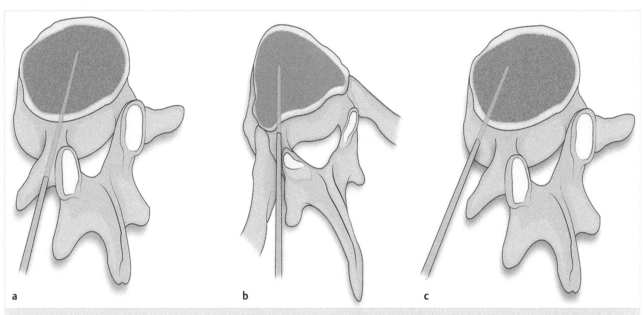

Fig. 32.4 Illustrations of percutaneous vertebral augmentation access approaches. The transpedicular approach is most commonly performed **(a)** and allows for easiest recognition of anatomic landmarks. If the pedicle is too small or infiltrated by tumor, parapedicular **(b)** or posterolateral **(c)** approaches can be performed; however, these approaches may be associated with a higher risk of paravertebral hemorrhage or lung injury.

A multicenter randomized controlled trial was published by Berenson et al[35] in 2011. In this study, there was a statistically significant reduction in pain severity scores in patients who received kyphoplasty compared to nonsurgical management of painful VCFs due to underlying metastatic disease. Similar results were reported in a smaller randomized controlled trial by Yang et al[36] in 2012 assessing vertebroplasty for painful multiple myeloma metastases, with pain relief lasting up to 3 years in the PVA treatment group.

6. *Does the current literature support combined treatment approaches with vertebral augmentation?*

Local tumor control is an important consideration in patients presenting with a VCF secondary to osseous metastatic disease. Most commonly, this is achieved through radiation therapy and/or systemic chemotherapy. Other methods for local tumor control are also available, including percutaneous RFA.

a) PVA and radiation therapy:

Studies assessing the use of PVA and palliative external beam radiation therapy (EBRT) are limited. To date, there are no randomized controlled trials assessing the combined efficacy or optimal timing of EBRT with PVA. Should EBRT be performed before or after PVA? What time interval is ideal for EBRT before or following PVA? The current data behind these questions is unclear at this time.

In a retrospective cohort study by Kasperk et al,[37] pain intensity scores at 1-month and 1-year follow-ups were similar for patients treated with PVA or palliative EBRT in the setting of painful multiple myeloma compression fractures. In addition, both PVA and EBRT were significantly better at pain control compared to systemic chemotherapy alone. Another prospective study by Qian et al[38] demonstrated rapid and sustained (24-hour and up to 2-year follow-up assessment) decrease in pain intensity scores with kyphoplasty followed by EBRT (external radiation was performed 1–2 weeks after kyphoplasty).

Stereotactic body radiation therapy (SBRT) involves multiple radiation beams at different angles and delivers ablative radiation doses to the tumor. SBRT to the spine is associated with higher risk of VCF following treatment, with reported risk of 0.7 to 40.5%.[39] In a recent systematic review, the overall risk of VCF following SBRT was estimated to be approximately 14%.[3] This systematic review also determined risk factors for VCF following SBRT, including tumor size, osteolytic disease, and preexisting compression deformity.[3] In a retrospective study by Gerszten et al,[40] kyphoplasty performed prior to SBRT was found to be effective in patients with preexisting VCFs. However, this treatment strategy has not become common practice and no further studies have assessed the efficacy of PVA prior to spinal SBRT.

In recent consensus guidelines by the American Society of Therapeutic Radiology and Oncology (ASTRO),[41,42] kyphoplasty and vertebroplasty are recognized as potentially useful treatments for osteolytic metastases. However, ASTRO emphasizes that PVA does not obviate the need for external beam radiation. They also suggest that additional prospective trials are needed to better define patients who would benefit from treatment with PVA, and if so, how those procedures should be best sequenced with EBRT.

b) PVA and RFA:

While it is common practice to perform RFA prior to PVA, data to support RFA efficacy are limited. To date, one randomized controlled study has been published with use of PVA and RFA. In this study by Orgera et al,[43] RFA with PVA was shown to be effective and safe, but without additional pain control benefit when compared to PVA alone in the setting of painful multiple myeloma metastases. Local tumor control was not assessed in this study.

Several additional observational studies[44,45,46,47,48] have shown that RFA is safe and may be effective for local tumor control in nonmultiple myeloma vertebral metastases; however, this has yet to be validated with a randomized controlled study. Regarding pain control for nonmultiple myeloma metastases, several observational studies have reported excellent reduction in pain scores following RFA; however, these results are obscured by concurrent treatment with PVA.

One current, ongoing multicenter prospective trial, the STAART study,[49] has begun to assess the effectiveness of RFA with PVA for the treatment of painful pathologic vertebral fractures in patients who have failed radiation therapy (group 1) or who are radiation naïve (group 2). Preliminary results from this study are promising, with nearly 80% of patients demonstrating adequate pain and local tumor control, as well as no major complications related to RFA.

c) Other methods of percutaneous local tumor control:
Multiple other adjunctive percutaneous local tumor control therapies are available for use, including microwave ablation, cryoablation, alcohol ablation, laser photocoagulation, radiofrequency ionization, and brachytherapy. In general, these techniques are less commonly used as compared to RFA, and not well assessed in the literature. There have been a few small randomized studies assessing the efficacy of PVA with ^{125}I brachytherapy. In their first study, Yang et al[50] reported statistically improved pain scores at 6-month follow-up for PVA plus brachytherapy (mean visual analog score [VAS] pain intensity 2.3) versus PVA alone (mean VAS pain intensity 5.4) for treatment of mixed spinal metastases. However, local tumor control was not statistically different between the two groups. In a subsequent study, Yang et al[51] reported statistically improved pain scores for PVA plus brachytherapy compared to external beam radiation, with interval clinical follow-ups over a 1-year period. Also, the EBRT group did not show a pain response until 1 month after treatment.

7. *In high-risk patients (neurologic symptoms, posterior vertebral wall defect, spinal canal compromise, or cervical compression fractures), is there a role for vertebral augmentation?*
Multiple small observational studies have demonstrated that vertebroplasty and kyphoplasty can be safely performed in high-risk patients. In a systematic review published in 2016,[9] a review of 14 studies evaluating vertebroplasty for compression fractures with posterior wall defects or spinal canal compromise reported 22 major complications (4.1%). No major complications were reported in 2 small observational studies (45 patients) for kyphoplasty performed for similar indications.

Cervical PVA can also be safely performed; however, it does require modified approaches for vertebral access (anterolateral or transoral). Two observational studies, 1 a multicenter study, reported no major complications following cervical vertebroplasty (97 total patients).[9]

32.4 Level of Evidence

PVA efficacy: Given the patient's clinical presentation and imaging findings, treatment with PVA is a reasonable approach for palliative pain control (Class II, Level of Evidence B).

PVA safety: With the patients imaging findings, we can expect a very low risk for major complication following PVA (Class II, Level of Evidence B).

PVA with radiation therapy: PVA can safely be performed with previous or future radiation therapy; however, the optimal sequencing of PVA with radiation therapy has not been assessed in the literature (Class III, Level of Evidence C).

PVA with RFA: RFA is commonly performed with PVA; however, its efficacy for pain relief or local tumor control remains inadequately assessed in the literature (Class III, Level of Evidence C).

PVA for high-risk patients: Should the patient develop a symptomatic cervical vertebral lesion or thoracolumbar lesion with posterior cortex destruction, PVA is a possible option with a highly skilled neurointerventionalist (Class III, Level of Evidence C).

32.5 Landmark Papers

Berenson J, Pflugmacher R, Jarzem P, et al. Cancer Patient Fracture Evaluation (CAFE) Investigators. Balloon kyphoplasty versus non-surgical fracture management for treatment of painful vertebral body compression fractures in patients with cancer: a multicentre, randomised controlled trial. Lancet Oncol 2011;12:225–235.

The Cancer Patient Fracture Evaluation (CAFE) study was the first randomized controlled trial that assessed PVA efficacy and safety in the setting of painful metastatic spinal lesions. This multicenter trial was performed at 22 institutions in Europe, the United States, Canada, and Austria. Cancer patients with painful VCFs were randomized to kyphoplasty or nonsurgical management. The primary outcome of the study was pain control and functional status from baseline at 1 month after treatment, as assessed by the Roland Morris disability questionnaire (a 24-point scale, with 24 being the most severe pain/disability).

One hundred and thirty-four patients were enrolled in the study, 70 randomized to kyphoplasty and 64 to nonsurgical management. The two groups were equally distributed in regards to age, sex, and cancer type. The most common cancer for both treatment groups was multiple myeloma; however, the study also included many nonmultiple myeloma cancers (>50% were nonmultiple myeloma cancers in both groups). A few patients either withdrew from the study, died (no procedure-related deaths), or were lost to follow-up, equally impacting both groups.

At 1 month, the mean Roland Morris disability score was improved for the kyphoplasty group (minus 8.4 points) and essentially unchanged for the nonsurgical group (minus 0.2 points), a statistically significant difference. At 1 month, the kyphoplasty group also had a significant improvement in KPS score compared to the nonsurgical group, which measures overall functional impairment status. After 1 month, 37 patients crossed over from the nonsurgical to the kyphoplasty group. No serious adverse events were attributed to the kyphoplasty treatment group. The overall death rate among the two groups was not statistically different.

One limitation of this study was allowing patients to cross over from the nonsurgical to kyphoplasty group after 1 month, preventing long-term follow-up in these patients. Also, chemoradiation was not specified in either of the groups and was left to the discretion of the treating physician. Lastly, funding for the study was provided by Medtronic Spine LLC.

32

Yang Z, Tan J, Xu Y, et al. Treatment of MM-associated spinal fracture with percutaneous vertebroplasty (PVP) and chemotherapy. Eur Spine J 2012;21:912–919.

In this single-center study, 76 patients with painful multiple myeloma-associated spinal fractures were randomized to either PVA plus chemotherapy or chemotherapy-alone treatment groups. The demographics for both groups were equally distributed with regards to age, sex, and multiple myeloma subtype. Clinical follow-up was performed every 2 months for the first year, as well as at 3 and 5 years.

At 1-year follow-up, patients in the combined treatment group (PVA plus chemotherapy) had lower visual analog pain (VAP) and Karnofsky performance status (KPS) scores compared to the group treated with chemotherapy alone (both statistically significant). Overall multiple myeloma response rate was also statistically higher at 1-year follow-up in the combined group versus the chemotherapy-alone group (65.8 vs. 50%).

At 3-year follow-up, the VAP and KPS score remained statistically different between the two groups, with persistent pain relief for the combined treatment group. In the chemotherapy-alone group, there were two cases of paraplegia, versus none in the combined treatment group. At both 3- and 5-year follow-ups, overall survival was statistically higher for the combined treatment group (68.4% survival for the combined group at 5-year follow-up vs. 42.1% in the chemotherapy group).

There were no serious complications attributed to kyphoplasty. Cement leaks along the anterior or lateral side of the vertebral body occurred in 20 patients; however, these were all asymptomatic. No cases of spinal cord or nerve root compression occurred in the kyphoplasty plus chemotherapy group. The authors also reported statistically significant improvement in vertebral body heights following kyphoplasty, though this was only reported to be an approximate 1-mm increase from baseline.

The authors in this article theorized that there may be benefit of kyphoplasty beyond pain control in the setting of multiple myeloma, accounting for the increased response rate and survival for the combined treatment group. Proposed mechanisms included cytotoxicity of the PMMA cement to tumor, heating of tumor in the polymerization phase, and compressive effects from cement solidification resulting in tumor necrosis.

Although the results were found to be statistically significant, a major limitation of this study is its small sample size and its generalizability to the general population, Nonetheless, the results of this study are promising, and show that kyphoplasty can be safely performed in multiple myeloma patients, with potential long-term pain control benefit.

Pron G, Holubowich C, Kaulback K; Health Quality Ontario. Vertebral augmentation involving vertebroplasty or kyphoplasty for cancer-related vertebral compression fractures: A systematic review. Ont Health Technol Assess Ser 2016;16:1–202.

This comprehensive systematic review analyzed 111 clinical reports, including 4,235 patients, regarding effectiveness of kyphoplasty or vertebroplasty for patients with mixed metastatic spinal cancers, multiple myeloma, or hemangioma. The authors concluded that both vertebroplasty and kyphoplasty rapidly reduced pain intensity in cancer patients with compression fractures (moderate level of evidence). They also concluded that PVA reduces the need for opioid analgesics and improves overall pain-related disability scores in patients with osseous meta-static disease. The authors reported that major complications related to PVA were uncommon and that most cement leaks were asymptomatic. Regarding local tumor control, there was insufficient evidence to determine appropriate methods of adjunctive procedures or the sequencing of radiation therapy with PVA.

Goetz MP, Callstrom MR, Charboneau JW, et al. Percutaneous image-guided radiofrequency ablation of painful metastases involving bone: a multicenter study. J Clin Oncol 2004;22:300–306.

The work by Goetz et al was one of the earlier studies that investigated the efficacy of RFA for pain relief in patients with osteolytic metastases. In this multicenter prospective study, 43 patients were treated with RFA. To be included in the study, patients had to have a pain score > 3 out of 10 and failed other standard treatments, such as radiation therapy or analgesics. The majority of osteolytic lesions were in the pelvis or sacrum (24 patients), with 4 treated vertebral lesions.

Following RFA treatment, 95% of patients experienced a clinically significant decrease in pain score by week 1 (average pain score 5.8 vs. baseline of 7.9). Clinical follow-up for 26 patients was available at 12 weeks, which also demonstrated significant reduction in pain scores (average pain score 3.0). Opioid usage also significantly decreased at weeks 8 and 12. Overall, there were only three complications, none of which were life-threatening, and none related to vertebral RFA.

The main limitations of the study are lack of randomized design and small sample size, particularly as it relates to spinal RFA, where there were only four patients. This study did, however, demonstrate that RFA could potentially provide pain relief to patients with osteolytic metastases that had failed standard treatment. This study did not assess local tumor control.

Bagla S, Sayed D, Smirniotopoulos J, et al. Multicenter prospective clinical series evaluating radiofrequency ablation in the treatment of painful spine metastases. Cardiovasc Intervent Radiol 2016;39:1289–1297.

In this prospective, multicenter, single-arm study, 50 patients (69 treatment levels) with painful vertebral metastasis were treated with RFA. Concurrent PVA was also performed at 96% of treatment levels. The study objectives were assessment of pain relief and procedure safety. Patients were assessed clinically at 3, 7, 30, and 90 days following RFA.

Following treatment, the study found significant ($p < 0.0001$) improvement in pain and disability scores from baseline at all time intervals. No procedural-related complications were reported. The authors concluded that RFA with cement rapidly reduces pain and improves quality of life in patients with painful vertebral metastases.

Similar to the study by Goetz et al, this study is limited by lack of randomized design. Also, although there was significant improvement in pain scores, almost all patients were also treated with PVA, so it is difficult to determine if the pain relief was related to PVA, RFA, or both procedures. Several other retrospective studies have reported similar pain relief with RFA with concurrent PVA.[45,47,48] Local tumor control was not assessed.

Orgera G, Krokidis M, Matteoli M, et al. Percutaneous vertebroplasty for pain management in patients with multiple myeloma: is radiofrequency ablation necessary? Cardiovasc Intervent Radiol 2014;37:203–210.

In this prospective study, 36 patients with painful vertebral metastases secondary to multiple myeloma were randomized to RFA and vertebroplasty or RFA-only treatment groups. The primary outcomes assessed in the study were pain relief, technical success, and procedure safety. Pain scores were assessed at 24 hours and 6 weeks following the procedure.

There was a significant decrease in pain scores for both groups compared to baseline; however, there was no statistical difference in pain reduction between the two treatment groups (RFA plus PVA or PVA-alone). The amount of pain medication was also reported to be equally decreased among the two groups. No major complications occurred in the study.

This study is limited by two factors: small patient sample size (only 18 patients in each treatment group) and lack of long-term follow-up (patient only followed until 6 weeks after treatment). However, within these limitations, the results of this study do suggest that RFA may not have added pain relief benefit in the setting of multiple myeloma vertebral metastases, with more studies needed to validate these findings. Local tumor control was not assessed.

32.6 Recommendations

Though radiation therapy remains the treatment of choice for uncomplicated metastatic disease to the spine, PVA can also be beneficial in carefully selected patients with recent pathologic compression fractures. Many studies, including two randomized controlled trials, have demonstrated that PVA provides for rapid pain relief of compression fractures related to osseous metastatic disease. Several studies have also suggested that pain relief from PVA can be maintained for years after treatment.

The safety profile of PVA has been well established, and there are very few serious complications associated with vertebroplasty or kyphoplasty. Operators need to be aware of cement leak, and vertebral cement injections should be closely monitored by real-time fluoroscopy. The majority of cement leaks are asymptomatic; however, <2% can be associated with neurologic compromise or symptomatic pulmonary embolism. Higher incidence of adjacent-level vertebral fracture from intradisc cement leak is controversial, although a recent randomized study, the VERTOS II trial, has suggested that there is no increased risk.

Local tumor control is an important consideration in patients with spinal metastases, which is most often achieved through chemoradiation therapy. However, there are potential limitations of radiation therapy, including delayed pain relief, higher risk of fracture progression in the setting of preexisting compression deformity, and radiation dose limits. Also, certain tumors may not respond well to radiation therapy. Taking these factors into consideration, there is a role for PVA with radiation therapy, but the sequencing of these combined treatment modalities remains uncertain and has yet to be evaluated in the literature.

Percutaneous local tumor control techniques, most notably RFA, are commonly performed with PVA in the setting of osseous metastases. Although technically successful RFA for vertebral tumors can be safely achieved, the literature supporting its efficacy for pain relief or local tumor control is limited. While RFA may be a reasonable approach in nonmultiple myeloma patients who have failed radiation therapy, more studies are needed to assess its efficacy, and RFA is not currently considered a first-line treatment for vertebral metastases.

32.7 Summary

1. PVA has been shown to rapidly alleviate pain associated with pathologic compression fractures and is a reasonable treatment approach in patients who have failed conservative management and/or radiation therapy.
2. The most common complication from PVA is cement leak, the majority of which are asymptomatic.
3. Current evidence is insufficient regarding pain relief and/or local tumor control when combining PVA with radiation therapy or PVA with RFA.

References

[1] Gangi A, Buy X. Percutaneous bone tumor management. Semin Intervent Radiol. 2010; 27(2):124–136
[2] Rhee WJ, Kim KH, Chang JS, Kim HJ, Choi S, Koom WS. Vertebral compression fractures after spine irradiation using conventional fractionation in patients with metastatic colorectal cancer. Radiat Oncol J. 2014; 32(4):221–230
[3] Faruqi S, Tseng CL, Whyne C, et al. Vertebral compression fracture after spine stereotactic body radiation therapy: a review of the pathophysiology and risk factors. Neurosurgery. 2017; 0:1–9
[4] Baerlocher MO, Saad WE, Dariushnia S, Barr JD, McGraw JK, Nikolic B, Society of Interventional Radiology Standards of Practice Committee. Quality improvement guidelines for percutaneous vertebroplasty. J Vasc Interv Radiol. 2014; 25(2):165–170
[5] Shaibani A, Ali S, Bhatt H. Vertebroplasty and kyphoplasty for the palliation of pain. Semin Intervent Radiol. 2007; 24(4):409–418
[6] Golob AL, Wipf JE. Low back pain. Med Clin North Am. 2014; 98(3):405–428
[7] Stallmeyer MJZG. Patient evaluation and selection. In: Mathis JM, Belkoff SM, eds. Percutaneous vertebroplasty. New York, NY: Springer-Verlag; 2002: 41–60
[8] Deramond H, Depriester C, Galibert P, Le Gars D. Percutaneous vertebroplasty with polymethylmethacrylate: technique, indications, and results. Radiol Clin North Am. 1998; 36(3):533–546
[9] Pron G, Holubowich C, Kaulback K, Health Quality Ontario. Vertebral augmentation involving vertebroplasty or kyphoplasty for cancer-related vertebral compression fractures: a systematic review. Ont Health Technol Assess Ser. 2016; 16(11):1–202
[10] Baroud G, Heini P, Nemes J, Bohner M, Ferguson S, Steffen T. Biomechanical explanation of adjacent fractures following vertebroplasty. Radiology. 2003; 229(2):606–607, author reply 607–608
[11] Lin EP, Ekholm S, Hiwatashi A, Westesson PL. Vertebroplasty: cement leakage into the disc increases the risk of new fracture of adjacent vertebral body. AJNR Am J Neuroradiol. 2004; 25(2):175–180
[12] Voormolen MH, Lohle PN, Juttmann JR, van der Graaf Y, Fransen H, Lampmann LE. The risk of new osteoporotic vertebral compression fractures in the year after percutaneous vertebroplasty. J Vasc Interv Radiol. 2006; 17(1): 71–76
[13] Hierholzer J, Fuchs H, Westphalen K, Baumann C, Slotosch C, Schulz R. Incidence of symptomatic vertebral fractures in patients after percutaneous vertebroplasty. Cardiovasc Intervent Radiol. 2008; 31(6):1178–1183
[14] Klazen CA, Venmans A, de Vries J, et al. Percutaneous vertebroplasty is not a risk factor for new osteoporotic compression fractures: results from VERTOS II. AJNR Am J Neuroradiol. 2010; 31(8):1447–1450
[15] Kelekis AD, Martin JB, Somon T, Wetzel SG, Dietrich PY, Ruefenacht DA. Radicular pain after vertebroplasty: compression or irritation of the nerve root? Initial experience with the "cooling system". Spine. 2003; 28(14):E265–E269
[16] Krueger A, Bliemel C, Zettl R, Ruchholtz S. Management of pulmonary cement embolism after percutaneous vertebroplasty and kyphoplasty: a systematic review of the literature. Eur Spine J. 2009; 18(9):1257–1265

32

[17] Kim AK, Jensen ME, Dion JE, Schweickert PA, Kaufmann TJ, Kallmes DF. Unilateral transpedicular percutaneous vertebroplasty: initial experience. Radiology. 2002; 222(3):737–741

[18] Sadeghi-Naini M, Aarabi S, Shokraneh F, Janani L, Vaccaro AR, Rahimi-Movaghar V. Vertebroplasty and kyphoplasty for metastatic spinal lesions: a systematic review. Clin Spine Surg. 2018; 31(5):203–210

[19] Dudeney S, Lieberman IH, Reinhardt MK, Hussein M. Kyphoplasty in the treatment of osteolytic vertebral compression fractures as a result of multiple myeloma. J Clin Oncol. 2002; 20(9):2382–2387

[20] Julka A, Tolhurst SR, Srinivasan RC, Graziano GP. Functional outcomes and height restoration for patients with multiple myeloma-related osteolytic vertebral compression fractures treated with kyphoplasty. J Spinal Disord Tech. 2014; 27(6):342–346

[21] Pflugmacher R, Kandziora F, Schroeder RJ, Melcher I, Haas NP, Klostermann CK. Percutaneous balloon kyphoplasty in the treatment of pathological vertebral body fracture and deformity in multiple myeloma: a one-year follow-up. Acta Radiol. 2006; 47(4):369–376

[22] Vrionis FD, Hamm A, Stanton N, et al. Kyphoplasty for tumor associated spinal fractures. Tech Reg Anesth Pain Manage. 2005; 9:35–39

[23] Calmels V, Vallée JN, Rose M, Chiras J. Osteoblastic and mixed spinal metastases: evaluation of the analgesic efficacy of percutaneous vertebroplasty. AJNR Am J Neuroradiol. 2007; 28(3):570–574

[24] Masala S, Anselmetti GC, Marcia S, Massari F, Manca A, Simonetti G. Percutaneous vertebroplasty in multiple myeloma vertebral involvement. J Spinal Disord Tech. 2008; 21(5):344–348

[25] McDonald RJ, Trout AT, Gray LA, Dispenzieri A, Thielen KR, Kallmes DF. Vertebroplasty in multiple myeloma: outcomes in a large patient series. AJNR Am J Neuroradiol. 2008; 29(4):642–648

[26] Tseng YY, Lo YL, Chen LH, Lai PL, Yang ST. Percutaneous polymethylmethacrylate vertebroplasty in the treatment of pain induced by metastatic spine tumor. Surg Neurol. 2008; 70 Suppl 1:S1–, 78–83, discussion S1, 83–84

[27] Pflugmacher R, Taylor R, Agarwal A, et al. Balloon kyphoplasty in the treatment of metastatic disease of the spine: a 2-year prospective evaluation. Eur Spine J. 2008; 17(8):1042–1048

[28] Bosnjaković P, Ristić S, Mrvić M, et al. Management of painful spinal lesions caused by multiple myeloma using percutaneous acrylic cement injection. Acta Chir Iugosl. 2009; 56(4):153–158

[29] McDonald RJ, Gray LA, Cloft HJ, Thielen KR, Kallmes DF. The effect of operator variability and experience in vertebroplasty outcomes. Radiology. 2009; 253 (2):478–485

[30] Zou J, Mei X, Gan M, Yang H. Kyphoplasty for spinal fractures from multiple myeloma. J Surg Oncol. 2010; 102(1):43–47

[31] Chew C, Ritchie M, O'Dwyer PJ, Edwards R. A prospective study of percutaneous vertebroplasty in patients with myeloma and spinal metastases. Clin Radiol. 2011; 66(12):1193–1196

[32] Mikami Y, Numaguchi Y, Kobayashi N, Fuwa S, Hoshikawa Y, Saida Y. Therapeutic effects of percutaneous vertebroplasty for vertebral metastases. Jpn J Radiol. 2011; 29(3):202–206

[33] Anselmetti GC, Manca A, Montemurro F, et al. Percutaneous vertebroplasty in multiple myeloma: prospective long-term follow-up in 106 consecutive patients. Cardiovasc Intervent Radiol. 2012; 35(1):139–145

[34] Korovessis P, Vardakastanis K, Vitsas V, Syrimpeis V. Is Kiva implant advantageous to balloon kyphoplasty in treating osteolytic metastasis to the spine? Comparison of 2 percutaneous minimal invasive spine techniques: a prospective randomized controlled short-term study. Spine. 2014; 39(4):E231–E239

[35] Berenson J, Pflugmacher R, Jarzem P, et al. Cancer Patient Fracture Evaluation (CAFE) Investigators. Balloon kyphoplasty versus non-surgical fracture management for treatment of painful vertebral body compression fractures in patients with cancer: a multicentre, randomised controlled trial. Lancet Oncol. 2011; 12(3):225–235

[36] Yang Z, Tan J, Xu Y, et al. Treatment of MM-associated spinal fracture with percutaneous vertebroplasty (PVP) and chemotherapy. Eur Spine J. 2012; 21 (5):912–919

[37] Kasperk C, Haas A, Hillengass J, et al. Kyphoplasty in patients with multiple myeloma a retrospective comparative pilot study. J Surg Oncol. 2012; 105(7): 679–686

[38] Qian Z, Sun Z, Yang H, Gu Y, Chen K, Wu G. Kyphoplasty for the treatment of malignant vertebral compression fractures caused by metastases. J Clin Neurosci. 2011; 18(6):763–767

[39] Chang JH, Shin JH, Yamada YJ, et al. Stereotactic body radiotherapy for spinal metastases: what are the risks and how do we minimize them? Spine. 2016; 41 Suppl 20:S238–S245

[40] Gerszten PC, Germanwala A, Burton SA, Welch WC, Ozhasoglu C, Vogel WJ. Combination kyphoplasty and spinal radiosurgery: a new treatment paradigm for pathological fractures. J Neurosurg Spine. 2005; 3(4):296–301

[41] Lutz S, Berk L, Chang E, et al. American Society for Radiation Oncology (ASTRO). Palliative radiotherapy for bone metastases: an ASTRO evidence-based guideline. Int J Radiat Oncol Biol Phys. 2011; 79(4):965–976

[42] Lutz S, Balboni T, Jones J, et al. Palliative radiation therapy for bone metastases: update of an ASTRO Evidence-Based Guideline. Pract Radiat Oncol. 2017; 7(1):4–12

[43] Orgera G, Krokidis M, Matteoli M, et al. Percutaneous vertebroplasty for pain management in patients with multiple myeloma: is radiofrequency ablation necessary? Cardiovasc Intervent Radiol. 2014; 37(1):203–210

[44] Goetz MP, Callstrom MR, Charboneau JW, et al. Percutaneous image-guided radiofrequency ablation of painful metastases involving bone: a multicenter study. J Clin Oncol. 2004; 22(2):300–306

[45] Anchala PR, Irving WD, Hillen TJ, et al. Treatment of metastatic spinal lesions with a navigational bipolar radiofrequency ablation device: a multicenter retrospective study. Pain Physician. 2014; 17(4):317–327

[46] Bagla S, Sayed D, Smirniotopoulos J, et al. Multicenter prospective clinical series evaluating radiofrequency ablation in the treatment of painful spine metastases. Cardiovasc Intervent Radiol. 2016; 39(9):1289–1297

[47] Reyes M, Georgy M, Brook L, et al. Multicenter clinical and imaging evaluation of targeted radiofrequency ablation (t-RFA) and cement augmentation of neoplastic vertebral lesions. J Neurointerv Surg. 2018; 10(2):176–182

[48] Zhao W, Wang H, Hu JH, et al. Palliative pain relief and safety of percutaneous radiofrequency ablation combined with cement injection for bone metastasis. Jpn J Clin Oncol. 2018; 48(8):753–759

[49] Jennings J, Robinson C, Wallace A, et al. Prospective, multicenter evaluation of targeted radiofrequency ablation (t-RFA) and vertebral augmentation (VA) prior to or following radiation therapy (RT) to treat painful metastatic vertebral body tumors (STARRT Study): Interim analysis. Paper presented at the Society of Interventional Radiology Annual Scientific Meeting; 2017 Mar 4–9; Washington, DC

[50] Yang Z, Yang Z, Xie L, et al. Treatment of metastatic spinal tumors by percutaneous vertebroplasty versus percutaneous vertebroplasty combined with interstitial implantation of 125I seeds. Acta Radiol. 2009; 50(10):1142–1148

[51] Yang Z, Tan J, Zhao R, et al. Clinical investigations on the spinal osteoblastic metastasis treated by combination of percutaneous vertebroplasty and (125)I seeds implantation versus radiotherapy. Cancer Biother Radiopharm. 2013; 28(1):58–64

32

Index